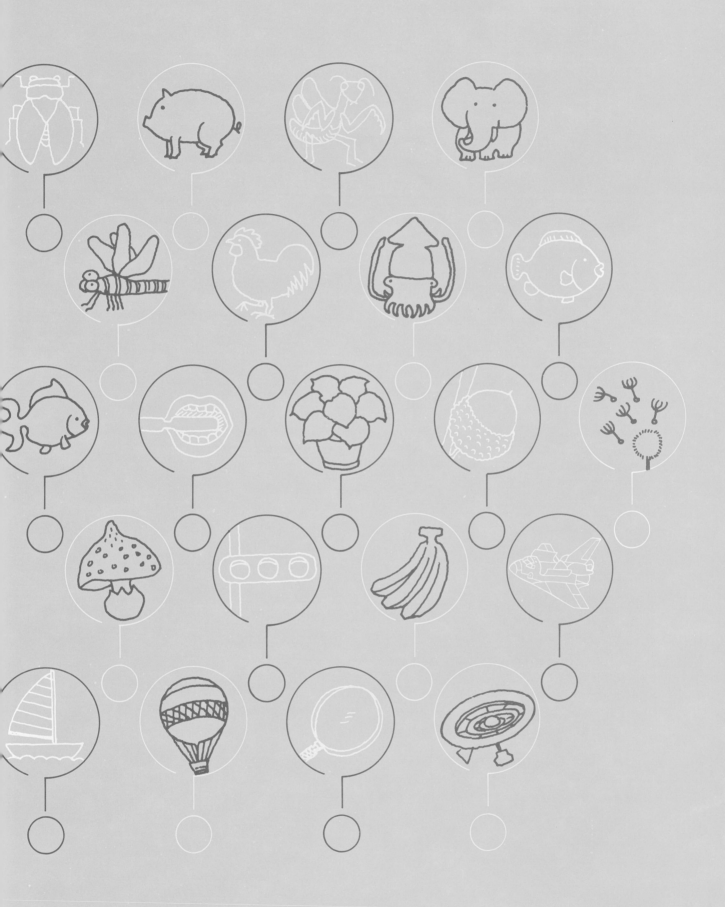

A Child's First Library of Learning

Health & Safety

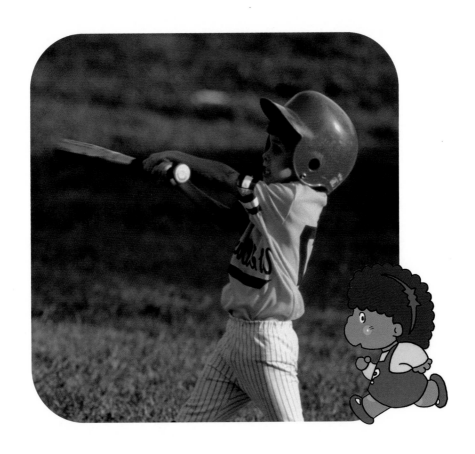

TIME-LIFE BOOKS • ALEXANDRIA, VIRGINIA

Contents

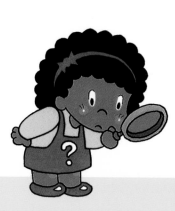
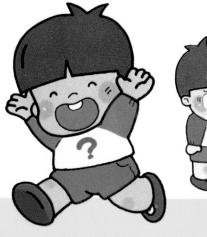
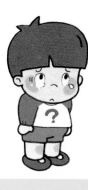

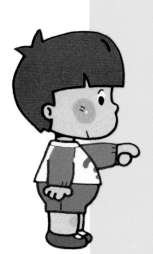
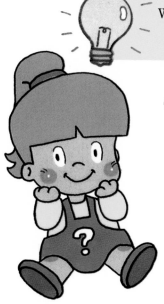
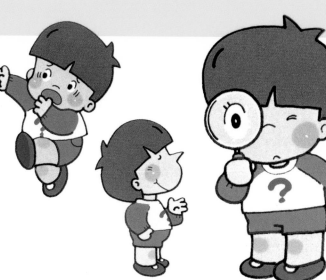
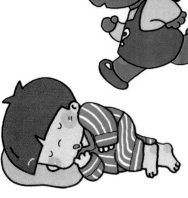

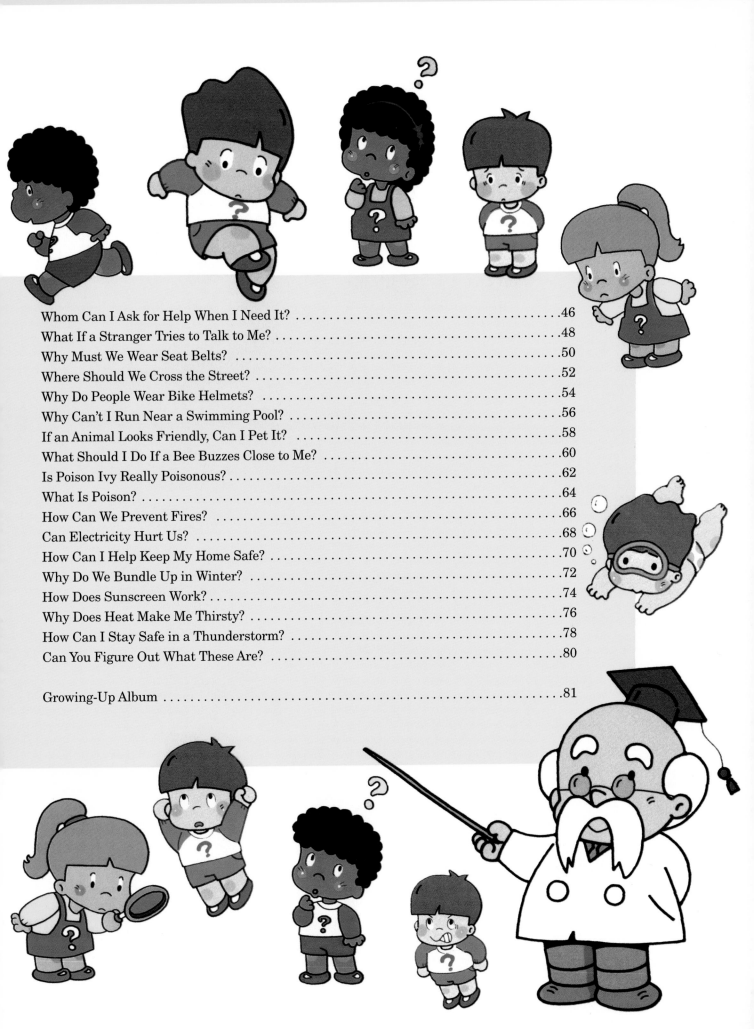

Why Do We Need to Eat Breakfast?

(ANSWER) The food you eat gives your body the energy you need to play and work and grow. While you sleep at night, you go many hours without food. In the morning, your body is low on energy, like a car that has run out of gas. So it's important to fill up with a good breakfast, which gives you the energy to start your day and keep going all morning.

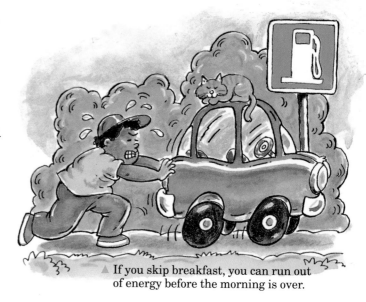

▲ If you skip breakfast, you can run out of energy before the morning is over.

■ A bunch of banana energy

The amount of energy stored in a food is measured in calories. A banana has about 80 calories. The more active you are, the faster you use up calories.

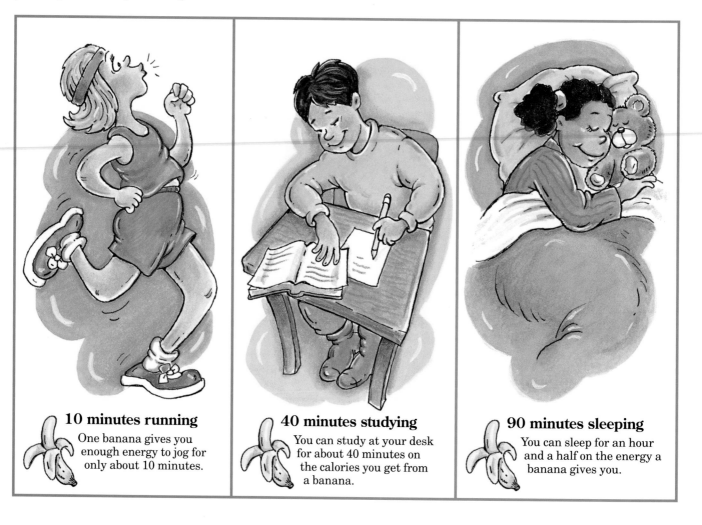

10 minutes running
One banana gives you enough energy to jog for only about 10 minutes.

40 minutes studying
You can study at your desk for about 40 minutes on the calories you get from a banana.

90 minutes sleeping
You can sleep for an hour and a half on the energy a banana gives you.

Why Is Water Important?

You can't live without water. In fact, about two thirds of your body is made of water. Water helps your body do almost all its work. For example, it helps you digest food and turn it into energy. When you sweat or go to the bathroom, you lose water. When you feel thirsty, your body is telling you it needs more water. Be sure to pay attention and have a good drink!

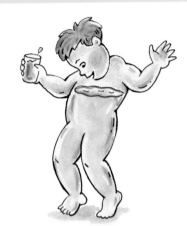

■ Breakfast around the world

What you eat in the morning may be very different from what a child in another country eats. Which of these breakfasts look good to you?

▼ The United States
A child in the United States might have pancakes with syrup, cereal with milk, and orange juice for breakfast.

▼ France
French children eat bread or rolls with butter and jam and drink hot chocolate for breakfast.

▼ Holland
In Holland, breakfast is a large meal that may include cold fish, cold meat, cheese, bread, boiled eggs, and tea.

► Guatemala
In Guatemala, children have corn tortillas, refried beans and sour cream, and apple juice or milk for breakfast.

► Japan
Japanese children have rice with nori (seaweed), miso soup, pickled vegetables, grilled fish, and tea for breakfast.

● To the Parent

Breakfast is an important meal for your child. Studies have shown that children who skip it are likely to become careless and inattentive by late morning. In fact, children who regularly skip any meal are more susceptible to infection and fatigue.

5

Do I Have to Eat Vegetables?

(ANSWER) Food contains ingredients called nutrients, which your body uses to grow strong and stay healthy. But no single food provides all the nutrients your body needs. So it is important to eat a number of different foods every day—and that includes vegetables.

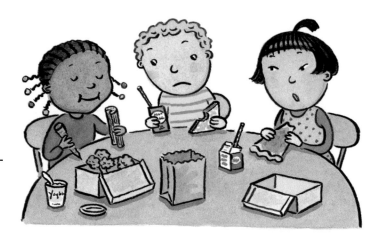

■ A tower of power

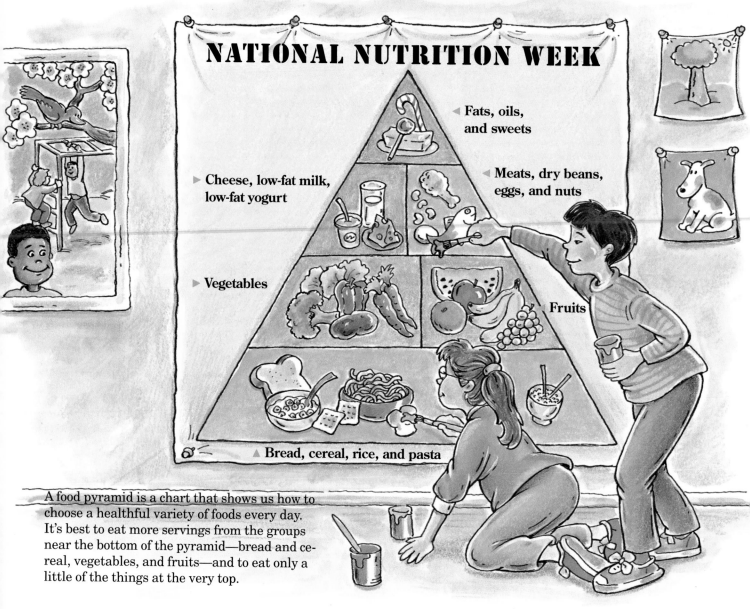

NATIONAL NUTRITION WEEK

◄ Fats, oils, and sweets

► Cheese, low-fat milk, low-fat yogurt

◄ Meats, dry beans, eggs, and nuts

► Vegetables

Fruits

▲ Bread, cereal, rice, and pasta

A food pyramid is a chart that shows us how to choose a healthful variety of foods every day. It's best to eat more servings from the groups near the bottom of the pyramid—bread and cereal, vegetables, and fruits—and to eat only a little of the things at the very top.

What Are Vitamins and Minerals?

Vitamins and minerals are nutrients found in many different foods. Some vitamins are named after letters of the alphabet. Each vitamin has its own special job that helps your body stay healthy. Your body also needs at least 14 minerals, including calcium and iron. Calcium builds teeth and bones. Iron makes blood.

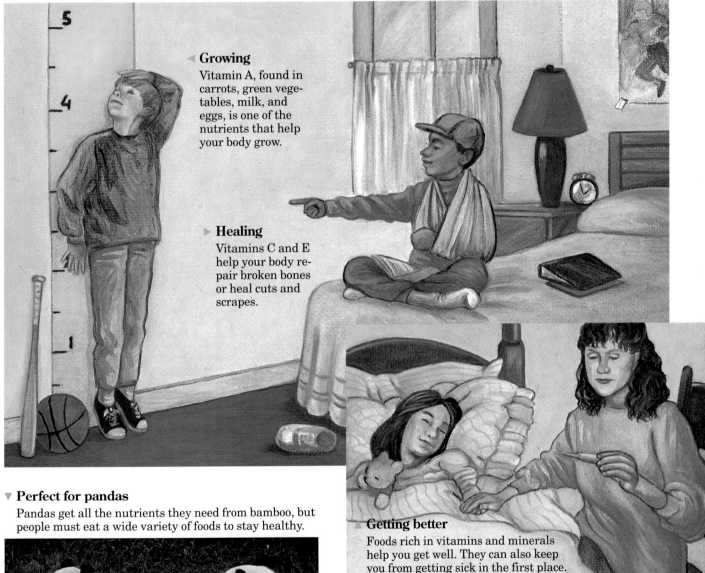

◄ **Growing**
Vitamin A, found in carrots, green vegetables, milk, and eggs, is one of the nutrients that help your body grow.

► **Healing**
Vitamins C and E help your body repair broken bones or heal cuts and scrapes.

Getting better
Foods rich in vitamins and minerals help you get well. They can also keep you from getting sick in the first place.

▼ **Perfect for pandas**
Pandas get all the nutrients they need from bamboo, but people must eat a wide variety of foods to stay healthy.

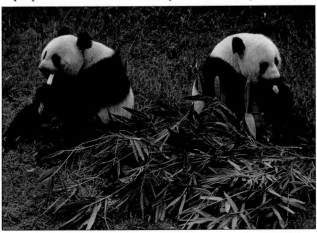

Why Are Some Foods Called Junk Food?

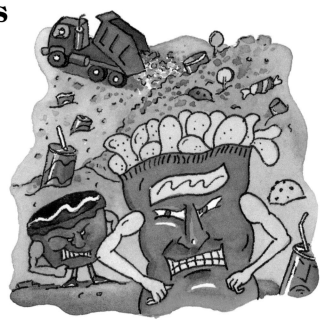

ANSWER Junk is the same thing as trash. People throw it away because they do not need it. Food that has a lot of calories but not many nutrients is called junk food because your body does not need it to grow and stay well. Junk foods are often full of sugar or fat or both.

■ The problem with junk food

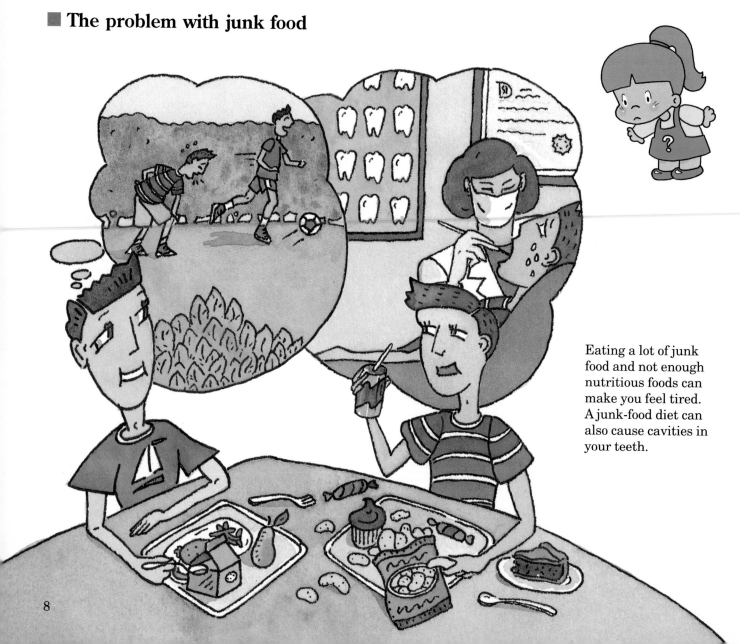

Eating a lot of junk food and not enough nutritious foods can make you feel tired. A junk-food diet can also cause cavities in your teeth.

Is It Ever All Right to Eat Sweets?

Snacking on sweets once in a while won't hurt you, as long as you eat enough of the foods your body really needs. Some sweets are better for you than others. Ice cream, for example, can be fatty, but at least it gives your body calcium. For an even healthier treat, try low-fat ice cream.

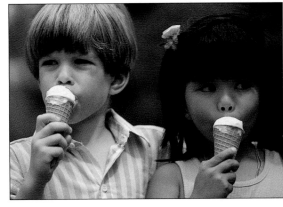

■ Choosing healthful snacks

When you feel hungry or thirsty between meals, it's best to fill up on fruits, vegetables, bread, pretzels, or non-fat yogurt. Drink fruit juice, water, or low-fat milk—that's what these boys and girls are doing.

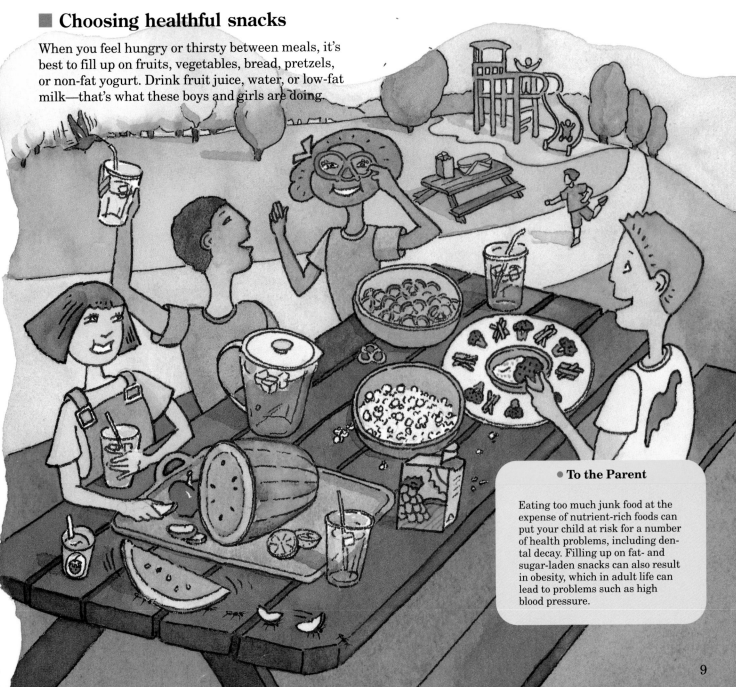

● **To the Parent**

Eating too much junk food at the expense of nutrient-rich foods can put your child at risk for a number of health problems, including dental decay. Filling up on fat- and sugar-laden snacks can also result in obesity, which in adult life can lead to problems such as high blood pressure.

9

Why Do I Have to Go to the Dentist?

ANSWER The dentist keeps your teeth clean and strong. When you eat, food gets caught in your teeth. Unless you brush right away, germs can grow in this food and make holes called cavities in your teeth. To keep that from happening, the dentist cleans your teeth and checks them to make sure they are healthy.

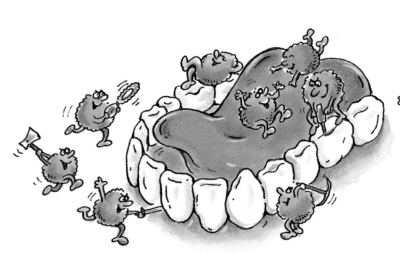

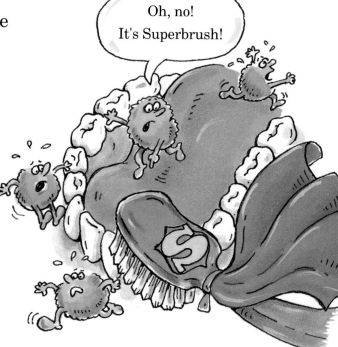

▼ **Brushing and flossing**

To fight germs, brush and floss after every meal. For upper teeth, brush downward from the gums; for lower teeth, brush up. Brush back and forth on the flat tops—they grind the food. Rinse well, then have a parent floss your teeth.

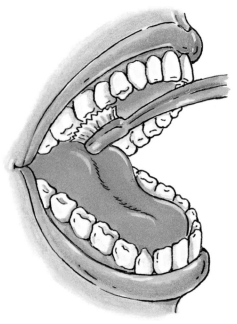

■ Who is this masked man?

Going to the dentist can make you feel like a Hollywood star: You sit in an easy chair under bright lights. The dentist wears a mask and gloves to keep germs out of your mouth. Using a mirror to see inside your mouth, the dentist chips away the food debris called plaque.

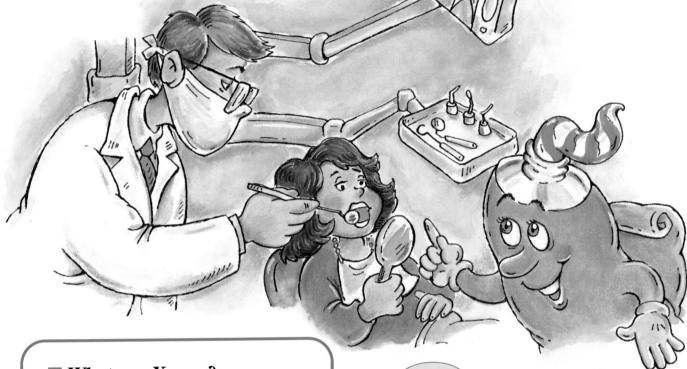

■ What are X-rays?

An X-ray machine *(below)* takes special pictures of your teeth. The X-rays *(bottom photo)* show cavities that need to be filled.

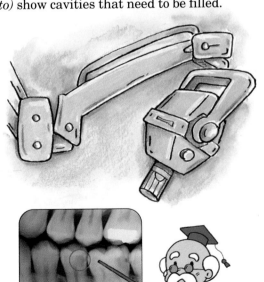

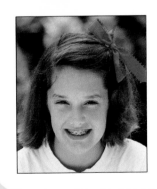

Have you ever wondered why some people wear braces? It's because their teeth grew in crooked. That makes it hard for them to chew. A dentist called an orthodontist puts metal braces on the teeth to straighten them over time.

● To the Parent

You can make your child's trip to the dentist a more positive experience if you prepare him for the visit. Describe what the office looks like, and how it feels to have your teeth cleaned. When you meet the dentist, ask her to watch your child brush his teeth. The dentist may give additional tips. You should floss your child's teeth until he is about 10 years old. Good brushing and flossing habits will help keep your child's teeth and gums healthy for the rest of his life.

Why Should I Wash My Hands?

ANSWER By washing your hands, you get rid of germs that could make you sick. Germs are too small to see, but they are everywhere. They stick to your hands when you touch something like a doorknob, a light switch, or money. Then, when your hands touch your face or your food, the germs can enter your body. But if you wash your hands with soap and warm water, the germs will be washed away. Always wash before eating or after you use the bathroom.

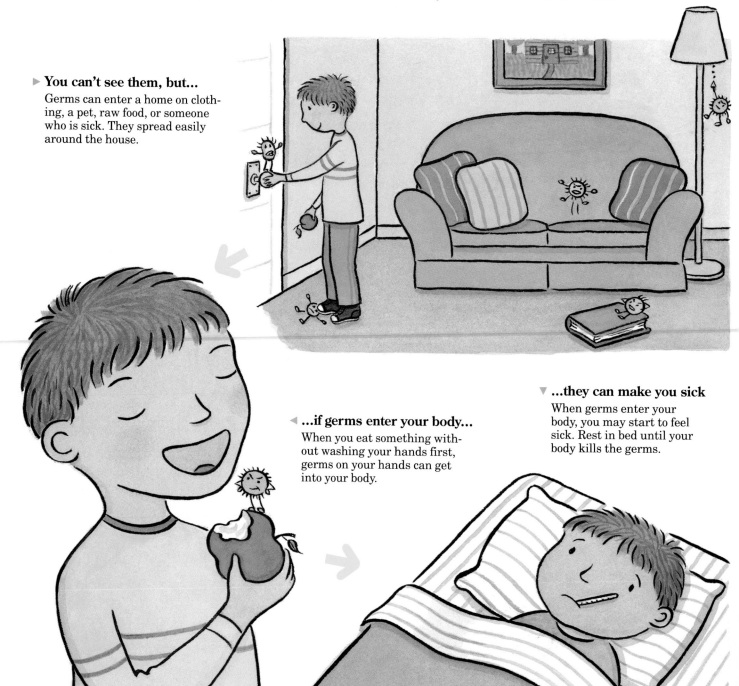

▶ **You can't see them, but...**
Germs can enter a home on clothing, a pet, raw food, or someone who is sick. They spread easily around the house.

◀ **...if germs enter your body...**
When you eat something without washing your hands first, germs on your hands can get into your body.

▼ **...they can make you sick**
When germs enter your body, you may start to feel sick. Rest in bed until your body kills the germs.

■ It pays to be wishy-washy

Washing hands means fighting germs. First, lather up with soap and warm water. Next, scrub your hands for 15 seconds. (Don't forget those fingernails!) Finally, rinse well, and dry with a clean towel.

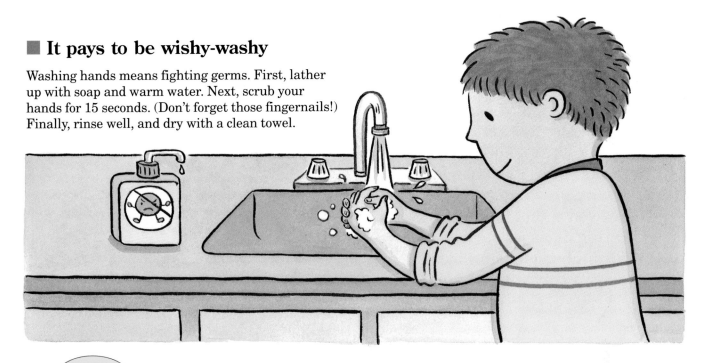

MINI-DATA

■ What are germs?

Germs are tiny living creatures. They are so small that 500 of them could fit on the point of a pencil. Some germs are called viruses; when they get inside your body, they can cause colds. Other germs are called bacteria; they can cause ear infections.

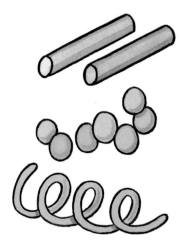

▲ **You guys make me ill!**
From bacteria to viruses, germs come in all shapes and sizes. This is how three types of germs look under a microscope.

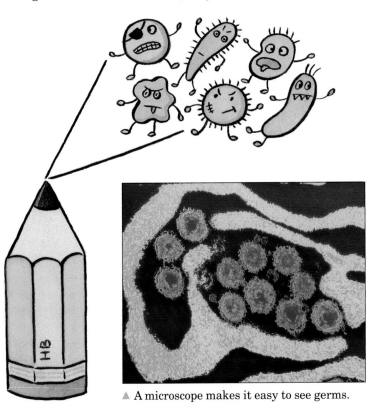

▲ A microscope makes it easy to see germs.

● **To the Parent**

Unwashed hands cause one fourth of all food-borne illnesses. They contribute to other infectious diseases as well. Teach children to scrub their hands and nails often during the day—especially before eating, after using the toilet, and after coming in contact with a pet, money, garbage, or a sick person.

What Does a Doctor Do?

ANSWER The doctor's job is to help you stay healthy. During a visit like the one shown here, the doctor checks your body to make sure you are growing well. She may give you a shot to keep you from getting diseases such as measles or mumps. Ask your doctor how you can stay strong and healthy.

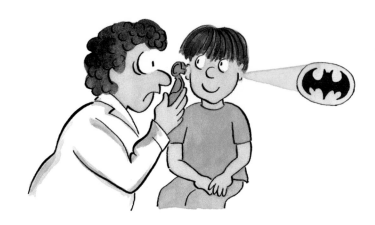

■ Check out this checkup

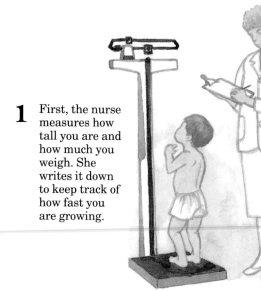

1 First, the nurse measures how tall you are and how much you weigh. She writes it down to keep track of how fast you are growing.

2 Next, the nurse takes your temperature. This tells whether you have a fever.

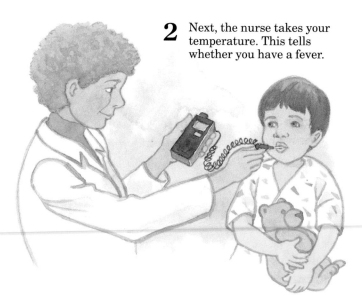

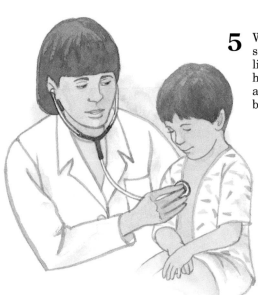

5 With a stethoscope, the doctor listens to your heart beating and your lungs breathing.

6 By pressing down on your stomach, the doctor can tell if your liver is healthy.

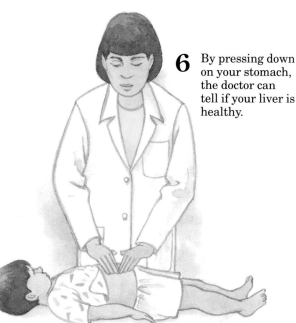

14

Why Do We Get Injections?

An injection causes special germ fighters, called antibodies, to go into your blood. The antibodies last for many years. They protect you from certain germs forever. Although it hurts to get a shot, it's over in a second; it feels like a quick pinch.

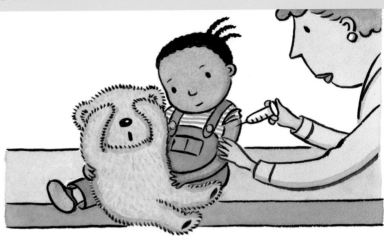

3 The nurse checks your blood pressure by using a special tool to listen to the blood moving through your arm.

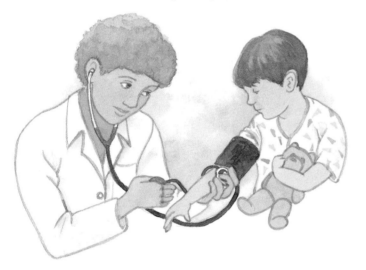

4 After you see the nurse, the doctor begins her checkup. She looks in your ears with a light called an otoscope.

7 The doctor may prick your finger with a tiny needle. The drop of blood is sent to a lab.

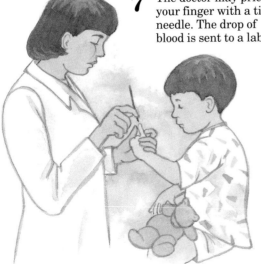

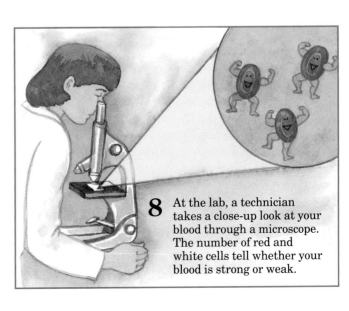

8 At the lab, a technician takes a close-up look at your blood through a microscope. The number of red and white cells tell whether your blood is strong or weak.

How Do We Catch Colds?

ANSWER A cold is spread from one person to the next by tiny germs. When someone with a cold sneezes, or coughs, or hands you something he has touched, the germs get into your throat and lungs. Once they are inside your body, the germs make you sneeze, sniffle, and snooze!

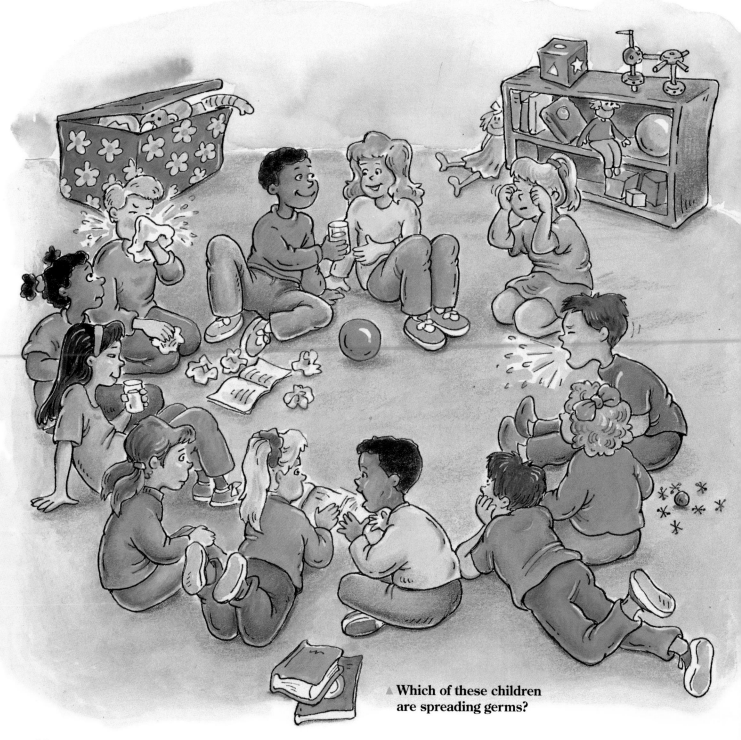

▲ **Which of these children are spreading germs?**

❓ What's the Best Way to Get Better?

If you have a cough, a sore throat, or a stuffy nose, or if you feel tired and achy, you probably have a cold. To get well soon, rest in bed and drink lots of water or juice. A cool-mist vaporizer and nose drops may help unclog your nose.

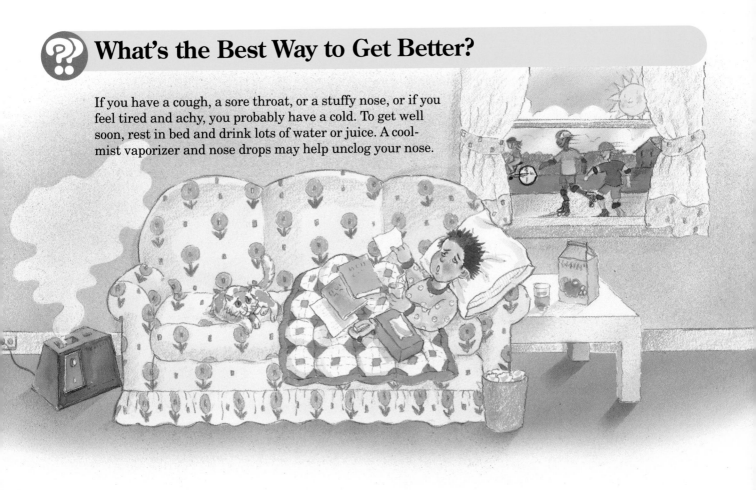

■ Got a cold? Keep it to yourself!

If you stay at home when you are sick, others will not catch your germs. To keep your germs from spreading, cover your mouth and nose with a tissue when you sneeze or cough. Throw away the tissue, then wash your hands.

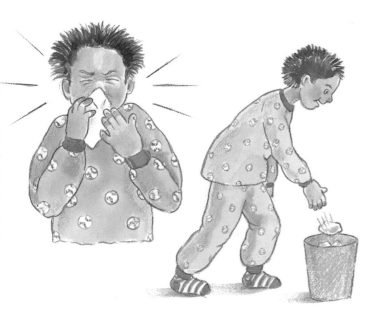

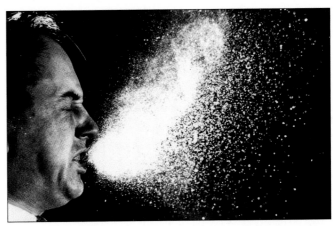

▲ Gesundheit! When you sneeze, your germs fly as far as 15 feet away. The germs can live in the air for several hours.

When Should We Take Medicine?

(ANSWER) When you feel sick, a doctor can find out why by examining you. He may tell you to take a medicine that helps your blood fight the germs that are making you sick. Medicine should be taken only if your doctor prescribes it, and only a parent or other adult should give it to you. Never take medicine on your own! Too much is dangerous, and could make you much sicker.

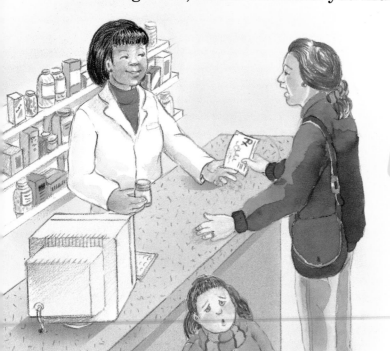

▲ **Getting a prescription**
The doctor writes the name of the medicine—plus how much you should take, and when—on a piece of paper. This is called a prescription. See if you can read it!

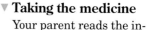 ▼ **Taking the medicine**
Your parent reads the instructions and gives you the right amount of medicine at just the right time.

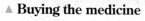 ▲ **Buying the medicine**
A pharmacist in a drugstore follows the doctor's instructions to prepare the medicine. The pharmacist then sells the medicine to your parent.

■ Nature's germ fighters

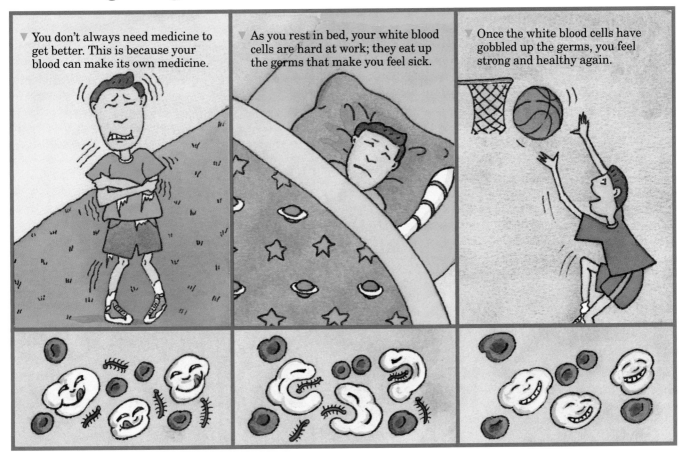

▼ You don't always need medicine to get better. This is because your blood can make its own medicine.

▼ As you rest in bed, your white blood cells are hard at work; they eat up the germs that make you feel sick.

▼ Once the white blood cells have gobbled up the germs, you feel strong and healthy again.

■ The talking medicine

Being upset about something can make you feel sick. When that happens, the best way to get well soon is to talk to someone you trust.

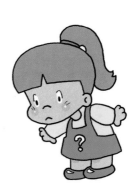

● **To the Parent**

Resist prescribing over-the-counter medications for your child yourself. Many medicines give only symptomatic relief, and some have side effects. The best treatment plan for a child's illness often consists of nothing more than rest, fluids, and TLC (tender loving care).

Keep all medicines out of reach, preferably under lock and key. Never ask a child to bring you medicine, and never refer to it as candy.

Why Are Some People in Wheelchairs?

(ANSWER) A person uses a wheelchair when his legs cannot carry his weight. Someone who is sick or injured may use a wheelchair for a few weeks. Other people use a wheelchair all the time because they were born with weak legs, or because they lost the ability to move their legs. Older people often use a wheelchair because it is too tiring to walk.

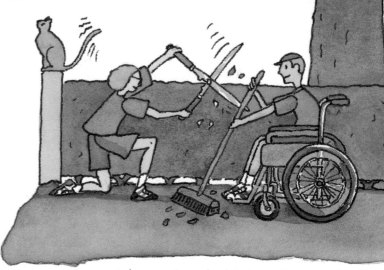

▲ A person in a wheelchair can do many of the same things that anyone else can.

■ Wheeling around

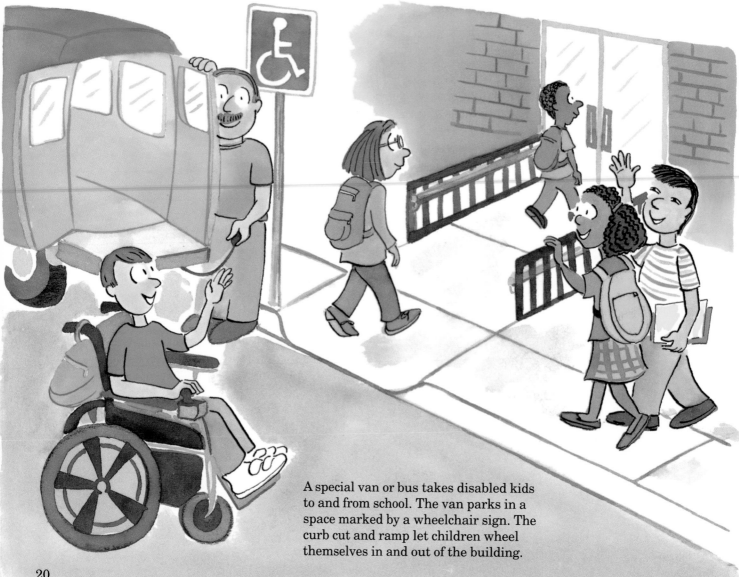

A special van or bus takes disabled kids to and from school. The van parks in a space marked by a wheelchair sign. The curb cut and ramp let children wheel themselves in and out of the building.

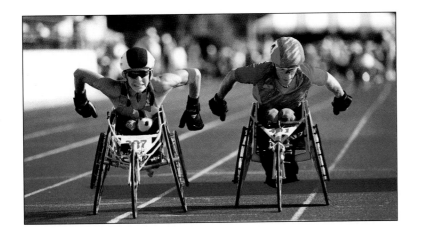

■ The race is on!

Two wheelchair athletes sprint for the finish. The most popular wheelchair sports are racing, basketball, and track and field events such as the shot put, the javelin throw, and the marathon (that's 26 miles!).

 ## How Do Wheelchairs Move?

A person in a wheelchair moves from place to place by turning the wheels with his hands. If the person cannot use his arms, special electrical devices let him move the chair with his hand or chin.

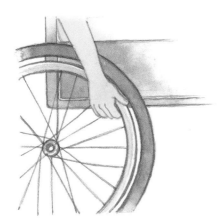

▲ A wheelchair has large wheels with rims. Pushing down on the rims turns the wheels.

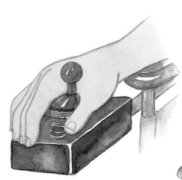

▲ Some wheelchairs are motorized. A joystick on one arm controls a motor that moves the chair forward and back.

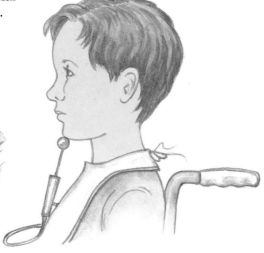

▲ Unable to use his hands, this boy drives his wheelchair by pushing a lever with his chin.

TRY THIS

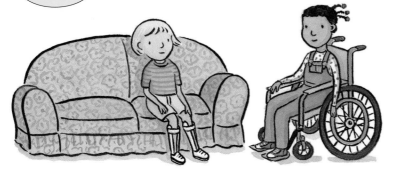

Using a wheelchair may look easy, but it's hard work. If you have a friend in a wheelchair, ask her to let you try it out. This will give you a good idea of what it's like to be disabled.

● **To the Parent**

Encourage your child to be considerate of those who are physically challenged. Discuss ways in which your child might help a person who uses a wheelchair. Emphasize that society values the contribution of everyone, regardless of disability, and this is why it makes special provisions such as wheelchair ramps and parking.

? Why Do People Go to the Hospital?

(ANSWER) A person goes to the hospital when she needs special care from doctors or nurses. She may need stitches to close a deep cut, or a cast to heal a broken bone. If she is very sick, she might need an operation. Mothers usually have their babies in a hospital. So even if you don't remember it, you've probably been to a hospital yourself!

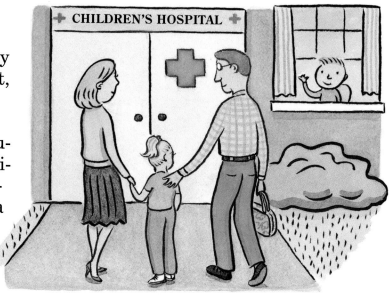

1 When you check into the hospital, a nurse gives you a plastic bracelet with your name and date of birth.

2 The nurse gives you a gown that ties in the back. You wear the gown until you go home.

3 The doctor examines you and asks you questions. (Feel free to ask him questions of your own.) The doctor decides what tests and treatment you need.

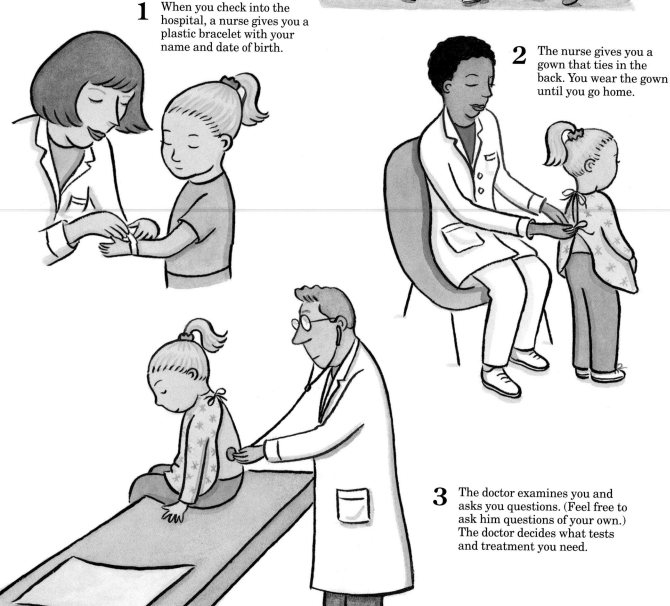

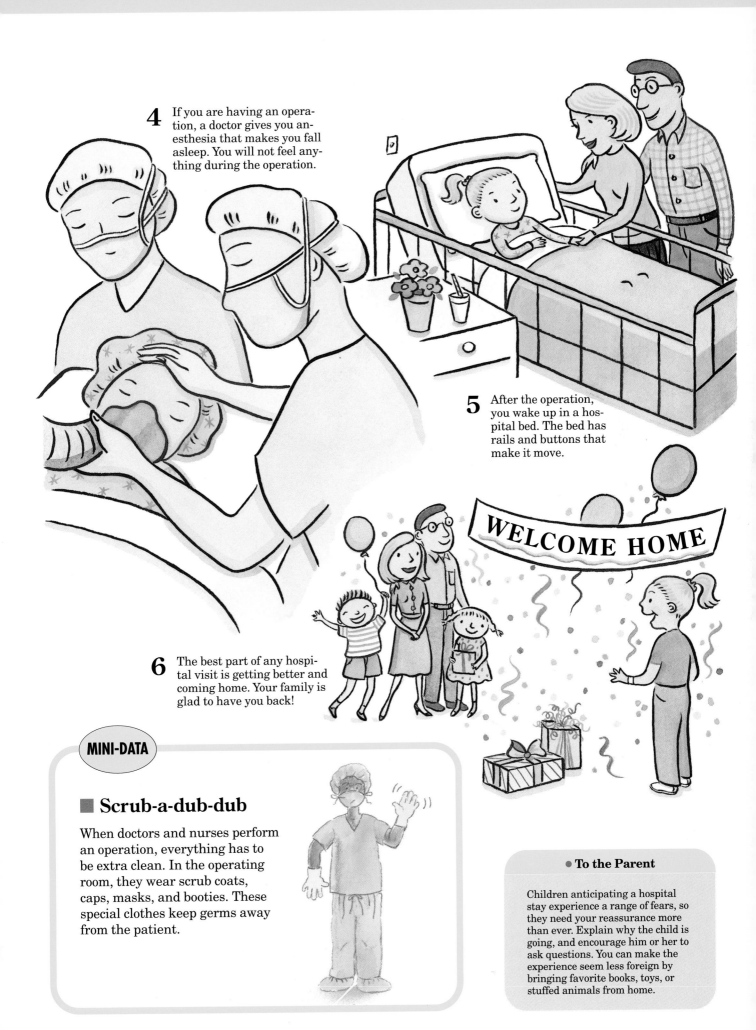

4 If you are having an operation, a doctor gives you anesthesia that makes you fall asleep. You will not feel anything during the operation.

5 After the operation, you wake up in a hospital bed. The bed has rails and buttons that make it move.

6 The best part of any hospital visit is getting better and coming home. Your family is glad to have you back!

WELCOME HOME

MINI-DATA

■ Scrub-a-dub-dub

When doctors and nurses perform an operation, everything has to be extra clean. In the operating room, they wear scrub coats, caps, masks, and booties. These special clothes keep germs away from the patient.

● **To the Parent**

Children anticipating a hospital stay experience a range of fears, so they need your reassurance more than ever. Explain why the child is going, and encourage him or her to ask questions. You can make the experience seem less foreign by bringing favorite books, toys, or stuffed animals from home.

Why Do Some People Smoke?

(ANSWER) Some people think that smoking is fun, or that it makes them look cool. But it's not, and it doesn't. Smoking hurts the human body. The smoke from cigarettes can damage the heart, lungs, and mouth. It can cause deadly diseases, such as cancer. Once a person starts smoking, it is hard to stop. That's because the body develops a need for the nicotine in cigarettes. Those who are smart don't start!

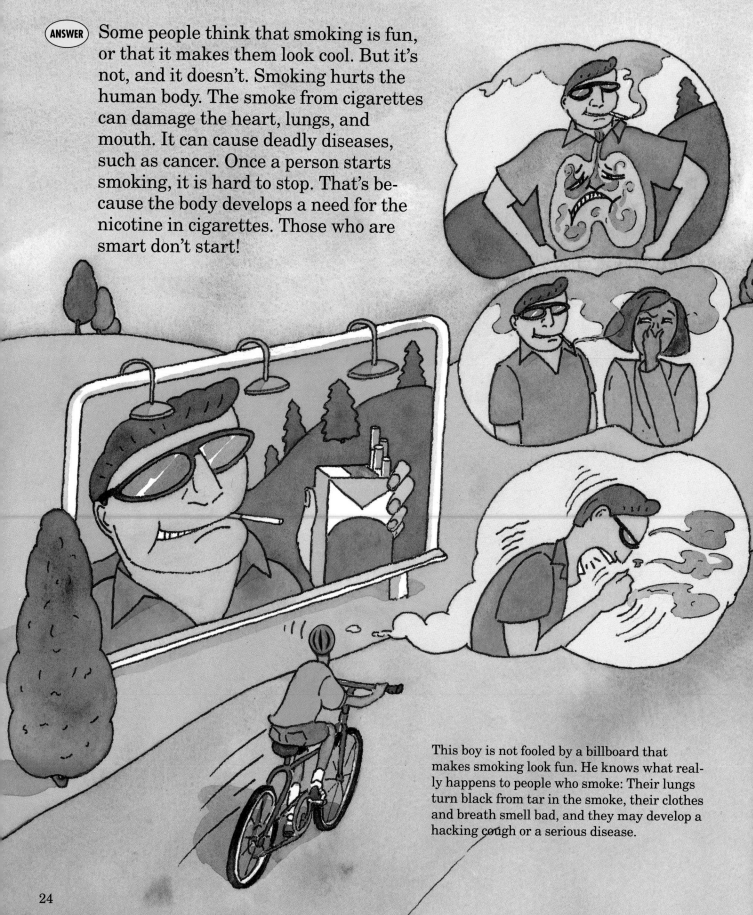

This boy is not fooled by a billboard that makes smoking look fun. He knows what really happens to people who smoke: Their lungs turn black from tar in the smoke, their clothes and breath smell bad, and they may develop a hacking cough or a serious disease.

■ Smoking is a drag

Have you ever wondered why people start smoking? Sometimes the habit begins when a person's so-called "friends" pressure him to smoke with them. It takes a smart and confident kid—like the young dragon at far right—to say "No!" to cigarettes. It's far better to disappoint your friends than to get a disease and die young.

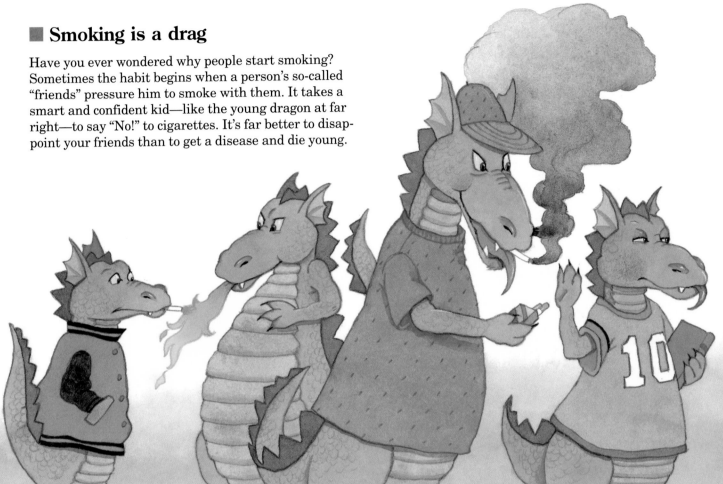

■ Second-hand smoke

Cigarette smoke is so poisonous that it can harm people who breathe in smoke from someone else's cigarette. For this reason, many restaurants and other public places say, "No smoking allowed!"

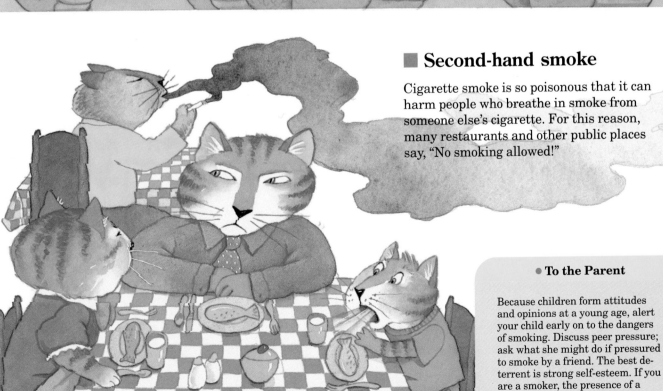

● To the Parent

Because children form attitudes and opinions at a young age, alert your child early on to the dangers of smoking. Discuss peer pressure; ask what she might do if pressured to smoke by a friend. The best deterrent is strong self-esteem. If you are a smoker, the presence of a child in the household can be just the incentive to stop.

? How Much Sleep Do I Need?

ANSWER When you were a baby, you slept most of the day. At the age of four, you need about 12 hours of sleep a day. Once you are eight, you need only about 10 hours.

Getting enough sleep is important because that's when your body rests and rebuilds its strength. Even animals need their sleep.

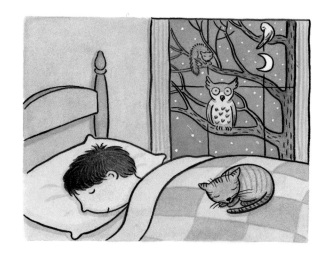

■ This is the way we hit the hay

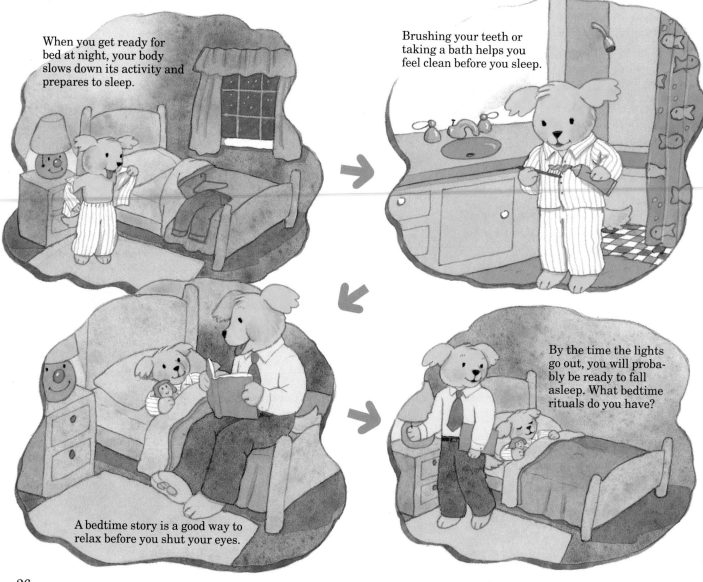

When you get ready for bed at night, your body slows down its activity and prepares to sleep.

Brushing your teeth or taking a bath helps you feel clean before you sleep.

A bedtime story is a good way to relax before you shut your eyes.

By the time the lights go out, you will probably be ready to fall asleep. What bedtime rituals do you have?

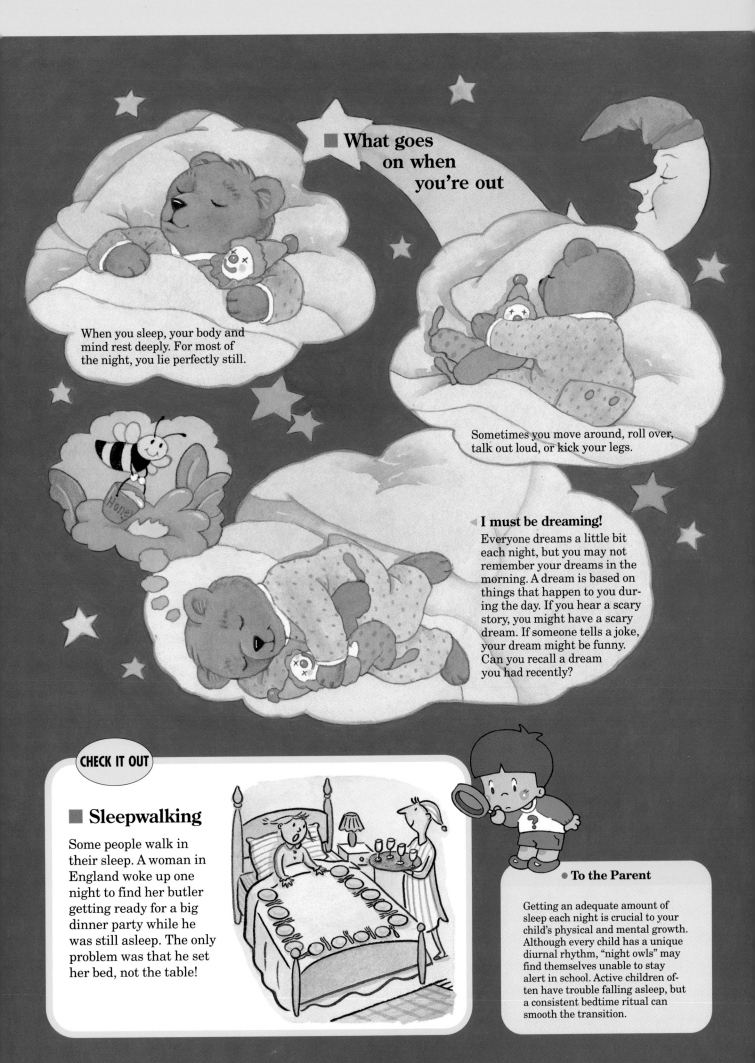

■ What goes on when you're out

When you sleep, your body and mind rest deeply. For most of the night, you lie perfectly still.

Sometimes you move around, roll over, talk out loud, or kick your legs.

◄ **I must be dreaming!**

Everyone dreams a little bit each night, but you may not remember your dreams in the morning. A dream is based on things that happen to you during the day. If you hear a scary story, you might have a scary dream. If someone tells a joke, your dream might be funny. Can you recall a dream you had recently?

CHECK IT OUT

■ Sleepwalking

Some people walk in their sleep. A woman in England woke up one night to find her butler getting ready for a big dinner party while he was still asleep. The only problem was that he set her bed, not the table!

● **To the Parent**

Getting an adequate amount of sleep each night is crucial to your child's physical and mental growth. Although every child has a unique diurnal rhythm, "night owls" may find themselves unable to stay alert in school. Active children often have trouble falling asleep, but a consistent bedtime ritual can smooth the transition.

Why Is It Good to Exercise?

ANSWER Exercise helps your body become strong, healthy, and flexible. Regular exercise is the best way to make your muscles grow. It's also a great way to feel good! There are many fun ways to get exercise. Which of the ones shown here do you like best?

▼ **Flexibility**
Exercise can keep your body flexible, or easy to move. A body that is flexible is less likely to get hurt.

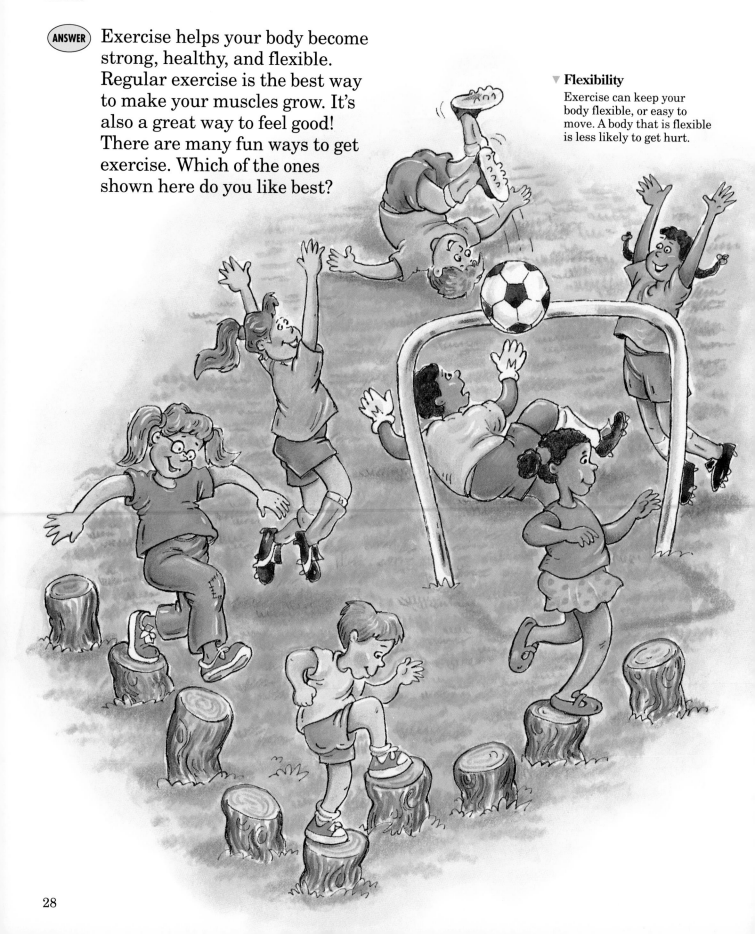

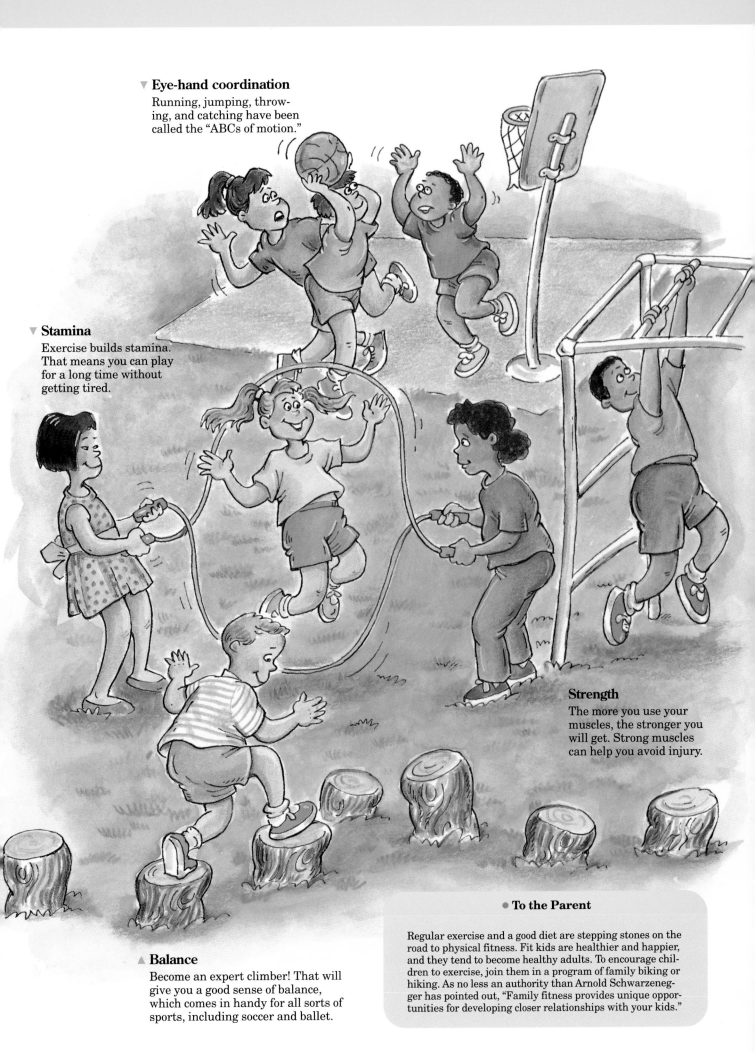

▼ Eye-hand coordination

Running, jumping, throwing, and catching have been called the "ABCs of motion."

▼ Stamina

Exercise builds stamina. That means you can play for a long time without getting tired.

Strength

The more you use your muscles, the stronger you will get. Strong muscles can help you avoid injury.

▲ Balance

Become an expert climber! That will give you a good sense of balance, which comes in handy for all sorts of sports, including soccer and ballet.

Is Watching TV Bad for Your Body?

ANSWER TV can be bad for your body if you watch too much of it. To stay healthy, you need to stay active. But how can you do that if you're sitting still and watching TV all the time?

People who watch a lot of TV also tend to snack on junk food. Not enough exercise and too much food is a double whammy; it can make your body weigh more than is healthy.

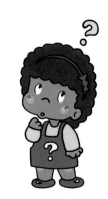

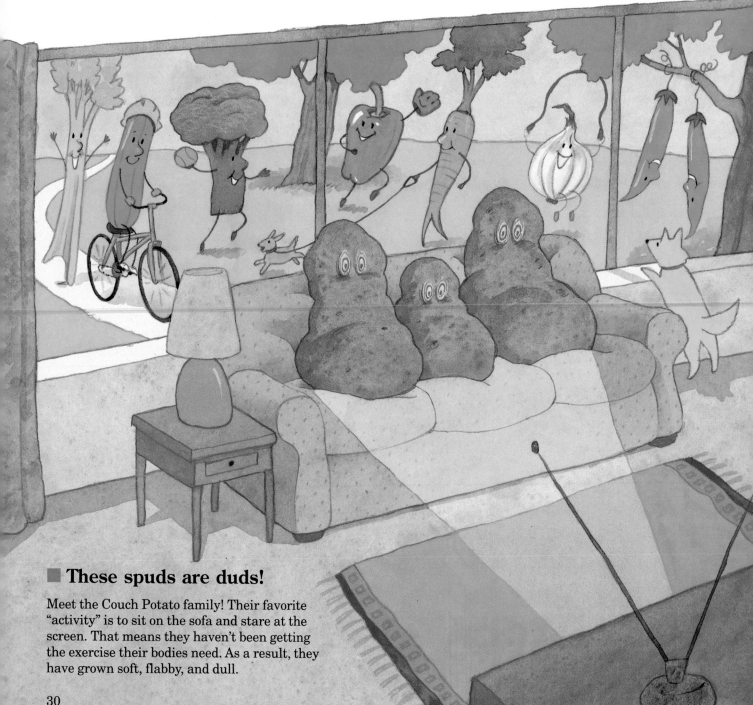

■ These spuds are duds!

Meet the Couch Potato family! Their favorite "activity" is to sit on the sofa and stare at the screen. That means they haven't been getting the exercise their bodies need. As a result, they have grown soft, flabby, and dull.

■ Set your dial to "Off"

The last week of April is "National TV-Turnoff Week." During this time, families agree not to watch television for seven days in a row. Instead, they read, talk, work, play, and do other fun things together. How can you tell that this household is taking part?

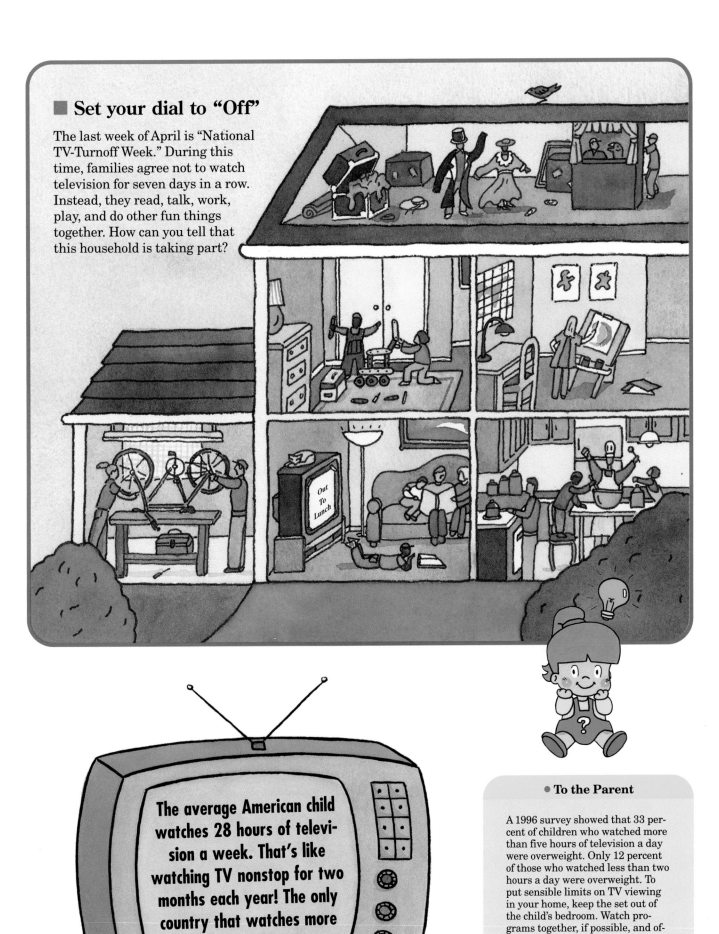

The average American child watches 28 hours of television a week. That's like watching TV nonstop for two months each year! The only country that watches more TV than the U.S. is Japan.

❓ What Is First Aid?

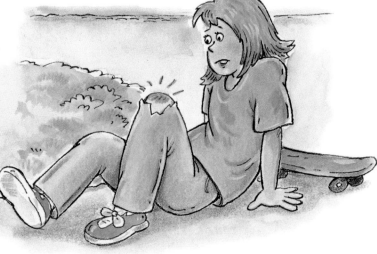

ANSWER First aid is the first thing you do to help someone who is injured. First aid can prevent the injury from getting worse. It can also help the person get better quicker. Although it is scary when you or someone you are with gets hurt, it's important to stay calm. If there are other people around, have one of them go get help; if not, you may have to go yourself.

■ What should I do if...

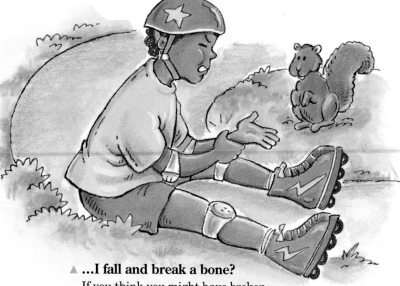

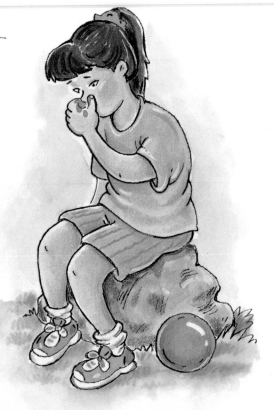

▲ **...I fall and scrape my knee?**
Firmly press a clean cloth against the scrape. When the bleeding stops, wash the cut with soap and water.

▲ **...I fall and break a bone?**
If you think you might have broken a bone, stay still. Don't move unless you are in a dangerous place. Send or call for help, and try to stay calm.

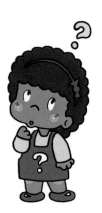

▶ **...my nose starts bleeding?**
To stop a nosebleed, pinch your nostrils closed and hold your head down. Don't tip your head back—the blood might run into your throat.

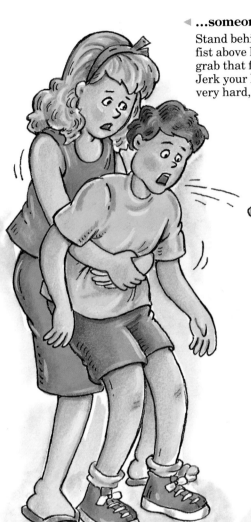

◄ ...someone is choking?

Stand behind the person. Put one fist above his bellybutton, then grab that fist with your other hand. Jerk your hands up and toward you very hard, six to 10 times.

▲ ...I burn myself?

Run the burn under cold water. Do not use ice or butter. Get help from a parent or other adult as soon as you can.

■ A first-aid kit

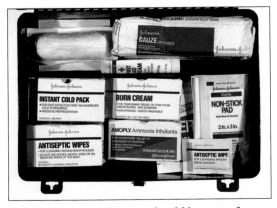

A first-aid kit like this one should be part of every home and car. The bandages let you treat injuries that do not need a doctor. They also let you treat more serious injuries until help arrives. Ask a parent to explain how each item should be used.

▲ ...I twist my knee or ankle?

If you have a bad sprain, RICE it. In other words, 1) **R**est the injury; 2) put **I**ce on it; 3) **C**ompress the injury by wrapping it tight; and 4) **E**levate it by propping up your leg.

● To the Parent

Each year in the U.S., some 13 million children suffer injuries requiring medical treatment. Ten million of these incidents involve an emergency-room visit, and 360,000 lead to hospitalization. Discuss emergency situations with your children so they will know what to do. Stress the basics: Stay calm, get help, do not endanger yourself, and do not move an injured person unless he or she is in immediate danger. Best of all, sign up for a course in first aid or CPR.

? What Are Allergies?

ANSWER If something you touch, breathe, or eat makes you sniffle and sneeze, you may have an allergy to it. Usually that "something" is not harmful, nor does it bother most people. If your eyes itch when cats are around, you are probably allergic to cats. The most common allergies are to pollen, dust, mold, and certain foods.

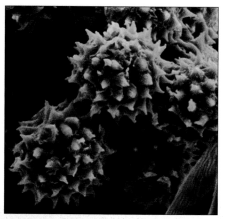

▲ Pollen looks like this in a microscope.

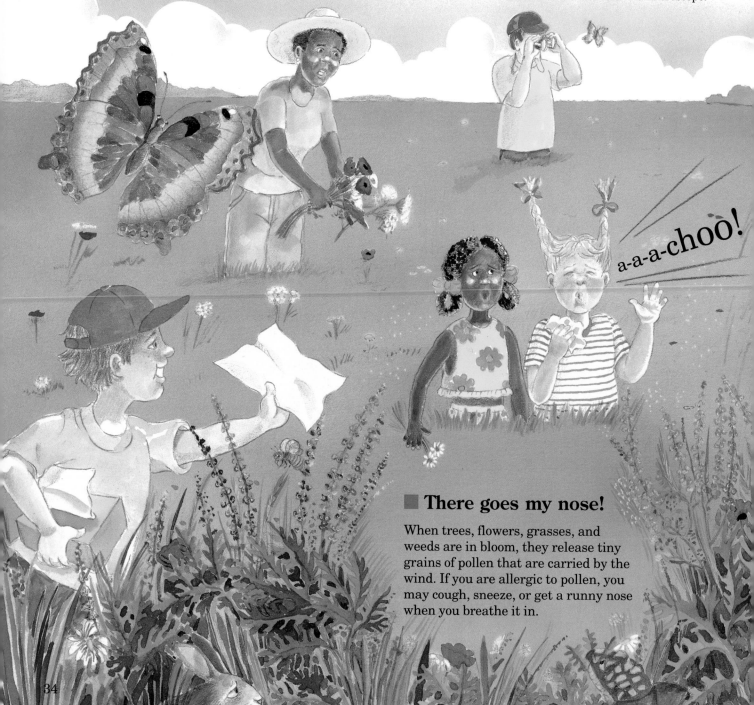

a-a-a-choo!

■ There goes my nose!

When trees, flowers, grasses, and weeds are in bloom, they release tiny grains of pollen that are carried by the wind. If you are allergic to pollen, you may cough, sneeze, or get a runny nose when you breathe it in.

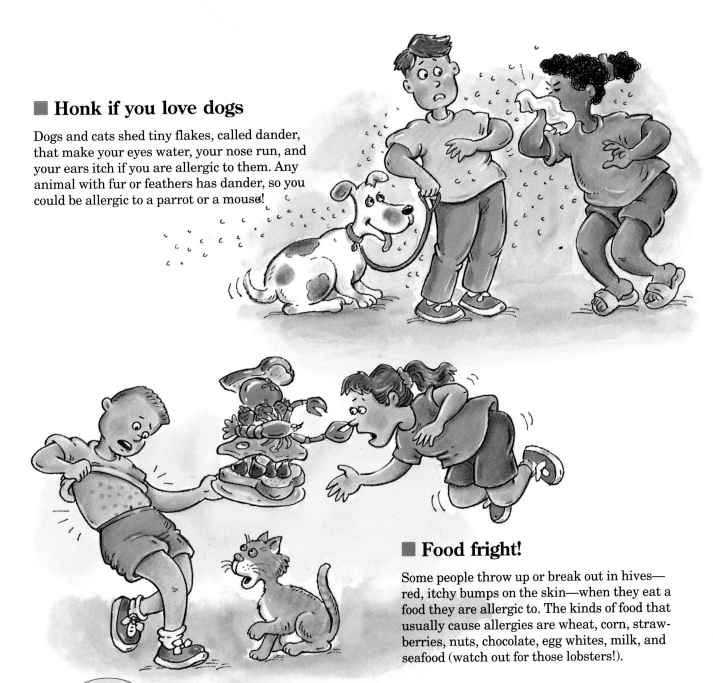

■ Honk if you love dogs

Dogs and cats shed tiny flakes, called dander, that make your eyes water, your nose run, and your ears itch if you are allergic to them. Any animal with fur or feathers has dander, so you could be allergic to a parrot or a mouse!

■ Food fright!

Some people throw up or break out in hives—red, itchy bumps on the skin—when they eat a food they are allergic to. The kinds of food that usually cause allergies are wheat, corn, strawberries, nuts, chocolate, egg whites, milk, and seafood (watch out for those lobsters!).

MINI-DATA

■ What is asthma?

Asthma, caused by allergies, affects three million American children. If you are one of them, you know that an asthma attack makes it very hard to breathe. Some children, like this baseball player, use an inhaler during an attack. It holds medicine that helps them breathe.

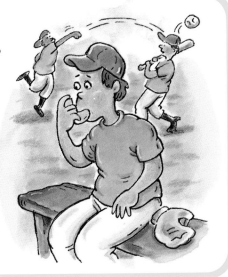

● To the Parent

One out of every five children has allergies. An allergy is an overreaction by the immune system to a substance, such as pollen, that is not harmful. When a virus, bacteria, or other foreign matter enters the body, the immune system orders certain cells to release histamines; these in turn produce runny noses, stomach aches, rashes, and other symptoms. Antihistamines provide safe but short-lived relief.

Why Do People Say "Laughter Is the Best Medicine"?

ANSWER Jokes and laughter can fix a lot of problems. When you feel sad, seeing something funny can make you feel better right away. In fact, many doctors think that jokes, laughter, and games really do help sick people heal faster.

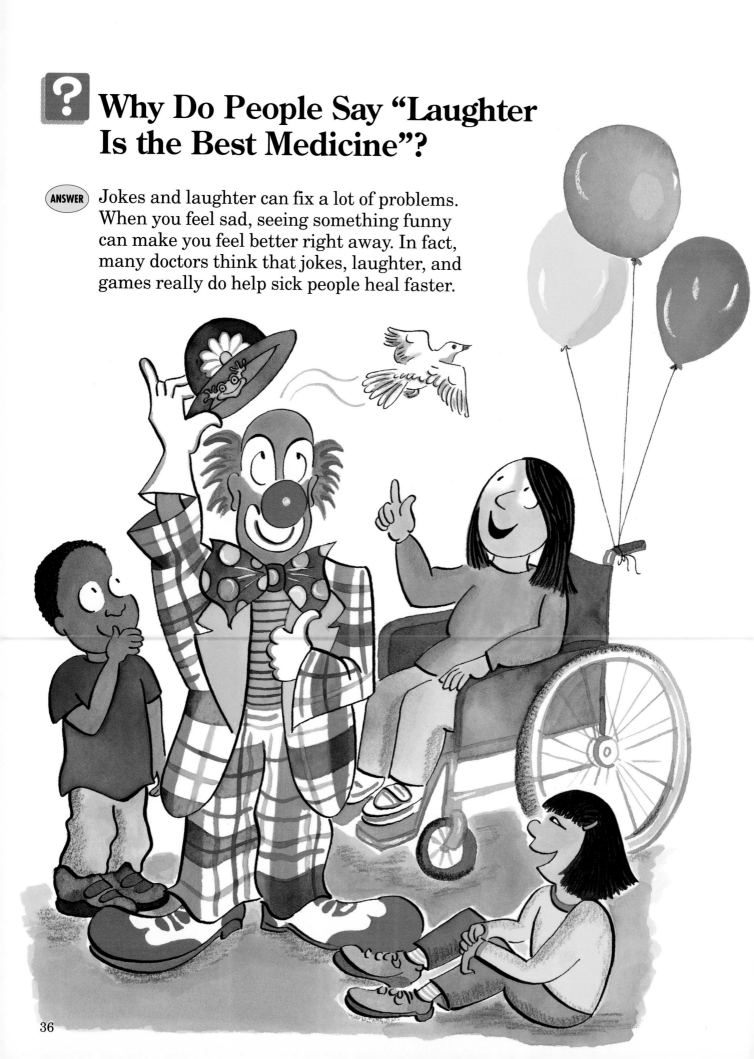

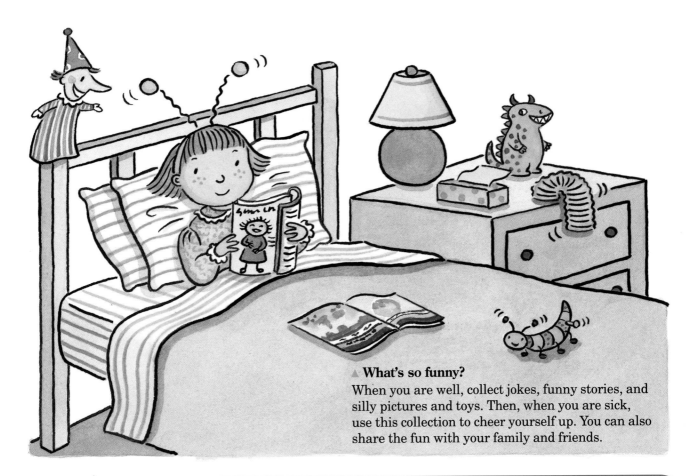

What's so funny?
When you are well, collect jokes, funny stories, and silly pictures and toys. Then, when you are sick, use this collection to cheer yourself up. You can also share the fun with your family and friends.

■ It takes patients to play

Some young cancer patients play computer games that show their bodies killing cancer cells. Doctors say the games make the patients feel better because they can beat their disease on the screen. In one hospital, kids with cancer invented a board game to help other patients deal with the disease. They used bandages and empty pill bottles for game pieces!

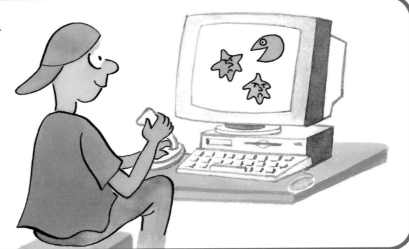

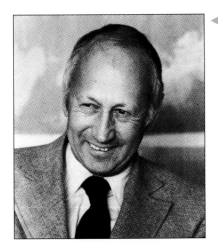

◀ Magazine editor Norman Cousins recovered from a crippling disease by watching funny movies, reading jokes, and taking Vitamin C. He wrote a book about his "laughter cure." Later on, he worked with hospitals to find ways to amuse very sick patients.

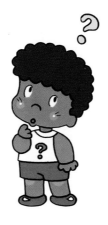

● **To the Parent**

The Biblical axiom that "a merry heart doeth good like a medicine" has a basis in fact: Medical researchers have shown that good old-fashioned belly laughter increases the heart rate, enhances respiration, and promotes the activity of disease-fighting immune cells. So try to keep your child's spirits up during an illness.

Is It Okay to Feel Sad or Angry?

(ANSWER) Everyone feels sad or angry sometimes. These feelings, or emotions, are a natural part of you. When you feel sad, or angry, or hurt, there are many things you can do to feel better. It's important to let the bad feelings out in a way that won't hurt anyone else. One good way is to tell your parents or friends what's bothering you, so they can help.

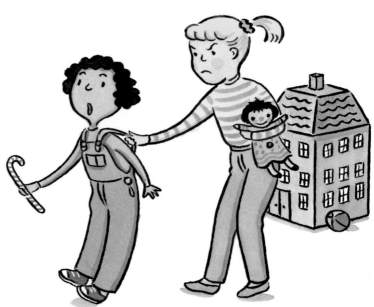

■ Gimme some candy!

Sometimes things just don't seem fair. But if you get into an argument when you're playing with a friend, no one has any fun. Ask a parent or another friend to help you work things out without hurting the other person's feelings.

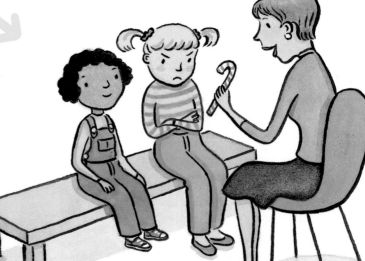

Did You Know That Crying Can Be Good for You?

Crying lets you and others know that something is wrong. You may be hurt, or you may just be sad. Going off alone to have a good cry gives you a chance to get away from the problem and express how you feel about it.

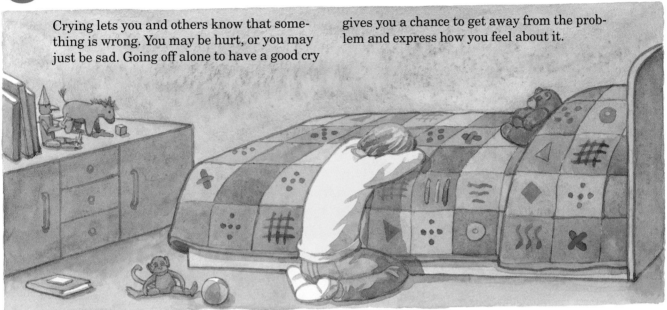

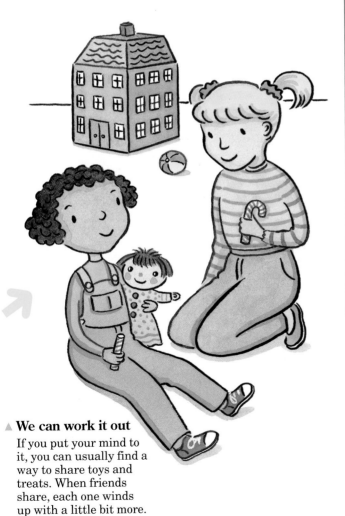

▲ We can work it out

If you put your mind to it, you can usually find a way to share toys and treats. When friends share, each one winds up with a little bit more.

■ Take that!

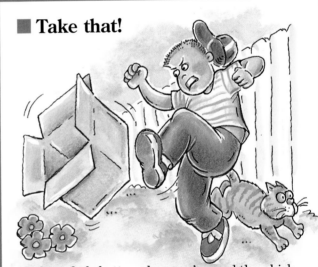

Nothing feels better when you're mad than kicking an empty cardboard box. Talk to a parent to choose a harmless way of letting off steam.

● To the Parent

Anger, sadness, resentment, and frustration are unpleasant but normal human feelings. You can help children cope with these negative emotions without denying them. Encourage children to name their feelings, then discuss them together. Acknowledge what they are going through; let them know you take their feelings seriously. Children who exhibit an unusual amount of anger, quarreling, or sadness may need the extra help of a professional counselor.

Why Do People Fight?

ANSWER Sometimes people try to settle their differences by fighting. A person who is angry at someone else, or unhappy with himself, may also try to pick a fight. And some people fight by yelling and hurting each other's feelings.

None of these is a good way to solve a problem. To work something out, talk it out—if not with the other person, with an adult.

▼ Many animals fight over food or territory. Have you ever seen two dogs play tug-of-war with a bone or a toy?

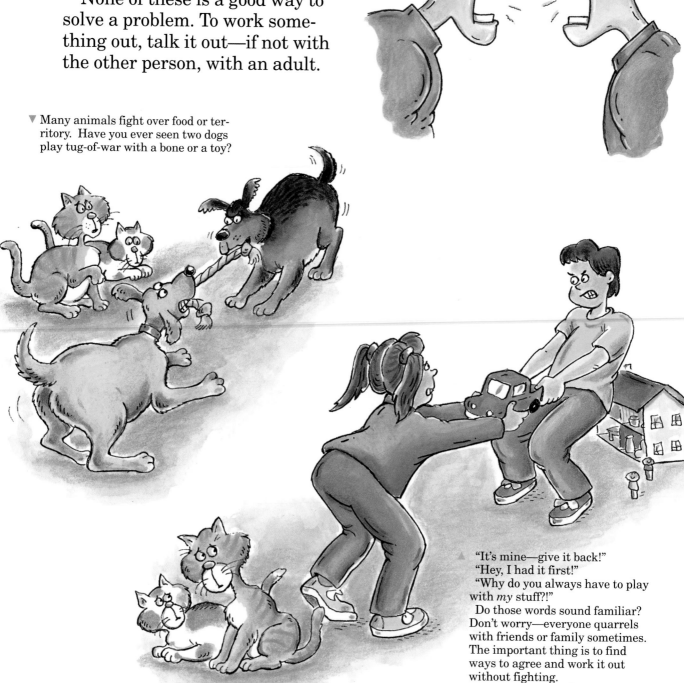

▲ "It's mine—give it back!"
"Hey, I had it first!"
"Why do you always have to play with *my* stuff?!"
Do those words sound familiar? Don't worry—everyone quarrels with friends or family sometimes. The important thing is to find ways to agree and work it out without fighting.

■ Three ways to avoid a fight

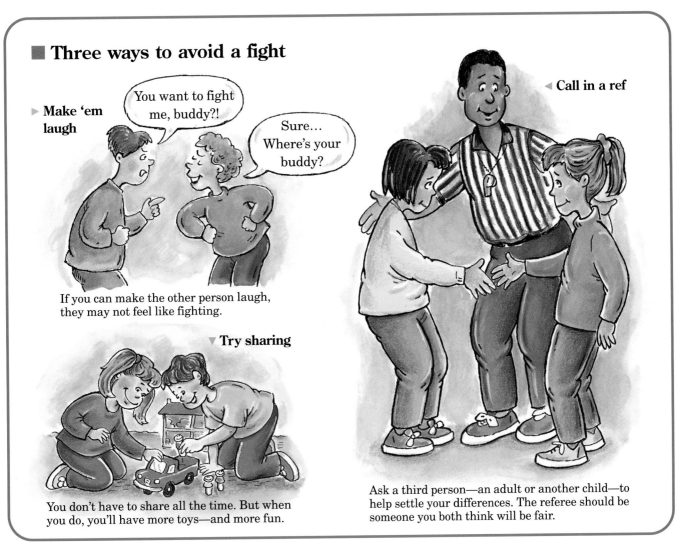

► **Make 'em laugh**

"You want to fight me, buddy?!"

"Sure… Where's your buddy?"

If you can make the other person laugh, they may not feel like fighting.

▼ **Try sharing**

You don't have to share all the time. But when you do, you'll have more toys—and more fun.

◄ **Call in a ref**

Ask a third person—an adult or another child—to help settle your differences. The referee should be someone you both think will be fair.

■ How to handle a bully

Bullies can be scary. One way to avoid them is to stay with a group of friends. If a bully frightens you, tell an adult about it. That way, both you and the bully can get help.

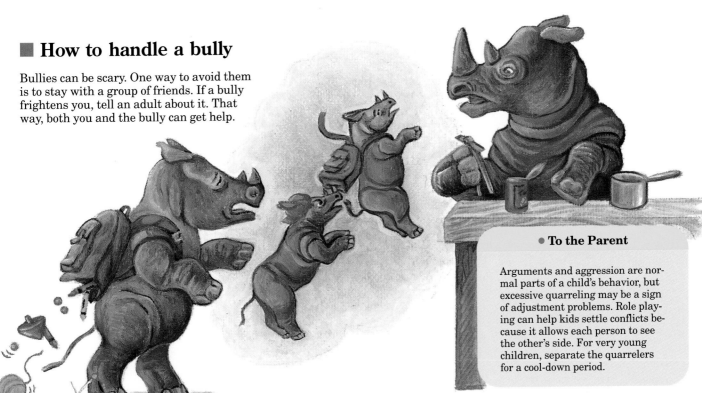

● **To the Parent**

Arguments and aggression are normal parts of a child's behavior, but excessive quarreling may be a sign of adjustment problems. Role playing can help kids settle conflicts because it allows each person to see the other's side. For very young children, separate the quarrelers for a cool-down period.

41

Why Do We Have Rules and Laws?

ANSWER Rules and laws help us get along with one another. Without them, life would be confusing—and dangerous! Traffic laws, for example, keep people safe. The laws tell all drivers to follow the same rules. Just imagine what would happen if everyone drove as they pleased—or followed their own rules!

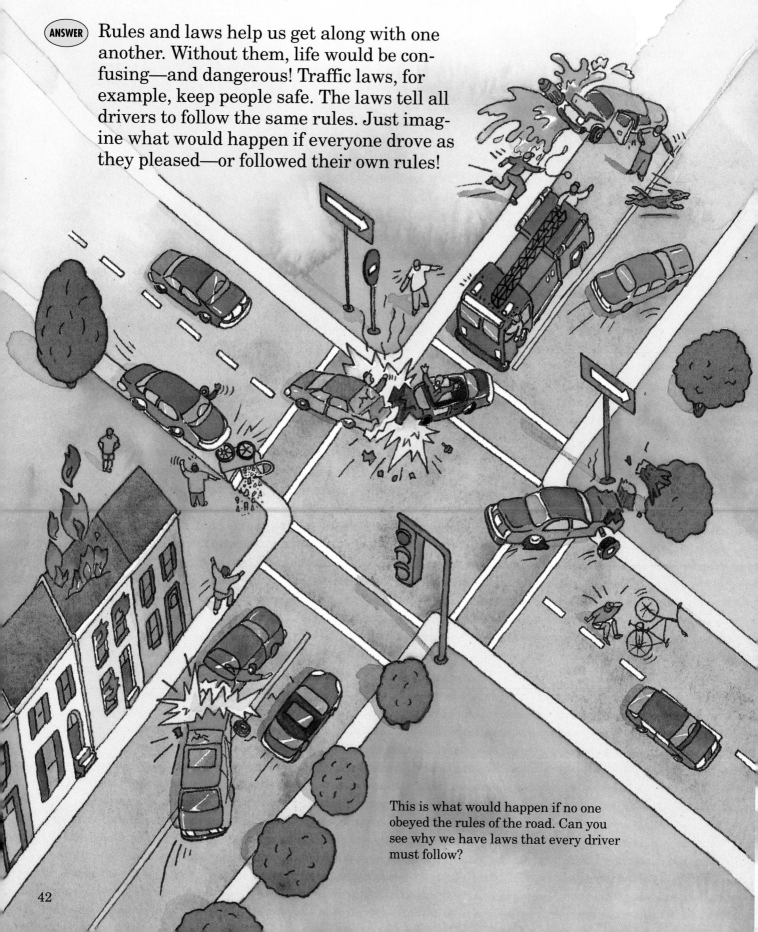

This is what would happen if no one obeyed the rules of the road. Can you see why we have laws that every driver must follow?

42

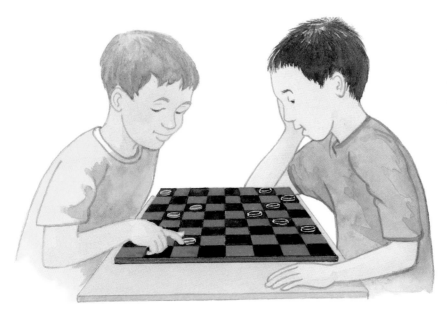

■ Rules to play by

Two boys enjoy a game of checkers because they both play by the rules of the game. Every game, from soccer to hopscotch, has special rules that all players must follow. The rules make the game both fair and fun.

■ Rules to learn by

Uh-oh...it looks like these kids forgot a few of the rules at school! One of those rules is "Take turns." What are some other rules they need to remember?

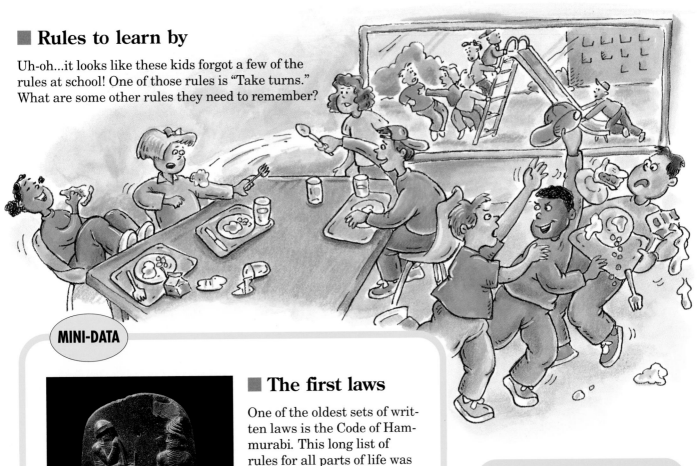

MINI-DATA

■ The first laws

One of the oldest sets of written laws is the Code of Hammurabi. This long list of rules for all parts of life was carved on a stone column *(left)* more than 3,700 years ago in a land called Babylon. It is named for the king who organized the laws. The top of the stone shows Hammurabi standing before the god of justice.

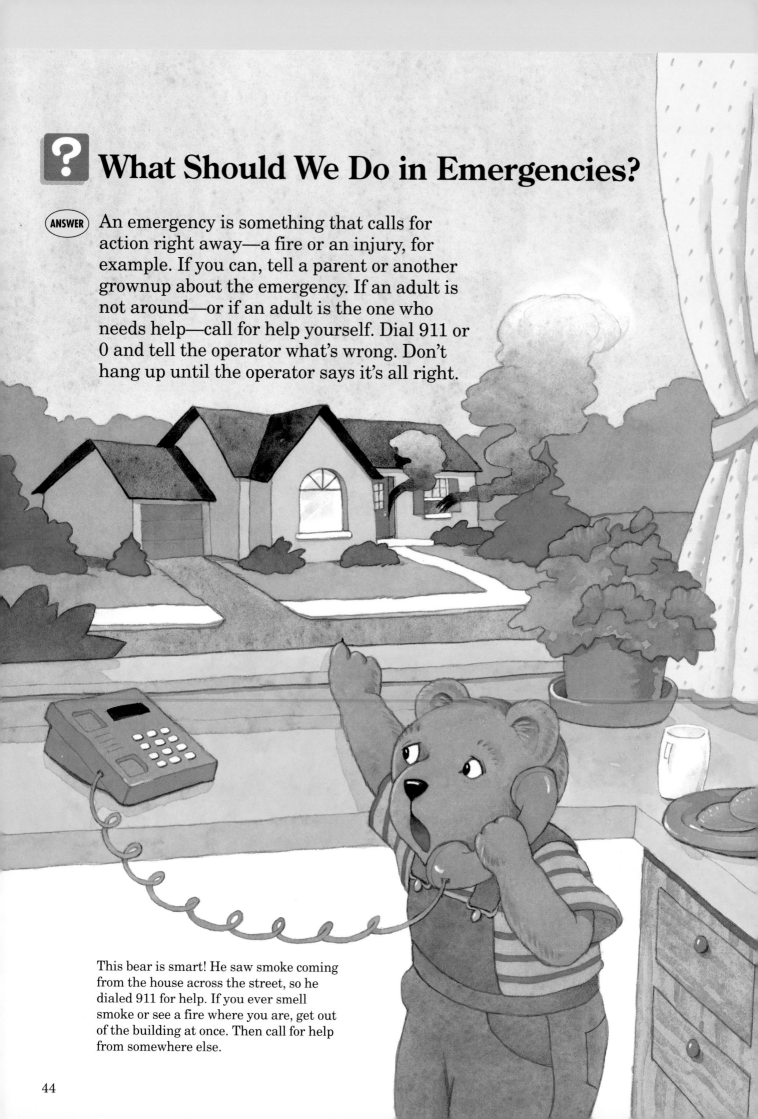

What Should We Do in Emergencies?

ANSWER An emergency is something that calls for action right away—a fire or an injury, for example. If you can, tell a parent or another grownup about the emergency. If an adult is not around—or if an adult is the one who needs help—call for help yourself. Dial 911 or 0 and tell the operator what's wrong. Don't hang up until the operator says it's all right.

This bear is smart! He saw smoke coming from the house across the street, so he dialed 911 for help. If you ever smell smoke or see a fire where you are, get out of the building at once. Then call for help from somewhere else.

What Should I Do If I Get Lost?

If you don't see your mom or dad, stay put! They will probably come back looking for you soon. In a store, you can go to a person at a cash register or behind a sales counter and ask for help. A police officer can also help you find your parent.

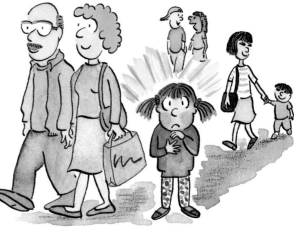

▲ Uh-oh! I don't see my mom anywhere. What should I do?

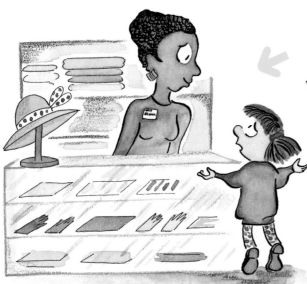

▲ I know! I'll go to a person who works for the store and ask her to help me find my mother.

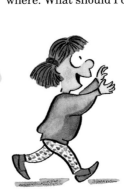

▲ There you are, Mom! I'm so glad you're not lost anymore!

■ Plan and practice

I can say my address and phone number! Can you say yours?

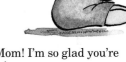 **● To the Parent**

Young children can learn how to get emergency assistance. Using an unplugged or toy phone, have your child practice dialing 911 (or 0, depending on your community). On shopping trips, point out sales clerks or cashiers and tell your child that these are the people to go to if he or she gets lost.

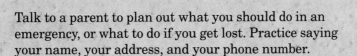

Talk to a parent to plan out what you should do in an emergency, or what to do if you get lost. Practice saying your name, your address, and your phone number.

Whom Can I Ask for Help When I Need It?

ANSWER All sorts of grownups care about you and can help you stay well and safe. Besides your parents, here are some of the people who can help you solve a problem: teachers, doctors, relatives, neighbors, police officers, fire fighters, and ministers, rabbis, or other religious leaders. Talk to your mom or dad about which people you should go to for help.

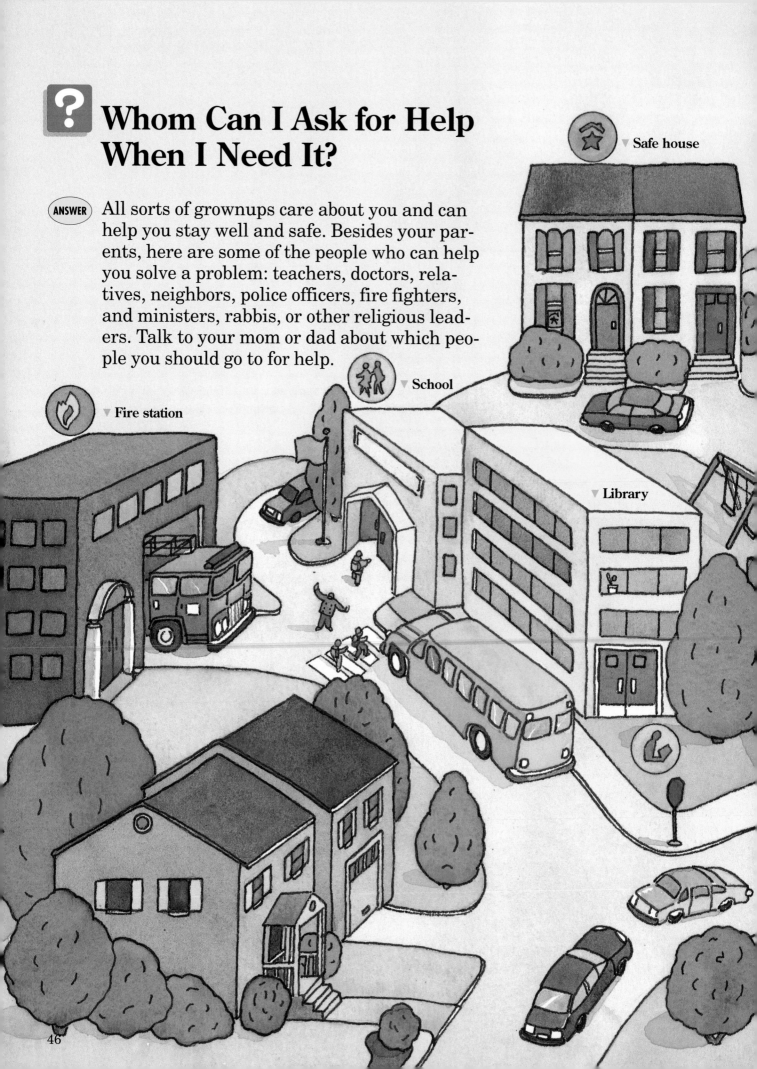

▼ Safe house

▼ School

▼ Fire station

▼ Library

46

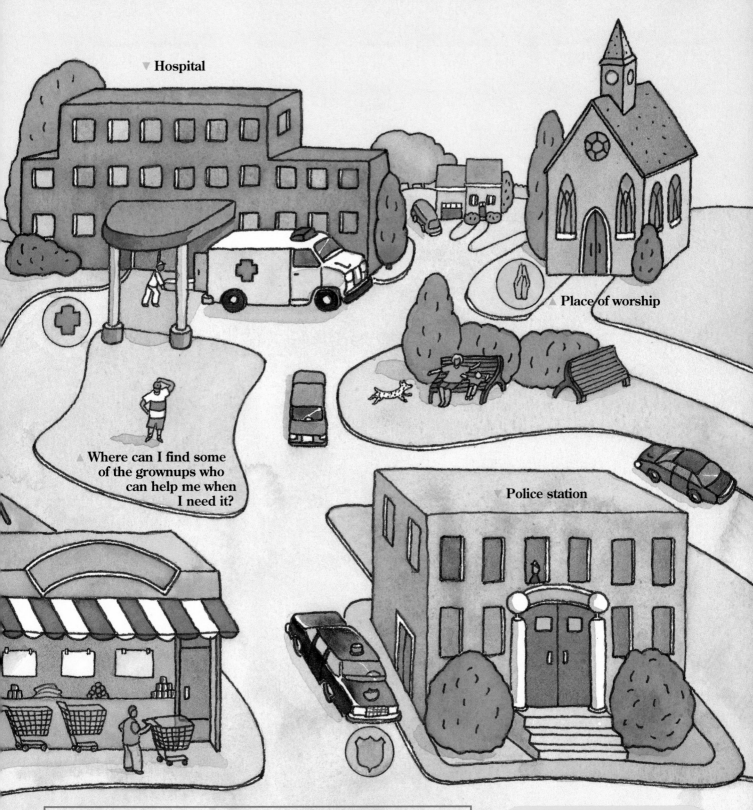

▼ Hospital

▲ Place of worship

▲ Where can I find some of the grownups who can help me when I need it?

▼ Police station

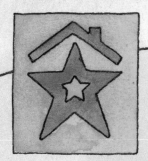

■ Block-parent program

In many neighborhoods, this sign on a house means it's safe to go there if you are hurt or frightened, or if you have another serious problem. The grownups who live there will help you. Ask a parent what sort of sign to look for in your community.

● **To the Parent**

Every community includes a collection of adults who care about the safety and well-being of children. Inform your kids who these people are; then, if they ever need to go to someone else for help, they will know whom it is safe to approach. Of course, you should also caution your children about the danger of strangers who approach them.

What If a Stranger Tries to Talk to Me?

ANSWER It's all right if a grownup you don't know smiles and says hello to you. But unless your parents are with you, you should not talk to that person—even if he or she seems friendly, and even if he or she knows your name. Never go anywhere with a stranger. If a stranger tries to talk to you, walk away and tell your parents.

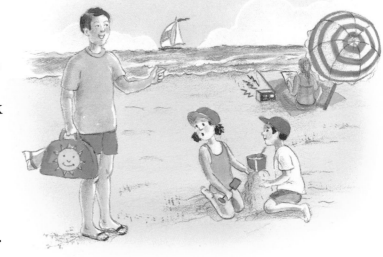

■ If someone offers you a treat

It is not okay for an adult you don't know to try to give you something. Say no and get away. Tell your parents, or another grownup you trust, what happened.

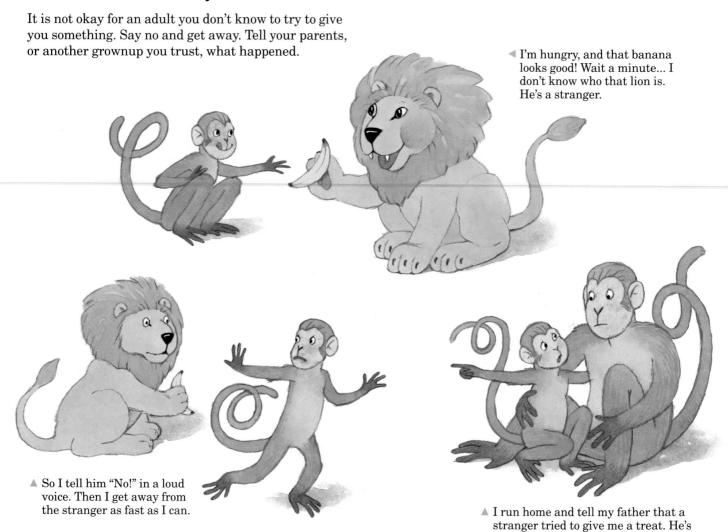

◀ I'm hungry, and that banana looks good! Wait a minute... I don't know who that lion is. He's a stranger.

▲ So I tell him "No!" in a loud voice. Then I get away from the stranger as fast as I can.

▲ I run home and tell my father that a stranger tried to give me a treat. He's glad I knew the right thing to do.

Are All Strangers Bad?

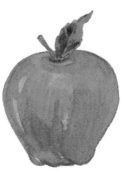 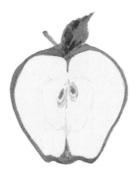 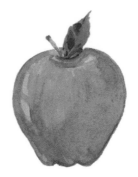 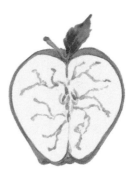

Apples are like people. They may look alike on the outside, but inside one may be good and the other one rotten. Most people are nice, but there are some people in the world who may not be nice to children. You can't tell just by looking at a person whether he is good inside.

■ What's the password?

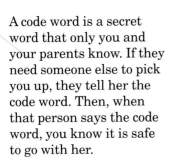

Do you and your parents
have a code word?
You should! Mine is—oops!
I can't tell anyone!

A code word is a secret word that only you and your parents know. If they need someone else to pick you up, they tell her the code word. Then, when that person says the code word, you know it is safe to go with her.

■ Saying no to a grownup

You can always say no to a stranger, but you can also say it to grownups you know. If anyone touches you in a way you don't like, you should tell them to stop.

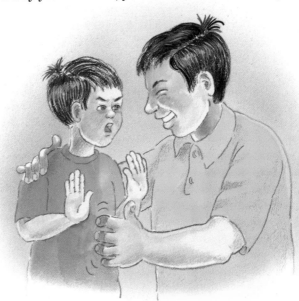

● To the Parent

Teaching children about inappropriate adult conduct helps them know what to do if they are ever faced with it. Emphasize that it is not okay for unfamiliar adults to stop and talk to children, to ask for their help, to try to touch them, or to offer candy, toys, or a ride. To help children remember what to do in such situations, teach them the "No, go, and tell" rule: They should say no, then go (run away), and then tell you. Children should also feel free to say no to anyone—friends and relatives included—who touches them in a way that makes them feel uncomfortable.

Why Must We Wear Seat Belts?

ANSWER Seat belts hold your body in place in a car. If the car stopped suddenly and you were not buckled in, your body would keep going forward. You might even be thrown from the car. That's why wearing a seat belt can keep you from getting badly hurt—or perhaps even killed—in an accident.

◼ Don't be a dumb cluck; buckle up!

See what happens to turkeys who don't wear their seat belts? If there's an accident, they may get thrown from the car—and seriously hurt. So always wear your seat belt.

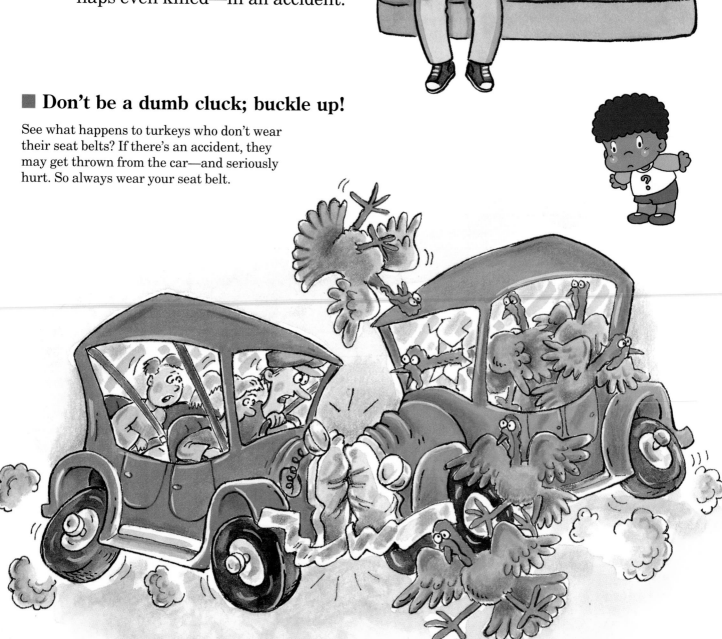

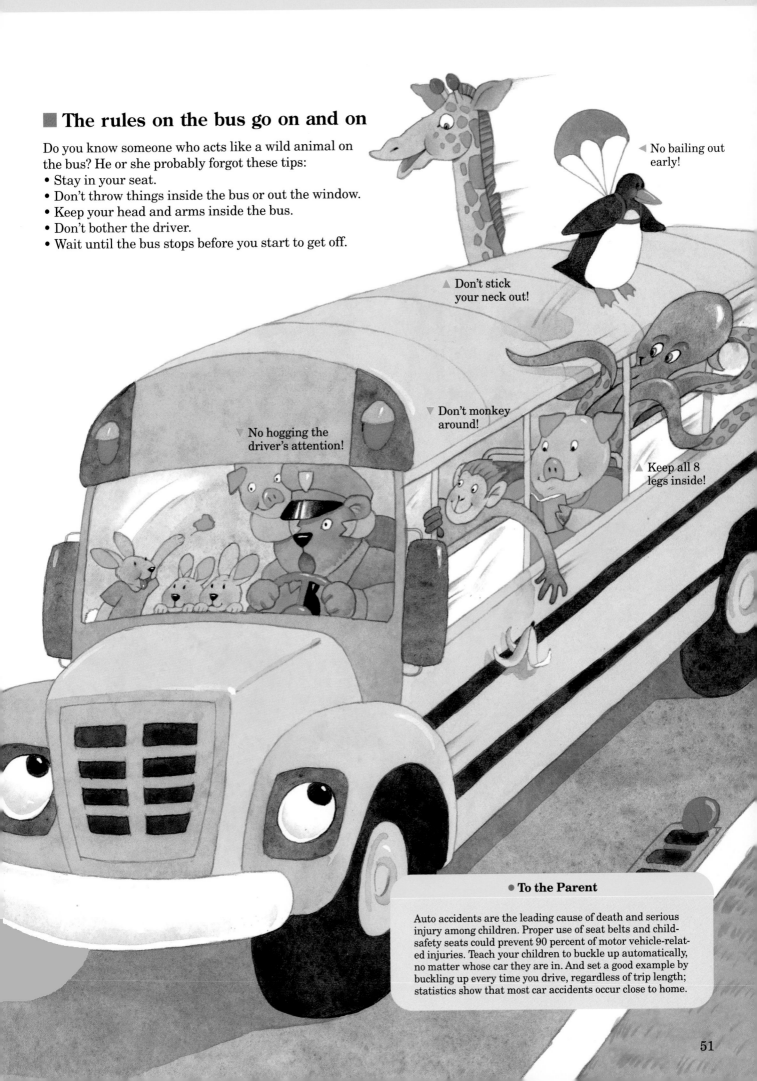

■ The rules on the bus go on and on

Do you know someone who acts like a wild animal on the bus? He or she probably forgot these tips:
• Stay in your seat.
• Don't throw things inside the bus or out the window.
• Keep your head and arms inside the bus.
• Don't bother the driver.
• Wait until the bus stops before you start to get off.

◄ No bailing out early!

▲ Don't stick your neck out!

▼ Don't monkey around!

▼ No hogging the driver's attention!

▲ Keep all 8 legs inside!

● **To the Parent**

Auto accidents are the leading cause of death and serious injury among children. Proper use of seat belts and child-safety seats could prevent 90 percent of motor vehicle-related injuries. Teach your children to buckle up automatically, no matter whose car they are in. And set a good example by buckling up every time you drive, regardless of trip length; statistics show that most car accidents occur close to home.

Where Should We Cross the Street?

ANSWER The only safe place to cross a street is at a corner or a crosswalk. Remember to "Stop, look, and listen":

1) *Stop* at the curb;

2) *Look* both ways and around the corner;

3) *Listen* for cars.

Wait to step off the curb until no cars are coming. If there is a traffic light, obey it. Cross with a grownup until you have permission to cross by yourself.

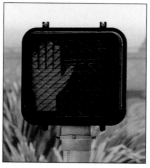

▲ When you see this sign, stay on the curb and out of the street. Don't walk!

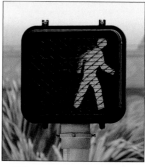

▲ When this sign lights up, look both ways; if it's clear, cross the street.

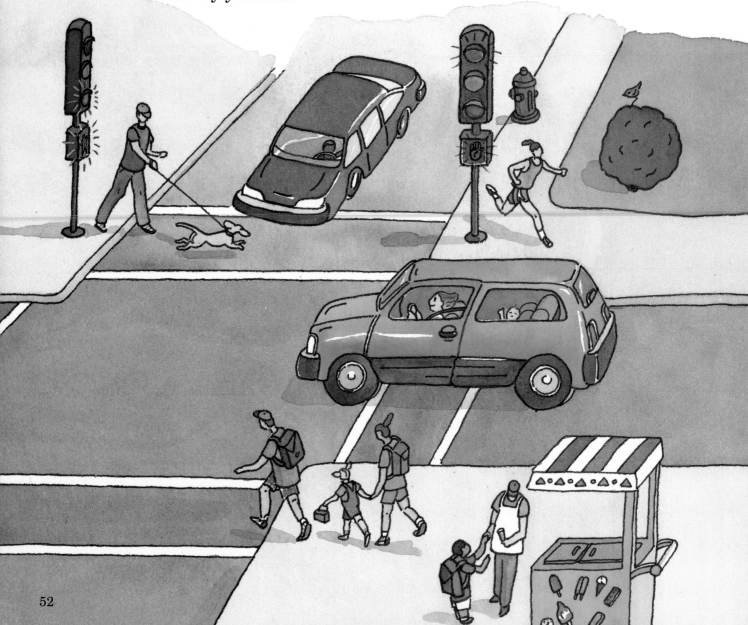

52

■ What should I do if...

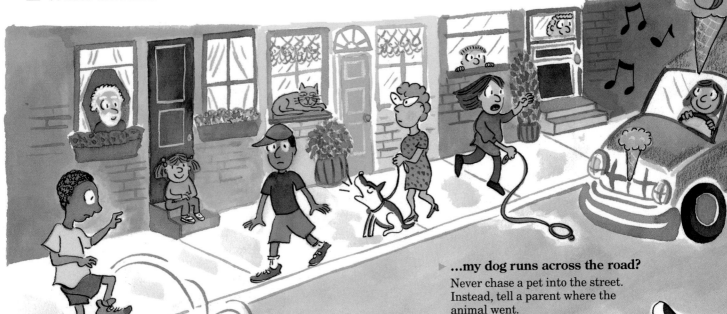

...my dog runs across the road?
Never chase a pet into the street.
Instead, tell a parent where the
animal went.

▶ **...my ball rolls into the street?**
Don't run after the ball, even if it
was your best one. (It's not worth
risking your neck to get your kicks!)
Let the ball go. Ask a grownup to
get it back.

▶ **...the ice-cream truck comes by?**
Do not run after the ice-cream truck,
no matter how much you want that
double scoop! Ask your parent to
take you.

■ Safety patrols

A school safety patrol, like the girl shown below, makes sure children
cross the street safely on their way to and from school.

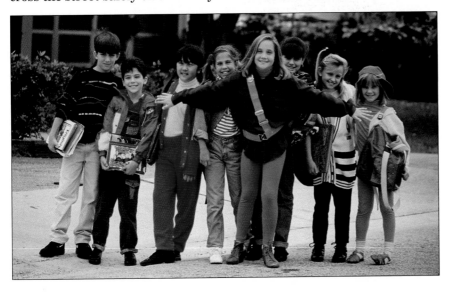

● **To the Parent**

Teaching your child the rules of
pedestrian safety at an early age
will make the rules second nature
by the time she is old enough to
cross the street alone. Safety experts recommend that children be
at least nine years old before they
cross the street or walk to school
without a grownup. You may also
want to caution your child that not
everyone drives predictably!

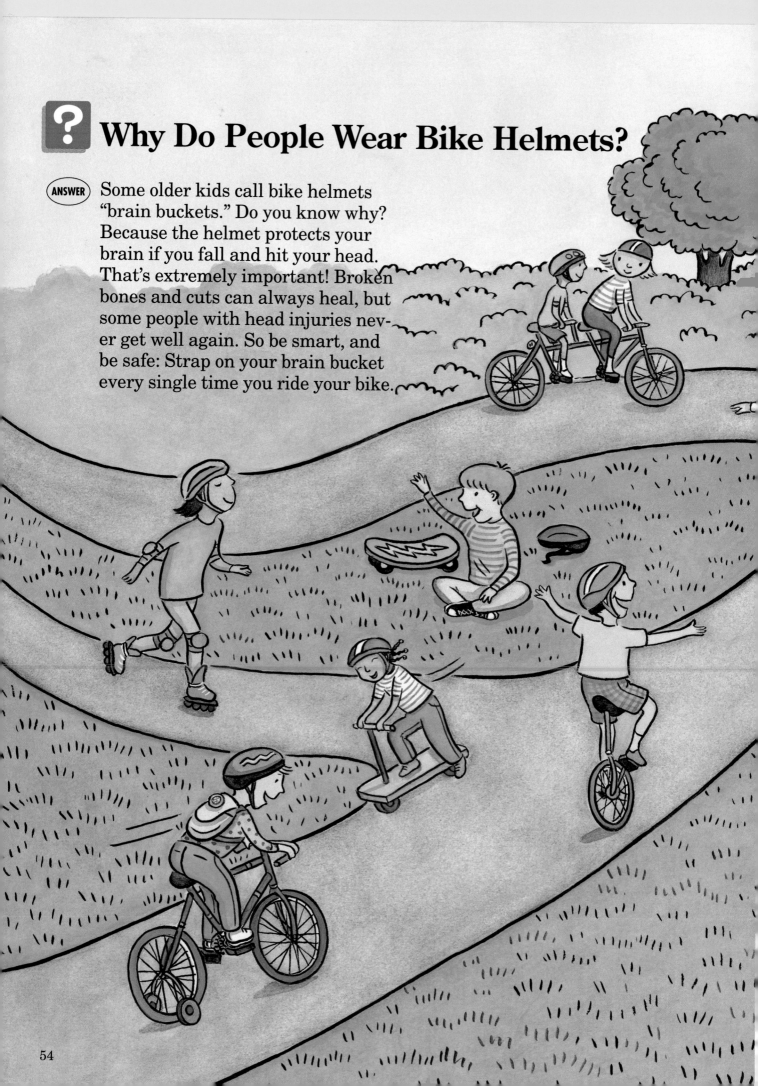

Why Do People Wear Bike Helmets?

(ANSWER) Some older kids call bike helmets "brain buckets." Do you know why? Because the helmet protects your brain if you fall and hit your head. That's extremely important! Broken bones and cuts can always heal, but some people with head injuries never get well again. So be smart, and be safe: Strap on your brain bucket every single time you ride your bike.

54

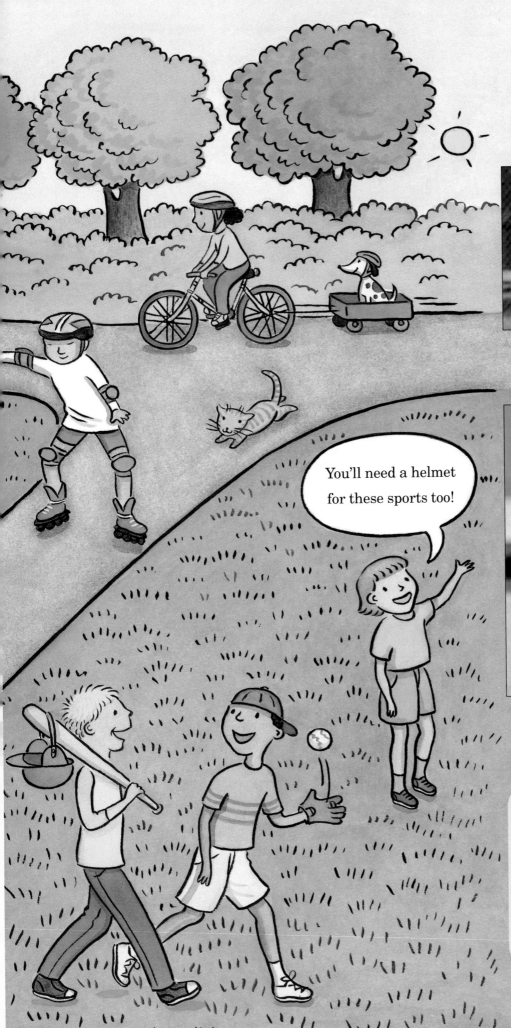

You'll need a helmet for these sports too!

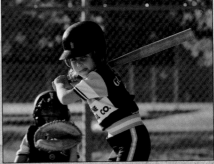

A good baseball player always wears her batting helmet when she steps to the plate. Watch out for wild pitches!

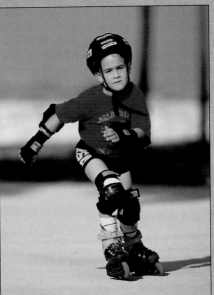

Before you put on your in-line skates, put on your helmet. Don't forget pads for your elbows, wrists, and knees.

● **To the Parent**

Each year, nearly 50,000 children suffer head injuries in bike accidents in the United States. More than 400 of them die. Wearing a bicycle helmet will reduce your child's risk of head injury by 85 percent. Insist that your child wear a helmet whenever she rides her bike. Other sports with high rates of head injury include skateboarding and in-line skating.

Why Can't I Run Near a Swimming Pool?

ANSWER The deck around a swimming pool gets splashed with water all day long. That makes it wet and slippery. If you run across this area, you could fall and get hurt. So always walk—do not run!—near a swimming pool. If you do run, you'll hear a loud "Phweet!" That's the lifeguard blowing his whistle to remind you to slow down.

■ What if someone is in trouble?

Yell and get help fast. Don't jump into the water yourself. Instead, throw something that will float, such as a life preserver, to the person who is in trouble. You can also find a pole or a rake and hold it out to the person.

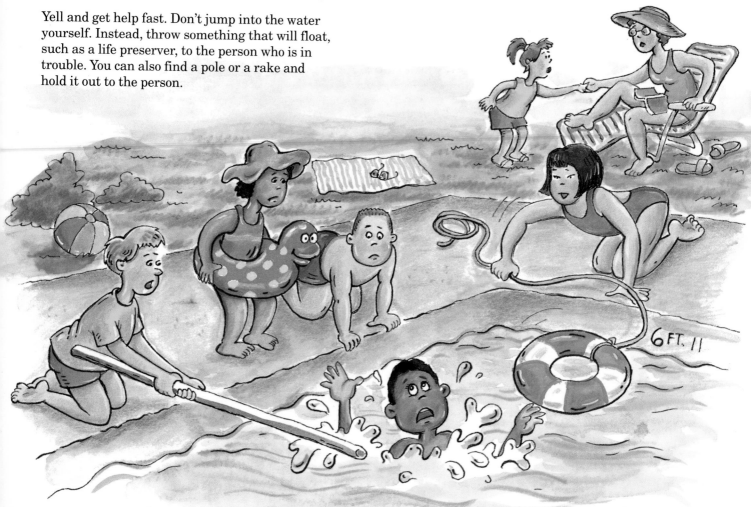

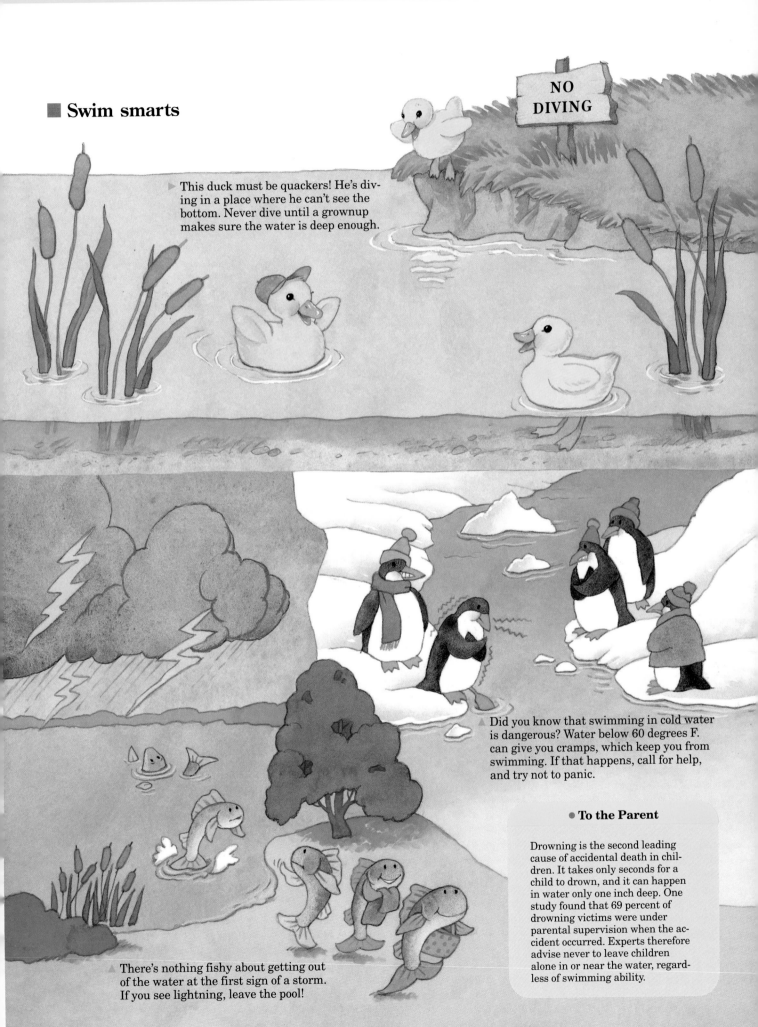

■ Swim smarts

NO DIVING

▶ This duck must be quackers! He's diving in a place where he can't see the bottom. Never dive until a grownup makes sure the water is deep enough.

Did you know that swimming in cold water is dangerous? Water below 60 degrees F. can give you cramps, which keep you from swimming. If that happens, call for help, and try not to panic.

● **To the Parent**

Drowning is the second leading cause of accidental death in children. It takes only seconds for a child to drown, and it can happen in water only one inch deep. One study found that 69 percent of drowning victims were under parental supervision when the accident occurred. Experts therefore advise never to leave children alone in or near the water, regardless of swimming ability.

There's nothing fishy about getting out of the water at the first sign of a storm. If you see lightning, leave the pool!

57

❓ If an Animal Looks Friendly, Can I Pet It?

ANSWER No! Sometimes a wild animal acts friendly because it has a dangerous disease called rabies. If the animal licked you or bit you, it could give you the disease. To be on the safe side, stay away from any animal you don't know—including stray dogs and cats.

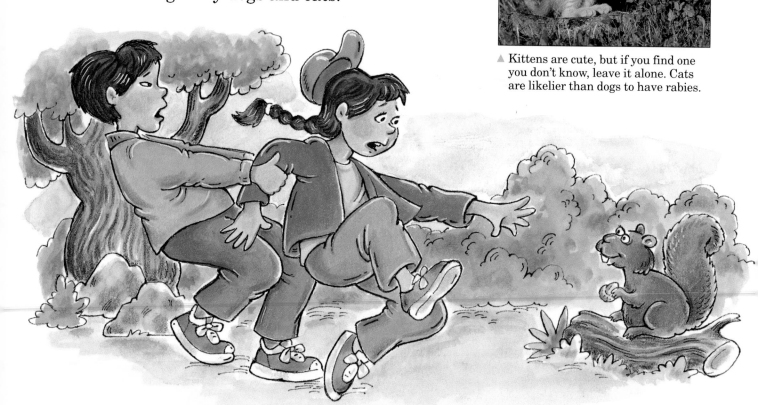

▲ Kittens are cute, but if you find one you don't know, leave it alone. Cats are likelier than dogs to have rabies.

■ Animals to avoid

These are some of the wild animals that can carry rabies. If you see any of these animals acting strangely, steer clear of them. Then tell your parents what you saw, so they can call the animal-control authorities or the police.

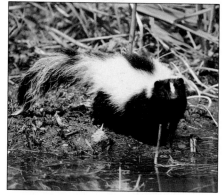

▲ One reason to avoid skunks is their smelly spray. Another reason is that they sometimes carry rabies.

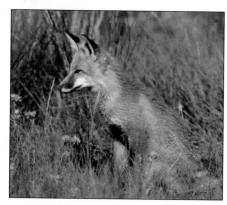

▲ Foxes are usually shy. If one comes toward you, it could be a sign that it has rabies—so keep your distance!

What If a Strange Dog Comes Near Me?

If a dog you don't know runs up to you, don't run or scream. Instead, keep calm, quiet, and still. The dog probably just wants to sniff you. That's how dogs get to know you. But even if the dog seems friendly, don't reach out to pet it. Don't look it in the eye, either. Dogs think that's a challenge. Let the dog walk away from you, then slowly back away. If you are riding your bike when a dog approaches, get off and hold the bike between you and the dog.

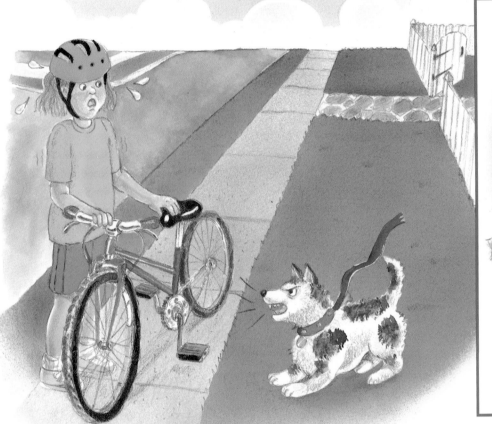

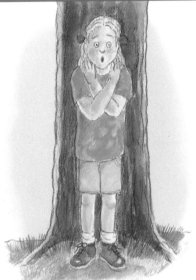

■ Be a tree

If you think a dog is about to attack, "be a tree." Cross your arms, put your hands around your neck, and stand as still as a tree.

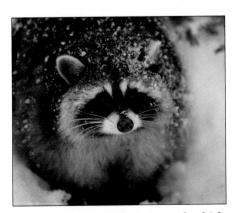

▲ Raccoons are mostly nocturnal, which means they come out at night. If one seems dizzy, it could be rabid.

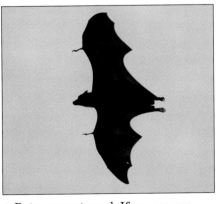

▲ Bats are nocturnal. If you see one during the day, it might have rabies.

● **To the Parent**

Each year, about 20,000 Americans are exposed to the deadly rabies virus. To safeguard your family, have your pets vaccinated annually. If you think your child has been exposed to rabies, wash the wound or lick site with soap and water for at least five minutes to reduce the risk of transmission, then seek medical help. To be effective, treatment must begin immediately.

What Should I Do If a Bee Buzzes Close to Me?

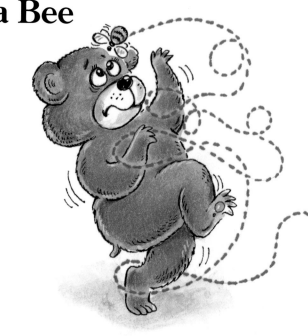

ANSWER If a bee or a wasp buzzes around your head, try to stay calm and still. It will probably fly away on its own. If the insect lands on you, brush it off gently and walk away. Don't swat at the air with your hands. The insect might think you are trying to hurt it, and that could cause it to sting.

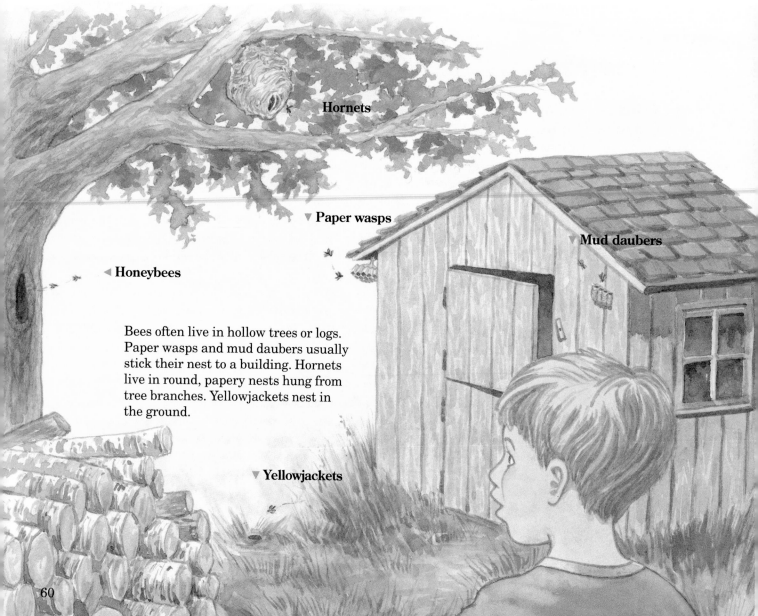

Hornets

Paper wasps

Mud daubers

Honeybees

Bees often live in hollow trees or logs. Paper wasps and mud daubers usually stick their nest to a building. Hornets live in round, papery nests hung from tree branches. Yellowjackets nest in the ground.

Yellowjackets

Why Do Bees and Wasps Sting?

Bees and wasps are social insects. That means they live in groups. They sting in self-defense—that is, to defend their nests or themselves. Some wasps use their stingers to stun other insects. Then they feed the insects to their larvae.

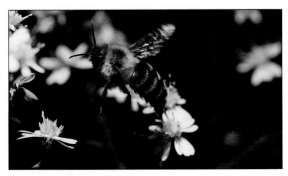

▲ A honeybee takes flight.

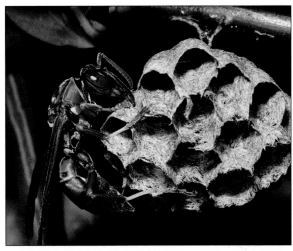

▲ A paper wasp crawls on its nest.

■ Take steps to avoid ticks

You can get sick from the bite of a tick, an insect that lives in woods, fields, and tall grass.

In the woods, keep ticks away by wearing a hat, a long-sleeved shirt, and long pants.

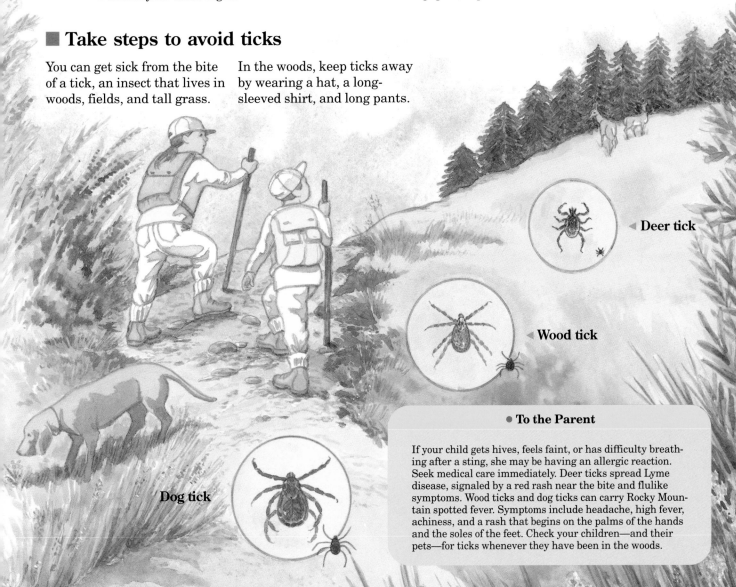

◀ Deer tick

◀ Wood tick

Dog tick

● **To the Parent**

If your child gets hives, feels faint, or has difficulty breathing after a sting, she may be having an allergic reaction. Seek medical care immediately. Deer ticks spread Lyme disease, signaled by a red rash near the bite and flulike symptoms. Wood ticks and dog ticks can carry Rocky Mountain spotted fever. Symptoms include headache, high fever, achiness, and a rash that begins on the palms of the hands and the soles of the feet. Check your children—and their pets—for ticks whenever they have been in the woods.

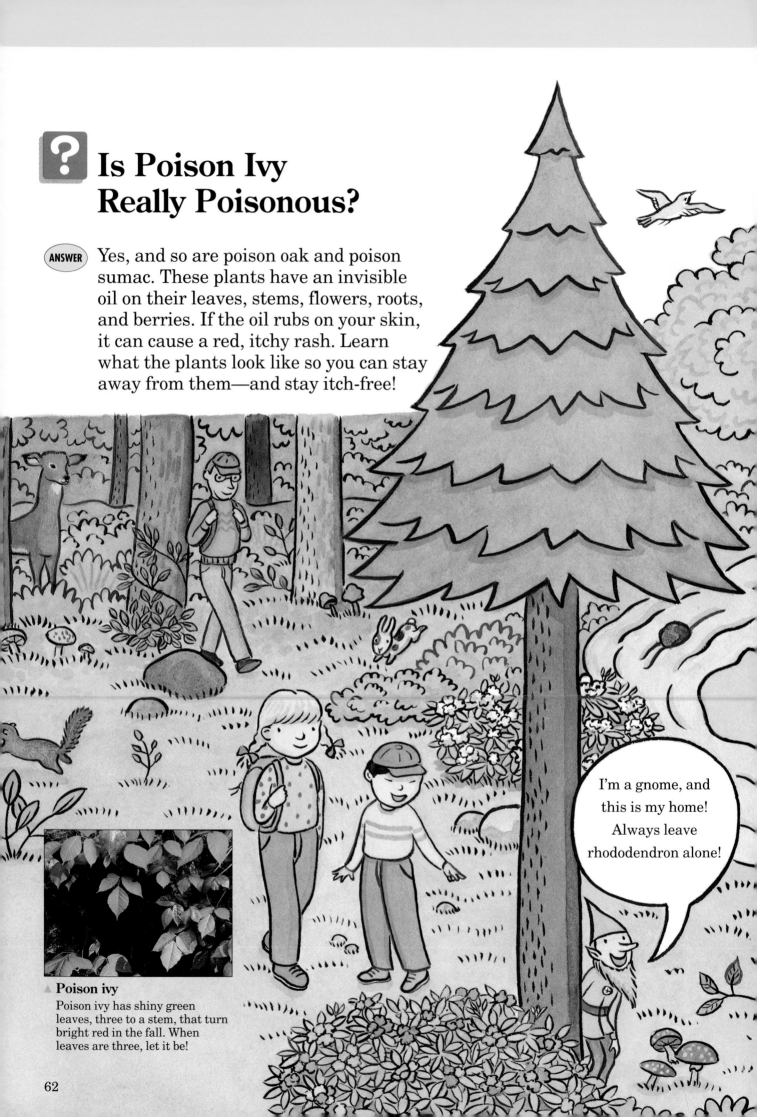

Is Poison Ivy Really Poisonous?

ANSWER Yes, and so are poison oak and poison sumac. These plants have an invisible oil on their leaves, stems, flowers, roots, and berries. If the oil rubs on your skin, it can cause a red, itchy rash. Learn what the plants look like so you can stay away from them—and stay itch-free!

I'm a gnome, and this is my home! Always leave rhododendron alone!

▲ **Poison ivy**
Poison ivy has shiny green leaves, three to a stem, that turn bright red in the fall. When leaves are three, let it be!

62

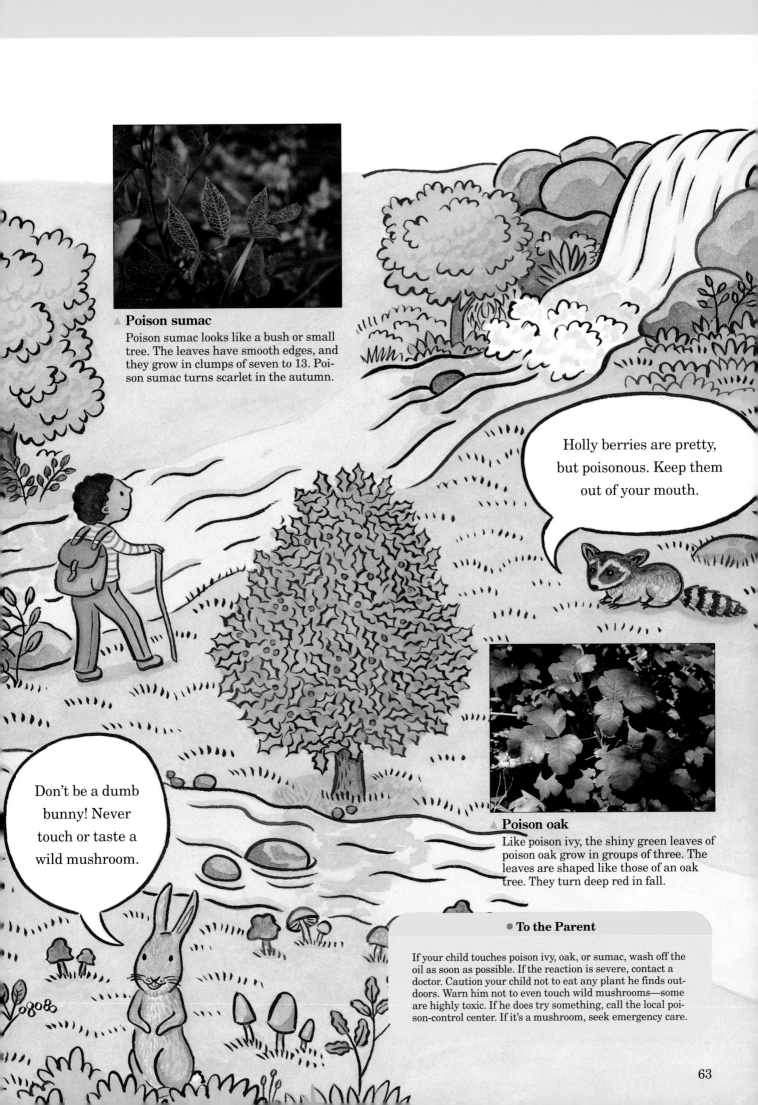

Poison sumac

Poison sumac looks like a bush or small tree. The leaves have smooth edges, and they grow in clumps of seven to 13. Poison sumac turns scarlet in the autumn.

Holly berries are pretty, but poisonous. Keep them out of your mouth.

Don't be a dumb bunny! Never touch or taste a wild mushroom.

Poison oak

Like poison ivy, the shiny green leaves of poison oak grow in groups of three. The leaves are shaped like those of an oak tree. They turn deep red in fall.

● **To the Parent**

If your child touches poison ivy, oak, or sumac, wash off the oil as soon as possible. If the reaction is severe, contact a doctor. Caution your child not to eat any plant he finds outdoors. Warn him not to even touch wild mushrooms—some are highly toxic. If he does try something, call the local poison-control center. If it's a mushroom, seek emergency care.

What Is Poison?

 ANSWER A poison is a solid, a liquid, or a gas that can hurt you or make you sick. Many ordinary items—even medicine!—can be poisonous if not used the right way. Soap, bleach, or paint thinner, for example, act as poisons if they get inside your body. Some plants—poison ivy, poison oak—are dangerous to touch. And certain gases in the air may be poisonous if you breathe too much of them.

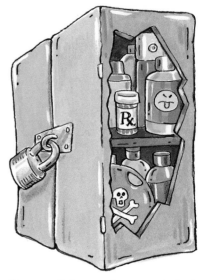

▲ Keep medicines and poisons locked up!

■ Can you spot the poisons in this picture?

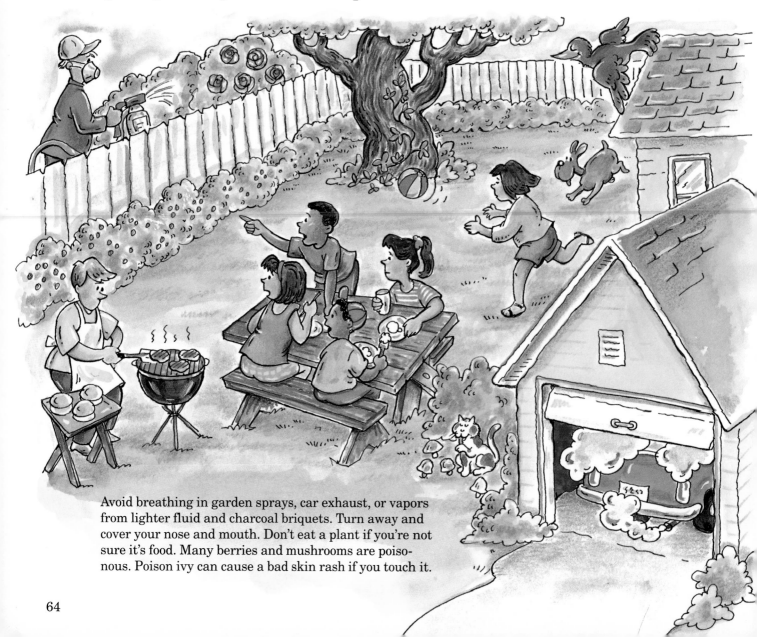

Avoid breathing in garden sprays, car exhaust, or vapors from lighter fluid and charcoal briquets. Turn away and cover your nose and mouth. Don't eat a plant if you're not sure it's food. Many berries and mushrooms are poisonous. Poison ivy can cause a bad skin rash if you touch it.

■ Put a lid on it!

Medicine bottles often have tops that babies and toddlers cannot open, no matter how hard they try. This is for their own safety. The tops keep children from eating or drinking the medicine by accident, which could make them very sick.

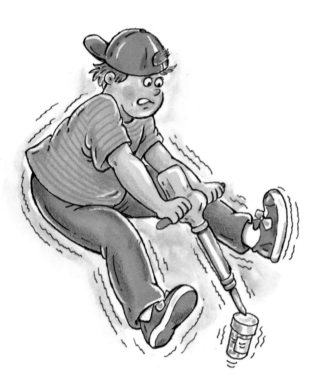

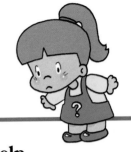

■ How to get help

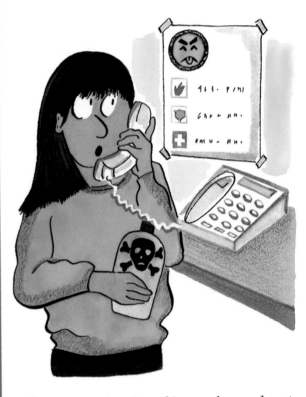

If someone gets poisoned in your house, do not panic. Staying calm, call the local poison control center, or dial 911, and ask for help. Tell these three things: 1) what the poison was; 2) who took it; and 3) how much was taken. An adult at the center will say what to do next.

■ Wash it off

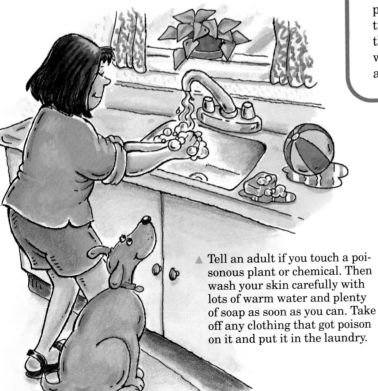

▲ Tell an adult if you touch a poisonous plant or chemical. Then wash your skin carefully with lots of warm water and plenty of soap as soon as you can. Take off any clothing that got poison on it and put it in the laundry.

● To the Parent

The increase of poisonous household products demands extra steps to protect children from accidents:
1) Post the number of your local poison-control center by the phone.
2) Label containers with Mr. Yuk stickers.
3) Keep medicines and chemicals locked up.
4) Teach children not to ingest any substance unless okayed by adults.

How Can We Prevent Fires?

ANSWER You can help keep your home safe from fire by never playing with matches or candles. Use appliances like the stove or a space heater only when an adult is around. Check electrical cords and plugs to make sure they are in good condition. You and your family should also practice what to do in case there is ever a fire.

■ **This home is safe...**

■ **...but this one is not!**

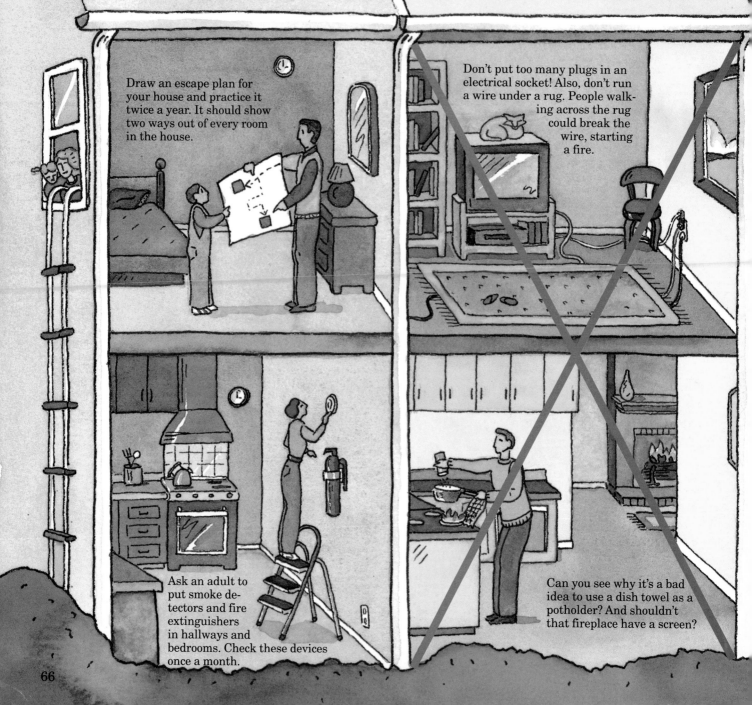

Draw an escape plan for your house and practice it twice a year. It should show two ways out of every room in the house.

Don't put too many plugs in an electrical socket! Also, don't run a wire under a rug. People walking across the rug could break the wire, starting a fire.

Ask an adult to put smoke detectors and fire extinguishers in hallways and bedrooms. Check these devices once a month.

Can you see why it's a bad idea to use a dish towel as a potholder? And shouldn't that fireplace have a screen?

Why Is Smoke So Deadly?

Most people who get caught in a fire are hurt by smoke, not flames. The smoke irritates their eyes so much they can't see. That makes it hard to escape from the fire. Smoke from a fire can even knock you unconscious. If you are ever in a fire, remember that smoke rises. You can crawl or roll under it to get away. If possible, cover your nose and mouth with a wet cloth.

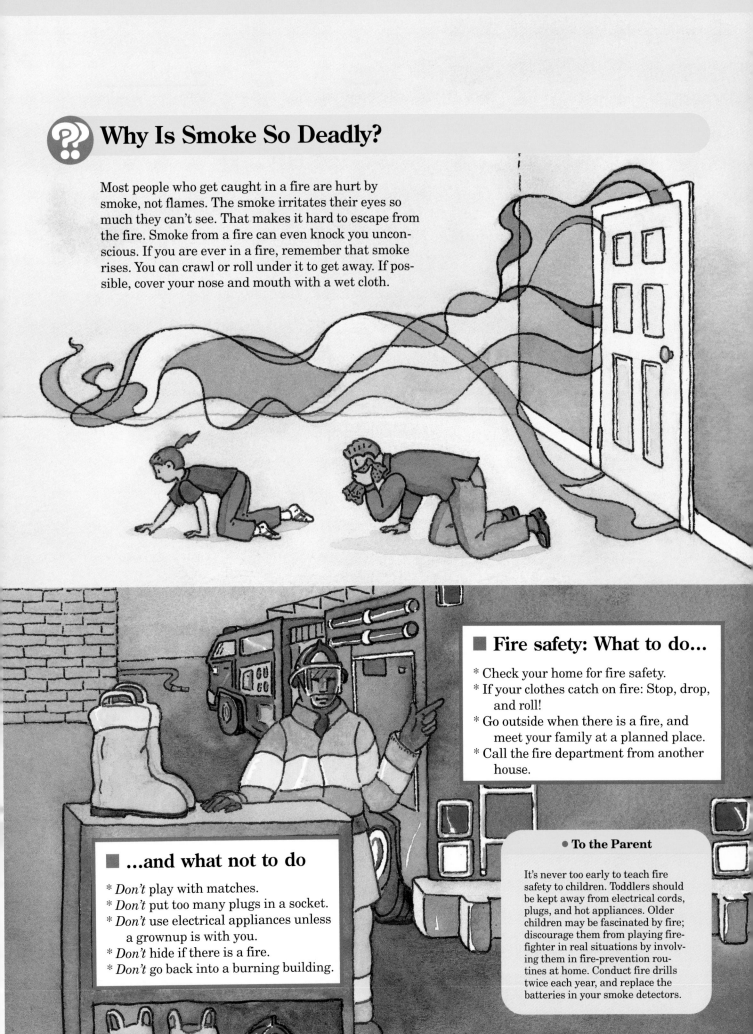

■ Fire safety: What to do...

* Check your home for fire safety.
* If your clothes catch on fire: Stop, drop, and roll!
* Go outside when there is a fire, and meet your family at a planned place.
* Call the fire department from another house.

■ ...and what not to do

* *Don't* play with matches.
* *Don't* put too many plugs in a socket.
* *Don't* use electrical appliances unless a grownup is with you.
* *Don't* hide if there is a fire.
* *Don't* go back into a burning building.

● **To the Parent**

It's never too early to teach fire safety to children. Toddlers should be kept away from electrical cords, plugs, and hot appliances. Older children may be fascinated by fire; discourage them from playing firefighter in real situations by involving them in fire-prevention routines at home. Conduct fire drills twice each year, and replace the batteries in your smoke detectors.

❓ Can Electricity Hurt Us?

ANSWER Electricity is safe when you are separated from it. But if you touch bare wires or use a broken electrical appliance, electricity can flow into your body and give you a shock. A shock could burn you, knock you out, or even kill you. Electricity from broken appliances or wires can also start a fire. Always use electricity safely.

▪ Danger: Power lines ahead!

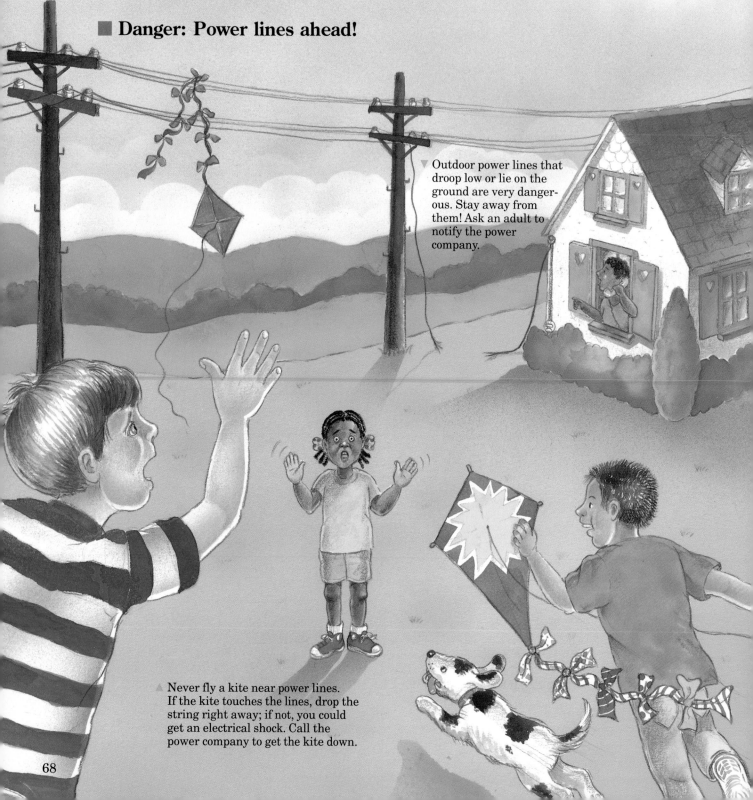

Outdoor power lines that droop low or lie on the ground are very dangerous. Stay away from them! Ask an adult to notify the power company.

Never fly a kite near power lines. If the kite touches the lines, drop the string right away; if not, you could get an electrical shock. Call the power company to get the kite down.

■ What is static electricity?

Rubbing certain materials—hair and fabrics, for example—causes electricity to build up on them. This is called static electricity ("static" is a fancy word for "standing"). Static electricity makes things cling together. It can also make hair stick to a comb or—as the girl at left found out—stand straight on end.

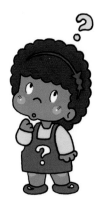

▲ Touching a Van de Graaff generator can be a hair-raising experience.

■ What should you do?

◀ If a piece of toast gets stuck, grasp the toaster's plug—never the wire!—and unplug it right away.

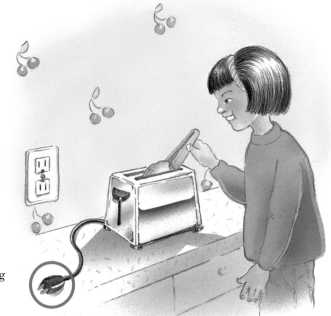

▲ With the toaster unplugged, use wooden tongs to remove the stuck toast. Touching the wires inside a plugged-in toaster could give you a bad shock.

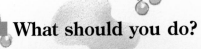

MINI-DATA

What is a shock?

When electric current from a wire or a battery flows through your body, it gives you an electric shock. A weak shock feels like a tingle. A strong one feels like a punch. Walk on a wool carpet, then touch a doorknob (or even someone else). Shocking!

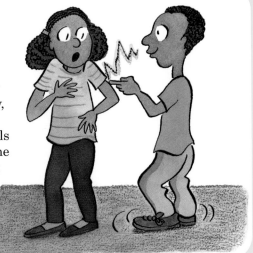

● **To the Parent**

Electricity is a common source of power in homes. Electric current forms circuits between power sources and the ground. If you get between electricity and the ground, you become part of the circuit, risking injury or death. Cover empty sockets to protect babies. Show children how to plug in and unplug appliances. Teach them not to touch anything electric when they are wet, and to call an adult if appliances are sparking or smoking.

How Can I Help Keep My Home Safe?

ANSWER Following a few simple rules will keep you and your home safe. When you are alone at home, make sure the doors and windows are locked. Learn how to make emergency phone calls for medical aid, or in case there is a fire or other danger. Ask your parents to help you set up a plan for what to do if you have an accident when they are not home.

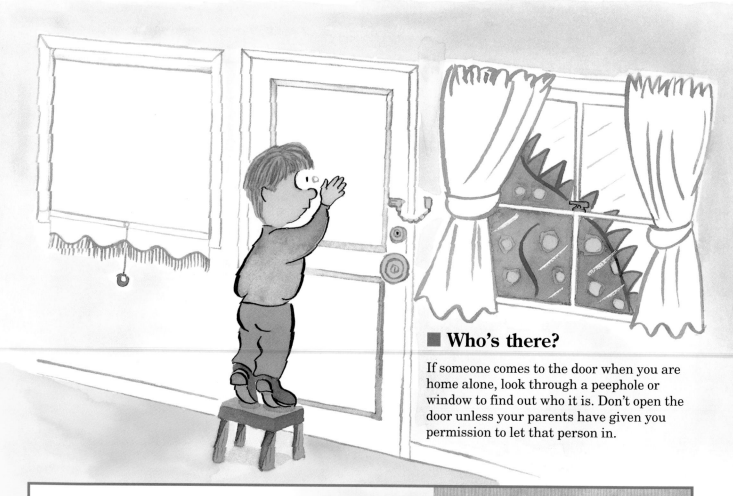

■ Who's there?

If someone comes to the door when you are home alone, look through a peephole or window to find out who it is. Don't open the door unless your parents have given you permission to let that person in.

■ Stay away from guns

Guns can seem interesting, but they are really very dangerous. Guns cause terrible accidents. You could shoot yourself, or a friend, by mistake. So if a gun is in your house, don't touch it. Stay away from any gun you might see at another person's home, too. Better yet, leave that place as soon as you can. If you ever find a gun, leave it alone and tell an adult about it.

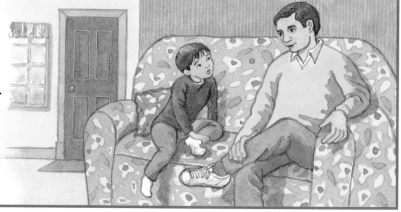

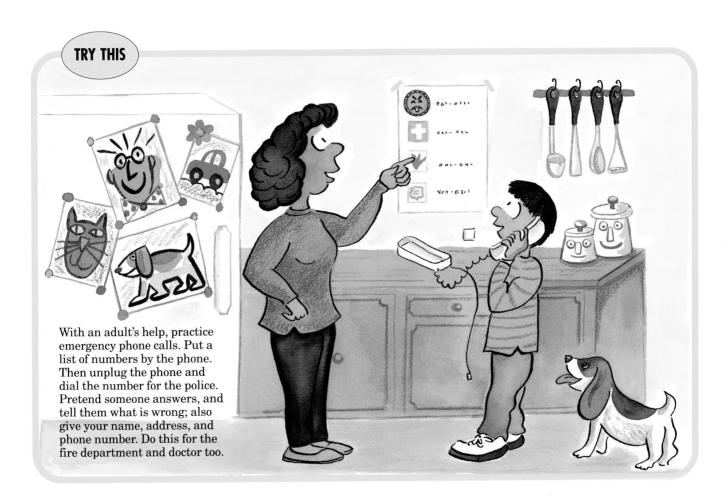

With an adult's help, practice emergency phone calls. Put a list of numbers by the phone. Then unplug the phone and dial the number for the police. Pretend someone answers, and tell them what is wrong; also give your name, address, and phone number. Do this for the fire department and doctor too.

■ Safety is a key issue

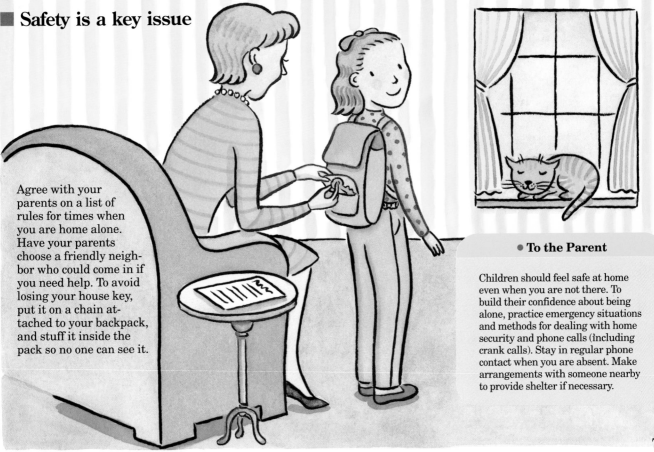

Agree with your parents on a list of rules for times when you are home alone. Have your parents choose a friendly neighbor who could come in if you need help. To avoid losing your house key, put it on a chain attached to your backpack, and stuff it inside the pack so no one can see it.

● **To the Parent**

Children should feel safe at home even when you are not there. To build their confidence about being alone, practice emergency situations and methods for dealing with home security and phone calls (including crank calls). Stay in regular phone contact when you are absent. Make arrangements with someone nearby to provide shelter if necessary.

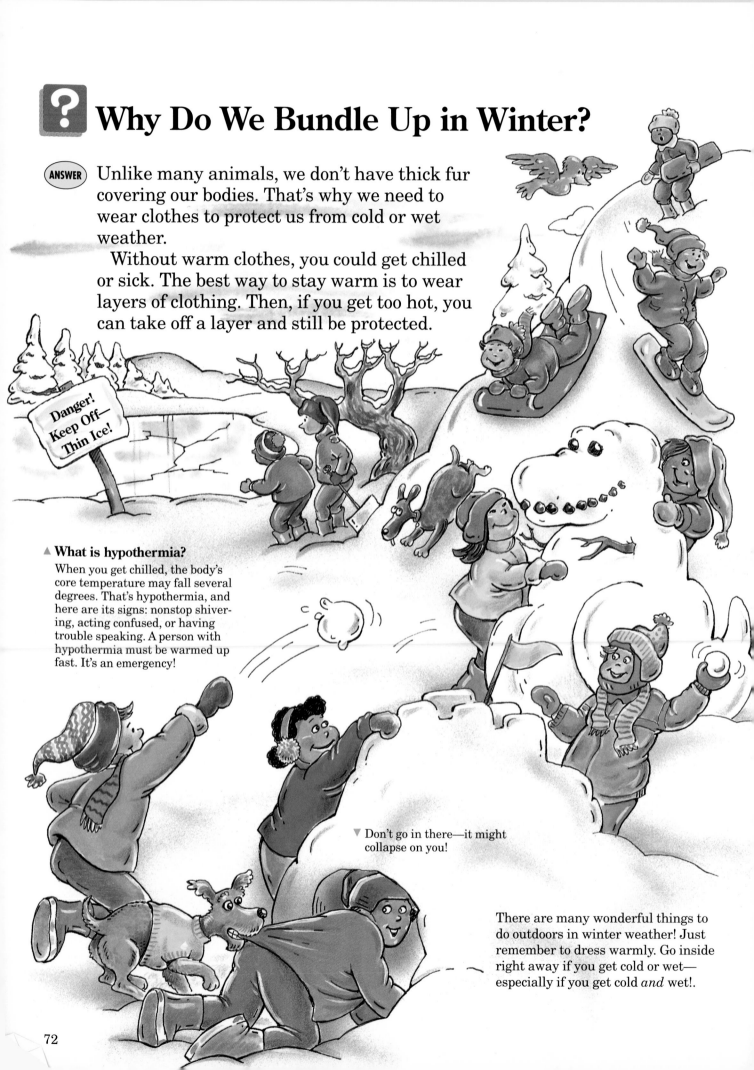

Why Do We Bundle Up in Winter?

ANSWER Unlike many animals, we don't have thick fur covering our bodies. That's why we need to wear clothes to protect us from cold or wet weather.

Without warm clothes, you could get chilled or sick. The best way to stay warm is to wear layers of clothing. Then, if you get too hot, you can take off a layer and still be protected.

Danger! Keep Off— Thin Ice!

▲ **What is hypothermia?**
When you get chilled, the body's core temperature may fall several degrees. That's hypothermia, and here are its signs: nonstop shivering, acting confused, or having trouble speaking. A person with hypothermia must be warmed up fast. It's an emergency!

▼ Don't go in there—it might collapse on you!

There are many wonderful things to do outdoors in winter weather! Just remember to dress warmly. Go inside right away if you get cold or wet— especially if you get cold *and* wet!.

■ Go for the layered look

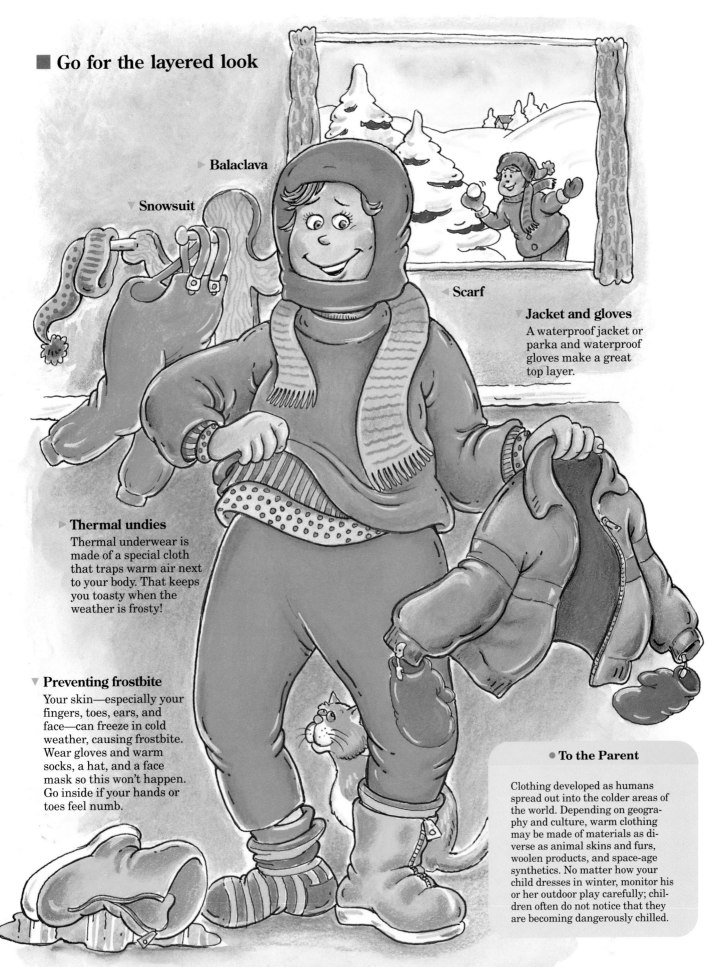

Balaclava

Snowsuit

Scarf

Jacket and gloves
A waterproof jacket or parka and waterproof gloves make a great top layer.

Thermal undies
Thermal underwear is made of a special cloth that traps warm air next to your body. That keeps you toasty when the weather is frosty!

Preventing frostbite
Your skin—especially your fingers, toes, ears, and face—can freeze in cold weather, causing frostbite. Wear gloves and warm socks, a hat, and a face mask so this won't happen. Go inside if your hands or toes feel numb.

● To the Parent

Clothing developed as humans spread out into the colder areas of the world. Depending on geography and culture, warm clothing may be made of materials as diverse as animal skins and furs, woolen products, and space-age synthetics. No matter how your child dresses in winter, monitor his or her outdoor play carefully; children often do not notice that they are becoming dangerously chilled.

? How Does Sunscreen Work?

ANSWER Ultraviolet (UV) sun rays cause sunburn. Sunscreen lotion contains chemicals that soak up many of these UV rays. It stops the rays from reaching your skin, just as if you were standing in the shade. Creams called sunblocks do an even better job. They stop all the light rays from reaching your skin.

■ How not to get burned

Here are some ways to play safely in the sun:
1) Make your own shade with a brimmed hat.
2) Wear light, loose clothes. 3) Cover bare skin with sunblock; repeat after swimming, or if you get sweaty. 4) Stay in the shade at midday, when the sun is strongest.

▲ Sunblock is like invisible armor. It protects you from UV (ultraviolet) sunlight, which can burn your skin.

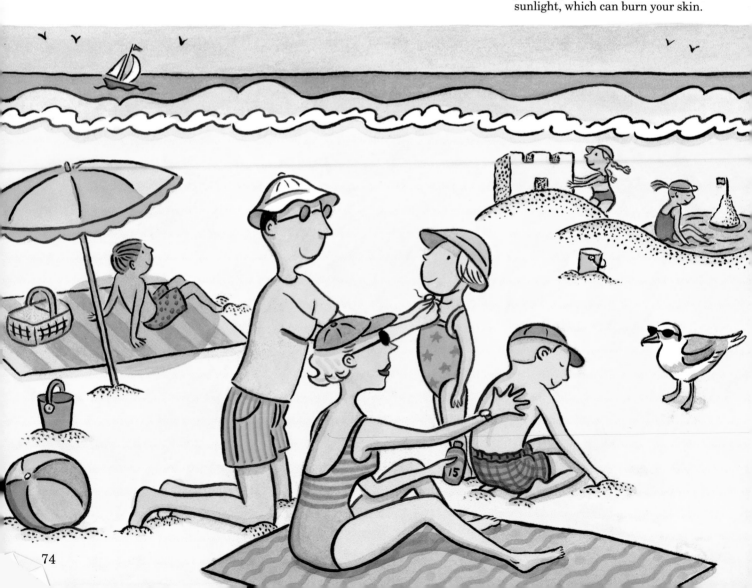

Can People of Any Color Get Sunburned?

Anyone can get sunburned, but people with dark skin don't burn as easily as light-skinned people. Skin contains little black grains, called melanin, that protect you from harmful sun rays. Dark skin contains more melanin, so it can stand more sun.

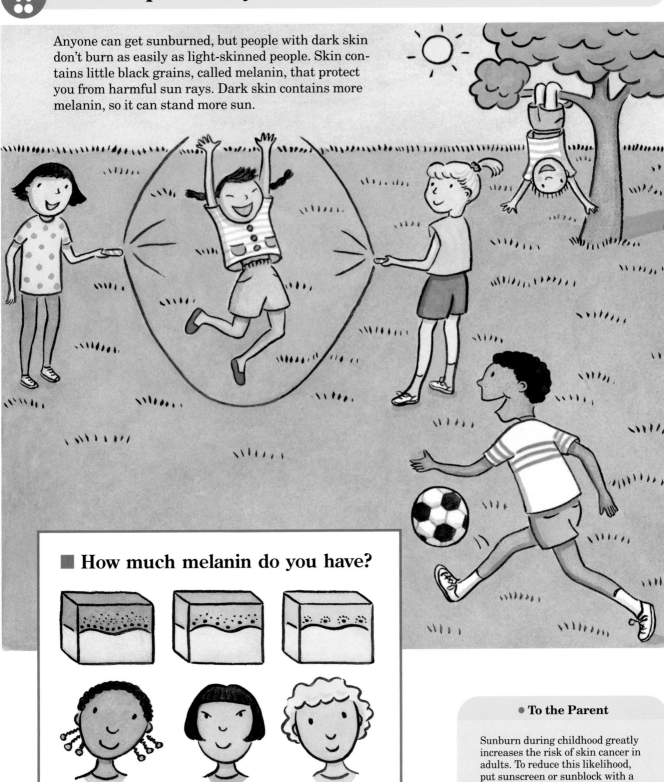

■ How much melanin do you have?

People whose ancestors evolved in Africa or southern India, where there is lots of direct sunlight, have the most melanin in their skin. Asian peoples have less melanin. Those whose ancestors came from the north, where sunlight is weak, have the least melanin.

● **To the Parent**

Sunburn during childhood greatly increases the risk of skin cancer in adults. To reduce this likelihood, put sunscreen or sunblock with a Sun Protection Factor (SPF) of 15 or higher on children more than six months old any time they play in the sun, winter or summer. Dress young babies in protective clothing, and keep them in the shade.

Why Does Heat Make Me Thirsty?

ANSWER When you get hot, your body sweats to cool you down. Little drops of sweat evaporate on your skin, making it cooler. But as you sweat, you lose liquid from your body. Your body therefore sends a signal to your brain: "I'm thirsty!" This tells you to drink enough to replace the liquid you lost as sweat.

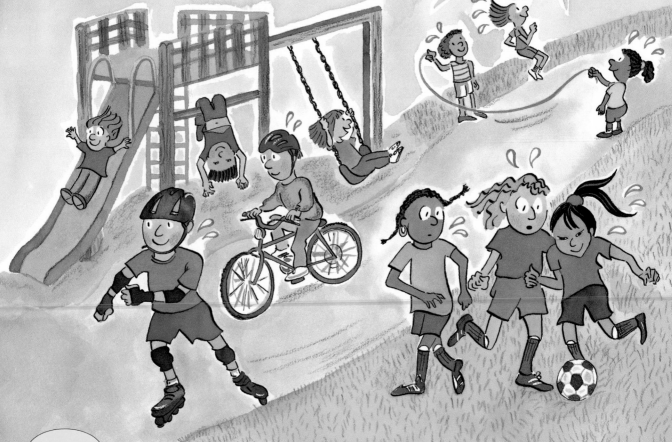

TRY THIS

■ Check your water loss

With an adult's help, put one hand inside a small clear plastic bag and tape it around your wrist. Wait 15 minutes. Do water droplets form in the bag? The drops are moisture that evaporated from your skin. Remove the bag. Are the drops salty?

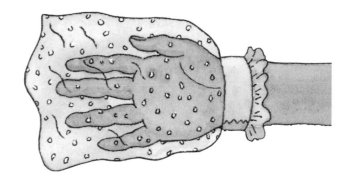

What Happens If We Get Too Hot?

If you exercise in the heat for a long time, your body may sweat so much it can't keep cool. You may lose so much liquid and salt that you feel faint, dizzy, or confused. You might also get a high fever and muscle cramps. This is called "heat stroke." A victim of heat stroke should lie down in shade while you call a doctor.

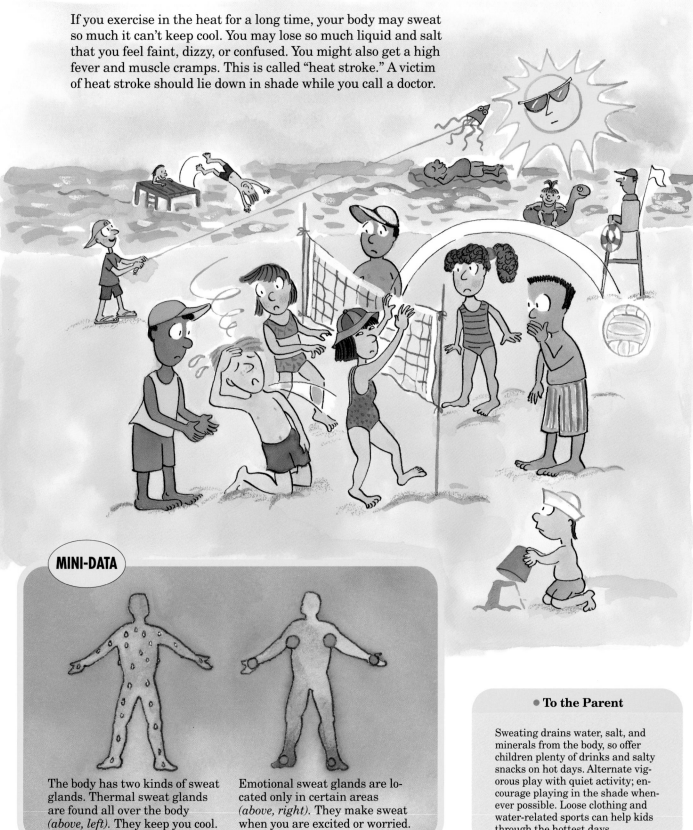

MINI-DATA

The body has two kinds of sweat glands. Thermal sweat glands are found all over the body *(above, left)*. They keep you cool.

Emotional sweat glands are located only in certain areas *(above, right)*. They make sweat when you are excited or worried.

● **To the Parent**

Sweating drains water, salt, and minerals from the body, so offer children plenty of drinks and salty snacks on hot days. Alternate vigorous play with quiet activity; encourage playing in the shade whenever possible. Loose clothing and water-related sports can help kids through the hottest days.

How Can I Stay Safe in a Thunderstorm?

ANSWER Thunder is scary, but it won't hurt you. Lightning, however, can hurt or kill people if it hits them. If you are outdoors when a thunderstorm comes up, go into a building or your family's car. If you are inside, stay away from windows, plumbing pipes, and the refrigerator. Don't use the telephone or an electrical appliance; lightning might travel down the wires.

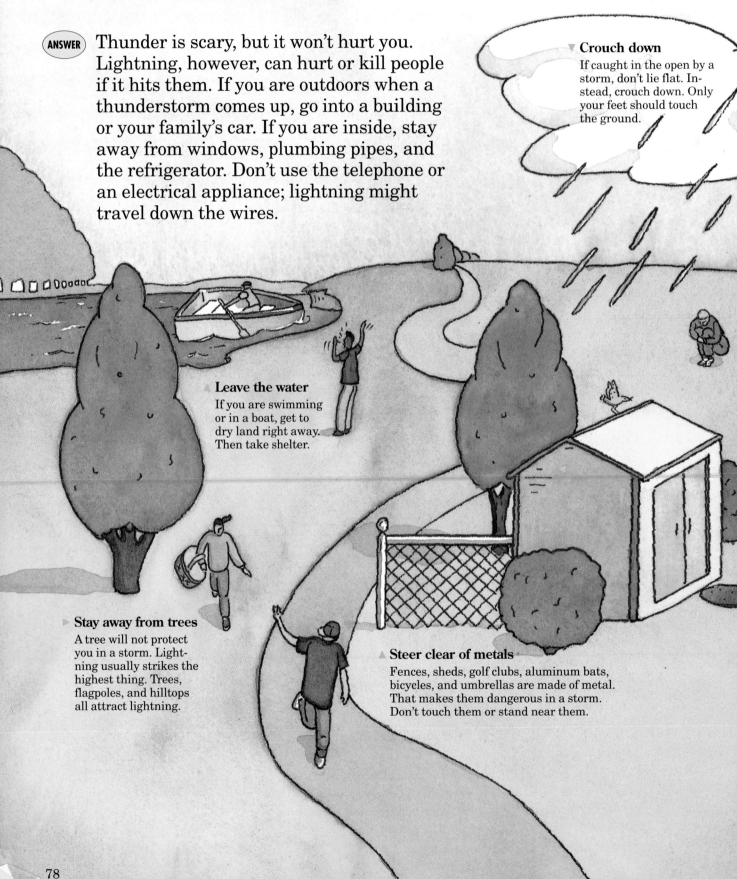

Crouch down
If caught in the open by a storm, don't lie flat. Instead, crouch down. Only your feet should touch the ground.

Leave the water
If you are swimming or in a boat, get to dry land right away. Then take shelter.

Stay away from trees
A tree will not protect you in a storm. Lightning usually strikes the highest thing. Trees, flagpoles, and hilltops all attract lightning.

Steer clear of metals
Fences, sheds, golf clubs, aluminum bats, bicycles, and umbrellas are made of metal. That makes them dangerous in a storm. Don't touch them or stand near them.

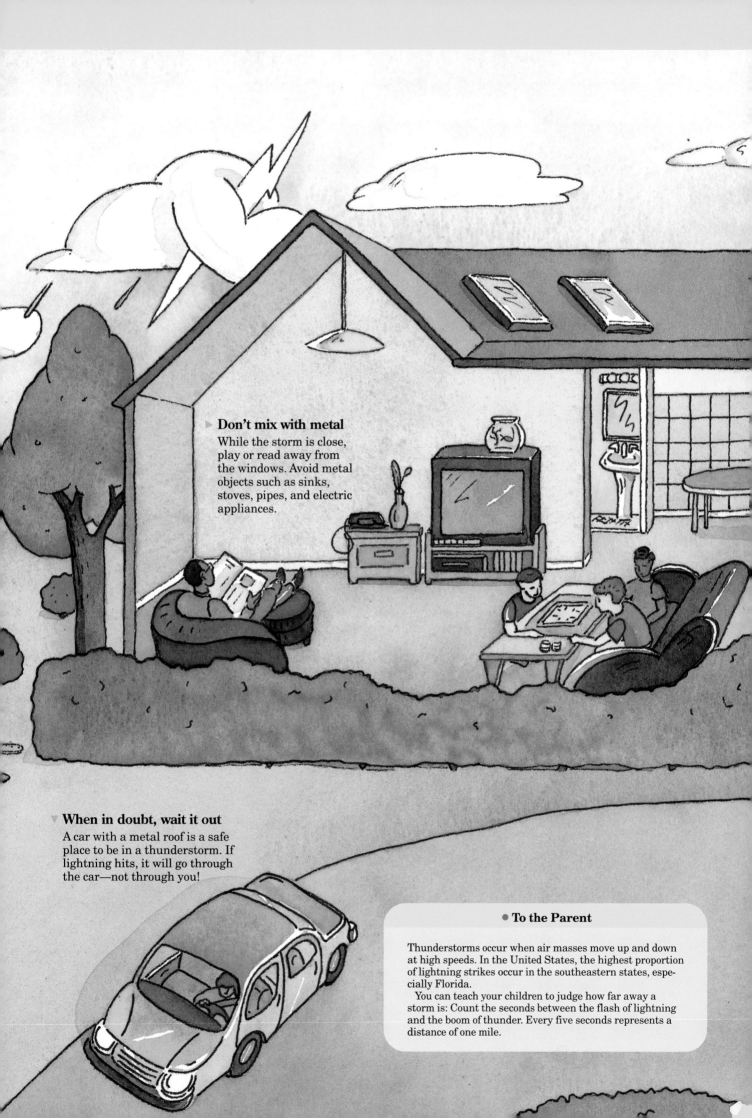

Don't mix with metal

While the storm is close, play or read away from the windows. Avoid metal objects such as sinks, stoves, pipes, and electric appliances.

When in doubt, wait it out

A car with a metal roof is a safe place to be in a thunderstorm. If lightning hits, it will go through the car—not through you!

● To the Parent

Thunderstorms occur when air masses move up and down at high speeds. In the United States, the highest proportion of lightning strikes occur in the southeastern states, especially Florida.

You can teach your children to judge how far away a storm is: Count the seconds between the flash of lightning and the boom of thunder. Every five seconds represents a distance of one mile.

Can You Figure Out What These Are?

A

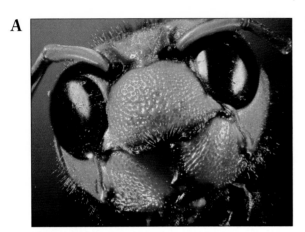

My face might *bug* you,
But my other end is a zinger of a stinger!

B

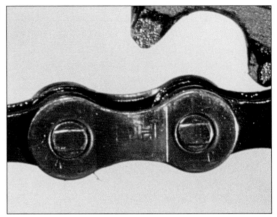

Riding a bike is easy, you think?
Try it with a missing _ _ _ _.

C

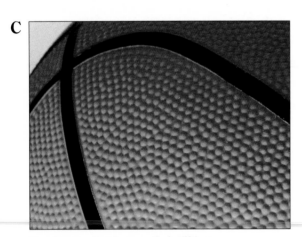

You know what I am called, I'll bet;
I'm most at home inside a net.

D

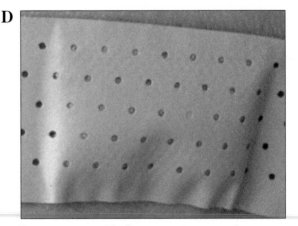

I come to your aid when you scrape your knee;
I'm full of holes—do you know me?

E

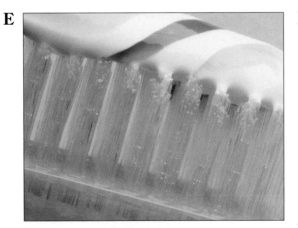

I keep your mouth clean,
I help your teeth gleam—what am I?

F

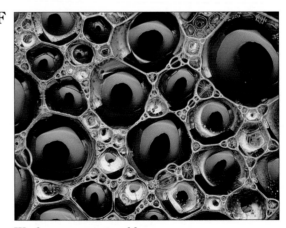

Wash away your troubles
With lots of soapy _ _ _ _ _ _ _.

Answers: A: Wasp, B: Link (Bicycle chain), C: Basketball, D: Band-Aid, E: Toothbrush with toothpaste, F: Bubbles.

80

Growing-Up Album

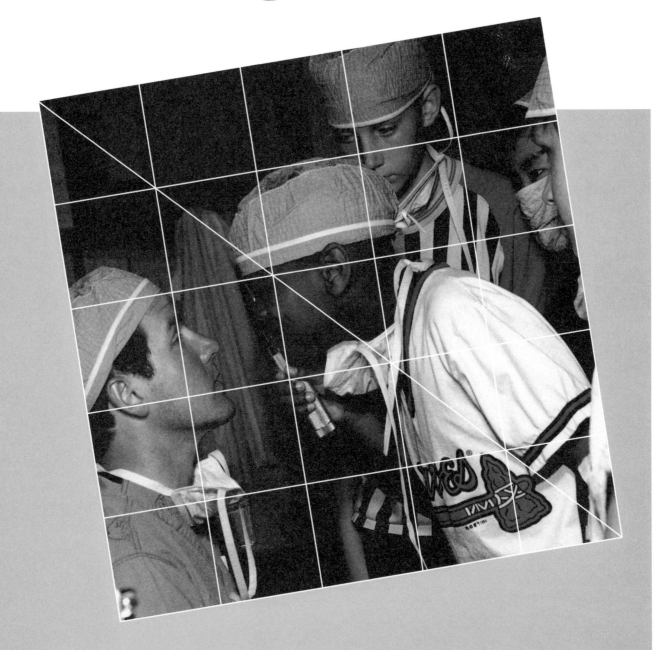

What's Wrong with This Picture?

From reading this book, you know that not all is right in the scene below. If you find only six things wrong, you're an accident waiting to happen. But if you find all 12 things wrong, you're a Health & Safety Expert!

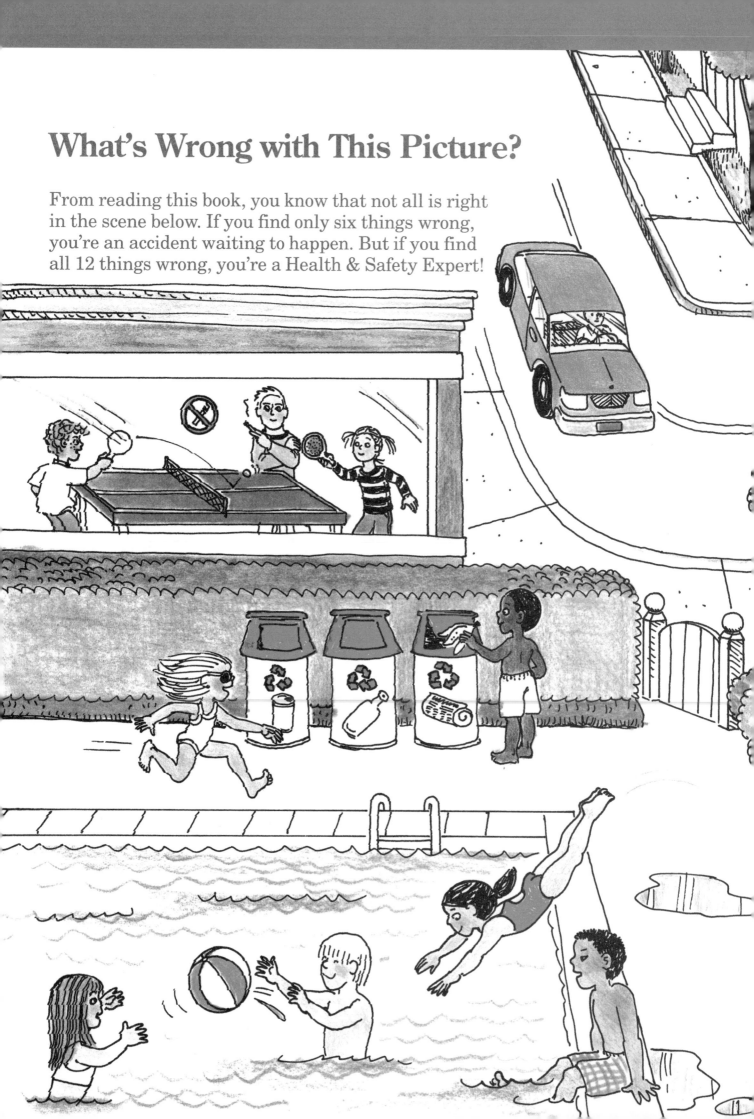

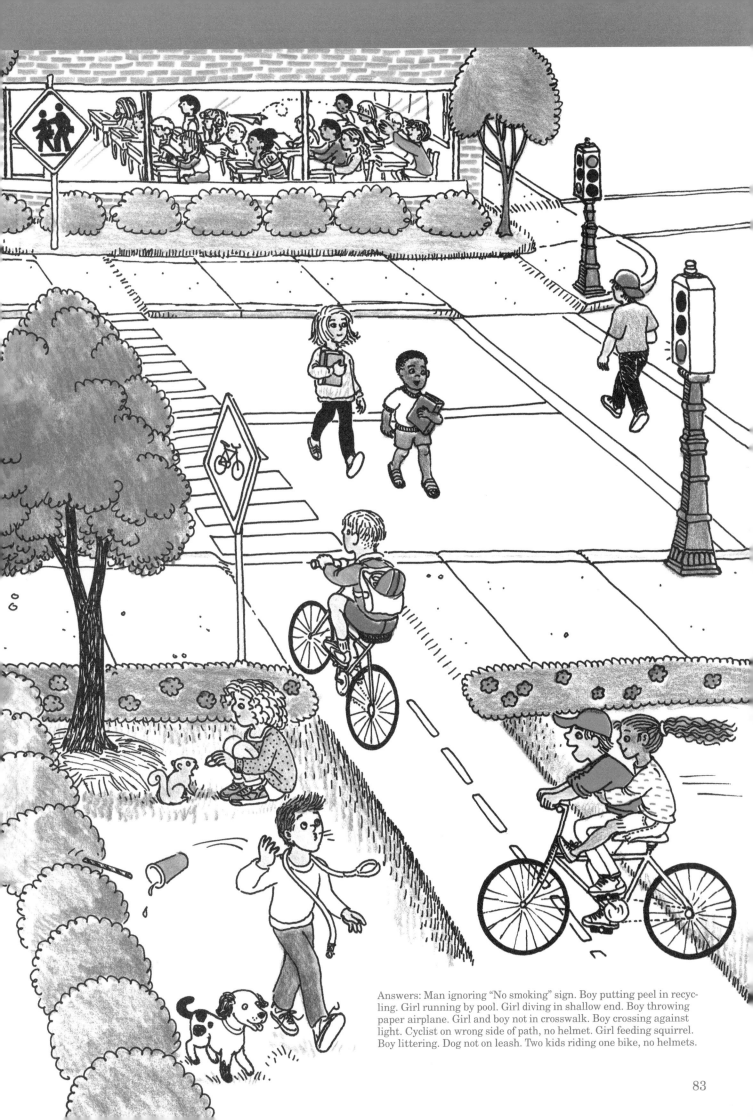

Answers: Man ignoring "No smoking" sign. Boy putting peel in recycling. Girl running by pool. Girl diving in shallow end. Boy throwing paper airplane. Girl and boy not in crosswalk. Boy crossing against light. Cyclist on wrong side of path, no helmet. Girl feeding squirrel. Boy littering. Dog not on leash. Two kids riding one bike, no helmets.

Build a Pyramid!

A balanced diet is like a pyramid made of blocks. Foods at the base of the pyramid are better for you than those at the top. The numbers suggest how many servings of each food group you should eat every day. Can you put each food in its proper group?

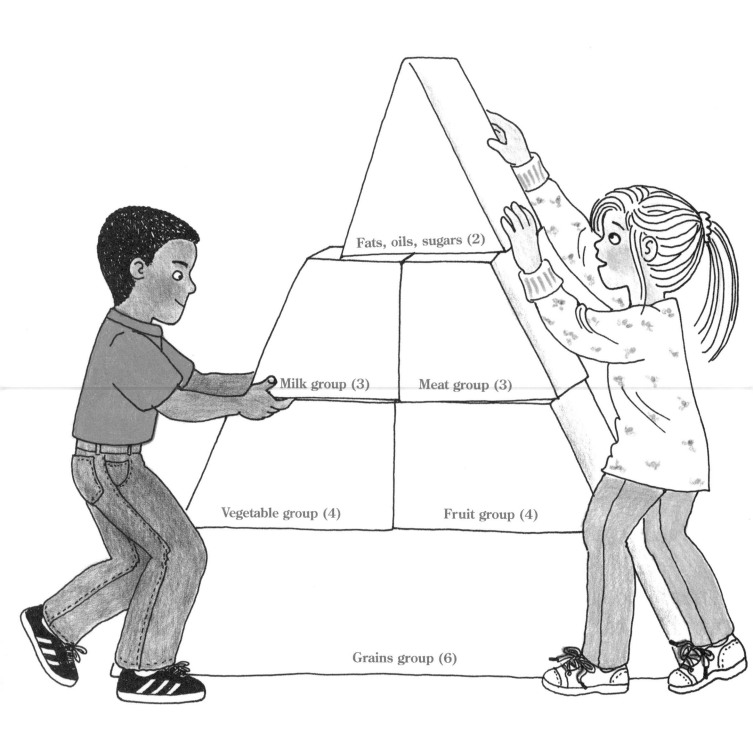

Fats, oils, sugars (2)

Milk group (3)   Meat group (3)

Vegetable group (4)   Fruit group (4)

Grains group (6)

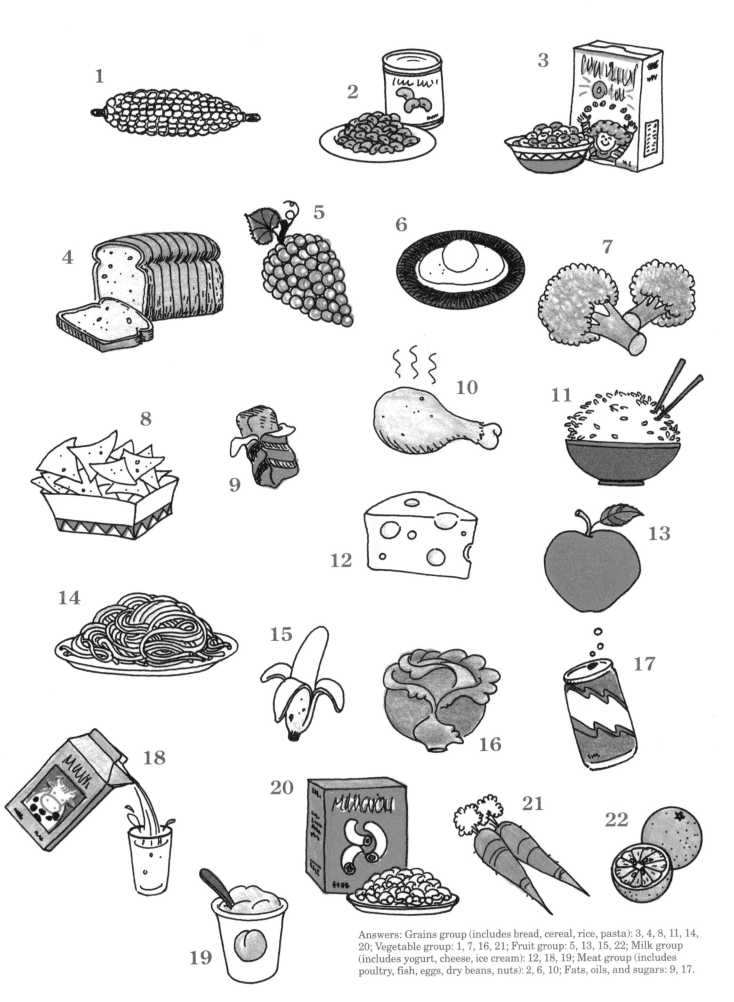

Answers: Grains group (includes bread, cereal, rice, pasta): 3, 4, 8, 11, 14, 20; Vegetable group: 1, 7, 16, 21; Fruit group: 5, 13, 15, 22; Milk group (includes yogurt, cheese, ice cream): 12, 18, 19; Meat group (includes poultry, fish, eggs, dry beans, nuts): 2, 6, 10; Fats, oils, and sugars: 9, 17.

The Case of the Missing Toys

These kids found a bunch of fun things to do instead of watching TV, but then their toys disappeared! Do you know which object belongs to each group of kids?

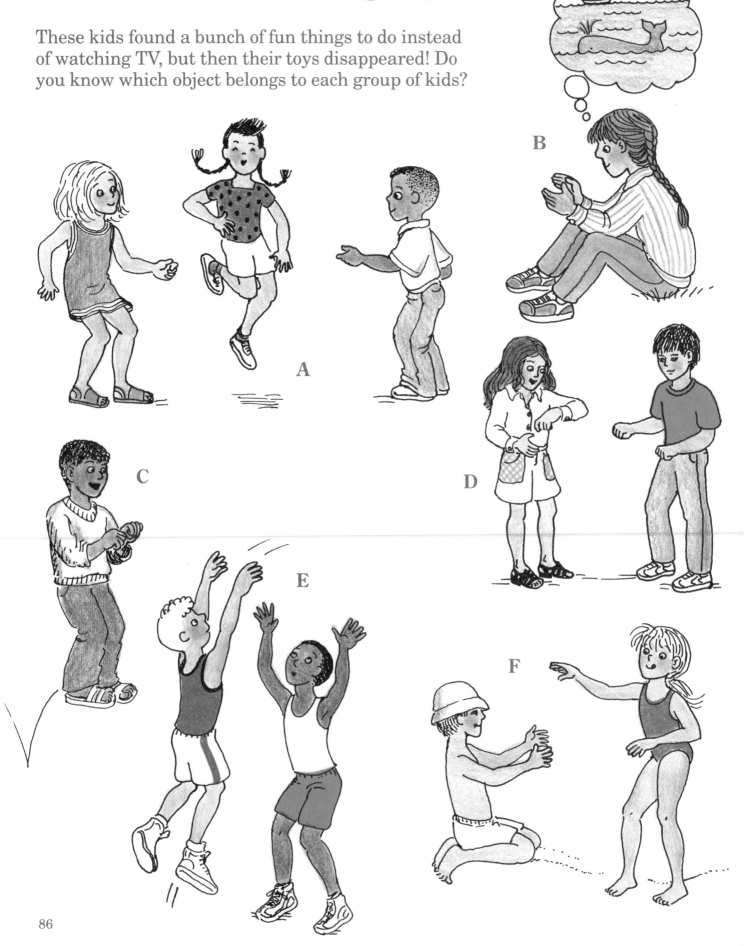

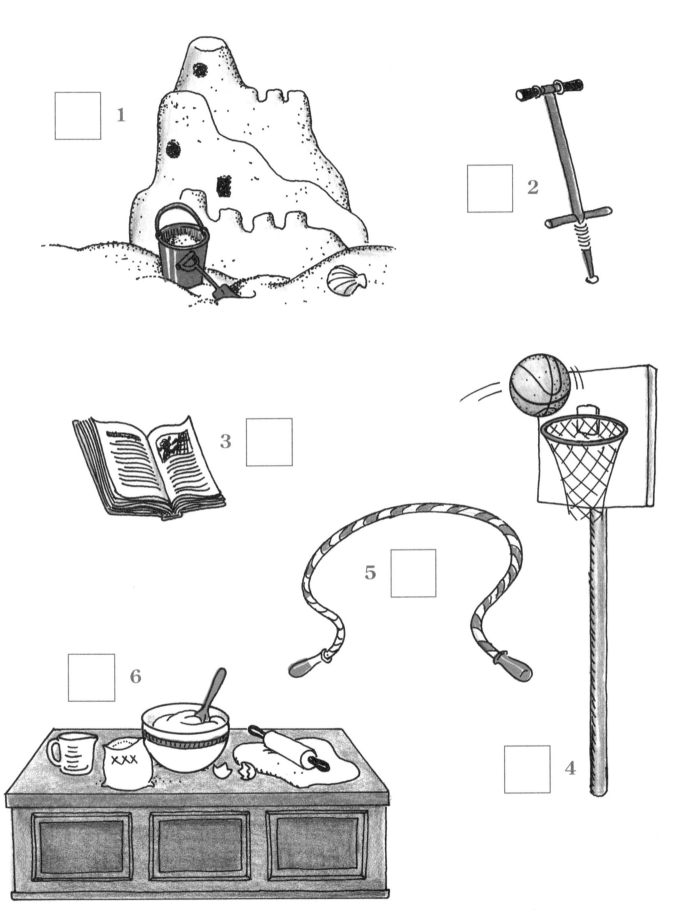

1

2

3

5

6

4

TIME®
LIFE
BOOKS

Time-Life Books is a division of Time Life Inc.

TIME LIFE INC.

PRESIDENT and CEO: George Artandi

TIME-LIFE BOOKS

PRESIDENT: John D. Hall
PUBLISHER/MANAGING EDITOR: Neil Kagan

A Child's First Library of Learning
HEALTH & SAFETY

EDITOR: Allan Fallow
DIRECTOR, NEW PRODUCT DEVELOPMENT: Elizabeth D. Ward
MARKETING DIRECTOR: Wendy A. Foster

Deputy Editor: Terrell Smith
Marketing Manager: Janine Wilkin
Picture Coordinator: David A. Herod
Picture Researcher: Mary M. Saxton

Design: Studio A—Antonio Alcalá, Sue Dowdall, Virginia Ibarra-Garza, Wendy Schleicher
Special Contributors: Vilasini Balakrishnan, Marfé Ferguson Delano, Jocelyn Lindsay, Elizabeth Thompson, Marike van der Veen (research and writing); Kristen Desmond (research)

Consultants: Steven Parker, M.D., a pediatrician in Boston, is writing the revised edition of *Dr. Spock's Baby and Child Care.* Eve Brouwer is a public-safety expert and a former elementary schoolteacher in Itasca, Illinois.

Correspondents: Maria Vincenza Aloisi (Paris), Christine Hinze (London), Christina Lieberman (New York).

Vice President, Director of Finance: Christopher Hearing
Vice President, Book Production: Marjann Caldwell
Director of Operations: Eileen Bradley
Director of Photography and Research: John Conrad Weiser
Director of Editorial Administration: Barbara Levitt
Production Manager: Marlene Zack
Quality Assurance Manager: James King
Library: Louise D. Forstall

Photography: Cover: © Markham Johnson. Back cover: © 1996 David Lissy, All Rights Reserved. Title page: © Jerry Wachter/Photo Researchers. 7: © Norman Myers/Bruce Coleman, Inc. 9: © Comstock. 11: Courtesy Sanford Brotman; © Anthony Edgeworth/The Stock Market. 13: © A. B. Dowsett, Science Photo Library/Photo Researchers. 17: Corbis-Bettmann. 21: © 1996, S'N'S/PVA, photo by Kurt Beamer. 33: © 1996, Custom Medical Stock Photo. 34: © 1994, Custom Medical Stock Photo. 37: Courtesy Mrs. Norman Cousins. 43: Photo RMN-H. Lewandowski. 52: © Henry Horenstein/The Picture Cube. 53: © Tom & Deeann McCarthy/The Stock Market. 55: © Lew Long/The Stock Market—© 1996 Allsport USA, Simon Bruty, All Rights Reserved. 58: © Alan D. Carey, The National Audubon Society Collection/Photo Researchers—© Leonard Lee Rue III, The National Audubon Society Collection/Photo Researchers; Paul Chesley/Photographers Aspen. 59: Images © 1996 PhotoDisc, Inc. 61: © Anthony Johnson/The Picture Cube; © Kenneth H. Thomas, The National Audubon Society Collection/Photo Researchers. 62: © Marilyn T. Wood/Photo/Nats. 63: © John A. Lynch/Photo/Nats—© Robert E. Lyons Photo/Nats. 69: Wisconsin Dells Visitor and Convention Bureau. 80: © 1994, Nile Root, RBP, FBPA, All Rights Reserved/Custom Medical Stock Photo; © David R. Frazier/Photo Researchers—© Garry Gay/The Image Bank; © Joseph Devenney/The Image Bank—© Stanley Rowin/ The Picture Cube; © Dr. Jeremy Burgess, Science Photo Library/Photo Researchers. 81: JoAnn Simmons-Swing.

Illustrations: **Loel Barr:** 4, 5 *(top)*, 6 *(bottom)*, 10-11, 16, 28-29, 32-33, 35, 39 *(bottom right)*, 40, 41 *(top)*, 43 *(middle)*, 50 *(bottom)*, 56 *(bottom)*, 58, 60 *(top)*, 64, 65 *(top left and bottom left)*, 72-73. **Leila Cabib:** 14 *(top)*, 20 *(bottom)*, 36, 37 *(middle)*, 45 *(top)*, 53, 56 *(top)*, 65 *(top right)*, 69 *(bottom)*, 70 *(top)*, 71 *(top)*, 76 *(top)*, 77 *(top)*. **Linda Greigg:** 5 *(bottom)*, 14-15 *(bottom)*, 19 *(bottom)*, 21 *(middle)*, 39 *(top)*, 43 *(top)*, 49 *(top)*, 60 *(bottom)*, 61, 70 *(bottom)*. **Annie Lunsford:** 25, 26 *(bottom)*, 27 *(top)*, 30, 44, 45 *(bottom)*, 48 *(bottom)*, 51, 57. **Gloria Marconi:** 17, 18, 23 *(bottom)*, 34, 48 *(top)*, 49 *(bottom)*, 59, 68, 69 *(middle)*. **Roz Schanzer:** 82-87. **Renee Gettier-Street:** 8-9, 19 *(top)*, 20 *(top)*, 24, 31 *(top)*, 42, 46-47, 52, 66-67, 76 *(bottom)*, 77 *(bottom)*, 78-79. **Bethann Thornburgh:** 6 *(top)*, 12-13, 15 *(top)*, 21 *(bottom)*, 22, 23 *(top)*, 26 *(top)*, 27 *(bottom)*, 31 *(bottom)*, 37 *(top)*, 38, 39 *(bottom left)*, 50 *(top)*, 54-55, 62-63, 71 *(bottom)*, 74-75. **Jeanne Turner:** 7, 41 *(bottom)*. **Stephen Wagner:** Cover illustrations.

First printing. Printed in U.S.A.
Published simultaneously in Canada.
School and library distribution by Time-Life Education, P.O. Box 85026, Richmond, Virginia 23285-5026.

TIME-LIFE is a trademark of Time Warner Inc. U.S.A.

Library of Congress Cataloging-in-Publication Data
Health & Safety.
    88 p.   cm.—(A Child's First Library of Learning)
    Summary: Answers basic questions about fitness, nutrition, and safety measures at home and at school.
    ISBN 0-8094-9479-5
    1. Health—Juvenile literature. 2. Safety—Juvenile literature. [1. Health. 2. Safety. 3. Questions & answers.] I. Time-Life Books. II. Series.
RA777.H38 1996
613—dc20   96-23704
                                                        CIP
                                                        AC

OTHER PUBLICATIONS:

COOKING
Weight Watchers® Smart Choice
   Recipe Collection
Great Taste–Low Fat
Williams-Sonoma Kitchen Library

TIME-LIFE KIDS
Family Time Bible Stories
Library of First Questions and Answers
A Child's First Library of Learning
I Love Math
Nature Company Discoveries
Understanding Science & Nature

SCIENCE/NATURE
Voyage Through the Universe

DO IT YOURSELF
The Time-Life Complete Gardener
Home Repair and Improvement
The Art of Woodworking
Fix It Yourself

HISTORY
The American Story
Voices of the Civil War
The American Indians
Lost Civilizations
Mysteries of the Unknown
Time Frame
The Civil War
Cultural Atlas

For information on and a full description of any of the Time-Life Books series listed above, please call 1-800-621-7026 or write:

Reader Information
Time-Life Customer Service
P.O. Box C-32068
Richmond, Virginia 23261-2068

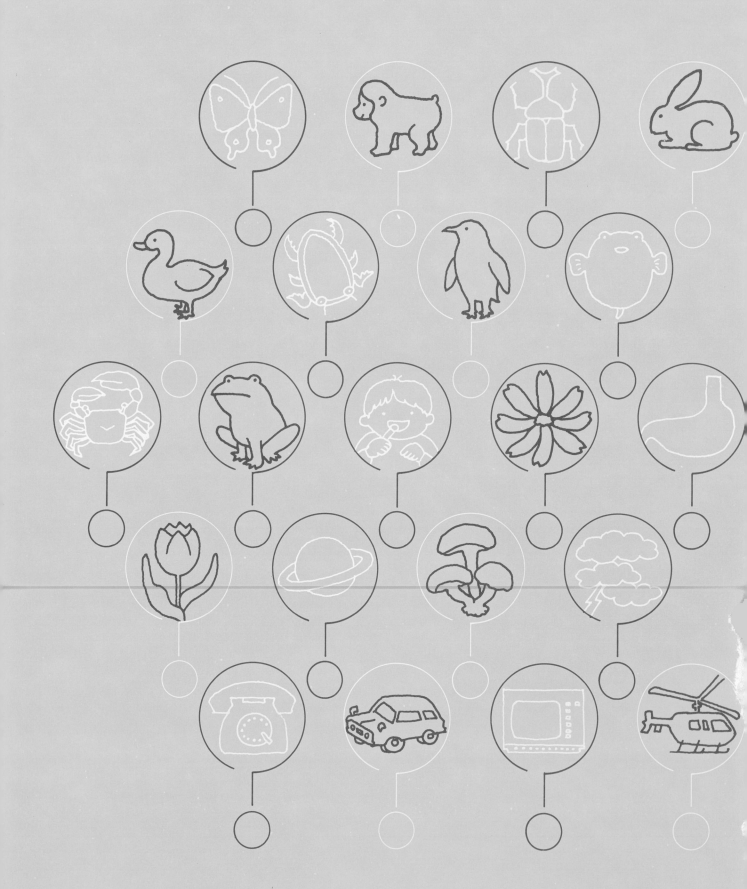

DEDICATION

To my four blondes:
Becki, my incredible wife, who allows me
to chase and accomplish my dreams;
Ryann, my oldest daughter, who was my steady
companion on the sideline for many years;
Sydney, my youngest daughter, whose constant vision
of what is real and what is not has kept me in line;
and my late mother—the ultimate teacher.

Sports Medicine Essentials

Core Concepts in Athletic Training & Fitness Instruction

2nd Edition

Sports Medicine Essentials

Core Concepts in Athletic Training & Fitness Instruction

2nd Edition

by Jim Clover, MEd, ATC, PTA

THOMSON

DELMAR LEARNING

Australia   Canada   Mexico   Singapore   Spain   United Kingdom   United States

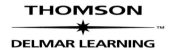

THOMSON
DELMAR LEARNING

Sports Medicine Essentials: Core Concepts in Athletic Training & Fitness Instruction, 2nd Edition
By Jim Clover

Vice President, Health Care Business Unit:
William Brottmiller

Director of Learning Solutions:
Matthew Kane

Managing Editor:
Marah Bellegarde

Acquisitions Editor:
Matthew Seeley

Marketing Director:
Jennifer McAvey

Marketing Channel Manager:
Michele McTighe

Technology Director:
Laurie Davis

Technology Project Coordinator:
Carolyn Fox

Production Director:
Carolyn Miller

Content Project Manager:
Kenneth McGrath

Senior Art Director:
Jack Pendleton

Library of Congress Cataloging-in-Publication Data
Clover, Jim.
  Sports medicine essentials : core concepts in athletic training & fitness instruction / by Jim Clover.—2nd ed.
    p. ; cm.
  Includes bibliographical references and index.
  ISBN-13: 978-1-4018-6185-8
  ISBN-10: 1-4018-6185-7
1. Sports medicine. 2. Physical fitness. I. Title.
[DNLM: 1. Sports Medicine. QT 261 C647s 2007]
RC1210.C5569 2007
617.1'027—dc22
                                        2007010385

Contents

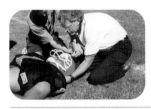
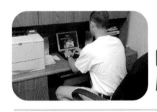

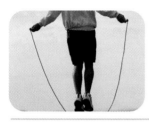

CHAPTER 3
Strength and Conditioning Specialist

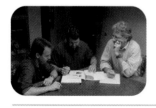

CHAPTER 4
Ethical and Legal Considerations

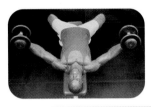

CHAPTER 5
Physical Fitness Assessment

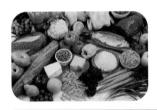

CHAPTER 6
Nutrition and Weight Management

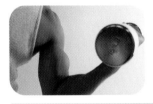

CHAPTER 7
Physical Conditioning

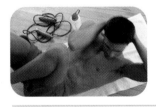

CHAPTER 8
Designing a Conditioning Program

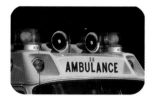

CHAPTER 9
Emergency Preparedness and Assessment

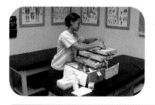

Chapter 10
Assembling the First Aid Kits and Equipment Bags

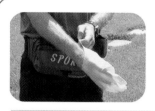

CHAPTER 11
Infection Control

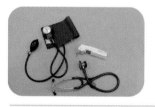

CHAPTER 12
Vital Signs Assessment

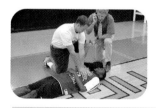

CHAPTER 13
Basic Life Support

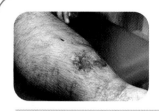

CHAPTER 14
Injuries to the Tissues

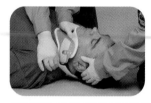

CHAPTER 15
Injuries to the Head and Spine

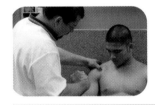

CHAPTER 16
Injuries to the Upper Extremities

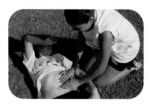

CHAPTER 17
Injuries to the Chest and Abdomen

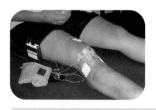

CHAPTER 18
Injuries to the Pelvis and Lower Extremities

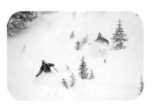

CHAPTER 19
Environmental Conditions

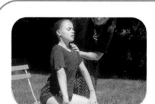

CHAPTER 20
Medical Conditions

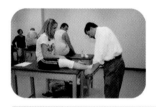

CHAPTER 21
Taping and Wrapping

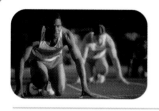

CHAPTER 22
Return To Play

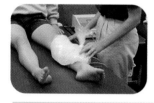

CHAPTER 23
Therapeutic Modalities

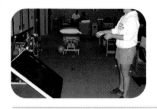

CHAPTER 24
Physical Rehabilitation

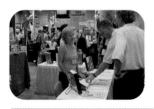

CHAPTER 25
The Selling Point: Promoting Fitness Products and Services

Preface

Sports Medicine Essentials: Core Concepts in Athletic Training & Fitness Instruction, 2nd Edition encompasses the fields of athletic training and fitness instruction. It is appropriate for high school and college level students interested in athletic training or fitness instruction.

Written by a National Athletic Trainers' Association (NATA)-certified athletic trainer, *Sports Medicine Essentials* provides students with the skills and knowledge they need to establish a career path in sports medicine in roles such as athletic trainer, physical therapist, strength and conditioning specialist, personal trainer, or medical salesperson. Topics include anatomy and physiology, emergency preparedness, vital signs, basic life support, treatment and prevention of injuries, nutrition and weight control, therapeutic modalities, and physical rehabilitation.

Students in sports medicine have to be multifaceted. All facets of sports medicine are included within the chapters. Additionally, *Sports Medicine Essentials* provides an introduction to injury evaluation, rehabilitation, fitness evaluation, strength and conditioning, taping and wrapping techniques, and medical sales.

The need for well-trained athletic trainers now and in the future is substantial in high schools as well as many other levels. With the changes in health insurance coverage, self-knowledge in health care is also very important. The goal of *Sports Medicine Essentials* is to ensure that the student is given a well-rounded view of the field of sports medicine.

TEXTBOOK ORGANIZATION

The book is divided into 25 chapters. The first part of the book establishes some of the available careers in sports medicine. Later chapters present the knowledge and skills needed in those careers. The chapters can be used in sequence, or because of the independent strength of each chapter, they can be used out of sequence. Although this book is designed to be used as a textbook, when the class is completed, it can easily be used as a reference book.

FEATURES

Each chapter begins with *Objectives* and *Key Terms* that will help focus the student on the concepts to be covered.

Student Enrichment Activities found at the end of every chapter provide review questions and activities so students can check their comprehension.

Each chapter also contains *Thinking It Through* scenarios that promote critical thinking skills that students can apply to real-life situations.

Full-color photos and illustrations bring authenticity to the content.

NEW TO THIS EDITION

All chapters have been revised for better readability and updated with changing information and new photos where applicable. Listed below are some of the highlights of those updates.

Chapter One was revised to reflect the changes in the career path to become a certified athletic trainer.

Chapter Two includes an updated definition of an athletic trainer to match NATA's description as well as new curriculum and certification guidelines set by NATA and the Board of Certification. In addition, Health Insurance Portability and Accounting Act

(HIPAA) regulations and how they relate to athletic training and other health care professions have been included.

Chapter Three now refers to the "strength and conditioning specialist."

In *Chapter Four,* the NATA Code of Ethics has been updated.

Chapter Five has updated fitness charts.

Chapter Six has updated nutritional charts based on changes to the Food Guide Pyramid and new information on creatine, steroids, and hydration has been included.

Chapters Seven and *Eight* have been updated as needed and *Chapter Nine* includes updated CPR standards.

Chapters Ten, Eleven, and *Twelve* include updated first aid kits, new standards for infection control, and new blood pressure standards.

Chapter Thirteen now includes the use of an automated external defibrillator (AED) and new CPR standards.

Chapter Fourteen has updated Occupational Safety and Health Administration (OSHA) guidelines and updated wound care, and *Chapter Fifteen* has new concussion guidelines.

Chapters Sixteen, Seventeen, and *Eighteen* have many new illustrations and include information on the Epstein-Barr virus.

Chapter Nineteen now includes lightning, one of the top-three causes of weather-related deaths.

Chapter Twenty has been updated to the new first aid standards; *Chapter Twenty-One* now includes elastic wraps; and *Chapter Twenty-Two* addresses managing sports injuries and determining return to play.

Chapter Twenty-Four continues to address physical rehabilitation.

Chapter Twenty-Five has been updated to match current sales conditions.

ALSO AVAILABLE FOR THE STUDENT

Student Workbook to Accompany Sports Medicine Essentials: Core Concepts in Athletic Training & Fitness Instruction, 2nd Edition, ISBN: 1-4018-6186-5

The workbook contains Assignment Sheets, Matching questions, True/False questions, Short Answer questions, Word Search puzzles, and Crossword puzzles all designed to test comprehension of chapter concepts.

ALSO AVAILABLE FOR THE INSTRUCTOR

Electronic Classroom Manager to Accompany Sports Medicine Essentials: Core Concepts in Athletic Training & Fitness Instruction, 2nd Edition, ISBN: 1-4018-6187-3

This CD package contains:

* **Instructor's Manual** containing tips for class instruction including topics for class discussion and learning activities. Also includes answers to *Thinking It Through* scenarios and answers to the *Student Enrichment Activities.*

* **Exam*View*® Computerized Test Bank** containing over 1,200 questions. You can use these questions to create your own review materials or tests.

* Over 280 **PowerPoint®** slides correlating to the chapters within the book. These easily can be customized to meet your needs.

ABOUT THE AUTHOR

Jim Clover, MEd, ATC, PTA, has been the coordinator of the SPORT Clinic in Riverside, California for over 25 years. The SPORT Clinic is part of Community Medical Group, a multi-specialty clinic made up of orthopedic surgeons, physical therapists, athletic trainers, a surgery center, and a family practice department. The SPORT Clinic reaches out to over 40 high schools and colleges, organizing the sports medicine coverage for over 3,000 events per year.

Mr. Clover has been an instructor of a regional occupational course "Sports Therapy and Fitness" for over 20 years, and has taught a tele-course on athletic training at Riverside Community College and University of California Riverside and an athletic training course at California Baptist College and Cal State San Bernardino.

Mr. Clover is the owner of Clover Enterprise, a corporation that provides athletic training coverage to 17 local high schools. He is also the inventor of the "Trainer's Angel," the first face mask removal tool; the inventor of the R.E.D. Book, a book that organizes sports medicine forms; producer of the athletic trainer's theme song "First to Come and Last to Leave;" author of five sports medicine videos for Cramer Products; past chair for the NATA District 8 Clinical Industrial and Cooperate Committee; past chair for the Job Development task force; District 8 representative for the NATA Foundation; a 25-year member of NATA; District 8 and NATA recipient of the "Most Distinguished Athletic Trainer's Award;" and past chair of the Riverside SPORT Hall of Fame.

In addition, Mr. Clover has authored several chapters of marketing books, EMP America's "Sports Medicine First Aid," and numerous articles; been a speaker at numerous events; and been an instructor for all first aid and CPR courses taught through EMP America.

Mr. Clover is coordinator of Practical Applications in Sports Medicine, a sports medicine conference that has been held for over 15 years, and coordinator of the Inland Empire All-Star Football classic for over 20 years (this event raised over $100,000 in college scholarships). He also coordinated Cramer Student Trainer camps in Riverside, California, and was a clinical coordinator for a sports medicine family practice fellowship for over 10 years.

Mr. Clover can be contacted at sportclinic@ earthlinic.net.

ACKNOWLEDGEMENTS

I would like to thank the following people: Jessica Bear, an undergraduate student at Wagner College; Jim Winn, MED, ATC, PTA; Todd Babcock, MS, ATC; Jim Elton, MS, ATC; Allen Boyd, ATC; the physicians and physical therapists at Community Medical Group and SPORT Clinic; Ellen Coleman for her expertise in sport nutrition; Carol Scott for her help with the editing; Jerome F. Wall, M.D. for his constant positive guidance and expertise; and my college instructors, Billy Hill, ATC; Linda Daniels, PT, ATC; and Mike Bordner, ATC. I also want to thank James B. Clover, Sr., a very talented teacher; Valerie Harris, who worked on the first edition; and my incredibly tolerant editors, Erin Curtis, Matthew Seeley, and Nikki Lee.

REVIEWERS

The following reviewers provided valuable feedback in the creation of this text. Their time, comments, and attention to detail are greatly appreciated.

Andrew E. Accardi, ATC/L, M.Ed.
　Newman Central Catholic High School, Sterling IL

Steven P. Broglio, MS, ATC
　University of Georgia, Athens, GA

James Buriak, ATC
　Roanoke College, Salem, VA

Dr. Lori Dewald, EdD, ATC, CHES
　University of Minnesota Duluth, Duluth, MN

Michael W. Goforth
　Virginia Tech, Blacksburg, VA

Pat Graman, MA, ATC
　University of Cincinnati, Cincinnati, OH

Birgid Hopkins, MS, L.ATC,
　Merrimack College, North Andover, MA

Barry Meier
　Riverside Community College, Riverside, CA

Randy McGuire, M.S., ATC
　Georgetown College, Georgetown, KY

Lisa T. Petruzzi, Med, VATL, ATC
　Mount Vernon High School, Alexandria, VA

Julie Rochester, MS, ATC
　Northern Michigan University, Marquette, MI

Karen Rossetter, RN, BSN, Personal coach
Tolles Career and Technical Center,
Plain City, OH

Patrick Sexton, EdD, ATC, ATR, CSCS
Minnesota State University Mankato,
Mankato, MN

Robert Stow, PhD, ATC, CSCS
Emporia State University, Emporia, KS

Edie Tagmir, M.Ed., R.N.
Mid-Del Technology Center,
Midwest City, OK

David Traylor, MSEd., ATC, LAT
Keller Central High School, Keller, TX

Richard B. Williams (Biff) PhD., ATC
University of Northern Iowa,
Cedar Falls, IA

We would also like to thank the following
reviewers from the previous edition:

Allen Felix, MD
Community Medical Group of Riverside,
Riverside, CA

Kevin Gerlach, MA, ATC/L
Crystal Lake South High School,
Crystal Lake, IL

Tricia Hernandez, MPT, ATC, CSCS
The SPORT Clinic, Riverside, CA

Brandon Johnson, MS, ATC, CSCS
Sierra College, Rocklin, CA

Mark Jones, CSMT
Lincoln High School/49er ROP,
Lincoln CA

Larry D. Monson, MPT, ATC, CSCS
Murray High School, Sandy UT

Bradford Smith, MS, Athletic Trainer
Apple Valley High School,
Apple Valley, CA

Jerome F. Wall, MD
Community Medical Group
of Riverside, Riverside, CA

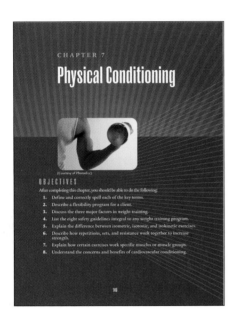

OBJECTIVES

Review this series of goals before you begin reading a chapter to help you focus your study. When you have completed the chapter, review these goals to see if you understand the key points.

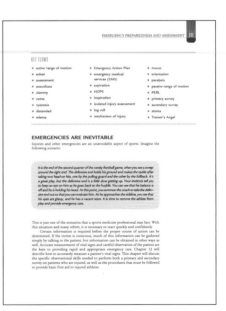

KEY TERMS

These are the critical vocabulary words you will need to learn for each chapter. These terms are highlighted within the text, and definitions are included in the margins. You will also find these terms listed in the glossary section at the back of the book. Use this listing as part of your study.

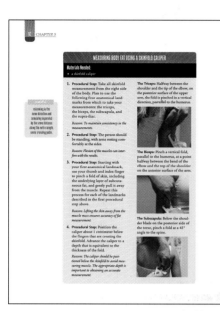

PROCEDURES

Review these step-by-step illustrated procedures by first reading the procedural step and then the rationale for performing the step. Use the illustrations to visualize the written procedure notes. This will give you the how and why of each step and deepen your understanding of the procedure described.

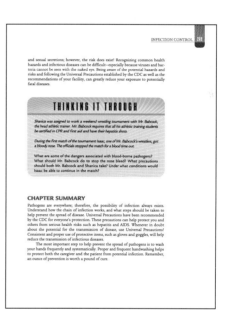

THINKING IT THROUGH

By reading the scenario and answering the questions, you will apply your knowledge of chapter concepts to actual situations while enhancing your critical thinking skills.

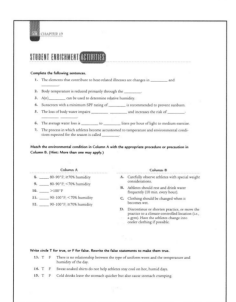

STUDENT ENRICHMENT ACTIVITIES

As a method of reviewing a chapter, answer this series of questions. These activities will stimulate your learning and allow you to synthesize and evaluate the knowledge gained when you study each section.

CHAPTER 1

Careers in Sports Medicine

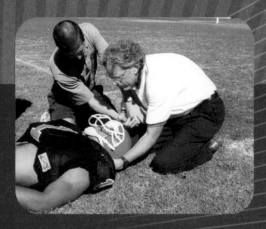

OBJECTIVES

After completing this chapter, you should be able to do the following:

1. Define and correctly spell each of the key terms.

2. Discuss the educational paths and employment opportunities for
   a. athletic trainers.
   b. physical therapists.
   c. strength and conditioning specialists.
   d. business opportunities in health care.
   e. other fields related to sports medicine and training.

3. Understand the personal characteristics, time involved, and education required for careers in sports medicine.

4. Describe the outcomes needed in each of these careers to be successful.

KEY TERMS

* athletic training
* Board of Certification (BOC)
* certified athletic trainer
* Health Maintenance Organization (HMO)
* National Athletic Trainers' Association (NATA)
* physical fitness program
* physical therapy assistant, aide
* sports medicine
* strength and conditioning specialist (SCS)
* therapeutic modality

SPORTS MEDICINE: THE CIRCLE OF CARE

Welcome to sports medicine, an exciting area of the health care system that is growing rapidly, creating many job opportunities for properly trained personnel. **Sports medicine** is the branch of medicine that deals with the prevention, evaluation, treatment, and rehabilitation of injuries that occur to athletes and the active population. When successful, sports medicine professionals bring their patients full circle with the care they provide. The circle of care begins with the athlete on the field or the individual in motion. If that person becomes injured, the requirement is immediate treatment, followed by rehabilitation. Upon successful rehabilitation, the individual returns to the activity or field of play with normal to near-normal abilities, completing the circle of care (see Figure 1-1).

sports medicine

the branch of health care that deals with evaluating athletes and preventing and treating injuries. These athletes will range from wheelchair basketball players to the extreme skier.

Those who work in sports medicine must draw from a vast array of disciplines including anatomy, physiology, strength training, psychology, and nutrition to help their patients or clients attain, regain, and maintain physical fitness. For example, if a patient sprains an ankle, putting that person on crutches is only the first step in treating the assessed injury. Other considerations include methods of controlling or eliminating pain, making the ankle strong enough to continue with the daily living activities, and decreasing the

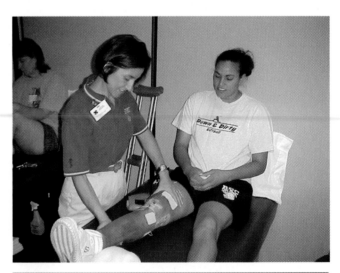

FIGURE 1-1 Sports medicine involves a circle of care that begins on the field of play, advances to treatment, progresses to rehabilitation, and returns to the field of play.

chance of reinjury. If the patient is overweight, becomes overweight while recovering from an injury, or has poor muscle tone, then these factors also must be addressed; in fact, these factors may even have contributed to the injury! Restorative treatment of the injury would revolve around the use of various **therapeutic modalities** and exercise. It is easy to see how the restoration of function and the prevention of additional injury depend upon a thorough understanding of the human body—in order to correct a dysfunction, one must first understand how the body functions normally.

CAREER OPPORTUNITIES

There are many career opportunities in sports medicine, many of which are clinical in nature. Physicians, physician assistants, nurses, physical therapists, physical therapy assistants, athletic trainers, and physical therapy aides may all find employment in hospitals, sports clinics, physician's offices, and other clinical environments. However, much of sports medicine takes place in the nonclinical environments in which sports are played and fitness is pursued.

Athletic training, a division of sports medicine, deals with the prevention, assessment, treatment, and rehabilitation of injuries and the management of the training methods used by professional or amateur athletes and the active population. The **athletic trainer** (Figure 1-2) mixes knowledge and hands-on skills to improve the athlete's physical safety within the athletic environment. This person is an important part of the sports medicine team. This course will introduce you to the career of athletic trainer. The certified athletic trainer is a college graduate professional who can find job opportunities in a variety of settings beyond the traditional environments of professional sports, colleges, and secondary schools. Athletic trainers have emerged in clinics, offices, and even industrial settings with excellent careers.

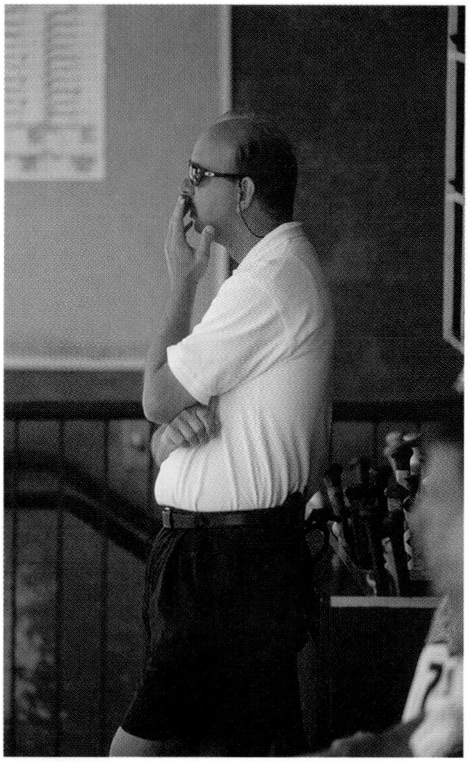

The **Board of Certification (BOC)** is the certifying organization for the athletic trainer. "The Mission of the Board of Certification is to certify athletic trainers and to identify for the public quality health care professionals through a system of certifications, adjudication, standards of practice, and continuing competency programs."—BOC Web site

The **National Athletic Trainers' Association (NATA)** is a not-for-profit organization dedicated to advancing, encouraging, and improving the athletic training profession. NATA represents and supports the 30,000 members of the athletic training profession through public awareness, education, and research. Athletic trainers are unique health care

FIGURE 1-2 Athletic trainers are responsible for the care and prevention of athletic injuries. Here, a certified athletic trainer is observing an athlete's return to play.

therapeutic modality

the use of heat, cold, or electrical stimulation to produce an increase or decrease in blood flow.

athletic training

the division of sports medicine that deals with the care and prevention of athletic injuries and the management of the training methods used by professional or amateur athletes and the active population.

certified athletic trainer

allied health care professional educated and trained in the prevention, assessment, treatment, and rehabilitation of injuries.

Board of Certification (BOC)

the certifying organization for the athletic trainer.

National Athletic Trainers' Association (NATA)

a not-for-profit organization, with more than 27,000 members nationwide, that is committed to the advancement, encouragement, and improvement of the athletic training profession.

providers who specialize in the prevention, assessment, treatment, and rehabilitation of injuries and illnesses that occur to athletes and the physically active.

The mission of the National Athletic Trainers' Association is "to enhance the quality of health care for athletes and those engaged in physical activity, and to advance the profession of athletic training through education and research in the prevention, evaluation, management, and rehabilitation of injuries."—BOC Web site

NATA >

As of 2007, over 30,000 professionals hold and maintain the ATC® credential "Certified Athletic Trainer." To hold the ATC® credential you must have completed an entry level athletic training educational program accredited by the Commission on Accreditation of Athletic Training Education (CAATE) and pass the BOC certificate exam. The current list of these CAATE-accredited programs can be found on the Web at www.bocatc.org by clicking the Store/Resources link and then FAQ.

"In order to qualify as a candidate for the BOC exam you must meet the following criteria.

* Have the endorsement of the Program Director of a CAATE-accredited program.

* Proof of a current certification in Emergency Cardiac Care (Note: The Emergency Cardiac Care certificate must be current at the time of the initial application and any subsequent exam retake registration).

* Students who have registered for their last semester or quarter of college are permitted to apply to take the exam prior to graduation providing all academic and clinical requirements of the CAATE Accredited Curriculum have been satisfied or will be satisfied in their last quarter or semester of college." BOC Exam Candidate Handbook

The certified athletic trainer is discussed in greater detail in Chapter 2.

strength and conditioning specialist (SCS)

a professional member of the sports medicine team who evaluates existing levels of fitness and athleticism, along with helping increase the strength and endurance of an individual or team while promoting a healthier lifestyle.

The **strength and conditioning specialist (SCS)** may have many different professional identities determined by the job setting. In a gym or clinic setting the classification may be a personal trainer, fitness instructor, or the strength and conditioning specialist, whereas in a high school or college setting SCS staff may be known as strength coaches (see Figure 1-3). The information provided will be the basic foundation of evaluating fitness and then setting up a conditioning plan.

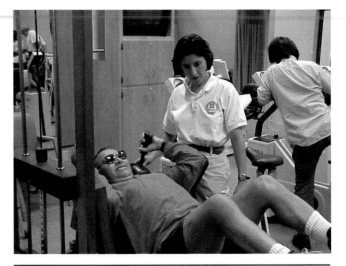

FIGURE 1-3 A fitness instructor helps individuals improve their health by developing effective physical fitness programs.

The SCS is an essential part of the sports medicine team not only in the prevention of injuries and conditioning of athletes but also the rehabilitation after an injury. SCS staff will be involved in the evaluation of existing levels of fitness and the alterations of the activities of everyday life to promote a healthier lifestyle. Motivation, direction, and health-related suggestions for individuals or teams of all ages will be provided by the SCS. They are there for a population interested in taking better care of their physical well-being. The SCS can work in health clubs, individual clients' homes, high schools, or with professional teams, to name a few sites.

Due to insurance controls, time restraints, equipment availability, and/or knowledge, the SCS can assist in strength enhancement of the individual for the prevention of injuries, return to activity, and rehabilitation of an injury. For example, many **Health Maintenance Organizations (HMOs)**, in order to control cost, have established a limit on physical therapy visits. For example, to fully rehabilitate a surgically repaired ACL of a knee, only 6 to 12 visits may be covered. For an athlete to be reinstated to active participation, it may take as long as 6 to 12 months of a continuous, professionally guided program. As in all sports medicine professions, the SCS must combine skills and knowledge to make sure the individual receives the best directions. Usually this is in conjunction with the athletic trainer, physical therapist, and/or physician.

The SCS must be familiar with risk factors, health status, fitness appraisal, and exercise prescription. Then the SCS must be able to incorporate activities that can improve the individual's functional capacity, along with the ability and knowledge to provide education about lifestyle modifications and individual fitness goal-setting.

As the American population continues to pursue more health-conscious lifestyles and seeks assistance in developing safe and productive **physical fitness programs**, the demand for strength and conditioning specialists will increase. Amateur and professional athletes will look to athletic trainers and other professionals to help prevent and care for their athletic injuries. Individuals who do not participate in sports on a regular basis, but would like to be in better health, may also seek the advice of the SCS. Further certifications from such organizations as American College of Sport Medicine (ACSM), www.acsm.org; National Academy of Sports Medicine (NASM), www.nasm.com; and/or the National Strength and Conditioning Association (NSCA), www.nsca-cc.org, are highly recognized and recommended. These organizations are recognized nationally and help to provide the credentials to help obtain positions and advancements in sports medicine careers.

Two other possible occupations are the **physical therapy aide** and the **physical therapy assistant**. The physical therapy aide works under the direct supervision of a physical therapist or a physical therapy assistant. The aide is there to help the physical therapist and physical therapy assistant by keeping the treatment area clean and organized while preparing for each patient's therapy.

Some duties of the aide might include clerical tasks, such as ordering supplies, answering phones, and filling out insurance forms and other paperwork. Because they are not licensed, aides do not perform clinical tasks like assistants are able to do. Students who complete this course will have the knowledge and skills necessary to become an aide.

Health Maintenance Organization (HMO)

group health care plan that provides a predetermined, prepaid medical care benefit package.

physical fitness program

a method of exercise designed to prepare an individual to become physically able to do the activities he or she wishes to do in daily life, without causing undue physical stress.

physical therapy aide

an individual who is not licensed but is able to perform clerical tasks under the direct supervision of a physical therapist or physical therapy assistant.

physical therapy assistant

an individual who has earned a two-year associate's degree and is involved in clinical tasks, such as patient care and recording treatments, under the direct supervision of a physical therapist.

A physical therapy assistant must attend an accredited program that will last two years while earning an associate's degree. These programs are divided into hands-on and academic study. Courses such as anatomy and physiology will be included in the degree. The assistant also works under the direct supervision of a physical therapist. The assistant will be more involved in patient care such as overlooking exercises and performing tasks like massage, electrical stimulation, and hot and cold treatment, to name a few. The assistant will keep records of the treatments and report outcomes of each treatment to the physical therapist.

The purpose of this text is to provide you with the information necessary to become an athletic trainer or SCS. What does it take to help someone who works at a desk ten hours a day become physically fit? What does it take to get an athlete into top condition? Do athletes have to follow different rules for fitness than everyone else? Who is qualified to set the guidelines for physical fitness? What type of training is required before one is qualified to work in these areas of sports medicine? These are just a few of the questions that will be answered in this text.

PERSONAL ATTRIBUTES REQUIRED FOR A CAREER IN SPORTS MEDICINE

Many times, certain bits of information are glossed over, assuming that everyone understands. Personal attributes of successful sports medicine practitioners may be one example of this. Health care careers aren't made for everyone. When the passion to help others is a trait, sports medicine could be the right career path.

An athletic training room filled with athletic training students wearing jeans, sandals, and skater hats will not convey the professional image needed in this profession. Although this may be stylish for a high school student, it is not the image needed to provide the athletes, coaches, administrators, and parents confidence in this profession. Personal attributes are important, and although every setting in sports medicine may have similarities and differences, these are some examples of essential personal attributes.

People Skills: Anyone working in health care must like people and like to be around them. Many situations will occur during which the health care professional may have to be the mediator in a problem.

Communication Skills: A person seeking a career in sports medicine must be able to explain important medical information to the patients, parents, coaches, and others in terms they can understand. Communication in sports medicine is verbally teaching information that must then be put into physical action wherein the patient/client/athlete will learn to take ownership of the situation.

Leadership Skills: When you are working a football game and Johnny has a possible broken neck, you must have skills to competently provide direction and control in the situation. You must walk the walk and talk the talk of a leader, being positive and sincere, without being patronizing. Leadership is confidence; confidence is acquired through knowledge.

Compassion: What if the starting guard on the basketball team blows her ACL and the athlete knows she is done for the season and maybe her career? The sports medicine professional needs to be there for the athletes—to be sensitive to the situation at hand, while being positive and at the same time being the voice of reason.

Good Listening Skills: In order to help others you must be able to listen to their needs and concerns. Remember: Your patients or clients will know where it hurts or what their personal needs are better than you will at first. Sometimes you have to work to get this information; patients don't always tell you everything you need to know. Information about preexisting injuries and illnesses is vital to learn from the patients.

Ability to Follow Directions and Work as a Sports Medicine Team Member: Time to throw out your ego and make your first priority that patient or client. Understand where you fit in the hierarchy of this team. If you are the athletic trainer, you work under the physician. This doesn't mean you never question anything, just that there is a right and a wrong time to do that.

Healthy Body: Working in health care is demanding. It takes its toll physically. In order to help your patients or clients become healthy, you have to stay healthy yourself. The athletic trainer may need to lift the water cooler or assist an athlete off the field.

Sincere Desire to Learn: In professional career choices you have to stay in tune with the latest literature. The only way to do that is to enjoy what you do enough to be eager to discover.

Positive Attitude: Although sports medicine focuses on preventing and overcoming physical setbacks, this is not always possible. Some injuries force drastic changes in a person's life. Be there and be truthful.

Working in sports medicine is exciting! It is also a big responsibility. You must be able to recognize the gravity of certain situations and respond appropriately in terms of both medical treatment and emotional support.

THINKING IT THROUGH

Sydney knew she wanted a career that allowed her to be around active people, maybe even athletes. She had played sports in high school, but she knew she wouldn't have the skills to play at the next level. During her playing days she had received injuries that were treated by the school's athletic trainer. She had been impressed by the athletic trainer's knowledge and noted how much he seemed to enjoy his job. Sydney thought that she might like to be an athletic trainer, but realized that becoming a strength and conditioning specialist, physical therapist, family practice physician, orthopedic surgeon, or nutritionist might be equally exciting.

What characteristics make a person well-suited to one of these careers? What types of classes should Sydney take that would benefit her in the pursuit of any one of these careers? How can she obtain information that will help her decide which career to pursue?

CHAPTER SUMMARY

The field of sports medicine is growing rapidly. This book provides information on the many career opportunities in sports medicine. In these jobs in sports medicine, there will be opportunities for advancement through a combination of additional education and on-the-job training.

As an athletic trainer, physical therapy aide, or strength and conditioning specialist, you will be an important member of the sports medicine team. You will provide valuable assistance to other team members. In doing so, you will participate in the exciting processes of healing patients' injuries, while restoring their physical functioning, maintaining their physical fitness, and preventing additional injuries.

Patients/clients are the most important people in a job as a health care professional in the field of sports medicine. They are top priority. Keep in mind throughout the learning process that you are on your way to one of the most rewarding careers you can imagine.

STUDENT ENRICHMENT ACTIVITIES

Answer the following questions.

1. It is now time to start a professional career. How many years of college does it take to become a:

   a. certified athletic trainer?

   b. physical therapist?

   c. physical therapy assistant?

2. What is needed to become a:

   a. physical therapy aide?

   b. enhanced personal trainer?

   c. certified strength and conditioning specialist?

3. In planning to go to or continue in college, what is the true cost of college per year? Include books, tuition, computer, housing, transportation, and incidentals.

4. What is the average starting annual salary of the following professions?

   a. high school certified athletic trainer

   b. college certified athletic trainer

   c. physical therapist working in a hospital setting

   d. physical therapist working in an outpatient setting

   e. physical therapy aide

   f. physical therapy assistant

5. What is the Internet site to find more information about being a certified athletic trainer?

Complete the following exercises.

6. Search an online business telephone directory and write down possible places for employment in the health care careers. Don't forget the selling of health care supplies and services.

7. Visit the following businesses and describe how the professionals dress for the job.

   a. local workout facility

   b. a physical therapist

   c. an athletic trainer

   d. a sporting goods salesperson

8. The strength and conditioning specialist could have a variety of other titles, depending on the work setting. What might some of them be called such as in a high school or local health club?

9. Which profession do you think you will pursue and why?

10. Goals

   a. It is now time to plan your career path. Write down a timetable, the cost to get to each step, how to or who will finance each step, some of the problems that could arise, how you will get by them, and what is the salary you expect at the end.

   b. Write down the ways you learn and remember best.

CHAPTER 2

Athletic Training

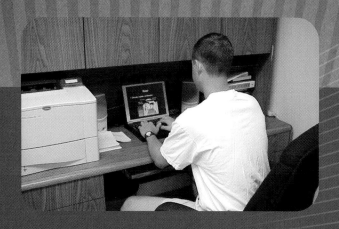

OBJECTIVES

After completing this chapter, you should be able to do the following:

1. Define and correctly spell each of the key terms.

2. List the members of the sports medicine team and describe their duties.

3. Describe the duties of an athletic training student, athletic training student aide, and a certified athletic trainer.

4. List the legal responsibilities of an athletic trainer.

5. Describe the record-keeping requirements involved in athletic training.

KEY TERMS

* assumption of risk
* athletic training
  student/aide
* hydrated
* liability

WHAT IS ATHLETIC TRAINING?

Athletic training is a division of sports medicine that focuses on the care and prevention of athletic injuries. Athletic trainers are the first to arrive and the last to leave at most practices and games. Although the job of athletic training requires many hours, the rewards are great. Athletic trainers fill many roles, from nutritionist to fill-in parent. They are responsible for making sure the athletes receive the care they need in order to perform at their best. In athletic training, as in other fields of sports medicine, many people must work together as a team to ensure a high quality in the level of care.

THE SPORTS MEDICINE TEAM

Like an athletic team, the sports medicine team must work together and support the team captain. The sports medicine team consists of the physician, the athletic trainer, the coach, the athletes, and, in some cases, the community health care facility. In school sports, the athletes' parents and school administration are also important members of the team. Additional members may include a nutritionist, sports psychologist, coach, and/or strength and conditioning specialist. These specialists all bring something to the table, such as what the athletes should eat before an event, how to get themselves mentally ready, and finally to work on specific aspects of their sport such as hitting, pitching, or increasing strength. No matter how many professionals put together one athlete or a team of athletes, they must work collectively with the athlete's best interest in mind.

The Team Physician

The captain of the sports medicine team is the team physician or the athlete's family physician. Most colleges, a few high schools, and all professional teams have a physician who oversees the team and who decides if an athlete is able to participate in a given game or practice. In cases where there is no team doctor, the family's physician or medical specialist will decide if the athlete may participate. No ancillary medical person, such as the athletic trainer, can overrule the physician.

If the sports team is fortunate enough to have a team physician (see Figure 2-1), it is the physician's job to coordinate the rest of the medical team. This involves making sure that everyone works together as a unit, rather than as a group of independent agents. If there is no team physician, the athlete's family physician or medical specialist will make the final decisions regarding the care of the individual athlete. However, since each athlete is likely to have a different family physician, a family physician cannot be expected to coordinate the efforts of the entire sports medicine team. In the absence of a team physician, this responsibility belongs to the certified athletic trainer.

The Certified Athletic Trainer (ATC®)

According to the National Athletic Trainers' Association (NATA), the certified athletic trainer (abbreviated as ATC® by NATA) is a health care professional who specializes in preventing, recognizing, managing, and rehabilitating injuries that result from physical activity (see Figure 2-2). Certified athletic trainers work as part of a complete health care team under the direction of a licensed physician and other health care providers as well as athletic administrators, coaches, and parents.

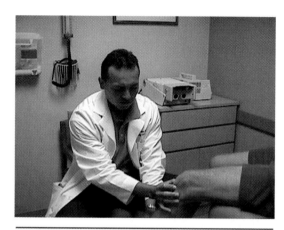

FIGURE 2-1 A physician makes all the final decisions about an athlete's medical care.

To become a certified athletic trainer, you must have a degree from an accredited institution with an athletic curriculum. Courses include areas such as first aid, injury prevention, human anatomy, physiology, nutrition, physical therapy, illness prevention, and emergency care.

Once you obtain a degree, you must also pass a comprehensive test administered by the Board of Certification. If certification is granted, you must continue to meet ongoing educational requirements to maintain your certification.

An athletic trainer also helps organize the sports medicine team by serving as a communication liaison, while staying within HIPAA (Health Insurance Portability and Accounting Act of 1996) guidelines. More information and updated information can be found at www.hhs.gov/ocr/hipaa, the Web site for the U.S. Department of Health and Human Services. The athletic trainer, while working closely with the school administration, must put these guidelines in place, especially for athletes under the age of 18. Parents or guardians must sign release forms so the medical and coaching staff can share confidential information about the athletes' health among themselves. Certain states and different participation levels may have different requirements, but it is important that the athletic trainer follow the legal policies of his or her employer.

The athletic trainer also is responsible for knowing the health

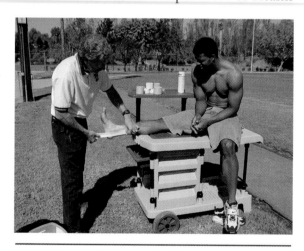

FIGURE 2-2 The certified athletic trainer is responsible for making sure the correct information is passed along to the people who need it.

history of all athletes and providing information to the sports medicine team so that they are aware of any preexisting injuries, conditions, and/or illnesses that could cause harm to the athlete or other athletes. This is also when the athletic trainer should list the items that athletes must have access to, such as an inhaler for asthmatics.

Certified athletic trainers can be found almost anywhere people are physically active. Athletic trainers work in secondary schools, colleges and universities, professional sports, sports medicine clinics, hospitals, the military, industrial and commercial settings, and in the performing arts, to name a few. These responsibilities will be discussed in more detail later in this chapter.

The Coach

The coach is a crucial part of the sports medicine team. It is the coach who teaches participants how to engage, improve, and excel in a particular sport without injury. To do this the coach must be knowledgeable about the injuries common in the sport and what actions to take to prevent them. In the event that an injury does occur, the coach should refer the athlete to the athletic trainer, or if one is not on staff, to the team physician or the athlete's family physician. In the case of student athletes, the coach should then contact the parent(s) or guardian(s) of the student and inform them of the situation. The coach must be certified in first aid and CPR. The coach should make sure the athletes receive the best of care and first aid in every situation (see Figure 2-3). It also is a coach's responsibility to help prevent further injury

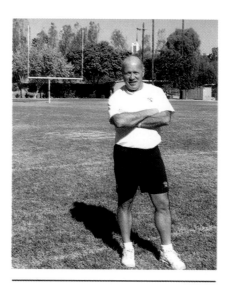

FIGURE 2-3 The coach must make the sport as safe as possible for the athletes.

to a player by not permitting the athlete to return to play until it is deemed safe to do so by the certified athletic trainer or team or family physician. This can be difficult when competition is fierce and the athletes are anxious to play. The coach must remember that athletes are not always the best judges of their own physical capabilities. A coach must not be influenced by the enthusiasm of the athletes, but instead support the instructions of the physician when making decisions that affect the athlete's physical well-being. Clear communication and respect among the coach, athletic trainer, and team or family physician ensures that the athlete receives the same message from each member of the sports medicine team.

In some settings coaches are responsible for maintaining equipment and protective devices for their sport, along with making sure that all gear is of appropriate quality. With personal safety equipment such as football helmets, coaches and athletic trainers must verify and constantly check to ensure equipment fits properly and stays in good condition. The coach may also be responsible for keeping injury records, consent forms, and health insurance information if a certified athletic trainer is not on staff. It also is the coach's responsibility to have all of the necessary medical forms, records, and reports at hand whenever the team leaves the campus for an event. The coach or athletic trainer, if there is one, should always ask the athletes at the beginning of the season if they have experienced any injuries in the off season and record the information. Only then can a coach decide, based on the physician's recommendation, whether the athlete can return to play.

The Athlete

The athlete's responsibilities are to carry out the instructions given by the doctor, athletic trainer, or coach. If an injury occurs during play, the athlete must make the appropriate person aware of it (see Figure 2-4). Furthermore, upon receiving written permission from a physician to return to play, the athlete must make both the coach and the athletic trainer aware of the treatment history, so that the appropriate measures can be taken to safely recondition the athlete to a competitive level. For instance, if an athlete sprains her ankle and is unable to participate in the sport for a period of two weeks, she may decondition during that time. This means she will not be able to resume the activity at the same level she performed immediately prior to the injury. Without reconditioning, she could face further injury.

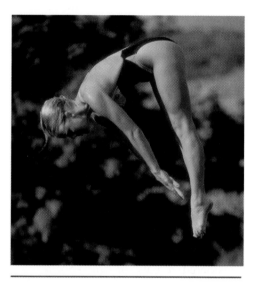

FIGURE 2-4 After an injury, athletes must be safely reconditioned to a competitive level.

The Athletes' Parents or Guardian

In school sports, the athletes' parents or guardian must always be treated with respect. Make sure to clearly establish them as special people in the athlete's life and as part of the sports medicine team. If the athlete is a minor, the parents or guardian must be informed in writing of any injury that may affect their son or daughter (see Figure 2-5). If an injury occurs, the parents or guardian must be informed immediately, either verbally or in writing. Parents and guardians should do whatever they can to secure proper medical treatment for their children. In an emergency, unless the legal guardians are present when the injury occurs, it will be necessary to

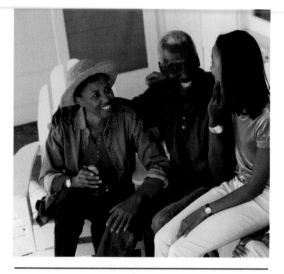

FIGURE 2-5 In school sports, the athlete's parents or guardian are an important part of the sports medicine team.

notify them by telephone, so they can meet their son or daughter at the health care facility or hospital. The time and date of this conversation must be recorded in the injury report.

The School Administration

The school administration must make sure each athletic event and practice is attended by someone who can provide proper first aid and CPR. This applies to home and away (events played away from the home field or campus) events. The administrator should be aware of any injury trends that are taking place in each sport. Once these trends are established, the administrators should do what they can to prevent these injuries from happening. For example, if there are documented trends stating volleyball athletes have an increased chance of spraining an ankle during participation, the administrator might seek funds for preventive ankle braces for the team. The administrator is responsible for approving the funding for field equipment. When making decisions regarding the purchase and use of equipment, the administrator must give the safety of the athletes the highest priority.

The Community Health Facilities

The community health care facilities (see Figure 2-6) can also be considered a part of the sports medicine team. They provide needed services such as rehabilitation, drug testing, physicians' services, education, or even athletic training support for practice or event coverage.

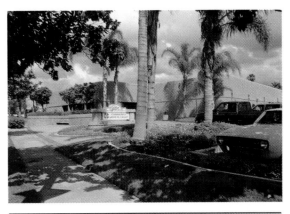

FIGURE 2-6 Community health care facilities provide treatment, rehabilitation, education, and, in some cases, athletic training support.

The key to being a responsible member of the sports medicine team is knowing when to "punt." This means knowing when the treatment of an injury is beyond your capabilities and that it is time to pass the case to someone with more medical experience. It is time to "punt" if skills are required that are outside of your training and expertise, or if you begin to feel uncomfortable with the situation.

WHAT DOES IT TAKE TO BE AN ATHLETIC TRAINER?

It takes a special person to be an athletic trainer. Athletic trainers work in a variety of settings and under many different conditions (see Figure 2-7). Events may be held indoors or outdoors. They may take place in blistering heat or freezing snow, and may be scheduled for day or night. Consequently, an athletic trainer must be prepared for any type of emergency that may occur in any of these settings. Therefore, an athletic trainer needs the following skills, knowledge, and characteristics.

Characteristics

- Dependability
- Adaptability
- Problem-solving/critical thinking skills
- Leadership ability
- Good judgment
- A sense of humor
- Good physical health
- Passionate about sports and helping others

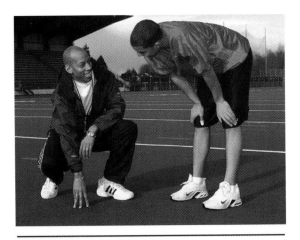

FIGURE 2-7 A successful athletic trainer is knowledgeable about the treatment and prevention of sports injuries, is in good physical health, has an interest in sports, and possesses a variety of organizational skills.

Athletic Training Curricula (from the NATABOC Web site)

- Assessment and evaluation
- Acute care
- General medical conditions and disabilities
- Pathology of injury and illness
- Pharmacological aspects of injury and illness
- Nutritional aspects of injury and illness
- Therapeutic exercise
- Therapeutic modalities
- Risk management and injury prevention
- Health care administration
- Professional development and responsibilities
- Psychosocial intervention and referral

Athletic Training Practice Domains

- Prevention
- Clinical evaluation and diagnosis
- Immediate care
- Treatment, rehabilitation, and reconditioning
- Organization and administration
- Professional responsibility

Employers of Athletic Training Services

* Professional and collegiate sports
* Secondary and intermediate schools
* Sports medicine clinics
* Hospital ER, rehab clinics, and wellness centers
* Occupational settings
* Fitness centers
* Physicians offices

Ideal Practices for Athletic Trainers as Physician Extenders

* Orthopedics
* Osteopathy
* Family practice
* Primary care
* Physiatry
* Occupational medicine
* Chiropracty
* Acupuncture

Other Related Skills

* Time management
* Communications
* Computer literacy
* Organization

Some of these qualities can be developed through training, education, and experience. Others must be part of the athletic trainer's unique personality. Do you have some of the characteristics necessary to become an athletic trainer?

THE RESPONSIBILITIES OF AN ATHLETIC TRAINER

Prevention, assessment, treatment, and rehabilitation of injuries are some of the responsibilities of athletic trainers. They can perform the initial evaluation, administer immediate care in the form of first aid, set up emergency action plans, establish and supervise the rehabilitation of the injured athlete, and purchase and organize all sports medicine equipment and supplies. Because it is not possible to be everywhere at once, it is the athletic trainer's responsibility to make sure all of the coaches are certified in CPR and first aid.

Because injury prevention is such an important part of the job, the athletic trainer should be a key advisor to all athletic programs in the development of conditioning programs—not just during the season, but year-round. Athletic trainers know important facts about various types of athletic exercise equipment and their proper use. The athletic trainer must also keep records of all injuries. These records provide the opportunity to look at injuries from past seasons, which also helps the coaching staff prevent injuries in the seasons to come. Injury records can also provide useful information regarding what the team has been doing right. If the coach has been using a certain conditioning program to prevent injuries, it is apparent that the program is working if the records show a decrease in injuries.

The athletic trainer must be skilled in protective taping, padding, and bracing. Proper use of any specialized padding or bracing can be used as protective equipment during rehabilitation programs.

Providing necessary medical assistance to visiting teams is another responsibility of an athletic trainer who works in a school setting. Athletic trainers administer first aid and provide any injury prevention measures needed by visiting teams if they do not have athletic trainers of their own.

The athletic trainer must set up an athletic training room. This room must be clean and look professional at all times; it should have the appearance of a medical facility. The floor must be vacuumed or mopped daily, and the counters and treatment tables must be cleaned with disinfectant after each use.

The athletic trainer also is involved with the rehabilitation of injured athletes. Athletic trainers must closely monitor any physical therapy prescribed by the physician that is administered to the athletes. The athletic trainer must make sure the therapeutic equipment is kept clean and in good working condition, and must keep records of all maintenance performed on this equipment. A calendar is helpful in keeping track of routine maintenance of the equipment (see Figure 2-8).

As you can see, organizational skills are extremely important in this field. The athletic trainer is responsible for keeping numerous records, such as the daily injury log, the treatment log, the rehabilitation progress reports, the insurance information, consent forms, health history forms, a statistical analysis of season-by-season injuries, and an inventory of athletic training supplies and equipment. The

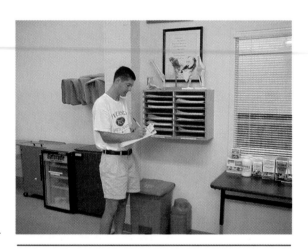

FIGURE 2-8 Maintaining accurate and up-to-date forms is one of the most important aspects of being an athletic trainer.

certified athletic trainer may be in charge of organizing a student athletic training program, teaching the **athletic training student** in the college setting, or the **athletic training student aide** in the high school setting, about their roles and responsibilities.

The athletic trainer must make sure every team has its own first aid kit, water, coolers, ice chest, and any other supplies that might be needed for both home and away events. What is ordered depends upon the type of sport, the number of participants, and the amount of money allocated to the athletic training program, but supplies can range from bandages to computers. The supplies can be obtained from a variety of places, such as pharmacies, medical supply stores, or sporting goods stores. There are also a number of online and mail order companies from which athletic trainers can place orders.

Finally, the athletic trainer, as a health care provider, is a patient advocate. This means that the athletic trainer acts on the athlete's or patient's behalf; the actions taken are intended to benefit the athlete's health and well-being. One of the steps that a responsible athletic trainer should take—one that often is overlooked—is to advise athletes and other interested parties to obtain proper insurance coverage. Without proper insurance, injured athletes may not receive the appropriate medical care. So, as a patient advocate, the athletic trainer should emphasize the importance of proper insurance coverage *before* the athlete becomes a patient!

ACADEMIC REQUIREMENTS AND PROFESSIONAL CERTIFICATION

The National Athletic Trainers' Association (NATA) was formed in 1950 as a paramedical profession. Students who want to become certified athletic trainers must earn a Bachelor's or master's degree in an athletic training curriculum accredited by the Commission on Accreditation of Athletic Training Education (CAATE) (www.caate.net) via the Joint Review Committee–Athletic Training (JRC-AT). Certification is granted by the Board of Certification (BOC).

A Certification for Emergency Cardiac Care Certification CPR/AED for the Professional Rescuer by the American Red Cross, or health care provider–level training by MEDIC First Aid International or BLS Healthcare Provider CPR by the American Heart Association is required. Providers are those adhering to the standards of the International Guidelines 2000 for Cardiopulmonary Resuscitation and Emergency Cardiac Care. The Emergency Medical Technician (EMT) card can be substituted for this requirement.

Entry-level athletic training education uses a competency-based approach in both classroom and clinical settings. Using a medical-based education model, athletic training students are educated to serve in the role of physician extenders, with an emphasis on clinical reasoning skills. Educational content is based on cognitive (knowledge), psychomotor (skill), affective competencies (professional behaviors), and clinical proficiencies (professional, practice-oriented outcomes).

Students must receive formal instruction in the following specific subject matter areas:

Foundational Courses

* Human physiology
* Human anatomy
* Exercise physiology
* Kinesiology/biomechanics
* Nutritional aspects of injury and illness
* Acute care of injury and illness
* Statistics and research design
* Strength training and reconditioning

Professional Courses

* Risk management and injury/illness prevention
* Pathology of injury/illness
* Assessment of injury/illness
* General medical conditions and disabilities
* Therapeutic modalities
* Therapeutic exercise; rehabilitative techniques
* Health care administration
* Weight management and body composition
* Psychosocial intervention and referral
* Medical ethics and legal issues
* Pharmacology
* Professional development and responsibilities

The ATC® Credential

The ATC® credential and the BOC requirements are recognized by 44 states (as of July 1, 2006) for eligibility and/or regulation of the practice of athletic trainers. Aggressive efforts are underway to pursue licensure in the remaining states.

BOC certified athletic trainers are educated, trained, and evaluated in six major practice domains:

* Prevention
* Clinical evaluation and diagnosis
* Immediate care
* Treatment, rehabilitation, and reconditioning
* Organization and administration
* Professional development

For more information, visit the National Athletic Trainers' Association Web site at www.nata.org and the Board of Certification site at www.bocatc.org.

Academic programs are accredited through an independent process by the Commission on Accreditation of Athletic Training Education (CAATE) via the Joint Review Committee on Educational Programs in Athletic Training (JRC-AT). The purpose of the CAATE is to develop, maintain, and promote appropriate minimum standards of quality for educational programs in athletic training.

THE ATHLETIC TRAINING STUDENT (ATS)

Athletic training students are college students who are enrolled in an athletic training curriculum and are supervised by a certified athletic trainer. They must be aware of their duties as assigned by the athletic trainer and must always be prepared to fulfill these duties calmly in circumstances that can be stressful. Knowing when it is time to get assistance from a more knowledgeable person is vital to learn. Understanding the limits of an athletic training student's responsibilities is just as important as being prepared to respond to the athlete's needs

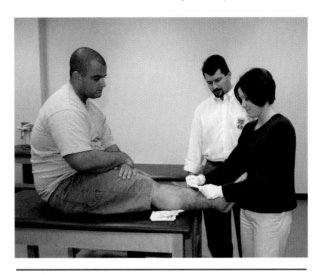

FIGURE 2-9 Athletic training students assist certified athletic trainers in a variety of duties.

(see Figure 2-9). These responsibilities must be discussed with the certified athletic trainer prior to the beginning of any sport season.

The athletic training student can help in any of the following areas, under the direct supervision of the certified athletic trainer:

* Taping, bandaging, or bracing the athletes and fitting any protective equipment

* Overseeing rehabilitation or use of therapeutic modalities, including anything from helping with an exercise program to a whirlpool treatment (see Chapter 22)

* Organizing insurance forms, parental consent forms, supply forms, or recording of any injuries

* Assisting with the daily record keeping so that injuries and rehabilitation may be tracked

* Ensuring that the athletic training room's facilities are clean, neat, and professional, and making sure that any practice or game site is clean and free of anything that may cause injury to the athletes

* Preparing the playing field by setting up water and first aid areas

The ATS may perform the following independent of athletic trainer supervision:

* Administering first aid to injured athletes after taking a recognized first aid course

* Activating the EMS (emergency medical services) (see Chapter 9)

In addition to these duties, the athletic training student must also help the certified athletic trainer by being aware of the athlete's concerns and bringing these concerns to the athletic trainer's attention. For instance, in football practice it is very important for the athletes to keep their heads up when tackling and blocking. Failure to do so may result in a cervical spine injury. The ATS can watch to make sure the athletes are keeping their heads up, thereby preventing the direct axial loading (compression) of the cervical spine that may result from a blow to the head.

Common sense and foresight are also very important in athletic training. A athletic training student's primary goal is to help provide the safest environment possible for the athletes. Therefore, the ATS must be able to anticipate and, if possible, prevent the circumstances that may result in hazardous situations for the athletes. Athletic training students can help by making sure that athletes are properly **hydrated** and by acting as observers during play to monitor occurrences that the certified athletic trainer or coach might miss, such as a player receiving a minor concussion. Sometimes athletes are unwilling to admit when they have received a minor injury, for fear of being removed from play. However, by refusing to admit they have been injured, even slightly, the athletes may unintentionally cause more-serious injuries to occur.

An athletic training student can also help with alternative exercises. These exercises are used, for example, when an athlete sprains an ankle and cannot run on it. The athletic trainer will create some activities to keep the athlete in condition while the injury heals, and the ATS will help supervise and encourage the athlete to perform the alternative exercises.

An ATS can provide valuable assistance in a number of ways; however, there are limits to the student's knowledge and skills.

THE ATHLETIC TRAINING STUDENT AIDE

Students with an interest in pursuing a career in sports medicine can begin the learning path right in high school. A school student who begins studying this field by assisting the athletic trainer or director at school is known as an athletic training student aide. Athletic training student aides work under the supervision of a certified athletic trainer. Thus, part of the athletic team will include students from high schools, colleges, or post-collegiate programs learning about sports medicine.

Athletic training programs are growing in popularity at high schools across the United States. These programs are often spread out over three years and usually contain a classroom, as well as a practical, component. In the classroom, students will study subjects such as first aid and CPR, nutrition, exercise and rehabilitation techniques, anatomy and physiology, kinesiology, biomechanics, and sports psychology. In practical sessions, students will have the opportunity to work with athletes in the training room.

The duties of an athletic training student aide may include stocking first aid kits and ice chests, covering practices, maintaining upkeep of the training room, record keeping, and even helping with treatment of injuries and taping under the direct supervision of the certified athletic trainer. As the student progresses through the program demonstrating knowledge and skill, duties and responsibilities can grow. These students must be respected as key members in the sports medicine team and work hard to earn this respect.

This is where students become familiar with the rest of the sports medicine team, from the athletes, coaches, administrators, and physicians to the rest of the rehabilitation team. Students should take advantage of this great learning opportunity and establish a foundation to build from, so when ready, they will be able to take a leadership role in the sports medicine team.

hydrated

possessing water or fluid, especially in the tissues.

RECORD KEEPING

Careful record keeping is an important aspect of athletic training for two reasons. First, information contained in the injury log is a valuable tool in the prevention of athletic injuries. This information can be used by both the athletic trainer and the coaching staff to determine the nature of the injuries that have occurred. If certain injuries seem to be occurring with any sort of regularity, additional protective equipment may be purchased, or the training and conditioning program may be altered to prevent those types of injuries in the future. Other records, such as the Pre-Participation Physical Evaluation and the Emergency Insurance Information and Consent forms, provide important information regarding an athlete's treatment in the event of injury. These records can be stored in other ways besides the filing cabinet. Specific athletic training software programs can store the information on a computer, PDA, or Web-based platform. This information can be shared once proper permission has been established via fax, e-mail, or written statement. Proper understanding of the Health Insurance Portability and Accountability Act (HIPAA) regulations (www.hhs.gov/ocr/hipaa) must precede the sharing of any information.

Second, but no less important, proper record keeping is necessary to protect you, the team, and the school from legal action in the event of a serious injury. Participation in sports involves certain risks. **Assumption of risk** means that an individual assumes responsibility for the risk taken while participating in the sport. A form must be signed indicating the athlete, parent, or guardian has assumed the risk of injury. This releases the school or organization from **liability**. In the case of minors, the athlete's parents or guardian must sign a form assuming the risk. By law, minors under the age of 18 cannot sign consents. You or the school (or club) may be held liable, however, if you cause additional injury to an athlete as a result of improper care; the assumption of risk does not cover negligence. The concept of negligence and other legal and ethical considerations important to those working in sports medicine or physical fitness are discussed in detail in Chapter 4.

Sports medicine differs from other branches of medicine in that it is "public medicine." Many times the first aid and care provided to an athlete will be done in front of a crowd, or even with cameras recording. This means there will often be witnesses to the care the sports medicine team provides. If the appropriate preventive measures are taken and skillful and competent first aid is provided, the evidence will show that.

The Risk Acknowledgment and Consent to Participate form (Figure 2-10) is used to inform the parents/guardian of any risks their son or daughter may take while participating in the sport. A parent meeting must be held at all school and club levels to provide information about being sport program participants and the risks of participation. The signing of the Risk Acknowledgment and Consent to Participate should be done at this face-to-face meeting between the athletic trainer, the athlete, and the parents/guardian. This provides the athlete and the parents/guardian with the opportunity to ask any questions.

The Emergency Insurance Information and Consent Form (Figure 2-11), when completed, will provide all the insurance information health care providers need to properly treat any injury that may affect one of the athletes. This form *must* be filled out and on file before any athlete is allowed to play in a game or participate in a practice session. It is vital that each athlete have a form on file. *There are no exceptions!* If a form is missing or incomplete, the athlete may not participate.

The Pre-Participation Physical Evaluation form (Figures 2-12A and 2-12B) is used prior to sports participation. The purpose of this form is to find out if the

assumption of risk

acceptance of responsibility for the risks involved in the participation in a given activity.

liability

legal responsibility to perform duties in a reasonable and prudent manner.

RISK ACKNOWLEDGMENT
AND CONSENT TO PARTICIPATE

(Please Print Legibly)

Participant's Name: _____   **Date of Birth:** _____

Address: _____   Telephone: _____

City: _____ State: _____ Zip: _____

Parent/Guardian Name(s): _____

Address: _____   Telephone: _____

City: _____ State: _____ Zip: _____

A.   INFORMED CONSENT

The above named participant wishes to participate in the sport of: _____ in the _____ sports program during the _____ season. I realize that there are risks involved in such participation, and I attended a meeting on _____ where these risks were discussed and explained. I watched the video entitled, _____, listened to presentations by administrators, coaches and sports medicine experts, and had all my questions answered. I am aware playing or practicing to play/participate in any sport can be a dangerous activity involving MANY RISKS OF INJURY. I understand that the dangers and risks of playing or practicing to play/participate in the above sport(s) include, but are not limited to death, serious neck and spinal injuries, which may result in complete or partial paralysis, brain damage, serious injury to virtually all internal organs, serious injury to virtually all bones, joints, ligaments, muscles, tendons, and other aspects of the muscular skeletal system, and serious injury or impairment to other aspects of my body, general health and well-being. I understand that the dangers and risks of playing or practicing to play/participate in the above sport(s) may result not only in serious injury, but in a serious and permanent impairment of my future abilities to earn a living, to engage in other business, social and recreational activities, and generally to enjoy life. I agree to accept these risks as a condition of participation in the above sport(s).

B.   AGREEMENT TO OBEY INSTRUCTION

Because of the dangers of participating in the above sport(s), I recognize the importance of following coaches' instructions regarding playing techniques, training and other team rules, etc. I agree to obey all such instructions, as well to comply with the recommendations of administrators, athletic trainers and doctors concerning injury prevention and care.

C.   RELEASE AND ASSUMPTION OF RISK

In consideration of the _____ Unified School District permitting me to try out for the sports at _____ High School and to engage in all activities related to the team, including, but not limited to, trying out, practice or playing/participating in that sport, I hereby assume all risks associated with participating and agree to hold the _____ Unified School District, its employees, agents, representatives, coaches, and all volunteers harmless from any and all liability, actions, causes of actions, debts, claims, or demands of any kind and nature whatsoever which may arise by or in connection with my participation in any activities related to the _____ High School team(s). The terms hereof shall serve as a release and assumption of risk for my heirs, estate, executor, administrator, assignees, and for all members of my family.

D.   CONSENT TO PARTICIPATE

_____   _____
Signature of Parent or Guardian   Date

_____   _____
Signature of Parent or Guardian   Date

_____   _____
Signature of Participant   Date

FIGURE 2-10 Sample Risk Acknowledgment and Consent to Participate Form

EMERGENCY INSURANCE
INFORMATION & CONSENT

(Please Print Legibly)

Emergency Contact Information

Athlete's Name: _____

Phone: _____

Address: _____

Parent or Guardian's Name: _____ (Father/Mother/Guardian)
                                                            Circle One

Address: _____

Employer: _____

Home Phone: (_____) _____ Work Phone: (_____) _____

E-mail: _____ Cell Phone: (_____) _____

Other Parent's/Guardian's Name: _____ (Father/Mother/Guardian)
                                                             Circle One

Address: _____

Employer: _____

Home Phone: (_____) _____ Work Phone: (_____) _____

E-mail: _____ Cell Phone: (_____) _____

Family Health Accident Insurance

Carrier: _____ Group: _____

Policy #: _____ Group#: _____ ID#: _____

Family Physician's Name: _____

Address: _____

Phone: (_____) _____ Alt. Phone: (_____) _____

Serious Medical Conditions: _____

_____

Allergies (list): _____

_____

* *

I/we hereby grant consent to any and all healthcare providers designated by _____
                                                                              School
to provide my child, _____, *any necessary medical care as a result of*
                          Athlete's Name
any injury/illness.

Insurance company, _____, *(does) (does not) cover football.*
                        Company   Circle One

_____   _____
Signature of Parent/Guardian   Date

_____   _____
Signature of Parent/Guardian   Date

FIGURE 2-11 Sample Emergency Information and Consent Form

PRE-PARTICIPATION PHYSICAL EVALUATION

Name _____ Age _____ Sex _____ Date of Birth _____
Address ___ _____ Phone _____
City _____ State _____ Zip _____
School _____ Grade _____ Sport(s) _____
Height _____ Weight _____ Personal Physician _____ Physician's Phone _____

Complete this form (including signatures) before your examination. Include dates of any problems and explain all "Yes" answers below.

	Yes	No			Yes	No
1. Are you currently under a doctor's care for any reason?...........	❑	❑	21. Has anyone in your family died of heart problems or sudden death before age 50?...................		❑	❑
2. Have you ever been hospitalized?................................	❑	❑	22. Do you have only one working organ of usually			
3. Have you ever had surgery?.......................................	❑	❑	paired organs (only one eye, kidney, etc.)?..................		❑	❑
4. Are you currently taking any medications or pills?..........	❑	❑	23. Have you ever sprained, broken, dislocated or had			
5. Do you have any allergies (medicines, bee stings, etc.)?........	❑	❑	repeated swelling or pain of any bones or joints?...........		❑	❑
6. Have you ever been dizzy or fainted during or after exercise?......	❑	❑	Head ❑ Neck ❑ Chest ❑ Shoulder ❑ Back ❑			
7. Have you ever had chest pain during or after exercise?............	❑	❑	Hand ❑ Wrist ❑ Elbow ❑ Forearm ❑ Hip ❑			
8. Have you ever had high blood pressure?........................	❑	❑	Thigh ❑ Knee ❑ Ankle ❑ Shin/Calf ❑ Foot ❑			
9. Have you ever been told that you have a heart murmur?...........	❑	❑	24. Are any of these bothering you currently?...................		❑	❑
10. Have you ever had racing of your heart or skipped heartbeats?..	❑	❑	25. Have you had any other medical problems?			
11. Have you ever had a head injury?	❑	❑	(asthma, mono, diabetes, etc.)		❑	❑
12. Have you ever been knocked out or unconscious?..............	❑	❑	26. Have you had any medical problems or injuries			
13. Have you ever had a seizure?..................................	❑	❑	since your last evaluation?		❑	❑
14. Have you ever had a stinger, burner or pinched nerve?..........	❑	❑	27. Were there any special instructions or precautions			
15. Have you ever been dizzy or passed out in the heat?...........	❑	❑	given by the Medical Practitioner?..............................		❑	❑
16. Do you have trouble breathing during or after exercise?...........	❑	❑	28. When was your last tetanus shot? _____			
17. Do you have any skin problems (itching, rashes, etc.)?	❑	❑	29. (Women only) Date of first menstrual period: _____			
18. Have you had any problems with your eyes or vision?...........	❑	❑	When was your last menstrual period? _____			
19. Do you wear glasses or contacts or protective eye wear?	❑	❑	What was the longest time between			
20. Do you use any special equipment (splints, neck rolls,			your periods during the past year? _____			
mouth guards, etc?	❑	❑				

Explain all "Yes" answers by question number and indicate dates for each item (include any special instructions):
_____
_____
_____

I/We hereby state that, to the best of my/our knowledge, the answers to the above questions are correct. I/We understand that by performing this examination, the undersigned physician does not assume responsibility for the medical care of this individual. I/We hereby grant consent to share this information to the sports medicine team (coach, athletic trainer, doctor, etc.).

Signature of Athlete _____ Date _____
Signature of Parent or Guardian (if athlete is under 18) _____ Date _____

-- **DO NOT WRITE BELOW THIS LINE** --

	Blood Pressure	HEENT	Skin	Heart	Lungs	Abdomen	Flexibility/Strength
NORMAL							
ABNORMAL							

While this does not constitute a complete physical examination nor replace the need for periodic health evaluations by a family physician, this individual appears to be physically capable of participation in interscholastic sports as of this date, except as indicated below.

❑ Cleared for sports without restrictions
❑ Cleared with the following restrictions: _____
❑ Cleared after completing evaluation/rehabilitation for: _____
❑ Not Cleared

At this athlete's screening exam the following is/are noted:
Condition/Sign/Symptoms with Simple Explanation/Recommendations
❑ Elevated (High) Blood Pressure. Increase in pressures in the artery during the beating and resting heart . Maximum normal (age group)__/__
❑ Heart Murmur. Flow of blood through the heart which is audible. In this case, it is: ❑ "Functional" (normal) ❑ Abnormal.
❑ Asthma. Blockage of small airways in the lung . ❑ Use inhaler as prescribed and 30 minutes before exercise.
❑ Allergic Reactions to Stings or Bites. Whole body swelling & shortness of breath when stung or bitten. ❑ Epinephrine injector should be available at all times.
❑ Diabetes. Abnormal sugars and sugar metabolism. Continue close monitoring with M.D.
❑ Scoliosis. Curvature of the spine. ❑ Continue close monitoring with M.D.
❑ Orthopedic Problem. Being seen by M.D. for this condition ❑ Should be cleared for play by M.D.
❑ Concussion: Further evaluation required before athletic participation permitted.
❑ Other _____

Physician's Name _____ Physician's Signature _____ Date _____

FIGURE 2-12A Sample Pre-Participation Physical Evaluation Form (front)

NOTICE TO ATHLETE

You have been identified as possibly having one or more of the following conditions. It is very important to have this confirmed and followed up by your regular family physician. For supplemental research, check www.webmd.com.

❑ HIGH BLOOD PRESSURE

Your blood pressure today was higher than normal. It is important to see your doctor to have this evaluated because high blood pressure can lead to stroke, heart disease, kidney failure and vision loss. While your condition is not life threatening at this time, your physician must clear you before you will be allowed to participate in sports.

What is high blood pressure? As blood flows from the heart out to the blood vessels, it creates pressure against the blood vessel walls. Your blood pressure is a measure of this pressure. When it goes above a certain point, it is called high blood pressure. It is common to not feel any symptoms with high blood pressure.

Many things can affect blood pressure, including certain medicines and the stress of a doctor's visit. Most high blood pressure, however, cannot be cured. The good news is it can be controlled by such things as weight loss, eating less salt, and exercise. If this isn't enough, medications can be added.

❑ ALLERGY/ANAPHYLAXIS

You have been identified as having either an allergy or an anaphylactic reaction to bee stings and/or insect bites. As this can be a life threatening condition, you will not be allowed to participate in sports until you have been further evaluated by your physician.

What is anaphylaxis? Anaphylaxis is a severe allergic reaction that happens rapidly and can cause diffuse swelling, flushing, hives, and difficulty breathing. It can progress to shock, collapse, seizures, or death if left untreated. There are medications that are used to treat this condition, and your doctor will determine what your condition requires.

❑ SCOLIOSIS

You have been found to have scoliosis on your exam today. Although this is not a life threatening condition, you will not be allowed to participate in sports until you have been further evaluated by your physician.

What is scoliosis? Scoliosis is also known as curvature of the spine. It is frequently discovered during routine physicals in children and young adults and is more common in girls. Some people will complain of low back aches or fatigue, while others will notice one shoulder looks higher than the other. Most cases can be treated with exercises and bracing.

❑ HEART MURMURS

A heart murmur was heard on your exam today. While most heart murmurs are not serious, some can cause fainting, heart failure, or even death. Therefore, it is important to be seen by your doctor to determine risks. You will not be allowed to participate in sports until your physician determines it is safe.

What is a heart murmur? A heart murmur is a sound produced by a change in the flow of blood within the heart. It can be caused by an increase in blood flow caused by a fever, which will go away with time. Many murmurs, however, are related to disease or damage of one or more of the heart valves. The valves can be too tight or too loose. Each will produce a certain noise that can be heard during an exam. If left untreated, this can produce too much stress on the heart and cause it to fail. Your doctor will decide what else needs to be done.

❑ ASTHMA

You have been identified as having asthma during your exam today. Many top athletes have asthma. You need to work with your doctor to come up with a treatment plan that allows you to breathe easy at all times. Because poorly controlled asthma can be life threatening, you will not be allowed to participate in sports until you are cleared by your physician.

What is asthma? Asthma is a disease in which airflow in and out of the lungs may be blocked by muscle squeezing, swelling, and excess mucus. This results in wheezing and/or coughing. An asthma "attack" is often triggered by things such as pollen, mold, dust, strong odors (perfume, paint), tobacco smoke, changes in weather, colds, and certain medications.

Exercise can also cause asthma symptoms. Many non-asthmatics can get chest tightness, coughing, and wheezing after exercise. These symptoms can be easily treated with an inhaled medication that helps to open up the airways. Even if you only have symptoms with exercise, it is important that you are tested for asthma because you may need medicines at other times as well.

❑ DIABETES

You have been identified as having diabetes during your exam today. Untreated, diabetes can lead to heart attacks, strokes, blindness, amputation, and kidney failure. It is important that you work closely with your doctor to keep your blood sugars under control. Because exercise can lower blood sugars, you will need to be seen by your physician before being allowed to participate in sports. Your doctor may need to make adjustments in your medications and monitor your body's response to exercise.

What is diabetes? Diabetes mellitus is a serious, chronic condition of high blood sugar. Some people are diagnosed in childhood, these people need insulin shots to control their sugars. More common is the adult-onset type of diabetes, which can sometimes be managed by oral medications alone. Important ways to control your sugars include following the diet prescribed, exercising, maintaining your weight, and seeing your doctor regularly.

Some symptoms of diabetes include frequent urination, unexplained weight loss, and extreme thirst. Early stages of the disease may be without symptoms. That is why it is important to be seen by a doctor.

FIGURE 2-12B Sample Pre-Participation Physical Evaluation Form (back)

athlete has any preexisting injuries or illnesses the medical or coaching staff should know about. Both the medical and coaching staff must be informed of any and all preexisting conditions an athlete may have. Once aware of an athlete's physical condition, the sports medicine team can work the athlete's special requirements into the training program or prepare for emergencies the athlete could encounter. The Pre-Participation Physical Evaluation form is filled out by the athlete (or in the case of a minor, the athlete's parents or guardian), and the medical portion of the form is completed by the physician.

Some conditions may prohibit an athlete from participating in certain sports. For example, an athlete having one eye or one kidney may not be permitted to participate in contact sports.

SPECIAL INSTRUCTIONS

Once a physician has performed a physical examination on the athlete, it is important to make note of any special instructions that may affect the athlete's health. These special instructions are based on the information obtained from the physical exam and can be recorded on a form like the one shown in Figure 2-13.

Special instructions for each athlete may be recorded on a single team roster or on individual forms. Although a copy of each form may be stored in the athletic director's office, original forms must travel with the coach to all practices and events, both home and away.

SPECIAL INSTRUCTIONS

Name: Sue Jones

Special Instructions: Type 1 diabetic. Sue self-administers daily blood glucose tests, and she will be given a periodic A1C blood test to check the level of sugar in her blood. If she complains of labored breathing, or gasps for air, has fruity smelling breath, shaking, nausea, vomiting, or mental confusion, the EMS should be called. Snacks scheduled around activities will help prevent the onset of symptoms. We have found Sue to be very responsible with the care of her diabetes.

Doctor: Robert Johnson, M.D. **Phone:** (101) 555-7777

Medication: Sue's health care team is prepared to administer her an insulin injection to prevent coma if her blood glucose is elevated as indicated by the above symptoms.

FIGURE 2-13 Sample Special Instructions Form

CHAPTER SUMMARY

Athletic training is an exciting profession. As an athletic trainer, you will have duties that require the ability to see "the big picture" and react in a responsible and appropriate manner. These duties span a wide range, from providing first aid to cleaning up the training room, but all are vital factors in providing efficient medical care to the athletes.

As in any medical profession, legal concerns and situations must be at the forefront of your mind as you make many of your decisions. You must remember that sports medicine is often performed while many people are watching, and the decisions you make will affect the well-being of the person you are treating. You will find that accurate record keeping and organized paperwork are important aspects of providing competent medical care that can also help protect you from liability in the event of a lawsuit.

The importance of obtaining more knowledge in any health care setting cannot be overemphasized. Education is a continuous process. Of course, a certain amount of education is required before you begin to work in the field, but you will find that as you work you will continue to learn new ways to improve your skills, while advanced education will bring even more success and additional growth.

Athletes and parents may want supplemental information on specific pre-existing illnesses. The following are some possible Web sites to refer them to.

* High blood pressure—www.americanheart.org

* Allergy/anaphylaxis—www.foodallergy.org; www.allergic-reation.com

* Scoliosis—www.scoliosis.org

* Heart murmurs—www.webmd.com; www.medhelp.org

* Asthma—www.webmd.com

* Diabetes—www.diabetes.org

STUDENT ENRICHMENT ACTIVITIES

Write the letter of the correct answer.

1. The captain of the sports medicine team is:

    A. the team physician.

    B. the athletic trainer.

    C. the coach.

    D. none of the above.

2. The athletic training student can help in the following areas:

    A. activating the EMS.

    B. organizing insurance forms, parental consent forms, and supply forms.

    C. preparing for practices and games by setting up water and first aid areas.

    D. all of the above.

3. The athletic trainer's primary responsibility is to:

    A. keep the necessary records organized.

    B. prevent and care for injuries.

    C. train the coaching staff in CPR.

    D. order equipment and supplies.

4. Proper record keeping:

    A. is important because information about past injuries can be an important tool in the prevention of future injuries.

    B. is important because thorough documentation can protect the athletic trainer and the team or the school from legal action.

    C. is not important because athletes assume the risk of injury when they participate in a sport.

    D. A and B are both correct.

Write T for true, or F for false. Rewrite the false statements to make them true.

5. T   F   An athletic training student may allow an athlete to return to play after an injury.

6. T   F   *Assumption of risk* means that an individual assumes responsibility for the risk he or she takes while participating in the sport.

Define the following terms.

7. assumption of risk

8. certified athletic trainer

9. hydrated

10. liability

11. NATA

Complete the following exercises.

12. Interview the athletic trainer at your local high school. Describe the school's procedures for risk management.

13. After your interview with the athletic trainer, list the personal characteristics you saw the athletic trainer had.

14. What characteristics do you have that would or would not make you a good candidate in becoming a certified athletic trainer?

15. Does your school have a parent/guardian meeting? If so, how is it organized? If not, how would you organize one?

CHAPTER 3

Strength and Conditioning Specialist

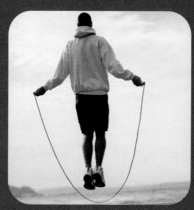

(Courtesy of Photodisc)

OBJECTIVES

After completing this chapter, you should be able to do the following:

1. Define and correctly spell each of the key terms.
2. Describe the duties of a strength and conditioning specialist.
3. List the characteristics required of a strength and conditioning specialist.
4. List the educational requirements for a strength and conditioning specialist.
5. Describe effective methods of working with clients to establish an effective working relationship.
6. Explain the difference between "subjective" and "objective" evaluations.
7. List the factors to consider when developing a fitness program.
8. Discuss ways of motivating clients in their pursuit of fitness and well-being.

KEY TERMS

* body composition
* cardiovascular endurance
* flexibility
* multitasking skills

* muscle endurance
* physical capabilities
* physical fitness
* physical limitations

* rapport
* strength

WHAT DOES PHYSICAL FITNESS MEAN?

In most areas of the United States, people have an avid interest and need for **physical fitness** and health. Whether motivated by studies that show the health benefits of exercise and proper dietary habits, or fueled by tantalizing images of attractive celebrities in magazines, movies, and television shows, Americans want to look and feel better than they do. They are flocking to fitness centers, health food stores, and sporting goods stores to plunk down their money for health and fitness products and services like no other society in the world (see Figure 3-1).

Despite the high interest in fitness, a surprising number of Americans cannot define what physical fitness means. Worse, they do not know how to evaluate their own levels of fitness or understand how those levels compare with the accepted standards in the health and fitness industries.

> **physical fitness**
>
> the ability to perform daily tasks vigorously and alertly, with energy left over for enjoying leisure-time activities and meeting emergency demands.

To put it simply, a person who is physically fit has the strength, endurance, and mental well-being to be comfortable in daily, recreational, and sports activities. However, even this definition is subject to a certain range of interpretation. As you might imagine, physical fit-

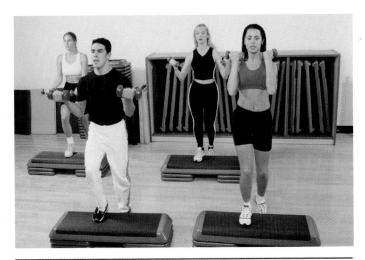

FIGURE 3-1 Aerobics classes are a popular means of achieving cardiovascular fitness. (Courtesy of Photodisc)

ness may mean something different to the average business person who works out a few times a week than it does to a professional athlete who has a rigorous training schedule. For instance, the business woman who works out at a gym three times a week and plays on the company's softball team requires different things from her body than an Olympic long distance runner. Yet, depending on a number of other factors, both individuals may be considered physically fit. So, even with a definition of physical fitness, a strength and conditioning specialist (SCS) needs to spend time with clients making sure both parties understand the client's needs and capabilities.

Fitness instruction is a very satisfying career choice because it enables a person to work regularly with clients and see how physical fitness dynamically brings about changes in their physical appearance and in their health. A strength and conditioning specialist is involved not only with training clients in terms of their fitness level, but also with the clients' personal growth and improved self-image. A strength and conditioning specialist can see clients change for the better, and will have the satisfaction of playing an important role in that positive change. So, when working as a strength and conditioning specialist at a health club, fitness center, sports clinic, or with a sports team, motivation of clients is a quest for better physical health. It is equally important to instruct clients on how to pursue fitness in a way that will be healthy and safe for them.

As already mentioned, American interest in fitness is high, and though it remains high throughout the year, the interest tends to peak at certain times. One peak occurs around the first part of January, when many people establish health-related resolutions for the new year. Interest in fitness peaks again at the beginning of summer when people spend more time outside, feel more like exercising, and usually wear clothing that exposes more of the body. A strength and conditioning specialist must be prepared for these surges in interest and help clients understand that a year-round, life-long fitness plan is the best way for them to both look and feel their best.

ARE YOU FIT FOR THE JOB?

A strength and conditioning specialist must be a very caring, knowledgeable, and motivational person. A good sense of humor and a good sense of fun are necessities. Leadership skills play an important role too; an SCS must be able to lead clients into a healthier lifestyle and a higher level of fitness, and it helps to demonstrate how to have fun while doing it.

The most important characteristic of an SCS is to be a "people person." A "people person" has the ability to anticipate the needs of others and express a sincere interest in those needs. This type of person has good listening skills. In order to anticipate a client's needs, listen to what the clients tell you about themselves. In fact, it is important to display those characteristics right off the bat because the first impression you make with clients will determine the relationship established with each client—a skill essential to success.

In addition, appearance will make a big difference in success. Clients will be much more likely to place their trust in people who look like they practice what they preach. They also will appreciate a well-groomed, professional appearance (see Figure 3-2).

A self-employed strength and conditioning specialist will also find the following skills necessary: billing/accounting skills, computer skills, marketing and advertising skills, and entrepreneurial skills.

Whether you become self-employed or work for an employer, **multitasking skills** will be of great value as an SCS. For instance, an SCS may want to instruct and monitor more than one person at a time in a fitness routine. And, as with many professions, SCSs are expected to be organized and dependable.

multitasking skills

skills that enable a person to competently perform more than one task at a time.

Educational Requirements

A person seeking a career in fitness instruction will have a variety of options from which to choose; job titles vary widely depending on the level of education attained and the type of certification sought. For example, positions are available for personal trainers, fitness specialists, exercise leaders, health/fitness directors, health/fitness instructors, strength and conditioning specialists, and more! The education and certification required for many of these positions will vary by state and facility; however, a universal requirement for all of these positions is CPR certification. To obtain specific information regarding educational requirements and exam preparation, contact the professional organization associated with your area of interest.

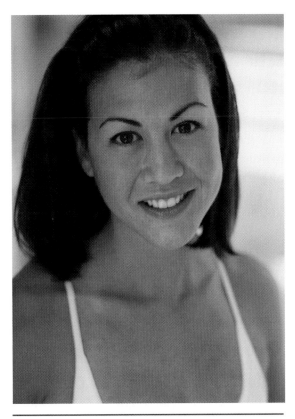

FIGURE 3-2 A positive attitude, a healthy body, and a solid education are key characteristics of a successful SCS.

The National Strength and Conditioning Association (NSCA) is one of the accredited certification programs in the fitness industry. Someone seeking a career as a personal trainer will benefit from courses in human anatomy and physiology as well as kinesiology. An NSCA-Certified Personal Trainer® (NSCA-CPT®) is awarded by the NSCA upon passing a challenging exam administered by an independent examination service. These credentials are widely respected and internationally recognized.

A Certified Strength and Conditioning Specialist® (CSCS®) must hold a bachelor's degree, be enrolled as a senior in an accredited college or university, and be CPR-certified to sit for the exam. Recommended courses for exam preparation include exercise physiology, kinesiology, biomechanics, and anatomy.

For further information regarding the NSCA and their certification programs, visit them on the Web at www.nsca-cc.org.

Another organization whose certifications are valuable in the health and fitness field is the American College of Sports Medicine (ACSM). The ACSM offers several certifications, depending on the candidate's level of education. The ACSM certified Personal Trainer™ (cPT) requires a high school diploma and a current adult CPR certificate to sit for the certification exam. To sit for the ACSM Health Fitness Instructor® (HFI) certification exam, a person must have an associate's or bachelor's degree in a health-related field from an accredited college or university, or be in the last term or semester of the program, and hold a current adult CPR certification. Exams are scheduled throughout the year at different locations across the United States and abroad. These exams are based on knowledge, skills, and abilities (KSAs) determined by the ACSM. The following is a list of the KSAs used as the basis for ACSM certification exams: functional anatomy and biomechanics, exercise physiology, human development and aging, pathophysiology/risk factors, human behavior/psychology, health appraisal and fitness testing, nutrition and weight management, exercise programming, program administration/management, electrocardiography, emergency procedures, and safety. Workshops to prepare for the certification exams are also available through ACSM.

For further information regarding the ACSM and their certification procedures, you can visit them on the Web at www.acsm.org.

Educational Materials

Your clients will appreciate brochures, pamphlets, and other handouts that tell them about you and about their fitness program. Promotional materials about you that include qualifications, fees, the services provided, etc., will be discussed in Chapter 24, but your clients will also need written information about a variety of other subjects. They will need to be informed about safety guidelines, injury prevention, legal liability, insurance coverage, health and nutrition information, and any other subjects that can affect the success of their fitness program. The following are some of the topics you might cover in handout sheets or brochures:

1. Informative Web sites

2. Injury prevention, including information on stress syndromes, such as carpal tunnel syndrome, which can result from improper postures used when typing or while exercising on the stair stepper

3. Correct weight and object lifting techniques

4. Insurance will facilitate the client's access to quality medical care. People who take fitness programs and their health seriously should be reminded that access to good physicians and specialists is important. Access to quality health care often depends on insurance coverage—not the physician. By encouraging clients to obtain adequate insurance, you will be providing them with a service that often is overlooked by other fitness professionals.

5. The client should sign an informed consent (liability release) (Figure 3-3) before you begin to provide services. This will help protect you from prosecution if your client gets injured while participating in your program. (See Chapter 4 for additional methods of preventing legal snares.)

WORKING WITH YOUR CLIENTS

Because working with people is an essential ingredient in the field of sports medicine, it is important to hone "people skills" so that clients develop trust. Developing a personal interest in each client is an enjoyable endeavor, one that can

Informed and Written Consent
for Fitness Program

Patient's Name: _____ **Date:** _____

1. Explanation of Fitness Program

You, hereby, consent to voluntarily take part in a physical fitness program to improve your present physical condition. Your fitness program will involve various types of physical exercise designed specifically for your condition. These exercises may include, but are not limited to, isometrics (tightening a muscle without moving the joint), isotonics (exercises with motion with and without weights), isokinetics (exercises on special machines with varying resistance and speed), and some exercises to improve cardiovascular endurance (stationary bicycling, rowing machines, treadmill, etc.). Initially, you will be started at a slow pace. The rate will be progressively increased as your tolerance will allow. At any time during your program you may ask to stop or request a change in your program.

2. Risks and Discomforts

Your fitness program will be designed to contain minimum risks and discomforts. Some of the normal reactions to a fitness program may include raising or lowering of blood pressure, increased or decreased heart rate, and fatigue. There is a possibility of muscle strain and increased joint stiffness at times. In very rare occasions fainting and/or heart failure may occur. Every effort will be made to minimize these situations by our professional staff. Emergency equipment and trained personnel are available to handle most situations if they should arise. If you suspect or know of any health condition which may adversely affect you, or if you feel uneasy or uncomfortable, please bring it to the attention of your instructor immediately. A doctor's release may be necessary for individuals with known health conditions.

3. Benefits to be Expected

The results of your fitness program are expected to improve your physical function and health.

4. Freedom of Consent

Your permission to engage in a physical fitness program is voluntary. You are free to deny consent if you so desire.

You have read this form and understand the general nature of the fitness program in which you will participate. You consent to engage in this fitness program and accept responsibility for any risks therein.

_____ _____   _____ _____
Signature of Participant   Date   Signature of Witness   Date

FIGURE 3-3 An Informed Consent (Liability Release)

become more personal with increased experience as an SCS. Below are some ideas to build upon.

Establishing Rapport

A good way to bring **rapport** into the client-SCS relationship is to learn and remember some personal information about the client. Learn the client's name and then use it regularly. For instance, check the client's file before the appointment, be sure to pronounce the client's name correctly, and use the name often so that the client feels special. Also, it's a good idea to learn something personal about the client, maybe a common interest. At the time the client mentions some personal anecdote, make that information part of conversation and bring that information up during the next meeting. For example, the clients may say something about their children or grandchildren, or they may mention something about their vacation or an event that has occurred in their lives. This information can help you relate to them personally and remember them as individuals.

Establishing Good Communication

Another important skill in working with a client is to establish clear communication. At times, this will mean that you have to stop moving, sit down, and listen to the client. Pay attention to the client's face, note the client's body language, and focus on what the client is saying.

When a client is talking, it is helpful to respond verbally or physically to the client's concerns when appropriate. This is called active listening. By responding in these ways, the client knows that you are listening. Keep in mind that if you don't listen to the client, some other strength and conditioning specialist will.

Active listening also will help identify the client's fitness challenges. As a result, you will see your client as an individual with unique fitness needs. Although this skill of stopping to listen seems simple, it is an important communication skill that is frequently overlooked by busy people.

If you are a very active person, which many SCSs tend to be, you might find it helpful to take notes while listening to your client; this technique is called active note-taking (see Figure 3-4). It helps you slow down and focus on the client. When taking notes, use a notebook with a section for each client, or make a daily notebook entry with the client's name listed and highlighted. While taking these notes, however, remember to listen to the client, respond to questions, and occasionally make eye contact.

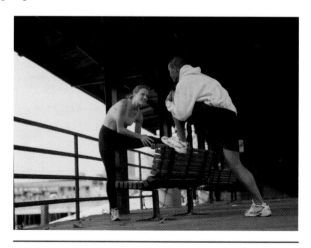

FIGURE 3-4 Having a partner to work out with is important to some people. If this is important to your client, add the information to your notes.

THE FIRST SESSIONS WITH YOUR CLIENT

Make Advance Contact

Let your clients know that they are important, even before the first meeting. It's a good idea to remind a client of the appointment by telephone, postcard, or e-mail prior to the meeting. At this time, mention the date, time, and place of the appointment and emphasize the importance of punctuality. Mentioning ways in which the client might best prepare for the visit with you is also a good idea. For example, suggest that the client wear loose workout clothing, eat lightly, and bring fresh water to the session. Advance contact makes the client less apt to forget or delay the appointment.

At the First and Every Meeting

Always greet clients with a handshake and a smile. Let them know that you are excited they have chosen you as their personal trainer. Let them see by your enthusiastic attitude and your attention toward them that they have made the right choice. As a result, clients will feel welcome and will feel motivated to return. Remember, every first impression is important.

Be on Time

Make sure to be ready for a client at least five minutes before the session begins. This way, you will feel prepared and ready for the client. Through actions and verbal cues, the client will also be encouraged to be on time. This will help keep you on schedule and will help clients feel that they have a commitment to their fitness training. For example, when reminding a client of the next appointment, say with enthusiasm, "You had a great session today! I'll see you at 3:00 sharp on Tuesday. We'll start out with a brisk 5-minute warm-up walk."

Your Appearance

A strength and conditioning specialist has to "look the look" and "walk the walk"; appearance is a vital tool in motivating clients. Your level of fitness, your exercise clothing, and your attitude will all influence the success of your career and your clients' fitness programs. So be fit, clean, healthy, and enthusiastic!

Dress appropriately for the type of activity in which you and your client will be participating. For instance, if you are showing your client how to do exercises correctly, you will be dressed in exercise clothing that is clean and sharp. Avoid provocative exercise outfits that are too tight or too revealing. Dress for success in fitness—for both you and your client.

Allow Extra Time for the First Session

The first session with a new client will last about $1^{1}/_{2}$ hours, so schedule and bill for that amount of time. It takes about 30 minutes to go over any disclaimers and other paperwork, such as insurance forms, with the client. Then have the client fill out personal information sheets and the materials that will help define fitness goals.

Generally, a regular conditioning session lasts approximately 30 minutes for minimum cardio-fitness. This will establish the base level of fitness. If the client has the desire and time available, there is the option to increase the level of fitness by adding 15-minute intervals to the program.

During this first day with a new client, walk the client through the technique for each exercise machine to be used during the early stages of the fitness program. It's best not to have a client do strenuous exercises on this first day because the client may get sore from the exertion and be too uncomfortable or discouraged to work out at the next session.

Be Organized

As an SCS, you will often work with large numbers of clients, so it is important to organize clients' records. You will need a system that allows you to have all your clients' paperwork and appointment opportunities ready and accessible. A good way to organize your clients' information is to create a chart, or folder, for each client. The chart should include all of the paperwork that was signed by the client at the first meeting, including the informed consent/liability release, payment agreement, etc. The client's chart will also contain written goals, weekly evaluations, bimonthly goal reviews, and any other written notes or documentation that pertains to that client. To protect clients' privacy, store their charts in a locked cabinet or some other secure area. Charts are confidential, and entries are made only by the SCS.

EVALUATING PHYSICAL FITNESS

Before starting a client on a fitness program, first evaluate the client's current level of fitness. Although the best type of evaluation to use is objective evaluation (based on measurable facts), a subjective evaluation (based on your client's perceptions) may be useful as well—particularly at the beginning of a program. Sometimes it is helpful to begin an evaluation with subjective information to get an idea of the client's fitness self-evaluation. Then follow up with an objective evaluation to see how that information compares with the client's impressions. Generally, the client's own assessment will be relatively accurate, but sometimes people think they are in better or worse shape than they really are. Use the results of both subjective and objective evaluations to motivate clients in their fitness program.

The form on the next page is the type of subjective evaluation an SCS could give to a prospective client. Once these questions are answered, review the results with the client.

In contrast, objective evaluations use observable and measurable factors to assess an individual's level of fitness. These measurable fators include height, weight, blood pressure, flexibility, and other physical aspects. The full details of performing an objective physical fitness assessment are described in Chapter 5.

Subjective Evaluation of Physical Fitness

	Yes	No
1. Do you wake up during the night before you are ready?	_____	_____
2. Do you feel tired when you wake up in the morning?	_____	_____
3. Do you tend to yawn throughout the day?	_____	_____
4. Do you become tired from tasks requiring little energy, such as climbing stairs or walking around in a shopping mall?	_____	_____
5. Do you run out of energy before the end of the day and often wish you could take a nap?	_____	_____
6. If you have children, are you unable to play active games with them without being sore the next day?	_____	_____
7. Do you wish you weighed less and/or had less fat in specific areas of your body?	_____	_____
8. Are there many chores you find yourself putting off until a day comes when you "feel more energetic"?	_____	_____
9. Do you often fall asleep in the evening while reading a book or watching television?	_____	_____
10. Are you frequently too tired to participate in leisure activities?	_____	_____
11. Do you experience frequent aches and pains?	_____	_____
12. Do you work in a high-stress job, or do you feel high amounts of stress in your life?	_____	_____
13. Do you purchase new athletic shoes because the old ones are dirty or out of style rather than worn out?	_____	_____
14. Do you lack energy and vitality?	_____	_____
15. Do you find yourself choosing activities that don't require much physical energy?	_____	_____

*Overall Evaluation—If more than five of your responses are "yes," then you are considered to have less than an adequate level of fitness or are working too hard.

Objective Evaluation of Physical Fitness

Objective information is obtained by evaluating the following:

1. Muscle strength and endurance
   * abdominal strength and endurance
   * upper body strength and endurance
   * lower body strength and endurance

2. Flexibility
   * hamstring/low back flexibility
   * back extension flexibility
   * upper extremity flexibility
3. Cardiovascular endurance
   * resting pulse
   * 1½ mile run test
   * Kasch pulse recovery test
4. Body composition (BMI = body mass index, a relative measure of body height to body weight for determining the degree of obesity.)
   * percent body fat
   * percent lean body weight
5. Special considerations
   * physical capabilities and limitations
   * blood pressure
6. Medical history (Figure 2-12A can be used to learn about preexisting illnesses or injuries.)

FACTORS TO CONSIDER WHEN DEVELOPING A FITNESS PROGRAM

There are two sets of factors to consider before developing a physical fitness routine for a client. The first set includes skill factors, such as skills needed to participate in rollerblading or the martial arts. The second set includes health factors, such as strength, cardiovascular endurance, muscle endurance, flexibility, body composition, and physical capabilities and limitations. Both skill and the health factors are objective—they can be observed and measured.

Skill Factors in Physical Fitness

Skill-related factors affecting physical fitness consist of eye-hand coordination, balance, coordination, speed, power, and a basic background in sports. For example, coordination is required for participation in the martial arts. Skill-related factors can help keep the client's interest level up by bringing some risk or challenge to a daily fitness routine. This can be helpful, as long as the risk level does not present a real danger to the client's health. Depending upon the skill required to participate, some activities might be better for some people than for others. For example, rollerblading requires a good sense of balance and proper coordination, so people who do not have those skills should probably choose a different activity.

Health Factors in Physical Fitness

strength

the ability of a muscle to exert a maximum force against a resistance.

Strength is probably one of the more familiar aspects of fitness. It is also one of the most visible aspects of fitness because the strength of a muscle is directly proportional to its size. Strength is the capacity of a muscle to exert a maximum force against a resistance. Strength training can result in some growth of the muscles and the ability to increase force against a resistance. Balance of strength is also important in fitness. Balance means that what you can do in the front or one side, you can also do in the back or the other side. For example, it is important to have balance of strength between the abdominal muscles and the lower back muscles. It is equally important to have balance of strength between the hamstrings and quadriceps muscle group in the upper leg muscles, and so on throughout the body. Therefore, to create balance of strength in the upper arms, if a client works the biceps for 2 sets of 10, the triceps should also be worked for 2 sets of 10.

Cardiovascular endurance is the most important aspect of physical fitness. The term *cardiovascular* refers to the heart, the lungs, and their associated structures. The heart is the muscle that pumps the blood, which carries oxygen and nutrients to the different cells of the body. Within the cells, oxygen is exchanged with carbon dioxide (CO_2); then the CO_2 is taken by the blood to the lungs, where it is expelled from the body. Cardiovascular endurance exercises, such as jogging, swimming, cycling, aerobics, and walking, enable a person to develop the ability to perform daily or athletic tasks without getting excessively tired. Since fatigue is often a contributing factor to injuries, the development of cardiovascular endurance can help prevent injuries.

Muscle endurance is the ability of a muscle or muscle groups to apply force repeatedly over a period of time. For example, the number of push-ups a person can do in a minute or the number of pitches a person can throw before fatigue sets in is a reflection of that person's muscle endurance (see Figure 3-5).

Flexibility is the ability to stretch a muscle through its full range of motion (ROM) without causing pain or muscle tearing. For most people, flexibility exercises are often overlooked or not done at all. Yet, for optimum fitness, flexibility exercises must be performed regularly in conjunction with strength training. Most importantly, stretching is an effective way to prevent many injuries, such as muscle strains.

Body composition refers to the amounts of water, fat tissue, and lean tissue that make up a person's total body weight. Body composition is much more useful than weight in determining a person's level of fitness. Because muscle is more dense than fat, weight alone can be

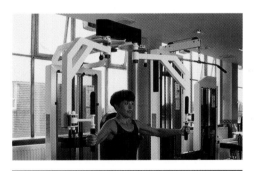

FIGURE 3-5 The number of repetitions a person can perform before muscle fatigue sets in is a reflection of that person's muscle endurance. (Courtesy of Photodisc)

a misleading reference in determining physical health. For instance, two men could each weigh 200 pounds. One of the men could be considered physically fit, while the other might be considered overweight. One factor might be body composition. If the percentage of fat is higher than it should be, it can literally weigh heavily on a person's physique. There is an increased risk of serious medical problems, such as cardiovascular disease and diabetes, if a person has excessive fat. Also, excess fat can limit a person's ability to perform work and other activities. Body composition will be discussed in more detail in Chapters 5 and 6.

Special considerations must also be assessed when evaluating a person's physical fitness. Does the client have high blood pressure? Is the client an athlete who possesses exceptional **physical capabilities**? Does the client have **physical limitations** such as back injuries, knee injuries, shoulder injuries, past operations, asthma, diabetes, or any other medical conditions that affect that client's

cardiovascular endurance
the ability of the heart, blood vessels, and lungs to perform efficiently during sustained physical activities.

muscle endurance
the ability of a muscle or a group of muscles to apply repeated force over a period of time until fatigue prevents the lifting or moving of the resistance.

flexibility
the ability to stretch a muscle through its full range of motion (ROM) without causing pain or muscle tearing.

body composition
the ratio between lean body mass and fat. Generally read as % body fat.

physical capabilities
physical health characteristics that increase one's physical abilities and that must be considered in the development of a fitness program.

physical limitations

physical health characteristics that inhibit one's physical abilities and that must be considered in the development of a fitness program.

level of fitness? These limitations, both temporary and permanent, *must* be considered in the development of an individual's physical fitness program. For instance, a client with asthma may have a very muscular body and may pursue a very healthy lifestyle in terms of diet and body composition, but may be limited in terms of cardiovascular endurance. Likewise, a client with a knee injury is not going to be able to perform any exercises that stress the area of the injury, but will be able to work on strength training, flexibility, and muscular endurance associated with other areas of the body, as well as on cardiovascular endurance and body composition.

Once a fitness routine that works is established for a client, it is important to keep giving the client guidance for continued improvement. As the client becomes more physically fit, alterations in the routine will be necessary to continue to increase the client's level of fitness. Changes in the routine can be done simply to keep it fun. It is up to the SCS to keep clients excited and motivated enough to make fitness a part of a daily lifestyle. The details of developing an individual conditioning program are discussed in Chapter 8.

MOTIVATING CLIENTS

As an SCS, it is vital to understand the benefits of exercise. However, it may take clients a while to understand how exercise changes their whole life for the better. So in many ways, the clients will depend upon the SCS to visually and verbally reinforce those benefits as part of a professional demeanor. As the clients' motivator, this is where the fun comes in for you!

Remember the SCS is the key to clients' success. By supplying the motivation to keep them striving for their goals, keeping them encouraged, and keeping them happy with their fitness program, the SCS can greatly enhance the accomplishments of the clients.

Helping Your Clients Set Goals

When your clients begin their fitness program, they will have some ideas about how a fitness program can benefit them; this is why they have sought out professional help. Some common goals are listed below:

* Weight gain or loss

* Increased strength

* Increased endurance

* Improved diet

* Rehabilitation of an injury

* Improved physical appearance

* Better job performance

* To have fun

* To socialize with others who are fit

* To start or learn a new sports activity

* To improve performance in a current sport activity

The clients' goals, depending upon their age, appearance, and health, may be very achievable, or sometimes may not be realistic at all. For instance, an overweight client may think that he can get fit within a very short time. As a result, he may want to exercise much more than is safe for his fitness level. It is the duty of the SCS to educate all clients to be flexible about their goals.

Sometimes people set goals for themselves that are realistic, but impossible to achieve alone (see Figure 3-6). They get frustrated and quit when they realize they can't do it. Many people find that it is much easier to be disciplined about a fitness routine when there is someone

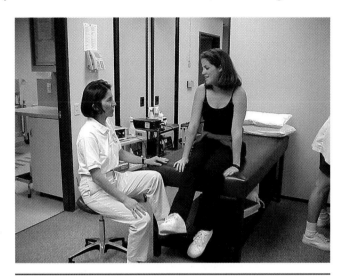

FIGURE 3-6 Personal one-on-one time spent in going over challenges and goals is important.

else involved to help keep them on track—like an SCS. Remember that nothing is more of a challenge for a client than not being able to reach a goal. So, take time to learn about the client's fitness needs, desires, and abilities. Use this information to help the client set reasonable and achievable positive goals.

Like most endeavors, getting fit has its ups and downs. As an SCS, helping clients set and attain *reachable, short-term goals* is a primary means of motivation. For example, encourage the client to write down a fitness goal, such as increasing the number of repetitions in a weight lifting exercise. Then, help the client to achieve that goal during the next two-week period by encouraging and working with her toward that achievement.

Another excellent short-term goal is a weight loss goal of say, 1 pound in one or two weeks, depending upon the client's ability. This is a reasonable, visible goal that the client can achieve. This way, the client sees results and feels motivated to continue getting fit. Losing weight gradually is a healthier goal and maintains weight loss over time.

The SCS will have to tactfully help clients set goals achievable within realistic time frames. These goals will also have to take into consideration the client's physical health, age, gender, and other factors, such as time limitations and family and job responsibilities. By helping clients to set and achieve *realistic, long-term goals*, they will stay motivated because as they achieve the short-term goals, they will see how the long-term goals are also achievable. For instance, a client may want to lose 48 pounds. This would be a good long-term goal, whereas a realistic short-term goal may be 1 pound per week for 12 months to achieve that goal.

Make sure the client understands that goals are always changing and evolving. Although someone's goal may be to have a body that looks like it belongs to a highly trained athlete, that may not be realistic. Or, even if it is realistic, it may take a very long time to achieve. Therefore, setting smaller, short-term goals will be much more rewarding for any client. This approach means that clientss will always be moving toward better health and fitness as they pursue long-term goals. For best results, clients should set aside about 1½ hours, three to four days per week to make steady progress in satisfying these goals.

Recent federal guidelines recommend 30 minutes of exercise daily to prevent chronic disease, 60 minutes a day to prevent weight gain, and 60 to 90 minutes a day to sustain weight loss, depending on your personal metabolism. The President's Council on Physical Fitness and Sports has a set of goals for all age groups and can be found at www.fitness.gov.

Sometimes, goals will not be met. This happens to everyone—particularly around the holidays. For instance, during the week of Thanksgiving, a client may not lose the 1 pound as set in the goal, and may even gain some weight. If this happens, stay positive. Provide encouragement by reminding the client of past successes, and help the client set a new short-term goal.

Although everyone fails to meet their goals at times, it is important to remember that when a goal is not met it may mean that the goal is not the client's first priority. This is an issue that must be addressed tactfully. It is crucial not to blame the client, because encouragement is always a better motivator than guilt. Understand how to set appropriate goals and motivate clients properly. Handling the topic of goals by using effective communication can make or break a fitness business.

Often, a strength and conditioning specialist will have clients keep their own goal and fitness files up to date. That way, they take ownership of their own fitness progress. So let the clients be active participants in keeping their files current. Have time set aside in each appointment during which the clients can update their goal review and fitness file.

Following are some examples of goal review and fitness progress records (Figures 3-7 and 3-8).

Name: Bill Smith — Goal: To do a 5K run in under 23 minutes				
	Weight	% Body Fat	Sit-ups	Bike
Date: 2/1/XX	195	36	30	20 min.
Date: 2/8/XX	195	36	40	25 min.
Date: 2/16/XX	192	35	50	25 min.
Date: 2/24/XX	190	35	60	30 min.

FIGURE 3-7 A Goal Review Record

Name: Bill Smith — Fitness Progress				
Date	Exercise	Duration/Sets	Repetitions	Weight
2-1	Curls	2	20	40#
	Triceps	2	20	40#
	Chest	2	20	150#
	Back	2	20	150#
	Shoulder/Int. Rot.	2	20	5#
	Shoulder/Ext. Rot.	2	20	5#
	Supra	2	20	5#
	Sit-ups	3	30	
	Back Ext.	3	30	40#
	Hamstring Flex	4	30 sec.	
	Bike	25 minutes		
	Treadmill	20 minutes		
2-3	Bike	25 minutes		
	Treadmill	20 minutes		
2-5	Curls	2	20	40#
	Triceps	2	20	40#
	Chest	2	20	150#
	Back	2	20	150#
	Shoulder/Int. Rot.	2	20	5#
	Shoulder/Ext. Rot.	2	20	5#
	Supra	2	20	5#
	Sit-ups	3	30	
	Back Ext.	3	30	40#
	Hamstring Flex	4	30 sec.	
	Bike	28 minutes		
	Treadmill	22 minutes		

FIGURE 3-8 A Fitness Progress Record

The fitness program that is set up with clients must be fun and should fit into their schedule. It should provide them with fitness and a healthier way of life. Also, after clients supply some basic information about their diet and eating habits, the knowledge obtained from Chapter 6 about nutrition will help you and your clients organize and set goals concerning nutritional fitness.

Positive Verbal Cues

Everything an SCS says while working with clients should be designed to encourage them, to reinforce their own efforts, and to add to their sense of enjoyment and fun. For instance, one might joke with a client when it looks as though they are about to give up during an exercise, all the while encouraging them by saying things like, "Just two more minutes on the stair stepper, then we can all collapse together."

Remember to praise the clients' efforts while they are working out. If clients want to discuss fitness trends during their sessions, use this as an opportunity to give them positive feedback. Be alert to any information they bring to a session and encourage them to keep learning about fitness. At the end of each session, evaluate how well they are coming along, give them encouragement, and show enthusiasm toward their progress.

Music as a Motivator

Music touches the spirit and moves the body! Use it to motivate and get the clients moving. Experiment with different kinds of music to find tunes that work best for each client. For instance, upbeat or fast-paced music may well move the hips of some clients, but may be too modern for others. On the other hand, classical music might help clients relax during stretching or cooling-down exercises, but offers little stimulation for cardiovascular sets. So try many different kinds of music—it may be surprising to see how much fun and how effective music is as a fitness tool.

The Appearance of the Facility

Use bright colors, good light, and informative posters in the workout facility to motivate clients positively. Posters illustrating proper posture and workout procedures, such as "Correct Lifting Techniques," help educate and motivate clients. Ideally, a workout facility should be a visual extension of the strength and conditioning specialist in its appearance and motivational atmosphere.

Are the Clients Having Fun?

A lively workout session, filled with good humor, fun music, and motivational verbal cues will help clients enjoy their fitness training (see Figure 3-9). An

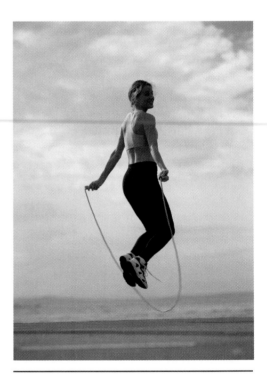

FIGURE 3-9 Fun is an important element in any fitness routine. (Courtesy of Photodisc)

energetic personality and sense of fun can make all the difference in how the clients perceive their fitness program. Needless to say, if the clients are not having fun, they probably won't feel motivated to continue their pursuit of fitness.

The strength and conditioning specialist is the motivator. This is not a day-to-day decision, but a necessary characteristic for all SCSs—they must be a motivational force for each client at every point in instruction. The ability to motivate clients can make or break you in the field of fitness. Fortunately, each SCS has a unique way of enthusiastically encouraging clients, and there are many books and DVDs available on this subject. Be creative! Find ways to make the hard work more fun. This will become easier as the relationship with the client grows. Most important, SCSs should *always* leave their clients looking forward to their next session.

THE LATEST TRENDS

Many times, when it comes to getting fit and healthy, people look for a quick fix. Sometimes clients may ask about a trendy concept from the latest fitness guru. Some clients may be swayed by these fads because the concepts are new and fascinating to them.

Fitness trends can be used to help motivate clients if the trends don't cause them any harm. Some people like gadgets—they feel like they are on the cutting edge when they use the latest devices and accessories.

Some fitness fads can be harmful to people. A strength and conditioning specialist must be able to gently explain to clients why some fads may not be good to try. Some diets can actually damage a person's health, and other fads require the purchase of products that can be a waste of a person's time and money. Become familiar with the current trends in fitness and really know the facts behind the fads. Avoid suggesting or recommending products if you are unsure or unfamiliar with their full effects.

Be careful not to embarrass clients with an unwanted reaction when approached with potentially radical ideas. Remember, clients must feel comfortable, or they will look for another SCS. Do not make them feel silly for being interested in fitness trends. Listen seriously to what they are saying, and respond with tact and diplomacy to their questions.

The field of strength and conditioning is exciting because many people are interested in becoming fit and healthy—and, like all things, the information about health and fitness is always changing. An SCS will need to be informed about the latest developments. Here are some Web sites that contain helpful information.

* www.acsm.org: American College of Sports Medicine

* www.webmd.com: resources for diseases, conditions, and wellness

THINKING IT THROUGH

Valerie, an SCS with over two years of experience, wants to inject new life into her business. Many of her clients don't seem as enthusiastic as she would like, and although the programs she designed for them should be effective, her clients are not making the progress she had envisioned. In short, she is afraid of losing their business. After analyzing her business practices she has concluded that she can make a number of changes to improve her business prospects. To keep current with the latest fitness trends and equipment, Valerie has enrolled in an upcoming seminar on strength training equipment and is considering enrolling in a sports nutrition class at a local college.

How might these changes help make workouts more enjoyable for her clients? How might these steps help her get new clients? What other changes can Valerie make to motivate clients and improve each workout session? How is continuing her education a positive step toward Valerie's goals?

CHAPTER SUMMARY

Being a strength and conditioning specialist is a fulfilling career in sports medicine because it allows the SCS to use many talents: good communication, organizational skills, fitness education skills, motivational talents, and active participation in good health and fitness habits. An SCS helps clients achieve physical fitness, defined as "the ability to carry out everyday tasks with vigor and alertness, without undue fatigue." The primary traits of physical fitness are strength, flexibility, muscle endurance, cardiovascular endurance, and body fat composition. The capacity of an SCS includes the ability to assess subjective and objective information regarding clients' physical fitness. It also involves assisting them in learning how to use exercise machines, routines, and fitness education so they can reach their fitness goals.

Good communication and organizational skills are essential to helping clients set realistic goals for their physical fitness program. Music, positive verbal cues, and variation in exercise routines can help ensure that clients are enjoying the experience of their fitness program. When clients are having fun, they are more likely to maintain fitness.

Don't forget the importance of first impressions. Punctuality, energy, and physical appearance reflect the potential for a positive rapport between the SCS and client. It can be very difficult to overcome a negative first impression, so make the first moments with clients especially positive!

STUDENT ENRICHMENT ACTIVITIES

Match the terms in Column A with the appropriate description in Column B. There is only one correct answer for each number.

Column A	Column B
1. physical fitness	A. muscle stretching without pain
2. strength	B. most important aspect of physical fitness
3. flexibility	C. cells, blood, fibroid tissue
4. muscle endurance	D. exerting a muscle against a maximum amount of resistance
5. cardiovascular endurance	E. physical disability
6. body composition	F. being able to carry out everyday tasks without fatigue
	G. ratio of fat to lean body mass
	H. muscle ability to apply repeated force over a length of time

Complete the following sentences.

7. _____ _____ and _____ _____ _____ are important elements of establishing good communication with clients.

8. You can motivate clients using _____, _____ _____ _____, and _____ _____.

9. For the strength and conditioning specialist, informed _____, subjective and _____ evaluations, and _____ review and _____ progress records are considered essential records.

Define the following terms and explain their significance in fitness instruction.

10. rapport

11. active listening

12. active note-taking

Complete the following exercises.

13. List 10 personal characteristics that are important to a strength and conditioning specialist.

14. List five important things to consider about the first sessions with a client.

15. List five questions you might ask in a subjective fitness evaluation and briefly describe the relationship between such questions and a client's physical health.

16. List five observable qualities included on an objective fitness evaluation and briefly describe the relationship between these observations and a client's physical health.

17. Explain why it is a good idea to do both subjective and objective evaluations.

18. Question an adult and a high school student about their concerns regarding health and fitness. Write a paragraph about the differences and similarities in their concerns.

19. Search a business telephone directory for possible jobs for a strength and conditioning specialist. Rank the top five jobs that interest you.

20. Think about how you would start your own business as a strength and conditioning specialist. Draft a simple business plan. Describe who your target clients will be and how you will advertise to reach them.

CHAPTER 4

Ethical and Legal Considerations

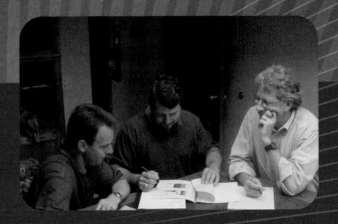

OBJECTIVES

After completing this chapter, you should be able to do the following:

1. Describe team ethics as they apply to different members of the sports medicine team.

2. Discuss the appropriate responses to failure to uphold ethical conduct and regulatory codes.

3. Understand the legal responsibilities associated with athletic training and fitness instruction.

4. List the elements of the Patient's Bill of Rights and explain their importance in sports medicine.

5. Discuss risk management in an athletic setting.

6. Establish a safety committee to protect the best interests of both the athlete and the team.

KEY TERMS

* battery

* ethics

* Health Insurance Portability and Accountability Act (HIPAA)

* malpractice

* negligence

* risk management

* standard of care

* tort

INTRODUCTION

All members of the sports medicine team are responsible for their actions and for conducting themselves in an ethical and legal manner. This chapter will expand upon many of the ethical and legal issues introduced in Chapters 2 and 3 and will emphasize each member's rights and responsibilities to achieve this goal. When a team member does not exhibit appropriate behavior, lawsuits often result. Even when everyone does everything right, athletes still get injured, and lawsuits may still arise out of desire for money or the need for someone to blame.

Never forget that sports medicine is often in the spotlight because sports are usually played in front of crowds and cameras (see Figure 4-1). Using appropriate preventive measures and providing skillful first aid in every incident provide confidence in ethical decisions and help to limit liability in legal matters. Witnesses and cameras will invariably bring attention to professional behavior.

This chapter will revisit the importance of proper record keeping to protect the involved parties from legal action in the event of a serious injury. In a legal matter, documentation is *everything*. One of the athletic trainer's most important responsibilities, with the help of the athletic administration, is to obtain and maintain current release forms, liability waivers, consent forms, and insurance documents. Such paperwork is extremely important because it establishes the athlete's assumption of risk and helps support **risk management** strategies used by the sports medicine team. These two concepts factor heavily in lawsuits that address **negligence** and appropriate **standards of care**.

risk management

reduction of the potential for injury.

negligence

the failure to give reasonable care or to do what another prudent person with similar experience, knowledge, and background would have done under the same or similar circumstances.

standard of care

the degree of care, skill, and diligence an equally qualified caregiver in the profession would provide in similar circumstances.

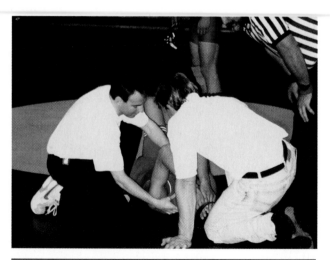

FIGURE 4-1 Sports medicine is often performed in full view of the public.

Failure to provide proper care can result in liability or negligence. The sports medicine team has certain responsibilities to ensure the safety of the athlete/client. Negligent torts may result from the following;

* Malfeasance—when the care provider performs an act that is not the care provider's responsibility or standard of care (for example, the athletic trainer relocates a dislocated ankle).

* Misfeasance—when the care provider commits an act that is the care provider's responsibility to perform, but uses the wrong procedures (for example, improperly stabilizing a dislocated ankle while waiting for paramedics).

* Nonfeasance—when the care provider fails to perform the care provider's legal duty of care (for example, all signs of an assessment indicate an ankle fracture and the care provider does nothing).

* Gross negligence—when the care provider has total disregard for the safety of others.

* Malpractice—when the care provider commits a negligent act while delivering care. Negligence on the part of the coach or medical professional may be called malpractice. This is professional misconduct or lack of professional skill that results in injury to the patient.

TEAM ETHICS

Ethics are morals; they are principles of right, wrong, and duty that guide our behavior. Some actions can be unethical but still be legal, and vice versa. Teams work better when the members work together and share the same ethics. Team ethics are essential to bring about the best experience for all participants both on and off the playing field. In their most basic sense, team ethics combine empathy and reason to guide important choices regarding interaction with others. The following are examples of good ethical behavior as it applies to individual members of the sports medicine team.

> ethics
>
> morals; a set of principles or values that influence behavior.

The Team Physician

The captain of the sports medicine team is the team physician or the athlete's family physician. If the team does not have a physician, the injured athlete's family physician will establish the plan of care. No ancillary medical person, such as the athletic trainer, should overrule or undermine decisions made by the physician. Accordingly, the team physician must exercise the ultimate in good conscience and integrity, not allowing decisions to be influenced by personal or professional motives, or by undue persuasion of other sports medicine team members, including an athlete. The athlete's long-term physical and mental well-being should never be compromised. The physician's behavior should be firmly founded on scientific judgements and compassionate understanding.

The Athletic Trainer

The athletic trainer is there daily for the care and prevention of athletic injuries (see Figure 4-2). The athletic trainer also helps organize the sports medicine team by serving as a communication link among all the individuals involved, making sure everyone has the necessary information. The athletic trainer plays one of the most pivotal and difficult roles in team ethics: keeping an athlete's confidential issues private. Remember, a large part of an athletic trainer's job is to keep the big picture in view and consider the long-term effects of short-term actions. At times, it may seem that the athletic trainer is more at odds with team members than in support; but his responsibilities to the athletes and the team will make confrontation necessary in certain situations. Again, it takes the cooperation of all members to make a team work well. The athletic trainer will enlist the help of other sports medicine team members as necessary to ensure the best possible care for each patient/athlete.

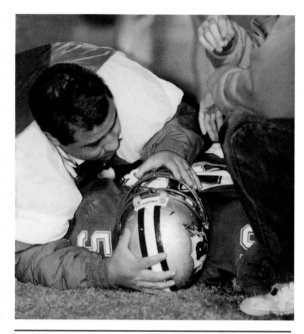

FIGURE 4-2 The athletic trainer is responsible for making sure all other members of the sports medicine team understand the nature of the injury and its treatment. Here the athletic trainer is communicating with the athlete.

The Coach

Naturally, the coach is a very important part of the sports medicine team. The ethical behavior of the coach will be recognized and reflected by all other members of the sports medicine team and their athletes (see Figure 4-3). The coach must emphasize commitment to providing a safe, unbiased, and positive environment in which all participants may excel. Perhaps the most difficult aspect of ethical behavior is the balance between the desire to win and the best interests of

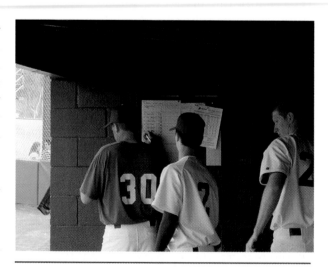

FIGURE 4-3 In addition to performing coaching duties, the coach must set a good example for the athletes in a competitive environment.

the athletes. The coach's ethics should include positive reinforcement, clear and accurate communication of expectations and problems, and, above all, the exhibition of honesty in the face of competitive interaction.

The Athlete

The athlete's responsibilities (Figure 4-4) to ethical behavior include understanding and complying with the team philosophy and written ethical codes, as well as demonstrating respect for parents, teachers, athletic trainers, coaches, and peers. In general, the athlete should not engage in behavior that is harmful or disrespectful to themselves or others. This ethical behavior should be extended to competitors as well as sports medicine team members.

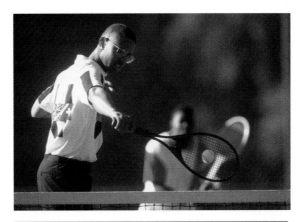

FIGURE 4-4 Athletes are responsible for good conduct and sportsmanship as well as delivering a strong performance.

The Athletes' Parents/Guardian

In school sports, the athletes' parents/guardian must always be treated with respect. Make sure to clearly establish them as special people in the athlete's life and as part of the sports medicine team. As integral members of the sports medicine team, parents have the responsibility to demonstrate ethical behavior by not disputing the coaching staff in front of athletes and refraining from overly enthusiastic support, such as insulting or getting physical with other parents, coaches, officials, or participants. Parents also contribute to team ethics by instilling values in their children that support the team philosophy, encouraging a team attitude in their children, and supporting the child's participation without exerting unreasonable expectations or pressure to excel.

The Administration

The school administration must also be ethical. The administration must know and adhere to state laws and policies and procedures of its athletic conference. School policies that promote athlete safety must be drafted and enforced, and appropriate funding must be provided for the purchase of necessary safety equipment. Damaged or worn-out equipment is not acceptable for team use. No team member should be allowed to play with substandard equipment. Furthermore, the administrative staff should practice what it preaches. If tobacco is prohibited for the team, it should not be used by the administration, coaches, or anyone on the sports medicine team. Likewise, the language, attitudes, and other behaviors expected of athletes should be demonstrated by the administrative staff.

EXPECTED CONDUCT FOR SPORTS MEDICINE PROFESSIONALS AND ATHLETES

Establishing a written set of guidelines and/or regulations is the best way to make sure that both the athletes and the sports medicine team fully understand and share expectations of conduct that is in the best interest of all members. Never count on verbal agreements or the assumption that "everyone just knows." These written standards for conduct, or behavior, and moral philosophy are known as a code of ethics. The National Athletic Trainers' Association (NATA) has a code of ethics that serves as an excellent example of the type of behavior expected of athletic trainers as well as other sports medicine professionals.

National Athletic Trainers' Association Code of Ethics

Preamble

The Code of Ethics of the National Athletic Trainers' Association has been written to make the membership aware of the principles of ethical behavior that should be followed in the practice of athletic training. The primary goal of the Code is the assurance of high quality health care. The Code presents aspirational standards of behavior that all members should strive to achieve.

The principles cannot be expected to cover all specific situations that may be encountered by the practicing athletic trainer, but should be considered representative of the spirit with which athletic trainers should make decisions. The principles are written generally and the circumstances of a situation will determine the interpretation and application of a given principle and of the Code as a whole. Whenever there is a conflict between the Code and legality, the laws prevail. The guidelines set forth in this Code are subject to continual review and revision as the athletic training profession develops and changes.

Principle 1

Members shall respect the rights, welfare, and dignity of all.

1.1 Members shall not discriminate against any legally protected class.

1.2 Members shall be committed to providing competent care.

1.3 Members shall preserve the confidentiality of privileged information and shall not release such information to a third party not involved in the patient's care without a release unless required by law.

Principle 2

Members shall comply with the laws and regulations governing the practice of athletic training.

2.1 Members shall comply with applicable local, state, and federal laws and institutional guidelines.

2.2 Members shall be familiar with and abide by all National Athletic Trainers' Association standards, rules, and regulations.

2.3 Members shall report illegal or unethical practices related to athletic training to the appropriate person or authority.

2.4 Members shall avoid substance abuse and, when necessary, seek rehabilitation for chemical dependency.

Principle 3

Members shall maintain and promote high standards in their provision of services.

3.1 Members shall not misrepresent either directly or indirectly, their skills, training, professional credentials, identity, or services.

3.2 Members shall provide only those services for which they are qualified through education or experience and that are allowed by their practice acts and other pertinent regulation.

3.3 Members shall provide services, make referrals, and seek compensation only for those services that are necessary.

3.4 Members shall recognize the need for continuing education and participate in educational activities that enhance their skills and knowledge.

3.5 Members shall educate those whom they supervise in the practice of athletic training about the Code of Ethics and stress the importance of adherence.

3.6 Members who are researchers or educators should maintain and promote ethical conduct in research and educational activities.

Principle 4

Members shall not engage in conduct that could be construed as a conflict of interest or that reflects negatively on the profession.

4.1 Members should conduct themselves personally and professionally in a manner that does not compromise their professional responsibilities or the practice of athletic training.

4.2 National Athletic Trainers' Association current or past volunteer leaders shall not use the NATA logo in the endorsement of products or services or exploit their affiliation with the NATA in a manner that reflects badly upon the profession.

4.3 Members shall not place financial gain above the patient's welfare and shall not participate in any arrangement that exploits the patient.

4.4 Members shall not, through direct or indirect means, use information obtained in the course of the practice of athletic training to try to influence the score or outcome of an athletic event, or attempt to induce financial gain through gambling.

Reprinted with permission of the National Athletic Trainers' Association.

School districts will usually have a written athletic philosophy that outlines the behavior expected of their athletes. Athletic trainers (Figure 4-5) who work in school environments may have the opportunity to help formulate such a philosophy for the athletic departments in their district. An example of a written set of ideals and expectations that may serve as helpful guidelines in the development of an athletic program philosophy begins on the next page.

Once such expectations and regulations have been written, a copy should be given to each member of the sports medicine team. In the case of minors, it is a good idea to have the parents/guardian sign a form indicating that they have read and accept the expectations described. This will help bridge communication gaps and enlist the support of one of the most influential, but usually least informed, members of the team—the parents/guardian. The athletic trainer must sure everyone is informed in writing of the rules regarding participation as well as the risks involved in the activity.

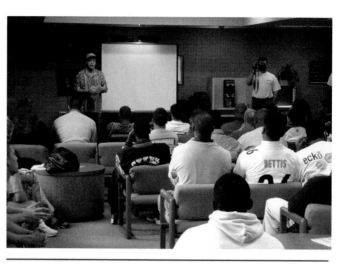

FIGURE 4-5 Here the athletic trainer is explaining the rules to the athletes while being digitally recorded.

Sample District Athletic Philosophy and Regulations

Philosophy

The athletic program of the School District endeavors to provide educational experiences through vigorous, specialized, and competitive activities, which will provide strong character values, healthy emotional dispositions, positive mental attitudes, and a high degree of personal health, vigor, and fitness.

Opportunities will be provided for every boy or girl who is interested and can qualify for participation. The school district endorses and incorporates the Constitution, Code of Ethics, and leadership of the C.I.F. Southern Section and the provisions as outlined in Title IX.

A. Code of Ethics

School District athletes should:

1. Strive to make this code a part of their character and use it daily in their relationship with others.
2. Maintain a constant positive attitude.
3. Strive for personal and team improvement through constant mental and physical performance.
4. Always keep themselves in physical and mental condition that allows them to give a 100% effort during practice and in competition.
5. Maintain a gracious attitude in victory or defeat.
6. Honor the uniform they wear and equipment they use.

7. Help develop team loyalty and spirit by:
   a. encouraging teammates at all times.
   b. maintaining a respectful attitude toward anyone trying to help them on the team.
   c. advancing on their own merits.
   d. never ridiculing or treating a team manager as a personal servant nor forgetting that the manager is an important part of the team.
   e. never pouting, sulking, or second-guessing a coach because they are not playing as much as other team members.
   f. never forming divisive or jealous groups within the team.
   g. never exploiting a team member, coach, or anyone else for the purpose of personal gain or achievement.
8. Remember that in athletics, as well as in life, you are owed nothing, and you will only benefit by constant efforts to improve physically, mentally, and socially.
9. Never make derogatory remarks about another individual, teammate, opponent, umpire, referee, manager, or coach.
10. Never openly criticize or degrade a teammate's abilities or actions.
11. Never offer excuses for their own, or another individual's, group's, or team's performance.
12. Never abuse the privilege of being allowed to participate in athletic competition.
13. Take all differences of opinion, criticisms, or suggestions to the team captain(s) or the coach.

B. Athletic Regulations

1. Scholarship
   a. Athletes must be eligible in accordance with the State, league, and District regulations.
   b. Athletes who drop below a 2.0 GPA will be dropped from competition until the next grade report.
   c. Athletes must be enrolled in at least four classes during the semester in session.
   d. Athletes who drop below four classes during the semester in session will be dropped from competition.
2. Citizenship
   a. Citizenship must be judged as satisfactory according to current standards in effect at the school.
   b. An athlete's past record may be taken into consideration in the determination of eligibility.
3. Appearance
   a. Athletes are expected to dress neatly and in good taste on trips or at any time they are representing the school or the team.
   b. Athletes who do not meet the standards set by the coach or the school may be suspended from competition.
4. Responsibilities to the Coach
   a. Each athlete is responsible to be at every practice called by the coach. Any time an athlete cannot attend practice, it is the athlete's responsibility to personally inform the coach before the time practice is to begin and explain the reason(s) for not attending.
   b. The athlete will practice the athletic code when dealing with all coaches.
   c. Any athlete who has a disagreement with the coach(es) should discuss the point(s) of disagreement with the coach(es).

5. Responsibilities to the Teachers
   a. An athlete's first responsibility is that of a student.
   b. Athletes are not to miss class(es) without making the teacher(s) aware that the athlete will be away from class and for what reason(s).
   c. Athletes are obligated to obtain assignments for class periods they must miss and are responsible for preparing the material and turning it in upon return to class.
   d. Athletes should conduct themselves as ladies and gentlemen at all times.
   e. Athletes should never expect or demand special treatment because of the fact that they are athletes.

6. Responsibilities to the School and Student Body
   a. Athletes are financially responsible for any equipment issued to them.
   b. Athletes must clear financial obligations from one sport before receiving equipment for another sport or team.
   c. Athletes will be financially responsible for the locker assigned to them and will maintain such in a clean and odor-free manner.
   d. Athletes will be responsible to assist in the maintenance of the team locker room or training room.
   e. Athletes are to represent the school and the student body on the athletic field in a sporting manner.

C. Training Rules and Standards

The training rules and standards for all athletes shall be announced to all potential squad members at the first regular meeting. It is recommended that coaches announce them and stress them again to athletes who have been selected as regular team members for the competitive season.

Coaches may set rules and standards for their teams, which may exceed those of the State, league, and District, but in no case may the rules and standards be less than those of the State, league, and District.

D. Scholastic Eligibility

Satisfactory scholastic achievement in terms of individual ability is of prime importance to students participating in athletics. To be scholastically eligible, a student must have passed 20 semester units of new work the previous report period, of which only one (1) class, or five (5) units may be in P.E., and achieved a 2.0 GPA overall.

If the student fails to achieve a 2.0 GPA, the student will be scholastically ineligible until the first subsequent grading period indicating that the 2.0 GPA standard has been met.

Receipt of the student's report card by the school will determine the date of eligibility determination for the 2nd, 3rd, and 4th quarters of the school year. The district may establish Scholastic Eligibility requirements that are more stringent than those set by the State, league, and District, but will never be less than the State, league, and District requirements.

E. Citizenship

As a member of a team, the athlete is a representative of the school and therefore expected to set a good example and to display high standards of conduct at school and while on trips away from the school.

An athlete while on or off campus and while a member of a school team, or while acting as a representative of the school, whose actions are considered to be exhibiting unsatisfactory citizenship will be referred to the school's vice principal. If the vice principal determines that the actions warrant discipline, the vice principal will administer discipline according to school policy and procedure. The vice principal may, at the case providers discretion, refer the athlete to the coach for discipline.

F. Team Tryouts

The head coach of each sport shall conduct tryouts for athletic teams in accordance with the rules as outlined in State, league, and District regulations. All coaches *must* be familiar with the rules that govern their sport.

All students will be given an equal opportunity to display their skills and abilities during this tryout period.

Members of another team still in season, or students missing the tryout period because of illness or other extenuating circumstances, will be given an opportunity to try out at a later date as long as it does not impede the progress of the team.

G. Dismissal from a Team

An athlete dismissed from a team for disciplinary reasons shall be ineligible for athletic competition for the remainder of that sport season, or until the disciplinary time period is completed. Dismissal from a team shall result in a loss of all honors and awards to be received in that sport.

H. Quitting a Team

All athletes should be encouraged to remain with a team until the close of the season for that sport. When an athlete quits a team, the athlete is to be athletically ineligible for participation in any other sport until the team completes its season. All awards and honors earned in the sport will be forfeited when an athlete quits a team.

If an athlete is released through an agreement between the coaches involved in the two sports and with the approval of the athletic director, the athlete will remain eligible and may try out for another team.

I. Travel Regulations

Athletes representing the district's high schools in interschool competition shall be neat in appearance and well groomed at all times when traveling with the school team.

Team and individual conduct when traveling by bus is expected to be exemplary. Immature conduct will not be tolerated and may result in disciplinary action by the school administrator. Bus drivers are to be treated with respect at all times. Excessive noise that could be distracting to the driver shall not be tolerated and athletes must be seated at all times when the bus is in motion.

The coach(es) shall be responsible for the conduct of the athletes on the bus and shall be held accountable for that conduct.

Athletic teams are to travel to and from games as a team whether in victory or defeat.

Athletes should not ask to be allowed to ride home or to the athletic event in private transportation when transportation is provided by the school. Requests for this type of permission will be denied except in extremely rare circumstances, and then only when prior arrangements have been made and approved.

Under no circumstances should an athlete be released to the parents/guardian of a teammate, friends, or other relatives for transportation, unless that was how the athlete arrived, without making prior arrangements with the administration.

J. Outside Competition

An athlete may not practice or play with any organized outside team or squad during the season of the school sport in which the athlete is participating, unless such outside participation or competition is specified in the current State, league, or District regulations.

K. Participation in Other School Activities

Athletes have a responsibility to their teammates and their coach during the season to fulfill their responsibilities and obligations. Attempts should be made by the athlete to schedule and limit outside activities so that conflicts of time and interests are kept to a minimum.

Whenever a school or outside function is scheduled and the athlete is involved, or wants to be involved, the athlete should contact the coach in advance of the event to ensure that there will be either no interference with the sport, or that the interference will be kept at a minimum.

Coaches should make their athletes aware of all special training conditions and regulations at the beginning of the sport season.

APPROPRIATE RESPONSES TO BREACHES OF ETHICAL AND REGULATORY CODES

Regulations and ethical codes are created to produce desirable behaviors. In sports, these behaviors are desired to protect the interests of everyone involved in the athletic experience: the athletes, the team owners and/or administration, family members, and of course the fans. Playing by the rules helps ensure the safety and well-being of the athletes, the job security of the sports staff and administration, and the enjoyment of the fans.

Unfortunately, not everyone plays by the rules. Therefore, it is important to enforce the existing ethical and regulatory codes and to report them when they are violated. As a member of the sports medicine team, "looking the other way" when rules are broken is not acceptable. This only leads to the breaking of more regulations and ultimately to the destruction of the team's effectiveness and spirit. Be prepared to deal with breaches of conduct swiftly, decisively, and effectively.

Feeling confident about reporting behaviors or breaches of conduct regarding health and safety is a "no brainer"; it is the athletic trainer's duty to notify appropriate sports medicine team members if athletes are observed putting their health or mental well-being in danger (see Figure 4-6). These dangers might include tobacco, alcohol, drugs, or unreasonable emotional stress. Likewise, if athletic trainers are aware of physicians, coaches, parents, friends, or any other people who are placing an athlete's health or well-being in danger, they should immediately, yet tactfully, bring such behavior to the attention of people who can help remedy the situation.

While the decision to report breaches of conduct is relatively easy to make when someone's safety is clearly at stake, it may be harder to break a confidence if it seems as if no one is being hurt by the violation. Make it easier on yourself by remembering that it really is not a question of deciding; regulations require reporting all breaches of conduct. Close relationships may develop between athletic trainers and athletes, and it may be tempting for athletic trainers to pretend they did not know about a violation. But the rules exist to protect *all* interested parties. Behaviors that don't conform to the rules can cause all kinds of damage. For example, if athletes are caught gambling on games, they may face suspension and possible expulsion from the team—maybe even the sport. This behavior not only damages athletes' reputations but also that of the institution for which they play. The team, school, or organization could be fined, penalized, or have sanctions placed against them because of the actions of one player. Any such activity must be reported to the administration immediately. Gambling is not only unsporting conduct, it is illegal and must not be tolerated. Such conduct may lead to criminal prosecution.

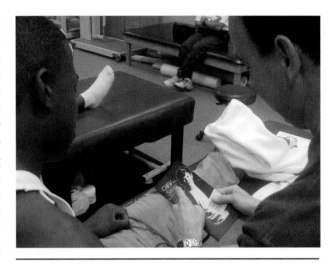

FIGURE 4-6 The athletic trainer is responsible for educating the athletes about a variety of health and safety issues.

Initiation rituals are another concern when considering appropriate behavior. An athletic trainer might witness or hear about various hazing rituals and initiation rites for new team members. While some initiation rituals are harmless and allowable, others are not. To protect the athletes, adopt a zero-tolerance policy for any rituals that involve unhealthy acts, controlled substances, or illegal activities. This policy means that any initiation ritual that involves a risk to a person's health and well-being is strictly prohibited. Any infractions of this rule must be reported to the administration. The consequences of such infractions can be very serious; student athletes have died as a result of poor judgement in this area.

LEGAL RESPONSIBILITIES

As already discussed, the athletic trainer's first duty is to act as an athlete's advocate. The complex process of deciding and acting in the best interest of the athlete while addressing the concerns of the rest of the sports medicine team can be one of the most demanding aspects of being an athletic trainer. It should be said that although other sports medicine team members may present goals that do not reflect concern for the athlete's well-being, it does not mean the concern does not exist. Each member of the sports medicine team has a different role to play, and although no one wants to see anyone get hurt, the fact that each person has a different set of responsibilities brings a variety of perspectives to a given situation (see Figure 4-7). It is the athletic trainer's job to recognize these different perspectives and to accommodate as many views as possible, always keeping the safety of the athletes as the primary consideration. By protecting the physical safety and emotional well-being of the athlete, the athletic trainer also enhances the entire sports organization.

Prevention of injuries has the utmost importance. Since not all injuries are preventable, injuries that do occur must later

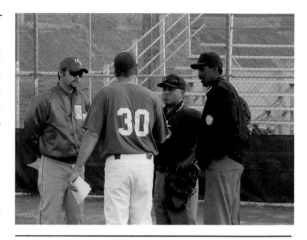

FIGURE 4-7 Although coaches and officials have different concerns, the safety of the athletes is the primary goal.

be reexamined to see if the injury could have been prevented, and if so, by whom. For minor injuries such examination will generally be conducted solely by the sports medicine staff; however, the cause of moderate to major injuries may be examined in a court of law. This is the purpose of litigation (a lawsuit). Litigation determines liability, the legal responsibility for any loss or damage that occurs as a result of one or more person's actions or inactions. If it is determined that someone is liable for an injury, then damages (financial compensation) may be awarded to the injured person. For example, a member of the sports medicine team who causes additional injury to an athlete is liable for that aspect of the injury and may have to pay for the athlete's medical bills as well as other miscellaneous fees and penalties such as for pain and suffering.

A **tort** is a wrongful act resulting in injury to another's person, property, or reputation, for which the injured party is entitled to seek compensation. Such wrongs may result from an *act of omission* or an *act of commission*. An act of omission is the failure to perform a legal duty, such as the failure to provide water for a practice period. An act of commission is an action that is performed illegally, such as the relocating of a dislocated shoulder without a medical license. **Battery** is an act of commission, such as hitting a player or inappropriately touching an athlete.

The majority of sports medicine lawsuits filed involve claims of negligence. Remember, negligence is the failure to give reasonable care or to do what another prudent person with similar experience, knowledge, and background would have done under the same or similar circumstances. To be a legitimate claim of negligence, a person's (or organization's) action or inaction must create an unreasonable risk or harm to others. For example, failing to provide appropriate supervision, allowing dangerous horseplay, returning someone to activity before the person is ready, or failing to recognize conditions that lead to heat stress are examples of exposing someone to unreasonable risk or harm. The law does not require health care professionals to be perfect, but in a negligence lawsuit their actions will be compared with the actions of others with similar responsibilities and training.

One of the best ways of preventing negligence lawsuits in sports medicine is to avoid issues of "failure to warn." This will only be useful in foreseeable risks. Failure to warn means failing to inform participants of the risks associated with the activity. This

tort

a wrongful act resulting in injury to another's person, property, or reputation, for which the injured party is entitled to seek compensation.

battery

the unlawful touching of an individual without consent.

risk of liability can be greatly reduced by having participants and the parents/guardian of minors sign the risk acknowledgment form discussed in Chapter 2. Make sure that all individuals who sign these forms understand what they are signing.

Sports medicine professionals such as physicians, nurses, and certified athletic trainers should carry **malpractice** insurance to prevent personal financial hardship in the event they are found liable for such negligence. Most employers carry liability insurance on employees who are working for them. When working outside of that job, a person should carry additional liability insurance.

> **malpractice**
>
> professional misconduct or lack of professional skill that results in injury to the patient; negligence by a professional, such as a physician, nurse, certified athletic trainer, or coach.

THINKING IT THROUGH

Sixteen-year-old Johnny was participating in a regular basketball practice with the rest of his team when Johnny slipped in a puddle of water during horseplay with another player and hit his head. This blow to his head caused Johnny to lose consciousness. As a result of this injury, he was taken to the emergency room and hospitalized for 24 hours. At the time of the injury, the coach was answering a telephone call in the physical education office, and therefore was not directly supervising the practice.

Was the coach negligent in his responsibility to supervise the team's practice? From a risk management standpoint, how could the athletic trainer have prevented the problem from occurring? What should the coach and athletic trainer do to prevent such problems in the future?

Specific laws for athletic training and fitness instruction vary from state to state, so it is important for professionals in these fields to know the laws of their state before beginning work. However, it is wise to assume that the sports medicine team has the following legal responsibilities:

* Knowledge of assessment and management of injuries

* Providing and maintaining safe and effective equipment and facilities

* Instructing the athlete or client in safety procedures and methods to minimize injury

* Planning an appropriate response for medical emergencies

* Taking reasonable steps to provide medical assistance when required

* Preventing the athlete or client from returning to participation if there is risk of aggravating the injury

* Maintaining confidential medical records

This is by no means a complete list of legal responsibilities. But, taking responsibility for these duties will help ensure the safety of the athletes or clients under supervision, thereby protecting the members of the sports medicine team and the employer.

Performing duties and responsibilities in a systematic manner will ensure that none are forgotten. An easy way to keep these responsibilities in mind is by remembering that the key concern is to keep the athlete S.A.F.E. through the following methods.

* Supervision from the locker room to the practice field. An injury can occur both on and off the field. Keep a close watch of the athletes before, during, and after practice.

* Aid the athletes when needed. This includes creating and practicing the emergency action plan; keeping proper records of physicals, injuries, treatments, insurance, parental releases, and equipment; making sure first aid kits are available and well-stocked; and checking to ensure that water and injury ice are available for the athletes.

* Facilities must be checked daily for possible hazards. If there is a hazard, the area must be clearly marked. A written work order must be filled out and a time frame for completion of the work must be established in writing on the work order. Make sure to keep a copy of the work order.

* Equipment in facilities should be checked daily. From the pitching machine to the modalities used in the athletic training room, all equipment should be well-maintained. This will ensure the equipment lasts longer and stays in proper working condition.

THINKING IT THROUGH

Stacy, Ridgecrest High School's overworked athletic trainer, had always felt it was too much work and that it was not her responsibility to give the coaches the medical information records for away games. She thought the coaches, especially Coach Bordner, would lose them, and then if she needed them for home games she wouldn't have the information to get the athletes the proper treatment.

Megan, a defender for Ridgecrest's varsity girls' soccer, suffered an open compound fracture of both the tibia and fibula in the second period, when she was kicked in the shin by an opposing player. Coach Bordner knew this was serious as soon as he rushed to Megan's side. He started to activate the emergency action plan for away games only to realize that he had no emergency medical records at all. When the EMS arrived Coach Bordner was given a choice of two local hospitals to which to take Megan. He asked the head athletic trainer from the home team for his suggestion, and Megan was off to General Hospital.

The hospital was not able to make immediate contact with the parents because of the lack of an emergency record. Knowing that Megan needed immediate medical treatment, Coach Bordner said he would act as the guardian and authorized treatment. The surgery required pins, screws, and plates to put Megan's leg back together.

Megan's parents finally arrived at the hospital and were very happy with the way Coach Bordner handled the situation, except for one thing. The hospital that Megan was brought to was not part of her health maintenance organization. Megan's parents would have to pay for all the services out of their own pockets.

Megan's parents had supplied all the information on the emergency medical record at the beginning of the season and had the right to sue for damages. They filed a lawsuit against Stacy and the school.

Is it Stacy's job to make sure the coach had the medical information records? Other than just giving the information records to the coach, what else could Stacy have done to make sure the coach had the necessary information and maintained her files at the same time? What are some possible outcomes of the trial? Is Stacy guilty of negligence? Why or why not?

THE RIGHTS OF THE PATIENT

When an athlete or client becomes injured, the athlete becomes a patient. As such, the athlete is entitled to certain patient rights during the course of treatment and rehabilitation (see Figure 4-8). Keep the Patient's Bill of Rights (Figure 4-9) in mind when providing first aid or participating in any form of rehabilitation.

Demonstrating respect for the patient is one of the most important aspects of the Patient's Bill of Rights. Try to empathize with what the patient is going through to help instill confidence for recovery. It is common for friends to casually talk about things that happen at work or gossip about other people. A patient's injury and treatment, in accordance with the **Health Insurance Portability and Accountability Act (HIPAA)**, is one area that must never be discussed in circles outside of the sports medicine team. The patient has the right to keep medical records confidential and that right must always be respected. Violating this right could lead to litigation.

However, athletes might discuss personal injuries among themselves or with others. Generally there is not a problem with this. This type of talk is common around the locker room. In some cases, such conversation could be beneficial. For example, Julie might share her knee-scoping experience with Tina, who is scheduled to have her own knee scoped in two days, or after the swelling has gone down. Conversations such as these

Health Insurance Portability and Accountability Act (HIPAA)

a federal regulation establishing national standards for health care information to protect personal health information.

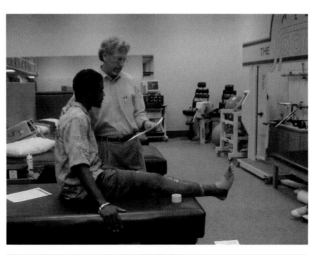

FIGURE 4-8 A patient's medical record is confidential.

Patient's Bill of Rights

1. The patient has a right to considerate and respectful care.

2. Patients have the right to obtain from their physician complete current information concerning their diagnosis, treatment and prognosis in terms they can be reasonably expected to understand.

3. An informed consent should include knowledge of the proposed procedure, anlong with its risks and probable duration of incapacitation. In addition, the patient has a right to information regarding medically significant alternatives.

4. The patient has the right to refuse treatment to the extent permitted by law, and to be informed of the medical consequences of his or her action.

5. Case discussion, consultation, examination, and treatment should be conducted discretely. Those not directly involved must have the patient's permission to be present.

6. The patient has the right to expect that all communication and records pertaining to his or her care should be treated as confidential.

7. The patient has the right to expect the hospital to make a reasonable response to his or her request for services. The hospital must provide evaluation, service, and referral as indicated by the urgency of the case.

8. The patient has the right to obtain information as to any relationship of his or her hospital to other health care and educational institutions, insofar as care is concerned. The patient has the right to obtain information as to the existence of any professional relationships among individuals, by name, who are treating him or her.

9. The patient has the right to be advised if the hospital proposes to engage in or perform human experimentation affecting his or her care or treatment. The patient has the right to refuse to participate in such research projects.

10. The patient has the right to expect reasonable continuity of care.

11. The patient has the right to examine and receive an explanation of his or her bill regardless of the source of payment.

12. The patient has the right to know what hospital rules and regulations apply to his or her conduct as a patient.

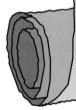

FIGURE 4-9 A Patient's Bill of Rights

may build stronger relationships between the two athletes and possibly bring a more positive attitude to the whole team. When taking part in a conversation between athletes that are discussing injuries, let discretion and common sense guide what is said.

RISK MANAGEMENT IN SPORTS

Risk management is the control of factors that produce some sort of risk. This means reducing the risks involved with participation in a given sport or exercise activity in whatever profession you pursue. Everyone involved in some type of sport lives with the risk of injury. To put the risk into perspective, participation in most sports is much safer than riding in a car—something most people do every day without being concerned about the risks involved. The ultimate goal in risk management is to make the activity as safe as possible for all participants by preventing situations that create opportunities for someone to file a lawsuit. Therefore, risk management involves injury prevention and the education of all members of the sports medicine team regarding emergency preparedness, proper procedures, and appropriate behavior.

To reduce the potential of litigation, the members of the sports medicine team must understand why lawsuits are filed. In general, athletes, their parents/guardian, and clients file lawsuits because they want compensation for some sort of personal damage or loss. In the fields of athletic training this damage or loss usually results from one of the following situations:

* Inadequate supervision of the athlete or client

* Inadequate training of the athlete or client

* Improper or inadequate medical treatment by one or more members of the sports medicine team

* Faulty equipment or facilities

* Sexual harassment, discrimination, or other inappropriate behavior by one or more members of the sports staff

These situations include two types of risk: the primary risk to the athlete or client of physical, mental, or emotional injury; and the secondary risk to the staff or organization of liability for the injury. A primary risk can be anything that negatively impacts the health of the athlete or client and that might diminish the quality of the life experience. It is unreasonable to think that all athletic injuries can be prevented; however, prevention of injury is the best way to reduce the secondary risk of liability for the sports organization or team staff.

Although liability is often loosely interpreted as financial compensation, a typical end result of liability, it is important to recognize that this legal responsibility is often accompanied by other damaging consequences as well. These consequences may include, but are not limited to, reduced social standing, damaged professional reputation, and potential loss of licensure or certification. Being well-informed and attentive can help to minimize both types of risk with proper documentation, ethical behavior, and active communication with appropriate team members.

Remember, lawsuits are better prevented than defended. Litigation is time-consuming and expensive, so it should be avoided whenever possible. Exercising ethics and good sense in every situation is the best way to avoid legal actions. Steps you can take to avoid legal wrong-doing include the following:

1. Do not allow a client or athlete to begin any program without obtaining a signed informed consent and liability release.

If working in private practice, have clients sign and date a form similar to the Informed Consent/Liability Release presented in Chapter 3 (see Figure 4-10). Likewise, athletic trainers should use a form similar to the Risk Acknowledgment and Consent to Participate introduced in Chapter 2. For athletes who are minors, a parent or guardian must sign the form. The athletes and the parents need an opportunity to ask questions, so it is important to be present when the forms are signed. This meeting can also be used as an opportunity to inform the athletes and parents of the precautions the sports medicine staff is taking to make the sport safe for the participants.

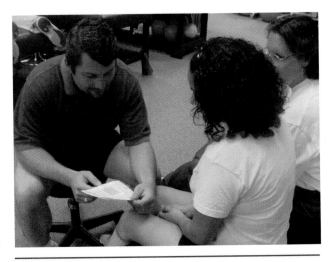

FIGURE 4-10 Signed informed consent forms are a vital aspect of risk management.

2. Agree upon fees/costs and put them in writing before the start of services.

Both parties should sign and date the agreement to avoid potential distortion of the facts, should the client become dissatisfied with the service in any way.

3. Make sure adequate facilities are available for women athletes in sports traditionally dominated by men, and vice versa.

If equal facilities are not available for both men and women, get creative in making appropriate and suitable arrangements to avoid the potential for charges of discrimination.

4. If possible, avoid being alone in a room with an athlete or client to avoid the suggestion of inappropriate behavior.

Please note that this rule of thumb applies to clients of the either gender, not just the opposite sex. A statement, gesture, or touch may be misinterpreted or even fabricated at any time. If possible, it can also be helpful to have another person present who is the same gender as the patient when an assessment, treatment, or procedure is being done. This can be used as a teaching moment for a student.

5. Keep detailed notes about all professional activities and those of the team.

The concept of documentation is emphasized repeatedly throughout this book, but its value cannot be overstated. Proper and thorough documentation provides the sports medicine team with important information that can be used to make decisions regarding the athletes' safety and in the event of a lawsuit may be used to support testimony.

6. Become familiar with the products and supplies used. Read all dealer's or manufacturer's warnings and disclaimers, and make sure the athletes or clients are aware of them.

Important warnings posted on exercise equipment in an athletic training room or gym may read, "Caution: Stop exercise if you feel pain, faint, or short of breath." Other equipment, such as football helmets, may also carry warnings or disclaimers. Football helmets generally have warning stickers placed inside them to warn players of inappropriate uses of the helmet as well as risks associated with its use. One example reads: "Do not use this helmet to butt, ram, or spear an opposing player. This is a violation of the football rules and can result in severe head, brain, or neck injuries, paralysis, or death to you and possible injury to your opponent. There is a risk these injuries may also occur as a result of accidental contact without intent to butt, ram, or spear. No helmet can prevent all such injuries."

7. Develop an Emergency Action Plan for every sport.

These plans should be practiced at *games and practices* and should include procedures for home and away events. Specific times (both day and evening) must be scheduled to practice the plans. These practice times must be recorded and all participants must sign a form stating that they participated in the exercise. Make sure everyone understands their role in the Emergency Action Plan so that they will be prepared to act when the need arises. Flexibility and adaptability should be key factors in any plan; expect the unexpected. These plans must be in writing and distributed to all plan participants; unwritten or undistributed plans are doomed to fail. Emergency Action Plans are discussed in greater detail in Chapter 9.

8. Consider *all* the sports involved in the athletic program, not just the ones that are conducted on a court or field, when developing emergency action plans.

Sports such as golf and cross-country can be difficult, but not impossible, to work into the plan because the distances covered in these activities complicates supervision of the athletes. You should also take into account the types of training involved in the various sports. For example, wrestlers are often sent out to run five miles, creating the same supervision challenges as golf or cross-country (see Figure 4-11).

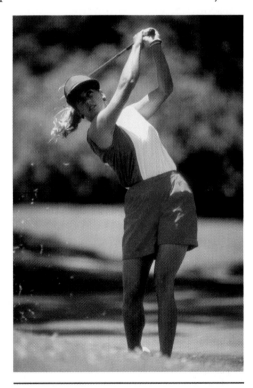

FIGURE 4-11 Distance sports, like golf and cross-country, can be difficult to supervise, but this aspect of risk management cannot be overlooked.

9. Follow appropriate procedures on all injury assessments.

Begin with the least invasive method of gathering information and progress to moving of the injury only if appropriate. Above all, avoid any actions that may increase the severity of the injury (see Chapter 9).

10. Ensure supervision of all athletes during treatment modalities, whether in the clinic or on the sidelines, and make sure those performing the treatment modalities are aware of any health problems or situations the athlete may have, such as diabetes or asthma (see Figure 4-12).

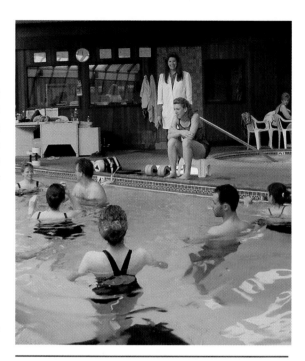

FIGURE 4-12 A physical therapist is supervising an aquatic therapy.

Preexisting health problems should be listed on the athlete's health history form. Having this information will allow preparations for emergencies by having the proper medications on hand. For example, if an athlete has asthma, make sure there is an inhaler available. When it is unknown what is wrong with an athlete, send the athlete to a physician for diagnosis. Then make sure the athlete returns with some written information from the physician. This will help with the continuity of care.

11. Make sure the coaches are up-to-date on all training techniques.

Any techniques that are found to have the potential to harm the athletes should be eliminated. Make sure the coaches are aware of the safety regulations pertaining to their specific sport. For example, in football the athletes may not lead with their helmet, in cross-country sports the athletes may not overtrain, and in basketball low bridging is prohibited. The coach is in charge of the playing strategy, so the coach must work together with the athletic trainer to ensure the safety of the athletes during training, practice, and games.

12. Conduct pre- and post-season reviews of past years and seasons, and learn from both the positive and negative events that occurred.

If a swimming coach has been coaching for 15 years and none of her swimmers have ever had any shoulder impingements, then that coach is doing something right and her training techniques should be shared with other coaches. Similarly, if the volleyball coach has the team run stairs on the first day of practice and one-third of the players suffer lower leg pain from the activity, the high rate of injury indicates that he needs to come up with a better off-season conditioning program—or a better method of making sure his athletes are following through with it.

13. Create a daily approach to safety. Make a daily checklist for key items of concern.

Walk around the fields and surrounding areas to check for any broken sprinklers that need to be fixed, glass or rocks that need to be picked up, and any gopher holes that need to be filled in before practices or games. A checklist will ensure those items will not be overlooked.

14. Create a safety committee.

A safety committee should consist of a group of individuals responsible for identifying safety measures and assuring their implementation. This group can be made up of administrators, coaches, parents, athletes, and sports medicine personnel. The diverse nature of the people on this committee will ensure a proper look from all perspectives. The athletic trainer's role is to help the committee focus on the things each team needs for safety, making sure that the committee emphasizes safety over winning. This may be difficult when the spirit of competition is high, but it can be vital to ensuring the safety of the athletes and protecting the coaching staff from lawsuits. Consider the following example:

THINKING IT THROUGH

In a New Jersey trial decision, a track athlete was recruited to play football. He had never played organized football before. He was recruited primarily because of his speed and was to be used as a receiver. Unfortunately, he was severely injured while tackling an opposing player after an interception. The athlete sued, contending that the injury was the result of insufficient training, conditioning, and supervision. Investigation showed that he had received only one practice session on tackling. Expert testimony stated that tackling can be an extremely dangerous skill and that proper technique and instruction is paramount to avoiding injury. The jury found the head coach to be 40% negligent and the line coach to be 60% negligent and awarded the plaintiff $6.5 million. The jury emphasized that the injured athlete was a senior who had trained primarily in track and did not receive adequate training and instruction in football. In addition, the jury believed that the attitude of the coaching staff indicated the emphasis was on winning and not on safety.

How could this situation have been prevented?

This is an example of the type of lawsuit individuals in sports medicine are most likely to face. The laws exist to protect the patient, client, or athlete. The laws help ensure that the proper steps are taken to prevent injuries, and that the best care possible is provided when injuries do occur.

15. Know personal limitations.

Always be aware of your scope of practice as defined by the laws of the state in which you are employed. It is also important to use good judgement in all activities; just because the law says you can do something doesn't mean you are the best person to do it. If you lack the training or education to put forth an informed opinion or perform a necessary skill, don't do it.

16. Be aware of changes in standards of care and any other changes that affect the field of work.

Work in the field of sports medicine requires ongoing education. Seminars, inservices, college classes, newsletters, Web sites, and networking with colleagues are all great ways of keep up-to-date. Never quit learning.

CHAPTER SUMMARY

Athletic trainers or sports medicine professionals are responsible for any negligent harm they may cause to another person. More importantly, a sports medicine professional may be held responsible for harm that results from a failure to resolve situations with a potential for injuries. A clear understanding of risk management and good judgement are essential to a successful career in sports medicine. Acting as a "prudent and reasonable" individual can minimize the risk of liability and improve the quality of care provided to the athletes/clients.

In addition to prudent and reasonable behavior, a well-written code of ethics, clearly defined consequences for failure to comply with ethical or safety regulations, and a supportive safety committee can go a long way in keeping athletic trainers or sports medicine professionals out of court. These components should always be documented (in writing) with nothing left to interpretation or chance. After creating a code of ethics, a list of consequences, and a safety committee, make sure that the rules and consequences are posted or distributed to all participants (and their parents/guardian in the case of minors). It is a good idea to have each participant sign a copy of these documents; these signed copies should be kept with other important legal documents such as insurance forms, waivers, and releases.

Above all, keep in mind that a positive experience for the athletes is the main objective of any athletic activity. If the athletes or clients are not enjoying themselves, something needs to change. Open and honest communication can help determine what changes need to take place. An equal blend of caution and compassion will help to effectively make those changes. The bottom line: The safety of the athlete is everyone's responsibility and should be treated as such.

STUDENT ENRICHMENT ACTIVITIES

Complete the following sentences.

1. _____ _____ _____ is the degree of care, skill, and diligence ordinarily exercised by other caregivers under the same or similar circumstances.

2. _____ determines liability.

3. The most common type of lawsuit involving athletic injuries is _____.

4. _____ _____ is the control of factors that produce risk.

5. _____ guide or influence our behavior.

6. Sports medicine is _____ medicine.

List the responsibilities that correspond to the letters in the acronym S.A.F.E.

7. S

8. A

9. F

10. E

Write T for true, or F for false. Rewrite the false statements to make them true.

11. T F Written standards for conduct, or behavior, and moral philosophy are known as a code of ethics.

12. T F Gambling on games is unsporting conduct, but is legal.

13. T F All initiation rituals are illegal.

14. T F Sports medicine professionals should have malpractice insurance.

15. T F The laws for athletic training and fitness instruction vary from state to state.

16. T F A patient's medical record is confidential.

Complete the following exercises.

17. If you were to set up a safety committee in your school, who would you ask to be involved?

18. Explain how the Patient's Bill of Rights might apply to an athlete.

19. Develop a set of ethical standards you would give to a team.

20. In small groups, form a safety committee and write down issues that your group feels are essential to risk management. Then discuss each safety committee's plan to minimize risk to the team, athletes, or clients.

21. Using the Internet, find the cost for liability insurance for a certified athletic trainer. Then describe what it covers and what it doesn't cover.

22. Evaluate two different sports and then put in writing any way the sport could minimize risk of injury.

23. Go to the NATA Web site (www.nata.org) and look at the injury breakdowns of two different sports. Comment on your findings. Discuss how the information might be used to prevent injuries.

CHAPTER 5

Physical Fitness Assessment

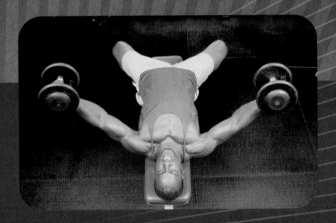

OBJECTIVES

After completing this chapter, you should be able to do the following:

1. Define and correctly spell each of the key terms.

2. Assess the capacity for extension and flexibility of the lower back and hamstrings.

3. Assess cardiovascular endurance.

4. Assess upper body, abdominal, and lower body strength.

5. Analyze the above assessments with respect to established fitness standards.

6. Measure body fat and make professional recommendations, based on those measurements, regarding weight ranges according to individual needs and goals.

KEY TERMS

* competitive fitness
* congenital
* essential body fat
* fat weight
* general fitness

* hamstrings
* lean body weight
* muscle contraction
* parallel
* range of motion

* recovery heart rate
* repetition
* resting heart rate
* trunk

FITNESS EVALUATION

As discussed in Chapter 3, when assessing a person's level of fitness, the following areas must be evaluated: muscle endurance, flexibility, cardiovascular endurance, body composition, and special considerations (e.g., physical capabilities or limitations and medical conditions). Evaluation of a client's physical fitness is very important because an individual's fitness baseline must be established before beginning an exercise program. Without this baseline measurement, it is impossible to evaluate the effectiveness of a client's exercise program.

The following pages present some basic methods of fitness evaluation that can be used to establish a baseline of fitness essential to measuring clients' progress and the effectiveness of their fitness program. Included in these evaluations is descriptive data regarding levels of fitness. In performing these evaluations, it is important to remember that although clients usually want to know how they compare to others, what really counts is how they perform and how they feel. Therefore, the tables included in this chapter offer clients a relative comparison to other members of the general public. The categories and ranges provided in these tables are solely for the clients' benefit. The measurements obtained in the evaluations are the only values significant to the athletic trainer or strength and conditioning specialist.

Although these evaluations can be used to assess anyone, the descriptive tables apply only to the general public. Thus a distinction must first be drawn between **competitive fitness** and **general fitness**. While the general public is normally evaluated according to standards of general fitness, athletes must meet the higher standards of competitive fitness; an athlete's daily tasks are typically more physically demanding than those of the general public. Therefore, measurement of performance in sport-specific activities is the goal of athletic assessment, in contrast with the less strenuous measurements used in general fitness. If a client has any specific pain or injury or if a specific test could increase the symptoms, the client should not perform that specific test. High blood pressure is another eliminator of tests unless the client's physician has approved.

---

competitive fitness

the strength, endurance, and mental well-being required to be competitive in sports activities.

general fitness

the ability to perform daily activities with vitality and energy, to withstand stress without undue fatigue, and to maintain physical health without medical intervention.

MUSCULAR ENDURANCE EVALUATIONS

Muscular endurance can be measured by how many **repetitions** are performed continuously over a period of time or by how long a **muscle contraction** can be held.

Bent-Leg Sit-Ups

Bent-leg sit-ups measure the muscular endurance of the abdominal muscles. Poor development of the abdominal muscles can contribute to lower back pain. Bent-leg sit-ups are recommended because they put less stress on the back than straight-leg sit-ups. Caution clients to not overstrain or hold their breath, but rather to breathe rhythmically, exhaling while sitting up and inhaling on the downward phase. The instructions for this test follow.

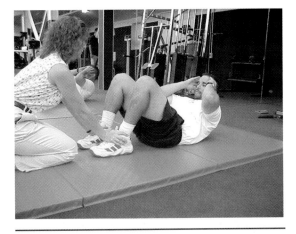

FIGURE 5-1 Start Position for the Bent-Leg Sit-Up

1. **Assume the Start Position.** The client must lie flat on the back with knees bent and the feet flat on the floor positioned approximately shoulder's width from one another (see Figure 5-1). Arms should be folded across the chest or held at the sides of the head. The chin should be tucked against the chest. Hold the client's feet flat on the floor.

2. **Begin the Sit-Up.** The client should lift the upper body away from the floor, curling toward the knees, until the elbows touch the thighs (see Figure 5-2).

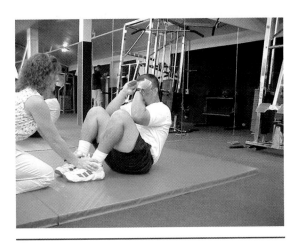

FIGURE 5-2 The client curls up until elbows touch the upper thighs.

3. **Complete the Sit-Up.** Release the curl slowly, contracting the abdominal muscles until the lower back comes in contact with the floor and the shoulders return to the start position.

4. **Repeat.** Perform steps 2 to 3 as many times as possible in 1 minute.

5. **Record the Results.** Write down the number of sit-ups performed in 1 minute. A comparison table is shown in Figure 5-3.

Bent-Leg Sit-Ups (1 Minute Timed)						
MEN	Age in Years					
	15–19	20–29	30–39	40–49	50–59	60+
Fitness Level*						
High	≥ 49	≥ 45	≥ 38	≥ 33	≥ 28	≥ 25
Med-High	42–48	37–44	31–37	26–32	22–27	19–24
Medium	38–41	34–36	27–30	23–25	18–21	15–18
Med-Low	32–37	28–33	21–26	17–22	12–17	9–14
Low	≤ 31	≤ 27	≤ 20	≤ 16	≤ 11	≤ 8
WOMEN	Age in Years					
	15–19	20–29	30–39	40–49	50–59	60+
Fitness Level*						
High	≥ 42	≥ 36	≥ 30	≥ 26	≥ 20	≥ 18
Med-High	34–41	29–35	23–29	19–25	13–19	12–17
Medium	30–33	25–28	19–22	14–18	8–12	7–11
Med-Low	24–29	19–24	13–18	8–13	4–7	3–6
Low	≤ 23	≤ 18	≤ 12	≤ 7	≤ 3	≤ 2

*Descriptive data based on compiled figures.

FIGURE 5-3 Abdominal Muscle Endurance Profile

Push-Ups

This test measures upper body endurance and allows the athletic trainer or SCS to evaluate muscular endurance in the arms, chest, and **trunk**. Because push-ups require a fair amount of upper body strength, this test is usually reserved for men, and modified push-ups are used to test women. This is not a generalization of women's capacity for strength, but a reflection of the fact that women often do not build their upper body mass as much as men do, and may not be as strong in that area. The push-ups should be smooth and without jerky movements. Caution clients to not overstrain or hold their breath, but rather to breathe rhythmically, exhaling on the upward phase and inhaling on the downward phase.

> **trunk**
>
> the torso; the area of the body on either side of and including, the spine, but excluding the arms and legs.

1. **Assume the Start Position.** The client should lie face down on the floor with the hands placed directly underneath the shoulders (see Figure 5-4). The legs should be straight and together with toes pointed toward the floor.

2. **Begin the Push-Up.** Keeping the upper body alignment as straight as possible,

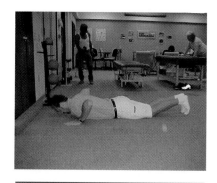

FIGURE 5-4 Start Position for the Push-Up

the client pushes the upper body off of the floor, until the arms are fully extended (see Figure 5-5).

3. **Complete the Push-Up.** The client lowers the body in a controlled motion until the chest is at a distance of one fist's width above the floor. The chest should not touch the floor (see Figure 5-6).

4. **Repeat.** Perform as many push-ups as possible. The client may rest in the up position if desired.

5. **Record the Results.** Write down the number of push-ups completed.

Modified Push-Ups

Because women do not typically develop their upper bodies as much as men do, they may have less strength in this area than men. Because of this potential difference, women and men with low upper body muscle mass may be tested using modified push-ups. This modified push-up requires less upper body strength to perform because less of the body is being lifted.

1. **Assume the Start Position.** The client should lie face down on the floor with the hands placed directly underneath the shoulders (see Figure 5-7). The legs should be together and bent at the knees. The body is kept straight from the top of the head to the knees.

2. **Begin the Push-Up.** Keeping the upper body alignment as straight as possible, the client lifts the body, pushing with palms against the floor until the arms are fully extended (see Figure 5-8).

3. **Complete the Push-Up.** Lower the body in a controlled motion until the chest is at a distance of one fist's width above the floor. The chest should not touch the floor.

4. **Repeat.** Perform as many push-ups as possible. The client may rest in the up position if he desired.

5. **Record the Results.** Write down the number of push-ups completed. A comparison table is shown in Figure 5-9.

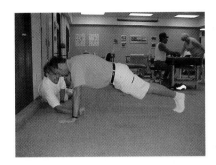

FIGURE 5-5 The client uses the arms to raise the body.

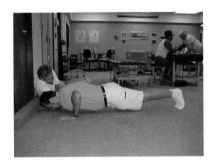

FIGURE 5-6 End Position for the Push-Up

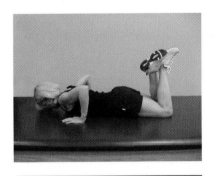

FIGURE 5-7 Start Position for the Modified Push-Up

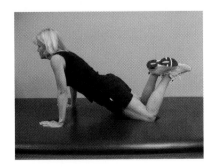

FIGURE 5-8 The client pushes the body up until the arms are fully extended.

Push-Ups (to Fatigue)

Men	Age in Years					
	15–19	20–29	30–39	40–49	50–59	60+
Fitness Level*						
High	≥ 42	≥ 38	≥ 31	≥ 25	≥ 22	≥ 20
Med-High	30–41	27–37	22–30	18–24	14–21	13–19
Medium	24–29	22–26	17–21	14–17	11–13	9–12
Med-Low	16–23	15–21	11–16	9–13	6–10	4–8
Low	≤ 15	≤ 14	≤ 10	≤ 8	≤ 5	≤ 3
WOMEN	Age in Years					
	15–19	20–29	30–39	40–49	50–59	60+
Fitness Level*						
High	≥ 32	≥ 29	≥ 28	≥ 24	≥ 20	≥ 18
Med-High	23–31	20–28	19–27	15–23	12–19	12–17
Medium	18–22	15–19	14–18	12–14	8–11	6–11
Med-Low	10–17	9–14	6–13	5–11	3–7	2–5
Low	≤ 9	≤ 8	≤ 5	≤ 4	≤ 2	≤ 1

*Descriptive data based on compiled figures.

FIGURE 5-9 Upper Body Muscle Endurance Profile

Bench Jump or Step

The bench jump test is used to determine the muscle endurance of the lower extremities. The test is performed by jumping from ground level to the top of the bench 16 inches high and back down again as many times as possible in a 1-minute period. If the client is unable to jump, the client may step up; however, stepping takes more time.

1. **Assume the Start Position.** The client should stand and face the bench with the arms held at the sides. The feet should be positioned at a distance that allows the client to jump or step up to the bench in one motion (see Figure 5-10).

2. **Begin the Jump/Step.** The client jumps or steps up to the bench and plants both feet on the bench. The arms may swing freely, but the hands may not be used to push against the thighs (see Figure 5-11).

3. **Complete the Jump/Step.** The client jumps or steps back into the start position, plant-

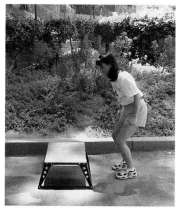

FIGURE 5-10 Start Position for Bench Jump/Step

ing both feet on the ground (see Figure 5-12). One repetition is completed each time the client both jumps (or steps) up on the bench with both feet and returns to start position. (One repetition = one jump up and one jump down.)

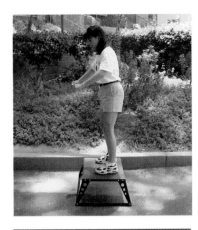

FIGURE 5-11 The client jumps to the bench, planting both feet on the bench.

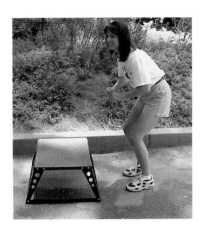

FIGURE 5-12 End Position for Bench Jump/Step

Bench Jump/Step (Repetitions in 1 Minute)			
MEN	Age in Years		
	< 30	30–50	> 50
Fitness Level*			
High	36–38	33–35	29–31
Med-High	33–35	30–32	26–28
Medium	29–32	26–29	23–25
Med-Low	26–28	23–25	21–22
Low	22–25	19–22	17–20
WOMEN	Age in Years		
	< 30	30–50	> 50
Fitness Level*			
High	26–28	24–26	21–23
Med-High	23–25	21–23	18–20
Medium	19–22	17–20	15–17
Med-Low	16–18	14–16	13–14
Low	12–15	10–13	9–12

*Descriptive data based on compiled figures.

FIGURE 5-13 Lower Body Muscle Endurance Profile

4. **Repeat.** Perform as many jumps/steps as possible in 1 minute.

5. **Record the Results.** Write down the number of bench jumps/steps completed in 1 minute. A comparison table is shown in Figure 5-13.

FLEXIBILITY EVALUATIONS

Flexibility is the ability to stretch a muscle through its full **range of motion (ROM)** without pain or muscle tearing. In general, a good rule of thumb is to measure the flexibility of the trunk, because the rest of the body usually is in similar condition. The following tests will help evaluate a client's flexibility or range of motion of the trunk.

Sit and Reach (Trunk Flexion)

The purpose of this evaluation is to measure the amount of forward trunk flexion as well as the amount of flexibility in the **hamstrings**. The client should be allowed to warm up the trunk muscles before doing the evaluation.

1. **Assume the Start Position.** A tape measure is extended on the floor. The client should remove both shoes and sit with the knees fully extended. A tape measure or yardstick is placed between the client's feet with the 15-inch mark positioned at the client's heels, and the zero mark toward the client's body (see Figure 5-14).

2. **Begin the Reach.** The client extends the arms forward with one hand on top of the other. The fingers are extended and held together.

3. **Complete the Reach.** The client reaches as far forward as possible and touches the tape measure (see Figure 5-15). Make sure the knees are straight, the head is down, and the arms extend evenly.

4. **Measure the Reach.** When the position can be maintained for 5 seconds, the measurement is taken at the point where the fingers touch the tape.

> **range of motion (ROM)**
>
> the maximum range through which a joint can move.

> **hamstrings**
>
> the muscles on the posterior aspect of the femur.

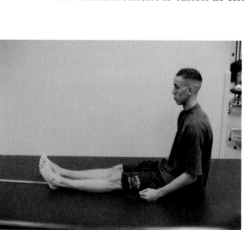

FIGURE 5-14 Start Position for Trunk Flexion Evaluation

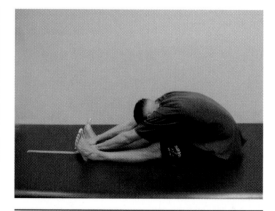

FIGURE 5-15 End Position for Trunk Flexion Evaluation

Allow the client to do this three times and record the highest measurement.

5. **Record the Results.** Write down the distance measured in the sit and reach. A comparison table is shown in Figure 5-18.

Back Bend (Trunk Extension)

This test helps the athletic trainer evaluate the ability of the abdominal muscles and the spine to extend backward. The client should be allowed to warm up the trunk muscles before performing this evaluation. Clients with back problems should not attempt this test.

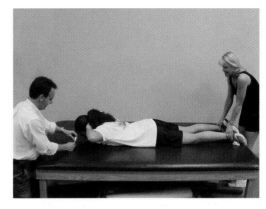

FIGURE 5-16 Start Position for Trunk Extension Evaluation

1. **Assume the Start Position.** The client lies face down on the floor or a flat surface with the fingers interlocked behind the neck, while another person holds the client's legs (see Figure 5-16).

2. **Perform the Bend.** Slowly and gently, the client raises the head and shoulders as far from the floor as possible. This position must be held for 5 seconds.

3. **Measure the Back Bend.** The bend is the distance measured between the floor and the client's chin (see Figure 5-17).

4. **Record the Results.** Write down the distance measured in the trunk extension in inches. A comparison table is shown in Figure 5-19.

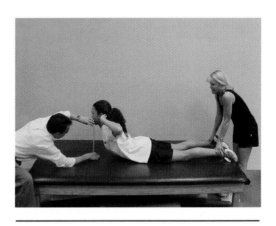

FIGURE 5-17 The Trunk Extension

resting heart rate

the number of times the heart beats in 1 minute when no physical activity is taking place.

recovery heart rate

the number of times the heart beats in 1 minute 60 seconds after completion of 3 or more minutes of exercise.

EVALUATING CARDIOVASCULAR ENDURANCE

Optimum muscular activity is possible only when the heart, blood vessels, and lungs are functioning effectively. The following test involves vigorous physical activity, which increases the demands on the heart and lungs. This exercise will enable the sports medicine professional to evaluate a client's cardiovascular endurance by measuring the **resting heart rate** and **recovery heart rate**.

Sit and Reach (in inches)

MEN	18–25	26–35	36–45	46–55	56–65	65+
Fitness Level						
Excellent	≥ 22	≥ 21	≥ 21	≥ 19	≥ 17	≥ 17
Good	20–21	19–20	18–20	16–18	15–16	14–16
Above Average	18–19	17–18	16–17	14–15	13–14	12–13
Average	16–17	15–16	14–15	12–13	11–12	10–11
Below Average	14–15	13–14	12–13	10–11	8–10	8–9
Poor	12–13	11–12	9–11	8–9	6–7	6–7
Very Poor	≤ 11	≤ 10	≤ 8	≤ 7	≤ 5	≤ 5

WOMEN	18–25	26–35	36–45	46–55	56–65	65+
Fitness Level						
Excellent	≥ 24	≥ 23	≥ 22	≥ 21	≥ 20	≥ 20
Good	22–23	21–22	20–21	19–20	18–19	18–19
Above Average	20–21	20	18–19	17–18	16–17	17
Average	19	18–19	17	16	15	15–16
Below Average	17–18	16–17	15–16	14–15	13–14	13–14
Poor	15–16	14–15	13–14	12–13	10–12	10–12
Very Poor	≤ 14	≤ 13	≤ 12	≤ 11	≤ 9	≤9

Adapted from YMCA Fitness Specialist Training Workbook, Third Edition (2000). Printed with permission of the YMCA of the USA.

FIGURE 5-18 Flexibility Profile (Sit and Reach)

Back Bend (in inches)

Fitness Level*	Men	Women
Excellent	≥ 23	≥ 26
Good	21–22	23–25
Above Average	19–20	21–22
Average	17–18	18–20
Below Average	15–16	16–17
Poor	13–14	14–15
Very Poor	≤ 12	≤ 13

*Descriptive data based on compiled figures.

FIGURE 5-19 Flexibility Profile (Back Bend)

Measuring the Heart Rate

In a fitness setting, the heart rate, or pulse, is determined by counting the number of heartbeats per minute. To get an accurate measurement of the heart rate, check the pulse for 30 seconds and multiply the number of beats by 2. This will determine the number of beats per minute (for example, $32 \times 2 = 64$ bpm). During exercise it may be easier to check the pulse for 10 seconds, and multiply this number by 6 (for example, $12 \times 6 = 72$ bpm).

There are two common places on the body used for checking the pulse. One is at the radial artery on the wrist, which can be done by placing a finger or fingers on the thumb side (inside) of the wrist. The second way is to check the carotid artery in the front of either side of the neck. (Never check both carotid arteries at the same time. The client will lose consciousness due to the restricted blood flow to the brain). Make sure to press firmly enough to feel the pulse, but not so hard that it interferes with the rhythm of the pulse. An evaluator should never use the thumb to check the pulse because the thumb has a pulse beat also. Use of the thumb to determine the heart rate may accidentally result in counting both pulses together, getting an inaccurate reading of the client's heart rate.

Determining the Resting Heart Rate

The resting heart rate provides a baseline with which to compare the client's physical fitness level. The client's resting heart rate should be taken while the client is sitting quietly, and never during or immediately after an activity. It should be taken several times to make sure that the measured numbers are accurate. The best time to have a client take a resting heart rate is in the morning after awakening. Have the client take a resting heart rate measurement for three days in a row; the average of those three numbers will give a reliable measurement. The resting heart rate for most adults should be 60 to 100 beats per minute (bpm). For conditioned athletes the rate should be closer to 40 to 60 bpm. If a resting heart rate is over 100 bpm, the individual is considered to be in poor condition.

The Pulse Recovery Step Test

This pulse recovery step test, also called the Kasch pulse recovery test or the 3-minute step test, measures a person's recovery heart rate following 3 minutes of exercise. To perform this test, first take and record the client's resting heart rate. Using a 12-inch-high step, have the client face the step with both feet flat on the ground. The exercise consists of stepping up onto the platform with both feet, one foot at a time, then stepping down with one foot at a time. The individual will need to perform the step exercise at a rate of 24 repetitions per minute for 3 minutes. A repetition is counted each time the full step is completed; a full step consists of stepping up with both feet and returning to start position. A metronome or pace beeping device set at 96 counts per minute can be helpful in maintaining a consistent pace.

Wait 60 seconds after completion of the 3-minute exercise, then take the client's pulse. Enter the result in beats per minute (bpm). A comparison table is shown in Figure 5-20.

Pulse Recovery Step Test

MEN	Age in Years					
	18–25	26–35	36–45	46–55	56–65	65+
Fitness Level						
Excellent	≤ 76	≤ 76	≤ 76	≤ 82	≤ 77	≤ 81
Good	84–77	85–77	88–77	93–83	94–78	92–82
Above Average	93–85	94–86	98–89	101–94	100–95	102–93
Average	100–94	102–95	105–99	111–102	109–101	110–103
Below Average	107–101	110–103	113–106	119–112	117–110	118–111
Poor	119–108	121–111	124–114	126–120	128–118	126–119
Very Poor	157–120	161–122	163–125	159–127	154–129	151–127

WOMEN	Age in Years					
	18–25	26–35	36–45	46–55	56–65	65+
Fitness Level						
Excellent	≤ 81	≤ 80	≤ 84	≤ 91	≤ 92	≤ 92
Good	93–82	92–81	96–85	101–92	103–93	101–93
Above Average	102–94	101–93	104–97	110–102	111–104	111–102
Average	110–103	110–102	112–105	118–111	118–112	121–112
Below Average	120–111	119–111	120–113	124–119	127–119	126–122
Poor	131–121	129–120	132–121	132–125	135–128	133–127
Very Poor	169–132	171–130	169–133	171–133	174–136	155–134

Adapted from *YMCA Fitness Specialist Training Workbook, Third Edition* (2000). Printed with permission of the YMCA of the USA.

FIGURE 5-20 Cardiovascular Profile

NOTE:

If the client cannot complete this test, enter the length of time the client was able to continue the test. Use this time as a baseline from which to measure progress as the client's endurance increases.

BODY COMPOSITION

lean body weight

the weight of a body after the fat weight has been subtracted.

To determine a person's **lean body weight**, first measure the amount of body fat (in terms of percent) at selected points on the body, using a skinfold caliper (a plier-like instrument used to measure thickness). To maintain accuracy and consistency in measurements and site selection, measurements should always be taken by the same person using the same caliper and measurement site. There are many different types of calipers, so the directions for use will vary. However, the basic procedure shown on pages 92 to 93 will apply to most calipers.

Once the percent of body fat has been determined, the amount of **fat weight** can be calculated:

Body Weight × % Body Fat = Fat Weight

The lean body weight is then determined using the following formula:

Body Weight − Fat Weight = Lean Body Weight (LBW)

For example, let's say that a 35-year-old man who is interested in fitness decides to have his lean body weight measured. He weighs 195 pounds. Using the caliper, the fitness trainer determines that the client has 15% body fat. The client's body fat weight is then calculated by multiplying the total body weight by the percentage of body fat, 0.15 (15%).

195 × 0.15 = 29.25 lbs

We see then, that this man has a body fat weight of 29 pounds (rounded off), which is then subtracted from his total body weight:

195 − 29 = 166 lbs

Thus, he has 166 pounds of lean body weight, and his body fat percentage of 15% falls well within the recommended range for males in his age bracket.

Recommended Ranges of Body Fat

Determining the correct or ideal percent body fat is difficult. The ideal percent body fat varies from person to person, depending on age, gender, heredity, and lifestyle. The important thing to remember is that a person's ideal percent body fat is the amount of fat at which that person performs and feels best. For athletes, the amount of body fat desired depends on the sport being played. However, the general guidelines in Figure 5-21 can be applied to most people in the general public.

It is important to realize that less body fat is not always better. A certain amount of body fat is necessary for proper protection of the internal organs. This minimum amount of body fat necessary for protection is known as **essential body fat**. Body fat requirements are different for males than for females. In males, the essential body fat is 3%. This means that no male, regardless of the sport he is in, should allow his body fat mass to fall below 3% of his total body mass. For females, the essential body fat is 12%.

Body Composition and Athletes

Now, what if the man used in the example for calculating lean body weight is also an athlete? The target body composition

Recommended Body Fat Percentage		
Age	Men	Women
<30	9–15%	14–21%
30–50	11–17%	15–23%
>50	12–19%	16–25%

Source: *How to Measure Your % Bodyfat: An Instruction Manual for Measuring % Body Fat Using Skinfold Calipers;* by Wallace C. Donoghue; Creative Health Products; copyright 1976, 1993. Used with permission.

FIGURE 5-21 Recommended Body Fat Percentage

---

fat weight

the weight of a body after the lean body weight has been subtracted; the weight of the adipose tissue of the body.

essential body fat

the minimum amount of body fat necessary for the proper protection of internal organs.

MEASURING BODY FAT USING A SKINFOLD CALIPER

Materials Needed:
* a skinfold caliper

parallel

extending in the same direction and remaining separated by the same distance along the entire length, never crossing paths.

1. **Procedural Step:** Take all skinfold measurements from the right side of the body. Plan to use the following four anatomical landmarks from which to take your measurements: the triceps, the biceps, the subscapula, and the supra-iliac.

   Reason: To maintain consistency in the measurements.

2. **Procedural Step:** The person should be standing, with arms resting comfortably at the sides.

   Reason: Flexion of the muscles can interfere with the results.

3. **Procedural Step:** Starting with your first anatomical landmark, use your thumb and index finger to pinch a fold of skin, including the underlying layer of subcutaneous fat, and gently pull it away from the muscle. Repeat this process for each of the landmarks described in the first procedural step above.

   Reason: Lifting the skin away from the muscle mass ensures accuracy of fat measurement.

4. **Procedural Step:** Position the caliper about 1 centimeter below the fingers that are creating the skinfold. Advance the caliper to a depth that is equivalent to the thickness of the fold.

   Reason: The caliper should be positioned below the skinfold to avoid measuring muscle. The appropriate depth is important to obtaining an accurate measurement.

The Triceps: Halfway between the shoulder and the tip of the elbow, on the posterior surface of the upper arm, the fold is pinched in a vertical direction, **parallel** to the humerus.

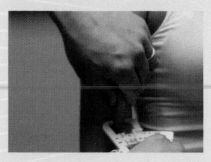

The Biceps: Pinch a vertical fold, parallel to the humerus, at a point halfway between the bend of the elbow and the top of the shoulder on the anterior surface of the arm.

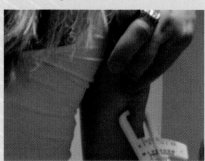

The Subscapula: Below the shoulder blade on the posterior side of the torso, pinch a fold at a 45° angle to the spine.

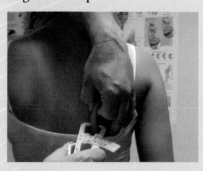

MEASURING BODY FAT USING A SKINFOLD CALIPER

The Supra-iliac: Pinch an approximately horizontal fold just above the iliac crest, the protrusion of the hip bone, on the anterior surface of the torso.

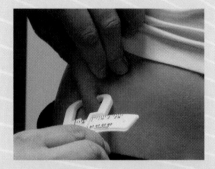

5. Procedural Step: Keep a firm hold on the fold with the fingers.

Reason: The calipers should only be measuring the thickness of the fold and not any of the forces required to keep the skin folded.

6. Procedural Step: Wait a few seconds for the calipers to "creep" a little.

Reason: The calipers may "creep" to a lower reading than when they are first applied. After a few seconds the creep will slow down markedly.

7. Procedural Step: Read the measurement on the caliper in millimeters.

Reason: Calipers are calibrated in millimeters.

8. Procedural Step: Repeat steps 3 through 7 for the remaining three skinfold sites, observing the recommended position of skinfolds for each site.

Reason: To obtain readings from several places on the body.

9. Procedural Step: Add the results the four measurements together.

Reason: The percent body fat can be determined from the total.

10. Procedural Step: Using the table in Figure 5-22, determine the percentage of body fat.

Reason: This will establish a body fat baseline from which you and the client can measure the effectiveness of the fitness program.

ranges are often different for athletes than for nonathletes. Whereas target ranges for nonathletes are often based on age, the ranges for athletes vary by gender, sport, level of competition, and sometimes, by the position played. The American College of Sports Medicine uses classifications to describe the body fat composition typical of athletes in various sports. For example, athletes who play hockey, women's basketball, tennis, volleyball, women's softball, and certain football positions typically fall in the "average" body fat range. According to ACSM classifications, *average* body fat for male athletes is 14 to 17%, whereas *average* body fat for female athletes is 21 to 25%. But, as mentioned earlier, the recommendations can vary by position played as well. Depending on the level of competition, football players may be told to strive for 14 to 22% body fat. Within that group, however, quarterbacks may be asked to maintain 14% body fat for optimal performance, while defensive linemen may perform better with 18% body fat.

It is important for athletes to make sure that their body fat does not fall below the low end of the range recommended for their sport. Body fat percentages that are too low will not provide adequate energy resources for high performance activities. This lack of resources can adversely affect both performance and health.

Skinfold Measurements and Percent of Body Fat

Skinfold (mm)	Male (age in years)				Female (age in years)			
	16–29	30–39	40–49	50+	16–29	30–39	40–49	50+
14	—	—	—	—	9.4	12.7	15.6	17.0
16	6.7	9.3	9.5	9.7	11.2	14.3	17.2	18.6
18	7.9	10.6	10.9	11.0	12.7	15.7	18.5	20.1
20	8.1	12.0	12.2	12.5	14.1	17.0	19.8	21.4
22	9.2	13.0	13.5	13.9	15.4	18.1	20.9	22.6
24	10.2	13.9	14.6	15.1	16.5	19.2	22.0	23.7
26	11.2	14.7	15.7	16.3	17.6	20.1	22.9	24.8
28	12.1	15.5	16.7	17.4	18.6	21.1	23.8	25.7
30	12.9	16.2	17.6	18.5	19.5	21.9	24.6	26.5
35	14.7	17.8	19.7	20.8	21.6	23.8	27.2	28.6
40	16.3	19.2	21.5	22.8	23.4	25.5	28.1	30.3
45	17.7	20.4	23.1	24.7	25.0	27.0	29.6	31.9
50	19.0	21.5	24.5	26.3	26.5	28.3	30.9	33.2
55	20.2	22.5	25.9	27.8	27.8	29.5	32.1	34.6
60	21.2	23.5	27.1	29.1	29.1	30.8	33.2	35.7
65	22.2	24.3	28.2	30.4	30.2	31.8	34.2	36.7
70	23.2	25.1	29.3	31.5	31.2	32.6	35.1	37.7
75	24.0	25.9	30.2	32.6	32.2	33.5	35.7	38.6
80	24.8	26.6	31.2	33.7	33.1	34.3	36.5	39.5
85	25.6	27.6	32.1	34.6	34.0	35.2	38.4	40.4
90	26.3	28.3	32.9	35.5	34.8	36.0	39.1	41.1
95	27.0	29.0	33.8	36.5	35.6	36.7	39.9	41.9
100	27.6	29.7	34.5	37.3	36.3	38.4	40.6	42.6
110	28.8	30.2	35.8	38.8	37.7	38.7	41.8	43.9
120	29.9	32.0	37.1	40.2	39.0	39.9	43.0	45.1
130	31.0	33.0	38.2	41.5	40.2	41.1	44.1	46.2
140	31.9	34.0	39.4	42.6	41.3	42.1	45.1	47.3
150	32.8	34.8	40.4	43.9	42.3	43.1	46.0	48.2
160	33.5	35.7	41.4	45.0	43.2	44.0	46.9	49.1
170	34.4	36.5	42.3	46.0	44.6	45.1	47.8	50.0
180	35.2	37.2	43.1	47.0	45.0	45.6	48.5	50.8
190	35.9	37.9	43.9	47.8	45.8	46.4	49.3	51.6
200	36.5	38.8	44.7	48.8	46.6	47.1	50.0	52.3

Source: *How to Measure Your % Bodyfat: An Instruction Manual for Measuring % Body Fat Using Skinfold Calipers* by Wallace C. Donoghue. Copyright Creative Health Products 1976, 1993. Used with permission.

FIGURE 5-22 Skinfold Measurements and Percent of Body Fat

Determining Muscle Gain or Loss

Measuring the amount of muscle gain or loss is one of the most important uses of the body fat measurements. Determining the amount of muscle gain or loss is very simple. Since muscle tissue is a part of the lean body weight that can change, the changes in lean body mass are going to be mainly caused by changes in the amount of muscle tissue. Find the weight of the lean body mass by measuring the percent body fat and total body weight. The person must be weighed and the body fat percentage calculated to find the ratio of current fat weight and lean body mass. After a period of exercise or diet programs the measurements are retaken. The amount of muscle gain or loss will be represented in the change of lean body mass.

For example, a woman weighs 145 pounds and has 27% body fat. Multiplying her total body weight by her percentage of body fat tells us that she has 39 pounds of body fat. Her lean body mass can then be calculated by subtracting 39 from her body weight of 145 to find that her lean body mass is 106 pounds. After the woman goes on a low-calorie diet for a month she discovers that she has lost 18 pounds, bringing her body weight down to 127 pounds. After measuring her with the calipers it is determined that her body fat is now 25%. Multiplying her new body weight by her body fat percentage tells us she now has 32 pounds of body fat. Subtracting this number from her total body weight gives her a lean body mass of 95 pounds. The results show that she has lost 11 pounds of lean body mass and 7 pounds of fat weight. She has lost roughly the same amounts of muscle tissue and fat. Results such as these reveal that her diet program is not a good one.

Before	After
Body weight = 145 lbs	Body weight = 127 lbs
Body fat = 27%	Body fat = 25%
145 × .27 = 39 lbs fat	127 × .25 = 32 lbs fat
145 − 39 = 106 lbs lean body mass	127 − 32 = 95 lbs lean body mass

Changes: 106 − 95 = 11 lbs lean body mass lost

39 − 32 = 7 lbs of fat tissue lost

In another example a man weighs 220 pounds. After measurements are taken, he finds that his body fat is 35%. Multiplying 220 pounds × 35% gives the man a total of 77 pounds of body fat. Subtracting 77 from 220 shows that this man has a lean body weight of 143 pounds. After a month of regular exercise and proper diet, the man's weight has dropped to 205 pounds and his body fat has dropped to 28%. Multiplying 205 pounds × 28% reveals that the man has 57 pounds of body fat. Subtracting his new body fat weight of 57 pounds from his new weight of 205 pounds gives him a new lean body weight of 148 pounds. This shows that he has gained 5 pounds of muscle mass and lost 20 pounds of fat mass. These are very good results; they mean that his exercise and diet program is working very well for him.

Before	After
Body weight = 220 lbs	Body weight = 205 lbs
Body fat = 35%	Body fat = 28%
220 × .35 = 77 lbs	205 × .28 = 57 lbs
220 − 77 = 143 lbs lean body mass	205 − 57 = 148 lbs lean body mass

Changes: 143 − 148 = 5 lbs of lean body weight gained

77 − 57 = 20 lbs of fat tissue lost

RECORDING

As discussed in Chapter 3, record keeping is essential to measuring individual progress in both athletic and nonathletic settings. Figures 5-23A and 5-23B illustrate a method of combining information obtained from an initial physical fitness assessment with follow-up assessments to measure progress. Alternatively, the progress information can be recorded on a progress record (see Chapter 3) or tracked on a computer. For example, some health clubs have magnetic cards that are swiped at each machine prior to beginning exercise. The card then tracks the number of repetitions, the weight used, etc., and data is fed to a computer where progress is calculated.

The methods described in this chapter may be used to assess a client's level of fitness at the beginning of and throughout the course of an exercise program. Progress is measured by improvement or in some cases, such as when the ultimate goal is reached, by maintenance.

SPECIAL CONSIDERATIONS

Frequently, professionals who perform fitness evaluations speak in terms of averages—average muscle endurance, average flexibility, and average cardiovascular endurance, to name a few. These averages provide a frame of reference for making individual comparisons. But the truth is, everyone is different. Every client that comes for a fitness evaluation will have a different set of circumstances affecting how the client will "measure up" on the fitness scale. For example, professional athletes have a higher standard than the average population in terms of the physical demands that are placed on their bodies, while others may have physical limitations that may effect their fitness, such as an injured knee or back.

When assessing a person's physical fitness, always consider the unique physical requirements of the person's daily activities. This involves evaluating the physical demands as determined by that person's career or lifestyle and considering what the person is physiologically capable of achieving from both short-range and long-range perspectives. Fitness potential can be influenced by a variety of factors that may be beyond a person's control or determined by profession.

Musculoskeletal Capabilities and Limitations

A different standard of fitness is applied to people with greater-than-average abilities and to those with decreased abilities. Even though physical fitness assessment focuses on objective, measurable data for strength, flexibility, and cardiovascular endurance, it is not realistic to hold everyone to the same standards of fitness. Clients will look elsewhere for guidance if there health care providers do not take this into consideration. For example, as mentioned previously, a professional athlete is likely to set a higher goal for fitness than the "average" person, because of the requirements of the profession. To stay competitive, such athletes must strive for constant improvement in the areas that are integral to this career. These areas may include aspects of fitness other than strength, flexibility, and cardiovascular endurance—such as speed and agility.

Physical Fitness Assessment Form

Name _____ Date _____

Sex M F   Birthdate ____ / ____ / _____

Address _____

City _____ State _____ Zip _____ E-mail _____

Phone (h) (_____) _____ (w) (_____) _____

Height _____   Weight _____   Target Weight _____

Medical Conditions Check all that apply

	Yes	No
1. Are you currently under a doctor's care for any reason?.............	❏	❏
2. Have you ever been hospitalized?...................................	❏	❏
3. Have you ever had surgery?...	❏	❏
4. Are you currently taking any medications or pills?.................	❏	❏
5. Do you have any allergies (medicines, bee stings, etc.)?..........	❏	❏
6. Have you ever been dizzy or fainted during or after exercise?......	❏	❏
7. Have you ever had chest pain during or after exercise?.............	❏	❏
8. Have you ever had high blood pressure?............................	❏	❏
9. Have you ever been told that you have a heart murmur?.............	❏	❏
10. Have you ever had racing of your heart or skipped heartbeats?..	❏	❏
11. Have you ever had a head injury?	❏	❏
12. Have you ever been knocked out or unconscious?	❏	❏
13. Have you ever had a seizure?	❏	❏
14. Have you ever had a stinger, burner, or pinched nerve?...........	❏	❏
15. Have you ever been dizzy or passed out in the heat?.............	❏	❏
16. Do you have trouble breathing during or after exercise?..........	❏	❏
17. Do you have any skin problems (itching, rashes, etc.)?	❏	❏
18. Have you had any problems with your eyes or vision?.............	❏	❏
19. Do you wear glasses or contacts or protective eye wear?	❏	❏

	Yes	No
20. Do you use any special equipment (splints, neck rolls, mouth guards, etc?)	❏	❏
21. Has anyone in your family died of heart problems or sudden death before age 50?................	❏	❏
22. Do you have only one working organ of usually paired organs (only one eye, kidney, etc.)?	❏	❏
23. Have you ever sprained, broken, dislocated or had repeated swelling or pain of any bones or joints?........	❏	❏
Head ❏ Neck ❏ Chest ❏ Shoulder ❏ Back ❏ Hand ❏ Wrist ❏ Elbow ❏ Forearm ❏ Hip ❏ Thigh ❏ Knee ❏ Ankle ❏ Shin/Calf ❏ Foot ❏		
24. Are any of these bothering you currently?................	❏	❏
25. Have you had any other medical problems? (asthma, mono, diabetes, etc.)	❏	❏
26. Have you had any medical problems or injuries since your last evaluation?	❏	❏
27. Any special instructions or precautions?	❏	❏
28. When was your last tetanus shot?_____		

Current medications

Additional notes

Page 1/2

FIGURE 5-23A Physical Fitness Assessment Form, Page 1

Evaluation   Score

	Week 1	Week 8	Week 20	Week 32
Musclar Endurance				
Bent-leg sit-ups (1 min)				
Push-ups (to fatigue)				
Bench jump/step (1 min)				
Flexibility				
Sit and reach (in)				
Back bend (in)				
Cardiovascular Endurance				
Recovery pulse (bpm)				
Body Composition				
Triceps (mm)				
Biceps (mm)				
Subscapula (mm)				
Supra-iliac (mm)				
Total (mm)				
Total % body fat				

FIGURE 5-23B Physical Fitness Assessment Form, Page 2

Limitations in strength, flexibility, and cardiovascular fitness can result from injuries or **congenital** conditions. Soft tissue injuries, surgeries, and illnesses often produce temporary limitations, whereas amputations, neural damage, and age may lead to permanent limitations. Consider a client who has been paralyzed from the waist down because of a traffic accident; the evaluation must be based on activities such a person is capable of performing and the areas of flexibility and endurance that can be maintained or enhanced. This person must focus on the aspects of fitness that can be maintained or improved rather than physical limitations; it is not fair or accurate to tell a paraplegic that optimal fitness cannot be achieved without the use of legs.

> **congenital**
>
> a condition present at birth.

Other Physical and Medical Conditions

Everyone starting a fitness program should have a physical exam performed by a physician to determine if they have any preexisting conditions. Clients with high blood pressure (hypertension) or low blood pressure (hypotension) require special considerations in their physical fitness assessments. Normal range for average adults is a systolic pressure of 100 to 139 mm Hg, and a diastolic pressure of 65 to 89 mm Hg (see Chapter 12). Readings outside these ranges indicate conditions that require evaluation and possible treatment by a physician. If blood pressure falls too low, there will be insufficient pressure to drive the blood through the small vessels and back to the heart. The brain needs a constant blood supply, and if blood flow is inadequate, consciousness will be lost. High blood pressure can exert extreme pressure on blood vessels, including the vascular regions of the brain. If the pressure goes too high, there is a danger of rupturing vital blood vessels, particularly those of the brain or heart. Do not even attempt to assess a client with abnormal blood pressure until the client has a physical exam and begins appropriate intervention. The physician can then recommend an appropriate level of exertion for that individual.

Pregnancy is another condition that requires special consideration. Because of the location of the fetus, pregnant women should not participate in activities such as sit-ups that put excessive strain on the abdominal muscles. Push-ups may also present problems; even if a physician clears a pregnant client for push-ups in the first trimester, the size of the client's belly may make push-ups impossible for her to complete in the second or third trimesters. Other activities may also be contraindicated for certain pregnant women. Therefore, a physician should always determine which activities are appropriate for a given pregnant woman before any testing takes place.

> **NOTE:**
>
> Since physical and medical conditions are not always easily apparent, *all* individuals should see a physician and be cleared for participation in strenuous activity before beginning a training program of any kind.

THINKING IT THROUGH

In working with Mark, a new fitness client, Bill knows he has his work cut out for him. Although Mark was an all-state basketball player in high school, that was a long time ago. He is now in his late forties, works long hours, has two kids, and wants to return to the same fitness level he was in high school in time for his class reunion.

Of course, Mark wants to get it all done in a week. But Bill has had clients like this before and knows that before they even begin to discuss time frames, he must do a physical fitness assessment. Once this is done, he can develop a plan that will help Mark meet his goal, but in a time frame that will be unlikely to cause injury.

What should Bill do first, even before testing Mark's fitness level? What are some tests Bill can use to assess Mark's level of fitness? How would Bill determine how much weight Mark needs to lose?

CHAPTER SUMMARY

Fitness industry standards and benchmarks will provide objective information on which to base a client's or an athlete's level of fitness. This information can be used to establish a baseline for the client from which to work. Without this baseline information, a fitness routine cannot be properly set up and the client's progress will be impossible to measure. The evaluation methods outlined in this chapter can be performed without expensive equipment, making it easier to establish a baseline in a wide variety of environments. A client's goal may be establishing a pre-season conditioning program, or training for a marathon, or simply toning up. In each case a baseline is useful for measuring progress. Remember that benchmarks are only used for comparisons; individual performance will vary greatly.

It is impossible to overemphasize the importance of record keeping; evaluation methods have no meaning if results are not properly recorded. Depending on the client's goals and the focus of the exercise program, the sports medicine professional or athletic trainer will find the forms in this chapter and Chapter 2 particularly useful. Client records not only help sports medicine professionals create effective exercise programs, they also help to keep the client and others informed of progress.

Remember that the tables and calculations in this chapter are general guidelines that may need to be modified to best serve the needs of individual clients. This is a particularly important consideration when working with clients who have very specific personal goals, preexisting medical conditions, and/or physical limitations. There is an extensive range of personal goals depending on gender, profession, and existing baseline—never attempt to apply the standards used for athletes to client's who are just trying to relax. Regardless of goals and baselines, *everyone* can benefit from consulting with a physician before beginning an exercise program.

STUDENT ENRICHMENT ACTIVITIES

Write T for true, or F for false. Rewrite the false statements to make them true.

1. T   F   In general, women should have a higher percentage of body fat than men.

2. T   F   Men and women should have the same amount of body fat.

3. T   F   The best time to take a resting heart rate is just before going to bed.

4. T   F   Endurance expectations can vary significantly according to age and gender.

5. T   F   When evaluating upper body strength for men with underdeveloped upper body mass, the modified push-up should be used.

Name the five areas of fitness that must be evaluated to establish a fitness level.

6.

7.

8.

9.

10.

Weigh four individuals and measure their body fat. Then use this information and their ages to record these baseline measurements.

11. Gender: M   F   Age _____   Total Body Weight _____

   % Body Fat _____   Fat Weight _____   LBW _____

   Acceptable range?   yes   no

12. Gender: M   F   Age _____   Total Body Weight _____

   % Body Fat _____   Fat Weight _____   LBW _____

   Acceptable range?   yes   no

13. Gender: M   F   Age _____   Total Body Weight _____

   % Body Fat _____   Fat Weight _____   LBW _____

   Acceptable range?   yes   no

14. Gender: M   F   Age _____   Total Body Weight _____

   % Body Fat _____   Fat Weight _____   LBW _____

   Acceptable range?   yes   no

List and describe the four anatomical landmarks where body fat is measured using skinfold calipers.

15.

16.

17.

18.

Complete the following exercises.

19. The football coach has asked you to supervise some physical evaluations in the gym while he teaches a class on strategy. You will assess the offensive team first. Without referring to the text, summarize on paper two of the following: Sit and Reach, Trunk Extension, Bent-Leg Sit-Ups, Push-Ups, and the Bench Jump.

    Explain how these physical evaluations will help this team.

20. Evaluate your own fitness level.

    Sit-ups _____   Push-ups _____

    Bench jump _____   Sit and reach _____

    Back extension _____   % body fat _____

    Lean body mass _____   Goal _____

21. Have five classmates fill out a copy of the Physical Assessment Form (Figure 5-23A), and then evaluate them on the items listed on Figure 5-23B.

22. Look in a business telephone directory to see where one might go to get a fitness evaluation. List three possibilities.

CHAPTER 6

Nutrition and Weight Management

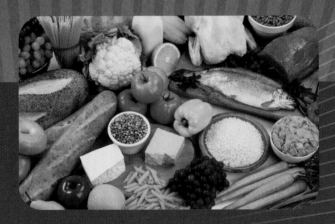

OBJECTIVES

After completing this chapter, you should be able to do the following:

1. Define and correctly spell each of the key terms.

2. Explain energy balance—how calories relate to weight maintenance, weight loss, and weight gain.

3. Define the six classes of nutrients, and explain their importance.

4. Identify the food groups, and list several food sources in each group.

5. Identify the leader nutrients that are supplied by each food group.

6. List five different physical activities, and discuss how they affect caloric expenditures.

KEY TERMS

* calorie
* carbohydrate
* dehydration
* dietary fiber
* Dietary Guidelines for Americans
* Dietary Reference Intakes (DRIs)
* energy expenditure
* energy intake
* fat
* Food Guide Pyramid
* metabolism
* minerals
* nutrients
* placebo effect
* protein
* vitamins
* water

THE HEALTHY DIET

When working with athletes and others needing guidance in achieving fitness, it is important to understand the essentials of nutrition and weight control. Proper diet planning and good weight management skills help athletes and others to set body weight goals and to achieve those goals successfully.

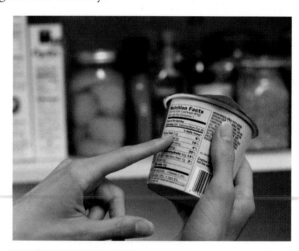

FIGURE 6-1 Reading food labels can help your clients plan a proper diet.

metabolism

the sum of all physical and chemical processes that take place in the body; the conversion of food into energy.

nutrients

substances that provide nourishment.

To create a healthy diet plan for clients and to help them properly manage their weight, one must understand how the human body uses food (see Figure 6-1). Food satisfies three basic needs: it supplies energy, it supports new tissue growth and tissue repair, and it helps to regulate **metabolism**. These three requirements are met by components of food called **nutrients**. The human body requires certain nutrients in order to achieve maximum levels of fitness, athletic performance, and/or injury and disease recovery.

There are six classes of nutrients: carbohydrates, fats, proteins, vitamins, minerals, and water. Each class has unique chemical characteristics suited to meet specific body needs. When balanced, these nutrients help promote optimum health and performance. However, an excess or deficiency of one or more may be harmful to health and may impair performance.

To create a healthy diet with the proper nutrients, two basic principles should be followed:

* Eat a variety of foods from each of the food groups daily, as well as different foods within each group. No one food or supplement provides all of the nutrients required for optimum health and athletic performance.

* Eat in moderation. Do not eat too little or too much of any one food or nutrient.

CARBOHYDRATES

Carbohydrates, such as starch and sugar (Figure 6-2), are the most readily available sources of food energy. During digestion and metabolism, all carbohydrates are broken down to the simple sugar glucose for use as the body's principal energy source. Glucose is stored in the liver and muscle tissue as a substance called glycogen, which is actually a long chain of glucose molecules. The body cannot store high amounts of glucose, so excess glucose not converted to glycogen is stored in the body as fat, where it can be used later for energy. A high-carbohydrate diet is necessary to maintain muscle glycogen, the primary fuel needed by athletes in most sports.

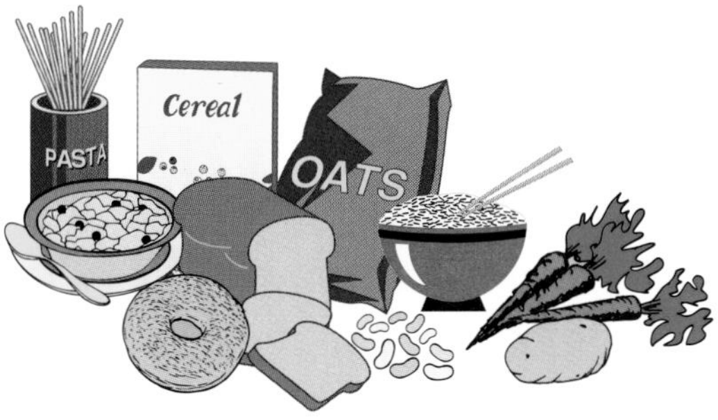

FIGURE 6-2 Carbohydrates are good sources of food energy.

> **carbohydrate**
>
> a complex sugar that is a basic source of energy for the body.

Sugar and complex carbohydrates (starch) are grouped together because they have a chemical similarity. All carbohydrates are made up of one or more simple sugars, the most common being glucose, fructose, and galactose. The simple sugar glucose, connected to the simple sugar fructose, forms sucrose, or table sugar. Starches or complex carbohydrates contain anywhere from 300 to 1,000 glucose units hooked together.

Although the body uses both sugars and starches for energy, a high-performance diet emphasizes complex carbohydrates. Foods high in complex carbohydrates such as bread, cereal, rice, beans, pasta, and vegetables also supply other nutrients such as vitamins, minerals, protein, and fiber. Sweet foods that are high in sugar (e.g., candy bars, cookies, and doughnuts) supply carbohydrates, but they also contain a high amount of fat and only insignificant amounts of vitamins and minerals.

Fruit contains the sweetest of all simple sugars—fructose. Since fruit is mostly water, its sugar and **calorie** content are relatively low. Like starchy foods, most fruits are rich in nutrients and are virtually fat free.

> **calorie**
>
> a unit of heat.

Athletes and Carbohydrates

For athletes and others in sports and/or fitness training, the glycogen contained in carbohydrates helps them maintain stamina and high energy during performance peaks or long-endurance aerobic events, such as the high activity periods that occur in competitive sports.

The idea is to have the athlete do "modified carbo consumption" prior to extended, strenuous activity periods to maximize glycogen storage. The American Dietetic Association (ADA) recommends that athletes should eat at least 800 milligrams of carbohydrates daily for three days before the anticipated high-energy-use sport activity. For example, the athlete, who needs to consume more carbohydrate calories than the body can use at that time, might do so by consuming large amounts of whole grain bread and pasta foods in those three days before a competitive running event. In this manner, when the active muscle tissue needs the converted sugar contained in the glycogen during the highly strenuous event the next day, that nutrient will be available.

Also, commercial carbohydrate products, such as liquid supplements, can be consumed during peak performance periods. An athlete choosing this method of carbohydrate intake should consume approximately 8 ounces of 5% carbohydrate liquid every 15 minutes during the peak activity time. Many of these products are on the market, and often the coach or athletic trainer selects those supplements based upon the choices most preferred by their athletes.

It may seem odd that athletes who consume larger portions of carbohydrates do not tend to gain weight, as happens in the general population. This is because the extra calories from carbohydrates are converted to energy, which is then expended during the next day's activity rather than stored as fat. From this process a "weight-energy balance" is achieved.

PROTEIN

protein

any of a class of complex, nitrogenous, organic compounds that function as the primary building blocks of the body.

Protein is a major structural component of all body tissue and is required for tissue growth and repair. Proteins are also necessary components of hormones, enzymes, and blood-plasma transport systems (see Figure 6-3). Protein is not a significant source of energy; however, the body will use protein for energy when a person doesn't eat enough calories or carbohydrates (during starvation or during a low-carbohydrate diet).

The proteins found in both plant and animal sources are composed of the same basic units, called amino acids. Of the 20 amino acids that have been identified, there are nine essential amino acids that the body cannot produce on its own and therefore must be provided in any diet. Meat, fish, and poultry contain all nine essential amino acids and are called complete proteins. Vegetable sources such as beans and grains, although valuable sources of proteins, do not supply the body with all the essential amino acids. For this reason they are called incomplete proteins.

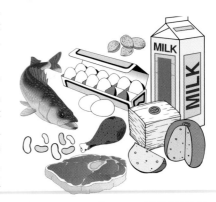

FIGURE 6-3 Protein is the primary building block of the body, but it provides little energy.

The body can make complete proteins if a variety of plant foods (such as beans, grains, vegetables, nuts, and seeds) and sufficient calories are eaten during the day. Because the body utilizes amino acids from foods eaten at different meals, vegetarians don't need to combine specific foods within a meal to achieve complete proteins. Well-balanced vegetarian diets can help decrease the risk of heart disease and cancer because they are lower in fat and higher in complex carbohydrates than the average American diet containing meat products.

In the construction of a proper diet, fat content is a significant factor to consider. When making food choices regarding proteins and other nutrients, it is important to understand that some foods contain a larger amount of fats than other similar foods. For instance, whole or 4% milk has a much higher fat content

High-Protein Foods and Fat Content

Food	Portion	Fat (grams)
Whole milk	8 oz.	8.0
Skim milk	8 oz.	0
Sour cream	3 tbsp.	7.5
Low-fat yogurt	1 cup	3
Cheddar cheese	1 1/2 oz.	13.5
Cottage cheese	1/2 cup	5
Tuna in oil	3 oz.	10.3
Tuna in water	3 oz.	1.1
Croissant	1 oz.	6.0
Whole wheat bread	1 slice	1.0
100% Natural cereal (Quaker)	1/4 cup	6.0
Rice Krispies (Kellogg's)	1 cup	0
Corn chips	1 oz.	10.0
Pretzels	1 oz.	1.0
Hash browns	1 cup	18.0
Baked potato (no butter or sour cream)	1 medium	Trace
Granola	1/3 cup	5.0
Grape Nuts (Post)	1/4 cup	Trace
Fried fish sticks	4 oz.	24.0
Flounder	4 oz.	1.0

FIGURE 6-4 High-Protein Foods and Fat Content

than 2% milk, and tuna in oil has more fat than tuna in water. Figure 6-4 provides examples of the difference in the fat content among similar high-protein foods.

Athletes and Protein

Although protein is essential to good health and the building of muscles, protein takes a lot longer to digest and convert into energy than carbohydrates. Also, foods high in protein often contain high amounts of fat too (e.g., cheese, ice cream, hamburgers, etc.). Therefore, athletes should consider the fat-to-nutrient ratio when choosing high-protein foods. Most importantly, they should remember their best source of quick energy comes from carbohydrates, whereas the energy from proteins, consumed days earlier, will increase stamina. This concept is discussed in greater detail in the "Pre-Exercise Meals" section toward the end of this chapter.

FAT

Fats, or lipids, are the most concentrated source of food energy. One gram of fat supplies about 9 calories, compared to the 4 calories per gram supplied by carbohydrates and protein. Calories are the units by which energy is measured; a caloric unit refers to the amount of energy taken in by food and expended with exercise. So, burning a gram of fat requires twice the amount of exercise that burning a gram of carbohydrates or protein does.

Fats are the body's only source of the essential fatty acids linoleic acid and linolenic acid, which are necessary for growth, healthy skin, and healthy hair. Fat insulates and protects the body's organs against trauma and exposure to cold. Fats are also involved in the absorption and transport of fat-soluble vitamins.

Fats are divided into two categories: saturated and unsaturated (including monounsaturated and polyunsaturated). As a general rule, saturated fat (e.g., butter and lard) is solid at room temperature and is derived mainly from animal sources. Unsaturated fat (e.g., safflower, corn, and canola oil), found mainly in plants, is liquid at room temperature.

Fats and Cholesterol

Dietitians recommend that when eating fatty foods, it's best to choose foods containing unsaturated fats because saturated fats contribute to the production of cholesterol, a white waxy substance found in the blood. When it builds up in deposits along the artery walls (a condition called atherosclerosis), cholesterol can inhibit blood flow and is a major risk factor in heart disease (see Figure 6-5).

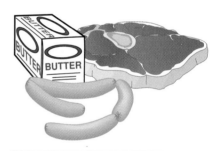

FIGURE 6-5 Consumption of saturated fats can increase the risk of heart disease.

However, some cholesterol is needed by the body for formulation of outer cell membranes and for providing "sheaths" that protect nerve fibers. Since the blood carries cholesterol to all parts of the body in the form of lipoproteins, the idea is to eat "good cholesterol," carried by high-density lipoproteins (HDLs), as opposed to eating "bad cholesterol," carried by low-density lipoproteins (LDLs). The HDLs, contained in monounsaturated fats (see Figure 6-6) found in canola oil, avocados, most nuts, and olive oil, appear to scavenge some of the cholesterol from the blood stream, and after further dissection in the liver, the bad cholesterol is disposed of in the urine. Polyunsaturated fats, found in salmon, sardines,

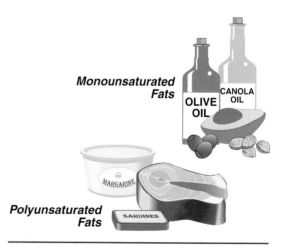

FIGURE 6-6 Unsaturated fats appear to lower the levels of cholesterol in the blood.

mackerel, and soft margarine, should be eaten in smaller quantities because though they eliminate the LDLs in the blood, they may also lower the amount of HDLs at the same time. Salmon in particular is also a good source for protein and omega-3 fatty acids.

Athletes and Fat

Some fat is stored in lean muscle tissue, which is the muscle tissue that is used in athletic activity. The majority of body fat, however, is subcutaneous fat and is "hoarded" by the body just under the skin. Because of this, athletes need to understand that severely restricting their calorie intake is not going to help them with weight control. The human body, once it realizes that the person is "fasting," will consume the lean muscle tissue in its search for energy nutrients—if no subcutaneous fat is available. So, for instance, during a high-performance activity, just when the athletic person needs that extra spurt of energy, the body will draw upon nutrients from the muscle tissue, thus diminishing the athlete's performance.

Athletes, then, need to watch their fat intake to be sure that it is adequate for their sports needs. At the same time, they need to closely watch the amount of fat they consume. For example, the American Dietetic Association advises that even for athletes, fat should contribute no more than 30% of total energy to the diet. Further, the ADA stresses that energy needs above this level should be derived from high-carbohydrate/low-fat food. So athletes, like the general population, need to monitor their fat intake carefully to avoid developing weight problems.

FIBER

Dietary fiber (roughage) is the portion of plant foods that cannot be digested. The soluble fiber found in fruit (especially apples, citrus fruits, and berries); vegetables (especially carrots); oat bran, dry beans and peas, and barley helps reduce the blood cholesterol level. The insoluble fiber found in wheat bran, whole grains (oats, rye, corn, brown rice), some vegetables (such as rhubarb), nuts, and seeds helps prevent constipation and other colon disorders. Fruits and vegetables contain both types of fiber. For optimal health it is important that patients and/or athletes include both types of fiber in their diet (see Figure 6-7). It is recommended that women try to consume 25 grams of fiber each day, and the intake for men should be 17 grams. Figure 6-8 provides the fiber content of some foods.

In certain cases, the possibility of "fiber overload" should be carefully monitored. If clients are not accustomed to eating fiber-rich foods, they

dietary fiber

material in food that resists digestion and adds bulk to the diet.

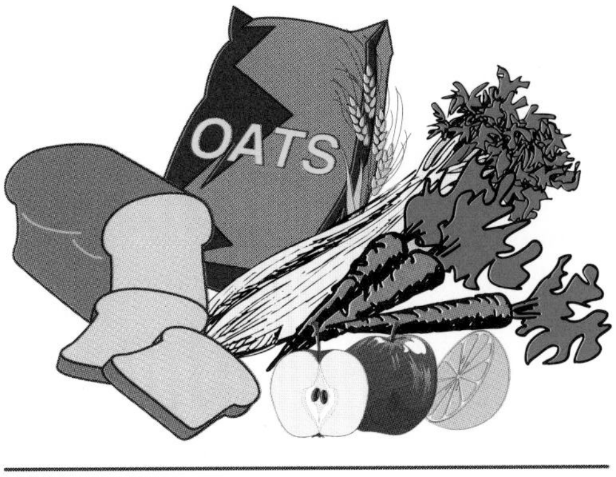

FIGURE 6-7 Dietary fiber is important in reducing levels of blood cholesterol and preventing constipation.

Fiber Content of Selected Foods

Food	Serving Size	Fiber (grams)
Apple (w/skin)	1 medium	2
Baked beans	¼ cup	3½
Baked potato (w/skin)	1 medium	2
Banana	½ medium	2
Blackberries	¾ cup	4½
Bran muffin	1 medium	3
Broccoli (cooked)	½ cup	3
Cabbage (raw)	1 cup	4
Cantaloupe	1 cup	4
Carrots (cooked)	½ cup	3
Corn (cooked)	½ cup	3
Dried prunes	3 medium	4
Green beans (cooked)	½ cup	2
Kidney beans	⅓ cup	6
Lettuce (raw)	½ cup	1
Navy or pinto beans	⅓ cup	3
Nectarine	1 medium	3
Peach (w/skin)	1 medium	3
Peas (cooked)	⅓ cup	4
Popcorn	3 cups	6
Rice (cooked)	½ cup	1
Strawberries	1¼ cup	4
Whole wheat bread	1 slice	2
White, pumpernickel, or rye bread	1 slice	1

FIGURE 6-8 Fiber Content of Selected Foods

need to increase the amount of fiber slowly to avoid abdominal distress. Also, they should drink plenty of water, which keeps the fiber moving through the intestines and helps the body to eliminate it efficiently.

Athletes and Fiber

Athletes should approach fiber intake in much the same way that nonathletes do. However, fiber should *not* be a part of the pre-exercise meal. Consumption of fiber in the hours prior to a sports activity can lead to the athlete having to interrupt the activity to have a bowel movement. Interruptions such as this are annoying during training and disastrous during competition! Therefore, it is a good idea for athletes to avoid eating fiber for approximately 6 hours prior to an event.

VITAMINS

Vitamins are organic (containing carbon) compounds that the body requires in small amounts but cannot manufacture (see Figure 6-9). These compounds are metabolic regulators that govern the processes of energy production, growth, maintenance, and repair. Thirteen essential vitamins have been identified. These vitamins are considered essential because each has a special function in the body and also works in complicated ways with other nutrients.

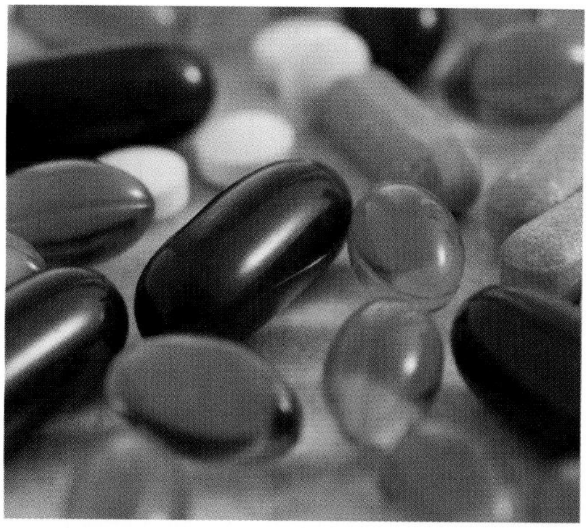

Fats, proteins, and vitamins do not provide the body with energy; however, some vitamins are involved in the release of energy from food. The daily vitamin needs of an athlete

FIGURE 6-9 The human body cannot manufacture vitamins; they must be obtained from foods or from dietary supplements.

> **vitamins**
>
> organic substances, other than proteins, carbohydrates, fats, and organic salts, that are essential in small quantities for normal body function.

are not significantly different than that of the general public. For this reason, it is unnecessary, and at times unhealthy, for an athlete to exceed the recommended levels of consumption of essential vitamins.

Vitamins are divided into two groups: water-soluble and fat-soluble. Fat-soluble vitamins include A, D, E, and K, which are stored in the fatty tissue, principally in the liver. Taking a greater amount of vitamins A and D than the body needs can produce serious toxic effects over a period of time.

Vitamin C and the B-complex vitamins are soluble in water and must be replaced on a regular basis. When more water-soluble vitamins are consumed than needed, the excess is eliminated in the urine. Although this increases the vitamin content of the urine, it does not enhance performance. As with the fat-soluble vitamins, consuming an excess amount of water-soluble vitamins, such as niacin, B_6, and C, can cause serious side effects if they are in the form of supplements. Vitamins—even the water-soluble type—that are consumed in the form of supplements tend to remain in the body longer than those that are obtained from food.

Athletes and Vitamins

According to the American Dietetic Association, athletes will not need vitamin and mineral supplements if they consume a variety of foods. However, supplements may be required if they are trying to lose weight or if they eliminate one or more food groups from their diet. However, it is common for many athletes to consume additional nutritional supplements because many believe that these extra nutrients will benefit them during high-performance activities. According to the ADA and other experts, it is scientifically proven that most athletes tend to eat nutritionally balanced, healthy diets, and as a result of their active physical lives, burn off any excess calories. Therefore, for most athletes, any vitamins more than the usual one-a-day type are not utilized by the body and are excreted in the urine.

MINERALS

minerals

inorganic compounds that are essential to body function.

Minerals are inorganic (carbonless) compounds that serve a variety of functions in the body. Some minerals, such as calcium and phosphorus, are used to build bones and teeth. Others are important components of hormones, such as the mineral iodine in thyroxin production. Iron is essential for the formation of hemoglobin, the oxygen-carrier within red blood cells. Certain minerals, called electrolytes, help regulate the contraction of muscles, the conduction of nerve impulses, and the regulation of normal heart rhythm.

Minerals are classified into two groups, based on the quantity needed by the body every day. Major minerals are needed in amounts greater than 100 milligrams (mg) per day. Calcium, phosphorus, magnesium, sodium, and chloride fall into this category. Minor minerals, or trace elements, such as iron, zinc, selenium, copper, and iodine are needed in amounts less than 100 mg per day.

Athletes and Minerals

Because an athlete eats more food than the average sedentary person eats, an athlete generally does not need to take mineral supplements. Two cautions to this guideline exist, however, which apply to all women, but should be emphasized for women athletes:

* Calcium intake should be 800 to 1,200 mg a day to help maintain bone strength and to help prevent osteoporosis.

* Iron depletion may result in reduced hemoglobin levels, leaving the athlete feeling tired. In such cases, increased iron intake can improve oxygenation throughout the body and boost energy.

WATER

water

H_2O; the odorless and tasteless fluid that is the principle chemical constituent of the human body.

Water is essential to life. **Dehydration** impairs athletic performance and increases the risk of heat-related illnesses, such as heat exhaustion and heat stroke. When at rest, people need at least 2 quarts (64 ounces) of fluid each day. An adequate supply of water is necessary for control of body temperature (particularly during vigorous exercise), energy production, and the elimination of metabolic waste products. In fact, water accounts for about 60% of the body's weight!

dehydration

the loss of water from a body or substance; to become dry.

Athletes and Water

Drinking water before and during exercise is neglected by many athletes because during vigorous activity, the "thirst mechanism" in the body is delayed. As a result, many athletes simply will not feel thirsty during their most active periods. Also, because water is readily available and has no caloric value, its significance often is overlooked. As a result, athletic trainers, fitness trainers, and others who work with athletes need to be sure to have ample water and/or sports beverages on hand. It's important to get athletes used to drinking sufficient amounts of fluid as part of their daily nutritional regime. According to the ADA, in moderate weather, athletes should consume 2 cups (8 to 16 ounces) of water 2 hours before vigorous physical activity. Then 15 minutes before exertion, they should drink another 2 cups of water.

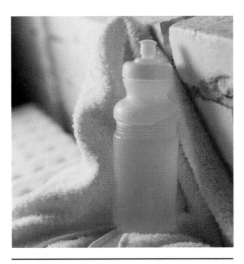

FIGURE 6-10 Water is the best fluid for replenishing lost body fluids.

Not only is it important for athletes to consume water prior to exercise, but it is equally, if not more, important for them to stay hydrated throughout physical activity (see Figure 6-10). A common and accurate method to determine proper hydration is by monitoring urine. People who consume sufficient water have pale yellow or clear urine, while dehydrated individuals tend to have dark yellow urine. If the athlete is taking vitamins, the color change may be caused by the vitamins, and this method will not work.

Because sweating can cause dehydration, an athlete must drink an appropriate amount of water during activity to keep their body properly hydrated. To do this, the athletes should begin drinking water early, and continue intake in regular intervals. Beware of many of the common symptoms of dehydration: headache, dizziness, fainting, fatigue, and vomiting.

During exercise, athletes should start drinking early and at a regular intervals in an attempt to consume fluids at a rate sufficient to replace all the water lost through sweating (i.e., body weight loss), or consume the maximum amount that can be tolerated.

DIETARY REFERENCE INTAKES

The **Dietary Reference Intakes (DRIs)** are a set of nutrient reference values used to plan and evaluate diets for good health. The goal of the DRIs is not just to protect the body against nutrient deficiency, but to also prevent diet-related diseases such as coronary heart disease, certain cancers, and osteoporosis. These standards are continuously being updated and published at www.healthymeals.nal.usda.gov. Go to this Web site for the most current information about DRI reports.

In general, consumption of different amounts of some nutrients can lead to different nutritional benefits. For instance, a given amount of a certain nutrient may reduce the possibility of deficiency, while another given amount of that same nutrient may reduce or influence the occurrence of chronic disease. At the very least, an individual should try to consume the amount of a nutrient

Dietary Reference Intakes (DRIs)

a set of nutrient reference values used to plan and evaluate diets for good health.

recommended by the Recommended Dietary Allowance (RDA) or Adequate Intake (AI). The RDA and AI are the amount of a nutrient that meets the estimated minimum nutrient needs of most people. To avoid toxicity, an individual should not exceed the Tolerable Upper Intake Level (UL) for a nutrient. Thus, it is easy to see why the subject of "nutrient adequacy" should be addressed according to an individual's needs or goals. It is for this reason that the DRIs are more extensive than the RDAs. Therefore, the DRI values require an expanded format that cannot be compressed into a simple chart or table.

For more information on the nutrient needs of a healthy body, including the results of deficiency and excessive consumption of common vitamins, minerals, trace elements, and electrolytes, see Figures 6-11, 6-12, and 6-13.

The **Dietary Guidelines for Americans** are recommendations for good health made by the U.S. Department of Agriculture and the U.S. Department of Health and Human Services. These guidelines are designed to help the American make dietary choices that meet national requirements and promote health. Current updates to Dietary Guidelines can be found at www.health.gov/dietaryguidelines and include the following recommendations:

> **Dietary Guidelines for Americans**
>
> recommendations for good health made by the U.S. Department of Agriculture and the U.S. Department of Health and Human Services.

* Eat a variety of foods. No one food can supply the body with all the essential nutrients. Therefore, an assortment of foods and drinks should contain a limited amount of saturated fats, added sugars, salts, and cholesterol. Choose a diet with adequate amounts of fiber-rich fruits, vegetables, and whole grains, while maintaining an appropriate caloric intake.

* The healthiest method of maintaining a healthy body weight is by balancing the amount of calories consumed to the amount of calories burned throughout exercise and daily actives. Slightly decreasing the amount of calories ingested and increasing exercise can prevent gradual weight gain. The prevention of weight gain is the first step in reducing the potential for obesity and risk of chronic disease associated with weight gain.

* Physical activity is vital for both weight control and good health. Regular physical activity is largely beneficial as it can improve physical and psychological health.

* Choose a diet low in saturated fats and cholesterol. Total fat consumption should provide 20 to 35% of total caloric intake.

* Chose a diet moderate in sugar and sodium. Diets high in sugar provide fewer nutrients that those high in nutrient-dense, complex carbohydrates. Also, high sodium intake can contribute to hypertension in sodium-sensitive individuals.

The Food Guide Pyramid

The **Food Guide Pyramid** serves as an educational tool to put dietary guidelines into practice. "My Pyramid Plan" can help individuals choose the foods and amounts that are right for them. This plan eliminates the one-size-fits-all plan from before. You get a quick estimate of what and how much a person needs to eat by entering age, gender, and activity level on the Web site www.MyPyramid.gov. The site supplies information on making smart choices from everyday foods, finding a

> **Food Guide Pyramid**
>
> educational tool that enables incorporating dietary guidelines into daily use.

Vitamins

Fat Soluble Vitamins	Food Sources*	Function*	Results of Deficiency*	Results of Excessive Consumption*
A	Liver; fish liver oils; carrots; eggs; whole milk products; dark green leafy vegetables; sweet potatoes.	Prevents night blindness; helps keep skin & mucous membrane linings healthy; promotes resistance to certain infectious diseases.	Frequent infections; night blindness; dry skin; retarded growth; respiratory, gastrointestinal, & genitourinary problems.	Nausea; headache; liver & spleen damage; joint pain; hair loss; dry, peeling skin.
D	Fortified milk; fish liver oils; oysters; butter; liver; egg yolk; salmon; sardines. (Also produced in the body in response to sunlight.)	Promotes strong bones & teeth; regulates calcium & phosphorus absorption.	Inadequate mineralization of bones.	Nausea; fatigue, bone pains; calcium deposits in soft tissues such as the kidney; loss of appetite; constipation.
E	Margarine; nuts; vegetable oils; green leafy vegetables; wheat germ.	Prevents oxidation of unsaturated fatty acids.	Lethargy; apathy; loss of concentration; loss of balance; anemia.	Generally nontoxic with doses up to 800 mg.
K	Spinach, broccoli & other green leafy vegetables; milk; eggs; cereals.	Assists in regulation of blood clots.	Impaired clotting; bruises; frequent nosebleeds.	Possible clot formation.
Water Soluble Vitamins				
B_1 (Thiamine)	Whole grains; dried beans; organ meats; yeast; seeds & nuts.	Assists in energy release from carbohydrates; necessary for efficient digestive & nervous systems.	Confusion; anorexia; weakness; peripheral paralysis; tachycardia; loss of coordination.	Generally nontoxic.
B_2 (Riboflavin)	Cheese; milk;, green vegetables; ice cream, enriched bread; cereals, fish; poultry & meats.	Essential for metabolism of carbohydrates, amino acids, & fats; maintains nerves & blood cells.	Mouth lesions; seborrheic-dermatitis; scrotal & vulval skin changes; anemia.	Generally nontoxic.
B_3 (Niacin)	Meat; poultry; fish; peanuts; whole grains; enriched cereals & breads.	Important in glycolysis, tissue respiration, & fat synthesis; necessary for cell reproduction & repair.	Irritability; depression; anxiety; sore mouth & tongue; gastrointestinal problems; pellagra.	Heartburn; nausea; burning, itching skin; flushing of the face.
B_6 (Pyridoxine)	Poultry; fish; kidney; liver; pork; whole grains; soy beans & peanuts.	Necessary for tryptophan metabolism; assists in use of other amino acids.	Anemia; nausea; convulsions; dermatitis around eyes & mouth.	Loss of muscular coordination & nerve sensation.
B_{12}	Animal foods, such as meat, fish, eggs, cheese, milk, & chicken.	Helps develop red blood cells & maintain nervous system.	Pernicious anemia; fatigue; sore tongue; memory loss; neurological symptoms.	Generally nontoxic.
Folate (Folic acid)	Liver; brewer's yeast; leafy vegetables; dried beans & peas; fresh oranges & whole wheat products.	Involved in synthesis of nucleic acid; prevents blood disorders; essential for growth.	Anemia; impaired cell division; alterations in protein synthesis; diarrhea; fatigue.	May interfere with anti-seizure drugs; stomach & sleep disturbances.
C (Ascorbic acid)	Citrus fruits & juices; spinach; broccoli; green & red peppers; potatoes & tomatoes.	Important to skin, tooth, & bone formation; promotes iron absorption; helps heal wounds.	Scurvy; bleeding gums; tender joints; nosebleeds; increased susceptibility to infections.	Diarrhea; possible kidney stones.

Note: Footnotes and sources appear on page 117.

FIGURE 6-11 Nutrient Needs of a Healthy Body—Vitamins

Selected Vitamins

	Food Sources*	Function*	Results of Deficiency*	Results of Excessive Consumption*
Pantothenic Acid	Liver; wheat germ; dried beans; eggs; nuts; lean meats; broccoli; milk.	Involved in proper skin growth & nerve function; maintains health of adrenal glands.	Headache; fatigue; nausea; muscle cramps; immune problems; mood changes; loss of coordination & sleep.	Generally nontoxic.
Biotin	Yeast; liver; egg yolks; nuts; soy flour; whole grains.	Assists in metabolism of fats & carbohydrates; essential for making protein & nucleic acid.	Anorexia; nausea; vomiting; pallor; hair loss; depression; inflamed tongue; dermatitis.	Generally nontoxic.

Minerals

	Food Sources*	Function*	Results of Deficiency*	Results of Excessive Consumption*
Calcium	Milk & milk products; leafy, green vegetables; salmon & sardines (with bones).	Essential to healthy bones and teeth; assists in nerve conduction & muscle contraction.	Abnormal heartbeat; muscle cramps; numbness & tingling of hands & feet; dementia.	Possible constipation or increased risk of kidney stones; possible kidney damage.
Phosphorus	Milk; fish; poultry; meat; eggs; cereal products; nuts; dried beans & peas.	Necessary for normal muscle metabolism, skeletal growth, & tooth development.	Bone loss; weakness; anorexia; malaise; bone pain.	Unknown.
Magnesium	Whole grain cereal; bananas; nuts; peas; beans; leafy green vegetables.	Important to bone structure; assists in nerve & muscle functioning; regulates heart rhythm.	Loss of appetite; nausea; diarrhea; muscle weakness; irritability; confusion.	Low blood pressure; fatigue; weakness; fluid retention; nausea; vomiting.
Iron	Red meat; fish; poultry; egg yolk; whole grain products; dark green vegetables.	Promotes formation of hemoglobin; contributes to energy release during metabolism.	Anemia; fatigue; impaired concentration; impaired immune function.	Constipation; possible increased risk of heart disease.
Zinc	Shellfish; beef; liver; lamb; pork; eggs; wheat germ; dried beans & peas.	Maintains senses of taste & smell; aids in healing.	Loss of appetite; slow healing of wounds; frequent infections; retarded growth; skin changes.	Depressed immunity; gastrointestinal distress; vomiting.
Iodine	Iodized salt; seafood; vegetable oil; seaweed.	Necessary for production of hormones that regulate growth, reproduction, & nerve & bone formation.	Fatigue; apathy; enlarged thyroid; weight gain; dry skin; intolerance to cold.	Thyroid problems; inflammation of salivary glands; elemental form can be fatal.
Selenium	Seafoods; kidney; liver; some whole grains & seeds.	Enhances immune function; helps prevent cancer & buildup of fatty deposits in arteries.	Muscular discomfort or weakness; predisposition to development of Keshan disease; heart problems.	Nausea; diarrhea; fatigue; hair loss; irritability; fingernail tenderness & loss.

Note: Footnotes and sources appear on page 117.

FIGURE 6-12 Nutrient Needs of a Healthy Body—Selected Vitamins and Minerals

Trace Elements

	Food Sources*	Function*	Results of Deficiency*	Results of Excessive Consumption*
Copper	Liver; kidney; crab; oysters; fruit; nuts; whole grain cereals.	Helps form red blood cells; acts as an antioxidant.	Anemia; skeletal defects; nerve degeneration; altered hair texture.	Unknown.
Manganese	Nuts; whole grain cereals; peas; beans & tea.	Normal bone growth; activation of enzymes used in carbohydrate & protein metabolism.	Retarded growth; poor reproductive performance; impaired glucose tolerance; bone & cartilage malformations.	"Manganese madness" (hysterical laughter; impulsiveness & sleeplessness; depression; muscle spasms & rigidity).
Fluorine (Fluoride)	Fish; tea; fluoridated water.	Increases resistance of teeth to disease; may help prevent osteoporosis.	Tooth decay; possible decreased bone growth.	Mottled tooth enamel; kidney damage; muscle & nerve damage; death.
Chromium	Liver; beef; poultry; wheat germ; thyme; broccoli; brewer's yeast.	Maintains normal glucose metabolism.	Nerve degeneration; diabetes-like symptoms; glucose intolerance.	Unknown.
Molybdenum	Milk; beans; breads & cereals.	Detoxifies sulfites; may also act as an antioxidant.	Rapid pulse; headache; rapid breathing; nausea; vomiting; night blindness.	Possible gout-like symptoms; loss of copper.

Electrolytes

	Food Sources*	Function*	Results of Deficiency*	Results of Excessive Consumption*
Sodium	Table salt & processed foods.	Regulates the body's fluid balance & acid-base balance; aids in the transmission of nerve impulses.	Loss of weight; loss of thirst; muscle cramping & weakness; nerve disorders; digestive disorders.	Edema & increased blood pressure.
Chloride	Table salt & processed foods.	Helps transport electrical charges through body; activates nerve impulses.	Constipation; inability to gain weight; electrolyte abnormalities.	Dehydration; increased blood pressure.
Potassium	Shellfish; most fruits & vegetables; beans; peanuts.	Promotes regular heartbeat; controls nerve conduction, muscle contraction; energy production.	Fatigue; weakness; abnormal heartbeat; drowsiness; muscle pain.	Muscle weakness; cold, pale skin; confusion; numbness & tingling of extremities; heart failure.

*May or may not be complete listings.

Source: Printed with permission from *Recommended Dietary Allowances: 10th Edition.* Copyright 1989 by the National Academy of Sciences. Courtesy of the National Academy Press, Washington, DC.

Additional information obtained from: *Taber's Cyclopedic Medical Dictionary, 20th Edition,* F.A. Davis Company, Philadelphia, PA, 2005; Ellen Moyer, *Vitamins and Minerals: Questions You Have . . . Answers You Need,* Wings Books, Avenel, NJ, 1993; Stanley Gershoff, PhD, *The Tufts University Guide to Total Nutrition,* Harper & Row Publishers, New York, NY, 1990.

FIGURE 6-13 Nutrient Needs of Healthy Body—Trace Elements and Electrolytes

balance between food and physical activities, and getting the most nutrition out of the calories you take in.

The USDA's MyPyramid (Figure 6-14) symbolizes a personal approach to a healthy eating and physical activity. The Pyramid has been designed to be simple and to remind consumers to make healthy food choices and to be active every day.

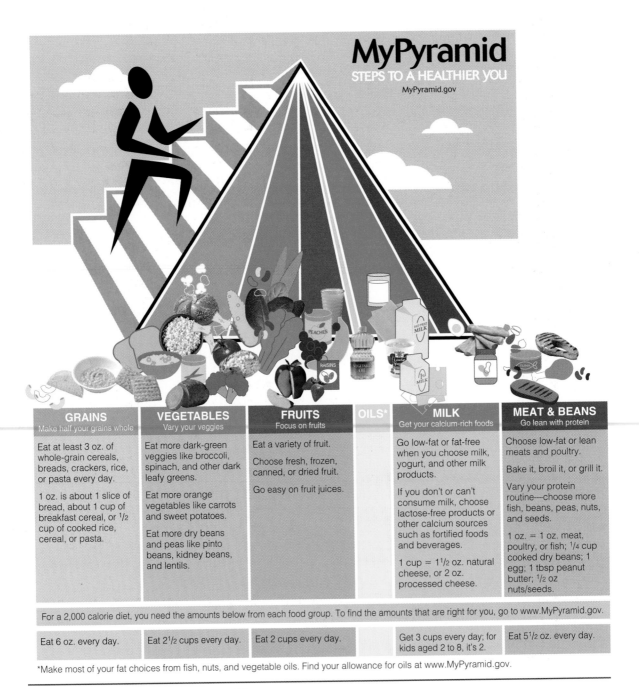

FIGURE 6-14 The Food Guide Pyramid

Notice that the various components of the Pyramid represent different aspects of a healthy lifestyle.

1. Activity is represented by the steps that will lead to the importance of daily physical activity.

2. Moderation is represented by the narrowing of each food group from the bottom to the top. The wider base stands for foods with little or no solid fats or added sugars. They are the best to select, whereas the narrower top dictates foods containing more added sugars and solid fats. The more active you are the more of these foods you can fit in your diet.

3. Personalization is shown by the person on the steps, the slogan, and the URL. Anyone can find the types and amounts of food each day at MyPyramid.gov.

4. Proportionality is shown by the different widths of the food group bands. The widths suggest how much food a person should choose from each group.

5. Variety is symbolized by the six color bands.

6. Gradual improvement is encouraged by the slogan. It suggests that individuals can benefit from taking small incremental steps to improve their diet and lifestyle each day.

The Dietary Guidelines describe a healthy diet as one that:

* Emphasizes fruits, vegetables, whole grains, and fat-free or low-fat milk and milk products

* Includes lean meat, poultry, fish, beans, eggs, and nuts

* Is low in saturated fats, trans fats, cholesterol, salt (sodium), and added sugars

The Well-Balanced Diet

The optimum diet contains adequate amounts of each of the six essential classes of nutrients. Of the 40 known nutrients, ten are considered "leader nutrients." If athletes obtain adequate amounts of these nutrients from the foods that they consume, they will probably obtain the other 30 nutrients as well.

The 10 leader nutrients are protein, carbohydrate, fat, vitamin A, vitamin C, thiamin, riboflavin, niacin, calcium, and iron. The food groups in the Food Guide Pyramid were developed based on these leader nutrients. The foods in the grain group are high in carbohydrate, thiamin, niacin, and iron. The fruit and vegetable groups contain foods high in vitamins A and C. Meat group foods are high in protein, niacin, iron, and thiamin. Foods in the milk group are good sources of calcium, riboflavin, and protein.

Since no one food or food group supplies all the nutrients needed, clients and/or athletes should choose a wide variety of foods from the groups in the pyramid. By eating a variety of foods from each food group daily, most people can obtain the nutrients needed for optimum performance.

USING NUTRITION FACT LABELS TO MAKE WISE FOOD CHOICES

To help consumers select foods that will be part of a healthy diet, the Food and Drug Administration now requires nutrition labeling for most foods (except meat and poultry).

On the label's "Nutrition Facts" panel (Figure 6-15), manufacturers are required to provide information about certain nutrients. The mandatory components include total calories, calories from fat, total fat, saturated fat, trans fat, cholesterol, sodium, total carbohydrate, dietary fiber, sugars, protein, vitamin A, vitamin C, calcium, and iron. The serving size is the basis for reporting each food's nutrient content.

The nutrients are declared as percentages of the Daily Values, which are label reference values. The amount, in grams or milligrams, of macronutrients (such as fat, cholesterol, sodium, carbohydrates, and protein) are also listed to the immediate right of these nutrients. The % Daily Values are based on a 2,000-calorie diet.

Declaring nutrients as a percentage of the Daily Values is intended to prevent misinterpretations that arise with quantitative values. For example, a food with 140 milligrams (mg) of sodium could be mistaken for a high-sodium food because 140 is a relatively large number. In actuality, however, that amount represents less than 6% of the Daily Value for sodium, which

Nutrition Facts		
Serving Size 1/2 cup (114g)		
Servings Per Container 4		
Amount Per Serving		
Calories 90	**Calories from Fat** 30	
		% Daily Value
Total Fat 3g		**5%**
Saturated Fat 0g		**0%**
Trans Fat 0g		
Cholesterol 0mg		**0%**
Sodium 300mg		**13%**
Total Carbohydrate 13g		**4%**
Dietary Fiber 3g		**12%**
Sugars 3g		
Protein 3g		
Vitamin A 80%	•	Vitamin C 60%
Calcium 4%	•	Iron 4%

* Percent Daily Values are based on a 2,000 calorie diet. Your daily values may be higher or lower depending on your calorie needs:

	Calories:	2,000	2,500
Total Fat	Less than	65g	80g
Sat Fat	Less than	20g	25g
Cholesterol	Less than	300mg	300mg
Sodium	Less than	2,400mg	2,400mg
Total Carbohydrate		300g	375g
Dietary Fiber		25g	30g

Calories per gram:
Fat 9 • Carbohydrate 4 • Protein 4

FIGURE 6-15 A Sample Nutrition Fact Label

is 2,400 mg. On the other hand, a food with 5 grams of saturated fat could be construed as being low in that nutrient. In fact, that food would provide one-fourth the total Daily Value because 20 grams is the Daily Value for saturated fat.

Daily Values and Dietary Reference Values

The new label reference value, Daily Value, comprises two sets of existing dietary standards: Daily Reference Values (DRVs) and Reference Daily Intakes (RDIs). Only the Daily Value term appears on the label, though, to make label reading less confusing. Note: Do not confuse the RDIs with the new Dietary Reference Intakes (DRIs) discussed on page 113.

DRVs have been established for sources of energy: fat, saturated fat, total carbohydrate (including fiber), and protein; and for cholesterol, sodium, and potassium, which do not contribute calories. DRVs for the energy-producing nutrients are based on the number of calories consumed per day and are calculated as follows:

* Fat based on 30% of calories

* Saturated fat based on 10% of calories

* Carbohydrate based on 60% of calories

* Protein based on 10% of calories (The DRV for protein applies only to adults and children over the age of 4. RDIs for protein for special groups have been established.)

* Fiber based on 11.5 g of fiber per 1,000 calories

Because of current public health recommendations, DRVs for some nutrients represent the uppermost limit that is considered desirable. The DRVs for total fat, saturated fat, cholesterol, and sodium are as follows:

* Total fat: less than 65 g

* Saturated fat: less than 20 g

* Cholesterol: less than 300 mg

* Sodium: less than 2,400 mg

A Word About "Fast Food"

It is recognized that in today's fast-paced society, many people do not have the time (or do not take the time) to prepare well-balanced meals for themselves or their families. In reality, it really takes no longer to run into a grocery store to buy a piece of fruit for lunch than it does to go to a burger place; however, many people still opt for the convenient drive-thru restaurant. Unfortunately, "fast food" is not only hard on the wallet—it can be hard on the body too. So, when clients choose convenience over cooking (or getting out of the car), advise them to take a moment before ordering an old favorite to see if there are any healthier items available on the menu.

Many fast-food restaurants are trying to raise the nutritional value of the foods they offer. Check out the nutritional content of the foods that are available through some of these eating establishments by consulting their in-store posted Nutritional Information or their Web sites.

Even those who do choose to eat at fast-food restaurants will benefit from the following advice:

* Stay away from menu items that say "fried," "crispy," "breaded," "creamed," "buttered," or "gravy." Healthy words to look for include "marinara," "steamed," "boiled," "tomato sauce," "poached," and "charbroiled."

* At Mexican restaurants, choose black beans instead of refried beans. Ask for soft corn tortillas instead of deep-fried shells. Use salsa instead of sour cream and guacamole—and watch the chips.

* If you choose Italian food, get the pasta with marinara, not the cream sauce. Pizza lovers should choose plain cheese or vegetarian.

* When going Chinese, choose stir-fried and steamed dishes, chicken, vegetables, and rice. Avoid deep-fried items such as egg rolls, wontons, and sweet and sour pork.

* At burger places the salad bars are great, but watch the dressing, eggs, and cheese. Look for grilled burgers, hold the mayonnaise, and go light on the cheese. Watch the French fry intake. (Go for the baked potatoes with margarine on the side). Drink low-fat milk rather than a milk shake.

WEIGHT CONTROL AND ENERGY BALANCE

energy expenditure

the total calories used for all activities over a given period of time.

energy intake

the sum of the caloric content in food ingested.

The energy that we obtain from food, as well as the body's **energy expenditure**, is measured in units of heat called calories. Carbohydrates and protein supply 4 calories per gram, fat supplies 9 calories per gram, and alcohol supplies 7 calories per gram.

Maintaining weight, gaining weight, or losing weight is a matter of energy balance. A person's body weight will stay the same when **energy intake** equals energy output (exercise); it will change when there is an imbalance between energy intake and energy expenditure. To gain weight, energy intake must be greater than energy expenditure; to lose weight, energy expenditure must be greater than energy intake (Figure 6-16). In short, people who need to lose body fat must eat less and exercise more.

Each person has a specific requirement for calories, which is determined by age, gender, body weight, and physical

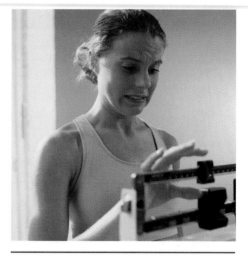

FIGURE 6-16 For a person to lose weight, energy output must be greater than energy intake.

activity. The average adult female requires about 14 to 17 calories per pound of body weight; the average adult male requires 15 to 18 calories per pound. Children, adolescents, and physically active people such as athletes, require more calories per pound of body weight.

Body Composition and "True Weight"

Often, people consume more calories than the body can use, but then expend those calories at a later time as a result of their exercise programs and other metabolic processes. So for most people, a slight fluctuation of body weight is normal. Also, many athletes will "carbo-consume" just before high-activity events—they may gain weight temporarily as a result. Therefore, for most people, athletes included, weighing in on standard weight scales reveals limited information because it does not reveal how much of the weight on the scale is body fat, as opposed to lean muscle tissue. As a result, weighing in on standard scales is only one way to evaluate body weight.

Because a standard weight scale cannot differentiate between fat weight and muscle weight, a more accurate method of measuring body fat is to assess one's body composition. This assessment divides weight into two categories: lean body mass (especially muscle) and fat. Many authorities in fitness agree that for athletes and others interested in fitness, determining the lean body weight (LBW) and the percent body fat is one of the best ways to measure the body's "true weight." The lean body weight is the weight that the human body has in its lean body mass after deducting the weight of the body fat mass. Using their lean body weight as a weight management guide is also helpful for athletes in a given sports activity, because it helps them to gauge their body weight accurately. As a result, they are able to perform at their best without damaging their health. For instance, when athletes are engaged in vigorous activity, they burn calories from fat tissues first. After the caloric energy the body needs is depleted from the fat tissues, the next source the body turns to is the lean muscle tissue. However, athletes and others do not want to burn lean muscle tissue because it is not an efficient source of energy, and it is not good for the health of the body.

The target percent of body fat for adult males is generally around 15%, and for females it ranges from 20 to 25%. For athletes, however, this figure can be different. For example, body fat in male baseball players often ranges from 10 to 12%, because any extra body fat can harm their performance. A person's ideal percentage of body fat is the percentage that allows that individual to perform at his or her best.

A body composition evaluation is recommended before and during a weight loss or weight gain program. When trying to lose weight, it is important to lose fat, not muscle; and when trying to gain weight, you want to gain muscle, not fat. The procedures for measuring body fat and calculating lean body weight to determine body composition were described in Chapter 5.

Losing Weight

If it has been determined either by a physician or by a body composition assessment that an individual needs to lose weight, that person is faced with dozens of weight loss methods from which to choose. Unfortunately for the people who try them, many of these methods do not work. An unbelievable number of weight loss gimmicks have been spawned by the obsession American consumers have about losing weight. Some of these gimmicks endanger the health of their victims, others merely thin wallets, and almost all fail to produce permanent weight loss—no matter what the marketing states. It takes a keen, well-educated eye to separate fact from fiction.

The most successful strategies for weight loss include calorie reduction (500 to 1,000 fewer calories per day), increased physical activity (moderate intensity activity of 30 minutes or more on most days of the week), and behavior therapy designed to improve eating and activity habits. The rate of weight loss should not exceed 2 pounds per week on a regular basis (1 pound of body fat equals 3,500 calories). A diet that reduces calorie intake by 500 to 1,000 calories per day will lead to a weight loss of about 1 to 2 pounds per week. Regardless of how much weight needs to be lost, consumption should not fall below 1,500 calories per day.

Eating fewer empty calories—foods high in fat, sugar, and alcohol—can decrease calorie intake. Eating habits can be improved by preparing smaller portions, eating slowly, and avoiding second helpings. Skipping meals early in the day can contribute to overeating later, so eating regular meals can also aid in weight control. Because fat is a concentrated source of calories, reducing fat intake helps to reduce caloric intake.

The timing of a weight loss program is critical. Avoid starting a client on a new diet around holidays when there is lots of tempting food around. Don't set a client up for failure!

Exercise should be included in every weight loss program, as it helps to counteract some of the negative effects of caloric restriction. Dieting decreases the body's use of calories, making it more difficult to lose weight. Combining exercise with caloric restriction decreases the amount of muscle that is lost. Furthermore, exercise burns fat; so to lose a certain amount of fat, caloric intake does not have to be reduced as much if exercise is part of the weight loss program.

Athletes, of course, have little problem with exercising regularly, but most other people who are interested in fitness and weight control have to make a place for exercise in their daily routines. Then, once they understand the relationship of the ratio of fat to muscle in their bodies, they will need to know these facts on the basics of exercise:

* One pound of fat (the body's densest fuel) = 3,500 calories.

* The average sedentary male (as an example) burns 2,000 calories a day.

* That leaves an excess of 1,500 calories a day that needs to be burned for every pound of fat that needs to be lost from the body.

As we age, our basal metabolic rate (the rate at which the body normally burns calories), decreases. Activity increases one's metabolic rate. In general, older people are less active than younger people. This is why it often is more difficult for people over the age of 35 to burn calories—their metabolic rate has decreased. However, by increasing activity through exercise and maintaining a proper diet, even those over 50 can build muscle tissue back up again, regaining the correct balance between body fat and muscle.

So, the answer to weight control and energy balance is to get moving, to burn fat away as energy—to exercise! When people exercise on a regular basis, they burn calories, and they keep burning those calories for hours after their exercise period is over. It works like this:

A. Active exercise makes a person breathe deeper.

B. Deeper breathing requires more oxygen, and transports more oxygen to the body's cells.

C. The more oxygen that is consumed and used in the cells of the body, the higher the number of calories that are burned.

Take, for example, the value of aerobic exercise. "Aero" refers to "air." Thus, when people perform aerobic exercises, they are breathing air (and more important, oxygen) deeply and quickly. Therefore, they are burning calories at a high rate.

Aerobic exercise (Figure 6-17) is the best method of losing body fat. However, weight training is also helpful, especially in increasing the proportion of lean weight. Remember these two primary facts about exercise:

1. The only way to create more of the enzymes needed to metabolize fat into muscle is through exercise.

2. The only way to build muscle is through exercise.

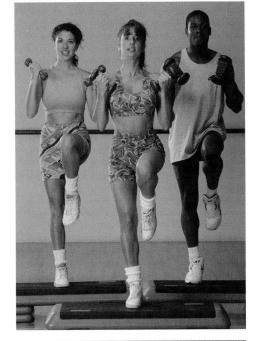

FIGURE 6-17 Get your clients moving; aerobic exercise helps burn fat.

A good rule of thumb for losing weight through aerobic exercise is to work the heart and lungs for 30 to 60 minutes, three to five times a week. For example, jogging 3 miles or riding a stationary bicycle for 30 minutes at a moderate intensity will burn off about 300 calories. Burning off less than 300 calories per session will not produce significant results.

Spot reduction exercises often are promoted to decrease body fat in specific areas of the body, such as sit-ups for the abdomen. But exercise, even when localized, draws from the fat stores of the entire body—not just from specific fat deposits in the target area. Therefore, sit-ups will increase the muscle tone of the abdomen and, thus, may reduce abdominal girth, but they aren't particularly effective in decreasing abdominal body fat.

Figure 6-18 is a chart that shows calorie expenditure for selected activities. Increased activity will help burn off extra calories. Most important, be sure that clients always do the following when exercising:

1. Medical Checkup. Consult a physician before beginning any exercise program.

Calorie Expenditure Chart

Activity	Calories Per Minute	Activity	Calories Per Minute
Archery	2.8	Lawn mowing (hand mower)	7.7
Badminton (singles)	6.0	Lying at ease	1.5
Basketball	12.0	Mopping floor	4.8
Bed-making	3.9	Mountain climbing	9.5
Bowling	3.2	Paddleball	10.7
Bricklaying	4.0	Painting at an easel	2.0
Calisthenics	6.0	Planting seedlings	4.8
Canoeing (15 min./mile)	7.0	Racquetball	10.7
Card-playing	1.8	Raking	5.4
Carpentry	6.8	Roller skating	11.2
Carpet cleaning	3.5	Rope-skipping (80 turns/min.)	11.3
Cleaning	4.2	Running (6 min./mile)	16.2
Climbing hills without load	9.5	Scrubbing floors	12.0
Climbing with 10 lb. load	10.1	Sitting quietly	1.7
Cooking	3.5	Skiing vigorously downhill	9.5
Cross-country skiing	14.0	Skin diving	12.0
Cycling (5 min./mile)	10.6	Sleeping (basal metabolism)	1.0
Dancing—Ballroom	5.4	Speed skating	15.0
Driving a car	2.	Soccer	12.0
Eating	1.7	Social dancing	6.0
Farm work in field	7.3	Softball or Baseball	7.2
Field Hockey	9.0	Square and Round dancing	7.0
Fly fishing (with waders)	4.6	Squash	10.7
Food shopping	4.5	Swimming (50 yds./min.)	9.1
Gardening	3.8	Table tennis	5.6
Golf (foursome—cart)	3.8	Tennis (singles)	6.0
Golf (foursome—carrying clubs)	6.0	Tennis (doubles)	4.0
Gymnastics	4.6	Tetherball	4.6
Handball	10.9	Trampolining	5.6
Ironing	2.7	Typing	1.8
Jogging (8 min./mile)	12.6	Volleyball (6 players)	3.6
Judo	12.0	Volleyball (2 players)	9.2
Knitting/sewing	1.8	Walking (17 min./mile)	5.4

FIGURE 6-18 Calorie Expenditure Chart

2. **Start Slowly.** Set modest goals, building up to difficult levels gradually. Try to keep from getting short of breath. A good rule of thumb to measure one's level of exertion is to attempt to carry on a conversation while exercising without getting short of breath.

3. **Warm Up and Stretch.** Always stretch and do a light cardiovascular warm-up to prepare the muscles for the stress of the coming exercises. Warming up and stretching help prevent injury and increase performance.

4. **Hydrate.** Drink at least one glass of water before exercising, hydrate every 20 minutes during the exercise period, and drink another glass of water immediately after exercising. Delaying hydration until one feels thirsty is not recommended. Once thirst sets in, the muscles are already beginning to dehydrate, and dehydrated muscles will fatigue quickly.

5. **Finish Cool.** Slow down exercises, and remember to stretch again, to cool down the body after exercising vigorously.

Gaining Weight

When weight gain is the goal, muscle gain is preferred to fat gain. Unlike fat tissue, muscle tissue can be used to produce force. So, the ideal weight gain program combines progressive weight training with increased caloric intake.

A safe goal for the gain of lean weight is 1/2 to 1 pound a week. To gain 1 pound of muscle, 2,500 additional calories are required, so a person who wants or needs to gain weight should increase caloric intake by 350 calories per day (see Figure 6-19). In addition, the caloric cost of weight training (about 200 calories per hour of conditioning) should be added each day. These calories are over and above what the individual normally requires to maintain body weight.

Caloric intake can be increased by eating larger servings of the foods already being consumed (the opposite of what is recommended for weight loss). Between-meal snacks can also be added. Some athletes use commercial liquid meals for convenient, between-meal snacks.

Many athletes take protein and amino acid supplements to gain muscle mass. Because the average American diet is high in protein, most people—even athletes—easily meet their protein needs through food and don't require supplements. If more protein than is needed is consumed, the excess will be burned for energy or converted to fat. Amino acids assist in the conversion of protein to energy, but because we get amino acids in most protein foods, additional amino acids generally are unnecessary.

NUTRITIONAL SUPPLEMENTS AND DIETARY FADS

In an ideal situation, we would get all of the nutrients we need directly from the foods we eat. Realistically, however, because a diet that accomplishes this requires careful planning, few people take the time and energy to do it. This is where nutritional supplements come in.

Nutritional supplements (Figure 6-20) are vitamins, minerals, amino acids, etc., that are consumed to help compensate for nutritional deficiencies in a diet.

Calories in Selected Foods

Food Description	Serving Size	Approximate Calories
BEVERAGES		
Lemonade	12 oz.	165
Milk (whole)	12 oz.	240
Milk (skim)	12 oz.	135
Orange juice	4 oz.	55
Soft drinks (carbonated)	12 oz.	150
Tea (no cream or sugar)	any size	0
BREADS		
Blueberry muffin	one 2½" dia.	140
Hamburger or hot dog bun	one bun	120
Hard roll	one aver. size	155
White bread	one slice	65
Doughnut (plain)	one aver. size	200
CEREALS AND GRAIN PRODUCTS		
Bran flakes	1 cup	105
Corn flakes	1 cup	100
Macaroni (cooked)	1 cup	190
Oatmeal (cooked)	1 cup	130
Pancakes	1 cake 4" dia.	60
Rice (cooked)	1 cup	225
Spaghetti (cooked)	1 cup	155
MEATS AND POULTRY		
Beef		
Hamburger patty (lean ground)	4 oz.	245
Hamburger patty (regular)	4 oz.	325
Roast beef	4 oz.	220
Steak (broiled, sirloin)	4 oz.	440
Pork		
Bacon	2 slices	90
Chops (lean)	4 oz.	300
Ham (baked)	4 oz.	325
Hot dog	2 oz.	170
Poultry		
Chicken, all meat (broiled)	4 oz.	150
Chicken (fried)	½ breast	155
Turkey (roasted)	4 oz.	220
SEAFOOD		
Fish sticks (breaded)	5 sticks, 4 oz. each	200
Halibut (broiled)	one 4 oz.	205
Lobster (meat only)	4 oz.	100
Trout (fried)	4 oz.	225
Tuna (canned in oil)	4 oz.	225
Salmon (baked)	one 4 oz.	205
EGGS, CHEESE, CREAM		
Cottage cheese (creamed)	4 oz.	132

FIGURE 6-19 Calories in Selected Foods

Food Description	Serving Size	Approximate Calories
Cottage cheese (uncreamed)	4 oz.	84
Egg, fried or scrambled w/fat	1 medium	110
Egg, soft or poached	1 medium	78
Processed American cheese	1 oz.	80
Whipping cream	1 tbs.	55
FRUITS AND VEGETABLES		
Apple	1 medium	70
Baked beans	1/2 cup	150
Banana	1 medium	100
Broccoli (chopped)	4 oz.	26
Cabbage (cooked)	1 cup	30
Carrots (cooked)	1 cup	45
Celery (raw)	8 in. stalk	5
Corn (canned)	1 cup	170
Corn on the cob	1 ear, 5 in.	70
Cucumber (raw)	6 slices	5
Grapefruit	1/2 medium	50
Green beans (cooked)	1 cup	30
Lettuce	3 large leaves	10
Onions (raw)	1 medium	40
Orange	1 medium	50
Peas (cooked)	1 cup	115
Peppers, sweet green (raw)	1 medium	15
Potatoes (baked—no butter or sour cream)	1 medium	90
Sweet potatoes (baked)	1 medium	155
Spinach (cooked)	1 cup	40
Squash, summer (cooked)	1 cup	30
Squash, winter (cooked)	1 cup	130
Tomato (raw)	1 medium	40
Tomatoes, canned (cooked)	1 cup	50
DESSERTS		
Apple pie (2 crusts)	1/8 of 9 in. pie	306
Chocolate chip cookies	one 2 in.	70
Chocolate pudding	1/2 cup	193
Custard	1 cup	305
Vanilla ice cream	1/2 cup	133
MISCELLANEOUS		
Cashews	1/4 cup	196
Catsup	1 tbs.	15
Mustard	1 tbs.	4
Margarine (regular)	1 tbs.	100
Peanut butter	1 tbs.	95
Peanuts	1/2 cup	210
Pickles, dill	1 medium	10
Pickles, sweet	1 medium	20
Popcorn, with oil and salt	1 cup	40
Potato chips	10 medium	115
Pretzels, thin twist	1 twist	25

FIGURE 6-19 Calories in Selected Foods (*Continued*)

Most experts agree that supplementing a diet with a multivitamin is acceptable, and in some cases recommended. However, the consumption of protein supplements, amino acids, creatine, and other dietary supplements should be evaluated on an individual basis by a registered dietitian.

A Word of Caution

Athletes and others who are interested in physical fitness often seek that "secret ingredient" or "shortcut" that will enhance their performance quickly. As a result, many of us

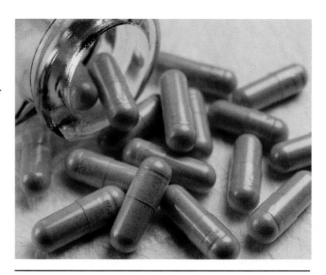

FIGURE 6-20 Although some dietary supplements, like multivitamins, can be helpful to some people, others should be avoided. Check with a registered dietitian.

are easy marks for nutritional faddism. Many nutritional supplements are available that supposedly relieve muscle soreness, boost stamina, speed healing, increase speed, improve muscle tone, improve memory, or reduce body fat. Sometimes, experienced athletes and other well-meaning people endorse such supplements. But sometimes these people are misinformed. Furthermore, some products are endorsed by nutrition quacks.

Nutrition quacks are people who claim to have skills, knowledge, or qualifications they don't possess. Because they have something to sell, these people make promises and exaggerated claims that they know the public wants to believe. Quackery can be very subtle. People who participate in it often capitalize on the understandable desire for a "quick fix" to a problem. They know that most people would like to believe that there is something that will boost performance faster and easier than a healthy diet. They may even display fraudulent degrees or diplomas to make themselves appear credible, or they may offer to perform various scientific-sounding tests, such as cytotoxic testing, applied kinesiology, or hair analysis to bolster their claims. Warn clients and athletes to be careful of this type of person—a quack is only after money!

A valid nutritional assessment should be part of a general health examination that requires the combined expertise of professionals such as physicians and registered dietitians. It usually involves a medical history, dietary history, and a clinical examination. If a physician or registered dietitian is not present, or valid credentials are not displayed, be suspicious.

Sometimes a nutritional supplement seems to work; a person takes a supplement and feels less tired, more alert, or less sore. It is important to understand that the **placebo effect** by itself is powerful enough to produce benefits. If a person believes that certain foods or supplements will improve performance, that belief can actually make the person perform better—even if there is nothing beneficial in the food or supplement.

placebo effect

a false sense of benefit felt by a patient caused by the psychological belief that a treatment is effective.

Ergogenic Aids

Ergogenic aids represent another trend in sports nutrition. Ergogenic means "work producing." Advertisers claim that these products enhance athletic performance. Many athletes believe that ergogenic aids such as amino acids, co-enzyme Q-10, and creatine will give them a competitive edge. Despite various claims, however, there is little scientific evidence that they offer any benefits, and they may be harmful. Therefore, it is probably best to avoid these products.

New ergogenic aids are continually being presented to athletic consumers. These products often are marketed without any scientific research to validate the benefits or reveal the harmful side effects. Some products go on and off the market before studies are done to establish or refute their claims. Worse, ingredient lists on some products occasionally are altered to support untruthful claims! Prosecutions and other legal actions for these practices on the behalf of consumers can take years, and the seller can reap their profits during the delay.

Nutritional faddism is more prevalent than ever. Traditional magazine advertisements, television infomercials, signs posted along the side of the road, and Web page ads all encourage the belief in wonderful nutritional discoveries. Promises of increased energy, improved endurance, and overnight weight loss are lavishly displayed to the public. Unfortunately, the fact of the matter remains: There are no quick and easy ways to do any of these things. But hope is not lost—performance and health can be improved by exercising, by eating a balanced diet, and by replacing fluid losses during exercise.

Steroids

Anabolic steroids are a class of natural and synthetic (manufactured) substances that are related to the major male sex hormone, testosterone. Anabolic steroids promote growth of muscles, and can make bones stronger and reduce body fat. In addition, all anabolic steroids are androgenic. This means they cause male characteristics, such as male patterned baldness, facial hair, and deepened voice. However, because of their chemical structure, steroid precursors can be converted into the major female hormone, estrogen. This can cause breast enlargement in men.

Steroids are illegal without a prescription in the United States. They can, however, be imported illegally or created in illegal labs. "Designer steroids" have been used orally (taken by mouth) and via injection (taken by needle). Anabolic steroids are listed in Figure 6-21.

Anabolic Steroids	
Oral	Injection
Anadrol	Boldenone
Danazol	Dihydrotestosterone
Dianabol	Nortestosterone
Winstrol	Testonsterone

FIGURE 6-21 Anabolic Steroids

Some substances were once legal and available as "dietary supplements," such as androstendione (a testosterone precursor), 19-norandrostenedione, and dehydroepiandrosterne (DHEA). These precursor steroids are rapidly converted into active hormones when taken, which can result in masculine (androgenic) traits, and are commonly used for their principal anabolic effects. These substances are related to hormones produced in the adrenal gland as well as the ovary and the testes. In October 2004, a bill voted on by Congress and signed into law by the President outlawed the sale of most of these substances in the United States.

Abusing anabolic steroids can lead to dramatic changes in one's body and emotional well-being. Some possible health effects include:

* Increased risk of liver, kidney, and prostate cancer, documented in laboratory animals

* High blood pressure, which increases the chance of heart attack and stroke

* Abnormal cholesterol levels, which increases the chance of heart attack and blood vessel disease

* Early stopping of bone development and linear growth (height)

* Damage to the liver, including the formation of blood-filled liver cysts that can rupture

* Acne

* Increased risk of HIV and hepatitis because of risks from sharing needles

* In males: shrunken testicles and temporary inability to father a child, breast formation, and baldness

* In females: smaller breast size, irregular mistral (monthly) cycles, masculine appearance (particularly facial and body hair), and deep voice

Psychological symptoms include:

* Mood swings

* Sleep disruption

* Aggressive behavior

* Extreme irritability

* Delusions

* Impaired judgement, because of feeling invincible

* Paranoid jealousy

* Euphoria (exaggerated feeling of well-being)

* Depression (after stopping steroids)

* Lack of sexual drive (after stopping steroids)

Creatine

Creatine combines with phosphate to form creatine phosphate (CP), a high-energy compound stored in muscles. Stored phosphocreatine (PCr) can fuel the first 4 to 5 seconds of a sprint, but another fuel source must provide the energy to sustain the activity. Creatine supplements increase the storage of PCr, thus making more adenosine triphosphate (ATP) available to fuel the working muscles and enable them to work harder before becoming fatigued. Research suggests that consuming 20 to 25 grams of creatine per day (5 grams consumed four to five times daily) for five to seven days increases CP stores in athletes by 20%, delays fatigue during explosive sprint performance, and facilitates ATP resynthesis following sprint-type exercise.

However, some studies have found that creatine does not improve strength, sprint performance, or body weight, while others state creatine supplementation offers short-term limited benefits. Whether or not it is harmful long-term has yet to be determined. (More information on this topic can be found in the book *Eating for Endurance*, 4th Edition by Ellen Coleman, RD, MA, MPH.)

PRE-EXERCISE MEALS

What a person eats several days before training or competition affects the amount of glycogen in the muscles. Therefore, the foods an athlete consumes on the day of training or competition do not really affect muscle performance because the glycogen has not had time to reach the muscles yet. So, although powering down high-protein foods on the day of an event won't enhance strength or endurance, it *is* important to plan to eat an appropriate pre-exercise meal on days when performance is critical.

A proper pre-exercise meal prevents hunger during exercise and helps maintain an adequate blood sugar level. If food is not consumed at appropriate times, the blood sugar level drops. Low blood sugar can inhibit concentration and hinder coordination and timing.

Exercising on a full stomach should be avoided because food that remains in the stomach during exercise can cause indigestion, nausea, and possible vomiting. So, athletes and others should plan to eat 1 hour before working out. It takes approximately an hour for the food to empty from the stomach into the intestines, although nervousness (such as pre-game jitters) can make this process take longer.

To avoid indigestion or nausea, the size of the meal should be reduced the closer to the time of the activity it is consumed. A big plate of pancakes is okay 4 hours before the event, whereas a small bowl of cereal with low-fat milk and juice or fruit is more appropriate an hour before exercise (see Figure 6-22). Athletes should try not to eat anything in the hour before they train or compete.

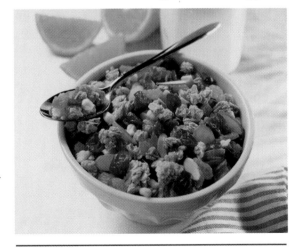

FIGURE 6-22 A person who wants to eat within the hour prior to exercise should select a small meal that is easy to digest, such as a bowl of cereal.

Some athletes who have problems eating before exercise may benefit from liquid or nutrition bar meals. Make sure that whatever they eat empties from the stomach quickly. It is a good idea to experiment with pre-exercise meals in a practice environment before trying them under event conditions.

High-fat, high-protein foods such as eggs, bacon, and hamburgers, and fried foods such as doughnuts and French fries are not digested quickly. Limit or avoid these in the pre-exercise meal. High-carbohydrate items such as cereal, pancakes, fruit, and pasta are the best choices because carbohydrates are quickly digested.

Some athletes eat sugary foods (candy or soft drinks) right before exercise for quick energy. Eating sugary foods won't help anyone run faster or hit harder. Most of the energy for exercise comes from foods people eat in the days leading up to an event.

Eating during practice or competition doesn't help performance, but it *is* vital to stay hydrated by drinking fluids before, during, and after exercise. There will be times when an event may last for hours. Sports bars, bananas, and sports drinks can be used to supplement the athletes' energy needs during periods of physical activity.

It is a tradition for some athletes to indulge in a pre-event meal of steak and potatoes. Although this type of meal will do little to affect the athletes' physical performance in a positive way, engaging in such a tradition may boost performance from a psychological standpoint. The psychological aspects of competition must never be ignored. So, if a meal of steak and potatoes is chosen as a tool to provide motivation a few hours before the event, that's okay—just make sure to trim off the fat, exchange the butter for margarine, and add some fresh fruit!

Recovery

After working out, a person will need carbohydrates to replace the glycogen in the muscles. A high-carbohydrate diet (50 to 60% of calories consumed per day) will help speed recovery from physical exertion. Interestingly, muscles are able to store more glycogen immediately after exercise than they are at other times. In fact, eating carbohydrates right after exercise will allow the muscles to store twice as much glycogen as they would if the carbohydrates are consumed 2 hours later! Recent research suggests grouping protein with carbohydrates. This combination increases the amount of glycogen that is stored. However, eating too much protein after physical activity can slow hydration and glycogen replacement. For this reason, carbohydrates and proteins should be consumed in a 4:1 ratio. For those who are not hungry immediately after exercise, sports drinks or sports bars can help supply this extra glycogen.

EATING DISORDERS

An eating disorder is a disturbance in eating behavior. These disorders are more commonly found in women, but they are also a problem for men. The most common disorders are anorexia nervosa and bulimia nervosa. Eating disorders are a serious problem; the longer the disorder exists, the more likely that some undesirable medical consequences will occur. It is estimated that the long-term death rate for those afflicted with anorexia nervosa or bulimia nervosa can be as high as 20 to 30%.

Because athletics involve a focus on the body, it is not uncommon to find athletes who, for one reason or another, have a problem with eating disorders. Some people are drawn to athletics to hide an existing compulsion for a thinner, more athletic looking body. However, men and women who participate in sports for the love of the game are also prone to developing eating disorders. In the quest for increasing athletic performance or proper athletic physique, the athlete may develop an eating disorder. An athletic trainer should watch for signs and symptoms of athletes with eating disorders and be aware of the weight qualifications for each sport—especially those that emphasize a lean body. Such sports include wrestling, gymnastics, long-distance running, crew, and swimming.

Bulimia Nervosa

Bulimia nervosa is a disorder that usually begins in adolescence and is more common in females than in males. Bulimia is characterized by binging on large amounts of food, followed by inappropriate behavior, such as purging (vomiting), fasting, overexercising, laxative abuse, or diuretic use to compensate for eating such huge amounts. The bulimic patient is generally within normal weight—not underweight. The bulimic has an abnormal concern about body size and a fear of becoming fat. Bulimics tend to overexercise and often alternate days of fasting with days of binging and purging. Many bulimics also use laxatives and diuretics. Laxative abuse can lead to irritable bowel disease or create an addiction to laxatives; diuretics may cause electrolyte imbalances and heart arrhythmias.

Because purging can cause other physical problems, bulimics may complain of sore throats and may have multiple dental problems. The constant purging causes destruction of tooth enamel by the stomach acids. This leads to dental erosion. Esophageal tears and gastric ruptures are not uncommon because of repeated vomiting, and swollen salivary glands also may develop. Bulimics often are dehydrated and have nutritional deficiencies, especially potassium. With repeated purging, they lose a significant amount of potassium, an electrolyte needed for the electrical activity of the heart. When potassium is depleted, it can cause cardiac arrhythmias and sudden death.

Treatment for bulimia nervosa includes monitored eating, evaluation by trained personnel, and individual and family therapy. Many health centers continue to work hard to find an effective treatment for bulimia, and some claim significant success. Often, bulimics require inpatient hospitalization.

Anorexia Nervosa

Anorexia means severe loss of appetite. Nervosa indicates this loss is related to emotional reasons. Actually, anorexic patients do not have a loss of appetite. They fight to keep from eating for other reasons, such as fear of weight gain, emotional distress, and so on.

A person with anorexia loses a great deal of weight. The label "anorexic" means the weight is less than 85% of the normal weight for the person's size. The individual refuses to eat a sufficient amount to maintain body weight and attempts to conceal skipping eating. The anorexic sometimes abuses laxatives and may exercise to extremes. Over half of the anorexic population also binges and purges.

Anorexics often weigh themselves several times a day, paranoid about gaining weight. They have an intense fear of becoming fat and see a distorted body image.

They are preoccupied with food and are obsessed about the number of calories they may be consuming and other food-focused thoughts.

As the disorder progresses, physical changes occur. The anorexic becomes hypothermic and wears sweaters in the summertime. Anorexics can develop hypotension, bradycardia, lanugo, electrolyte imbalance, and edema; females can experience amenorrhea. The anorexic may have difficulty thinking because of lack of nutrition. Many develop cardiac arrhythmias that may cause sudden death. When this disorder is not recognized and treated, the anorexic eventually starves to death.

As with bulimics, treatment of the anorexic includes monitored eating, evaluation by trained personnel, individual and family therapy. The immediate goal for the treatment of an anorexic is weight gain. It often requires hospitalization and intravenous feeding.

The Psychological Consequences of Eating Disorders

From a psychological perspective it can sometimes be difficult to decipher what problems have arisen as a result of the eating disorder versus what psychological conditions might have been precursors to the development of anorexia or bulimia. This is particularly true with the most prevalent psychological state, depression. With severe nutritional imbalances and starvation, depression is a general consequence. Therefore, these issues may need to be addressed prior to determining if there was an undiagnosed depression that contributed to the eating disorder. Brain function may be affected, as exhibited by the lack of ability to concentrate. Obsessive and compulsive behavior traits may be exhibited for the first time, or there may be a worsening of obsessive/compulsive disorders. In general, most of the psychological consequences will not be permanent. Therapy and appropriate medications are effective in addressing these issues.

THINKING IT THROUGH

After synchronized swimming practice Talia asked Marty, the athletic trainer, about losing some weight. Talia said she had already spoken with the coach about it and that she thought it might improve her performance. Marty asked Talia to keep a written diary of everything she ate, which she did on a daily basis for a week. He also scheduled her for a body composition assessment to determine if she really needed to lose any body fat.

A week later, after reviewing the results of the body composition analysis with Talia, Marty told her that although she was at a competitive level of fitness, her body composition analysis indicated that her body fat was down a little. On reviewing her diary with her, Marty noted that her activities included swimming for 2 hours per day. She was skipping breakfast and lunch, but eating a large, late dinner. Marty had noticed *her snacking at times and could not find any reference to these snacks in the diary. After asking her about it, Talia confessed to omitting the snacks from the diary because she would later stick her finger down her throat, causing her to vomit up the food.*

What eating disorder is Talia most likely suffering from? Should Marty contact anyone to help Talia with her disorder? What are the steps to determining if Talia really needs to lose weight?

CHAPTER SUMMARY

Basic nutrition and weight control are key factors in the body's ability to obtain optimum health and performance. An excess or a deficiency of essential food nutrients can be harmful to health and may impair fitness and/or athletic performance.

The key to proper nutrition and weight management is to follow good nutrition guidelines by eating a variety of foods chosen with knowledge from the Food Pyramid Guide. Eating in moderation and eating a balanced diet help to control caloric intake and body fat composition. At times, athletes and others who engage in vigorous physical activity will need to maintain optimum health by eating more carbohydrates, observing lean body weight guidelines, and drinking generous amounts of water during strenuous activities.

Because eating disorders frequently involve a distorted body image and physical deterioration, it is important that athletic trainers and other sports medicine professionals become familiar with the signs and symptoms of these disorders. Eating disorders like anorexia and bulimia can cause serious physical effects such as electrolyte imbalances and heart arrhythmias. In the long run, if undetected and untreated, people suffering from this type of disorder can experience serious depression, permanent physical damage, or even death.

STUDENT ENRICHMENT ACTIVITIES

Complete the following exercises.

1. Eating food helps the body perform what three essential functions?

2. Name the two basic principles to follow when choosing foods that supply a healthy diet.

3. List four foods that are composed of complex carbohydrates.

4. Generally, saturated fat is _____ at room temperature and is derived mainly from _____ sources. Examples of foods that contain saturated fat are _____.

5. Usually, unsaturated fat is _____ at room temperature and comes mainly from _____ sources. Examples of foods containing unsaturated fat include _____, _____, and _____.

6. List the three complete protein foods that contain all the essential amino acids needed by the body.

7. Vitamins are metabolic regulators that govern the processes of _____, _____, _____, and _____ in the body.

8. State what function the following minerals perform in the body: calcium and iron.

9. List three functions that water performs in the body.

10. Name and give examples of the foods in the different food groups that make up the latest Food Guide Pyramid.

Write the letter of the correct answer.

11. Deficiency of vitamin E can result in all of the following except:

    A. dry skin.
    B. frequent nosebleeds.
    C. frequent infections.
    D. retarded growth.

12. Which of the following activities expends the most calories per minute?

    A. volleyball
    B. square dancing
    C. mountain climbing
    D. field hockey

13. Based on equal serving sizes, which food contains the least calories?

    A. whole milk
    B. broiled halibut
    C. roasted turkey
    D. cottage cheese

14. You are making a sandwich for lunch. Which of these protein fillers is lowest in calories?

    A. bacon (4 slices)
    B. roast beef (4 oz.)
    C. hot dog (2 oz.)
    D. hamburger (4 oz. patty)

15. Which of the following is a characterization of bulimia nervosa?

    A. 85% of *normal* weight
    B. amenorrhea in females
    C. hypothermia
    D. gastric ruptures

Write T for true, or F for false. Rewrite the false statements to make them true.

16. T   F   Minerals need to be taken sparingly, always less than 100 mg daily.

17. T   F   Athletes overall need more vitamin supplements than normal less-active people do.

18. T   F   Athletes should refrain from drinking water when engaged in vigorous activity—it can cause painful stomach cramps.

19. T   F   The American Dietetic Association recommends that athletes should consume large amounts of complex carbohydrates before extended periods of strenuous activity.

20. T   F   The term "LBW" stands for lower body weight.

Complete the following exercises.

21. Write down everything you eat for two days. Then, answer the following questions. (If you have trouble obtaining the information you need for the foods you consumed, try searching the Internet for "calories" to find Web sites that can help. One Web site you can try is www.calories.com.)

    a. How many calories did you consume each day?

    b. How many calories from fat did you consume each day?

22. Go to MyPyramid.gov and compare your diet to the one that comes up in your search. How can you improve your diet?

CHAPTER 7

Physical Conditioning

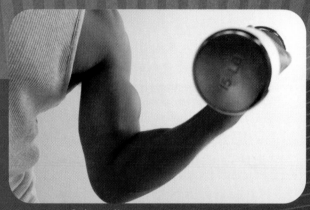

(Courtesy of Photodisc)

OBJECTIVES

After completing this chapter, you should be able to do the following:

1. Define and correctly spell each of the key terms.

2. Describe a flexibility program for a client.

3. Discuss the three major factors in weight training.

4. List the eight safety guidelines integral to any weight training program.

5. Explain the difference between isometric, isotonic, and isokinetic exercises.

6. Describe how repetitions, sets, and resistance work together to increase strength.

7. Explain how certain exercises work specific muscles or muscle groups.

8. Understand the concerns and benefits of cardiovascular conditioning.

KEY TERMS

* concentric contraction
* conditioning
* eccentric contraction
* isokinetic contraction
* isometric contraction
* isotonic contraction

* muscle mass
* muscle tone
* overload principle
* power
* proprioception
* resistance

* set
* specificity principle
* stretching
* variable resistance
* variation principle

INTRODUCTION

Conditioning prepares the body for optimized performance. It is achieved through building muscle strength and endurance, increasing and maintaining flexibility, and by exercising the heart and lungs. A healthy diet and proper hydration assists in this process by supplying the body with the fuel it needs to improve and maintain its level of fitness. Most effective when approached year-round, a good conditioning program addresses all of the health factors in fitness discussed in Chapter 3: muscle strength, muscle endurance, flexibility, cardiovascular endurance, body composition, and individuals' special considerations. The information in this chapter and Chapter 8 will help you understand how to help a client or an athlete achieve and maintain a healthy and productive level of fitness through the development of an ongoing conditioning program.

Effective conditioning programs require careful planning and consideration of certain fundamental rules. These "Rules of Conditioning" affect both the safety and success of the program and should be used in the development of all phases of every conditioning program. A discussion of these rules follows.

> **conditioning**
>
> the process of preparing the body for optimized performance.

Rules of Conditioning

1. **Safety.** Proper techniques should be used in all conditioning programs. Such techniques include the use of proper body mechanics, the correct use of equipment, and compliance with physician's instructions. Furthermore, the training area and all equipment should be inspected daily to make sure they are safe for use.

2. **Motivation.** Motivation is a prime conditioning factor for everyone. Without motivation, maximum effort won't be put forth. Most athletes are self-motivated by the prospect of competition, but even the best players respond well to external motivation in the form of enthusiasm and encouragement. Positive comments will help to motivate the client or athlete and reinforce the desired goal. When a conditioning program is working well for someone, periodic review of the goals and benefits of the program can also provide motivation.

3. **Specialization.** Exercises for strength, flexibility, and cardiovascular fitness should be included in the conditioning program. These exercises should be geared to condition the body to meet the demands of the specific sport or activity in which the athlete or client participates.

4. **Warm-up/Cooldown.** Adequate warm-up and cooldown periods are an essential part of the conditioning program. A warm-up should be done even before stretching; it prepares the large muscles for exercise and helps keep injuries from occurring. Warm-ups should last 5 to 10 minutes, and consist of any low-intensity total body cardiovascular activity such as bicycling, brisk walking, or jumping rope. Athletic trainers must keep up to date with any new warm-up procedures that pertain to an athlete's individual sport and make sure the coach is aware that one warm up time may not be adequate for the entire practice or game. For example, at the end of the half-time of a football game, the athletes will have to warm up again before the third quarter. Similarly, baseball players who don't go in until the fifth inning will have to rewarm up before they enter the game. Equally important, cooldowns should consist of flexibility exercises to allow the heart rate to gradually return to the resting pulse rate and to prevent the muscles from tightening up following the workout.

5. **Diet.** A healthy diet is vital to any conditioning program. Without the proper fuel, the body won't perform. Make sure athletes stay hydrated to avoid overheating and muscle cramping, and to achieve optimal performance during the workout.

6. **Hydration.** Individuals need to drink 17 fluid ounces 2 hours before exercise. During exercise, athletes should start drinking early and at regular intervals in an attempt to consume fluids at a rate sufficient to replace all the water lost through sweating (i.e., body weight loss). This comes from The American College of Sports Medicine position on hydration.

7. **Intensity.** The intensity of the work determines the results. Working out too hard breaks down the muscles and leaves them vulnerable to injury. Working out too little will not produce the desired benefits.

8. **Capacity.** Capacity means maximum capability. The client or athlete's performance should push physiological limits as far as health and safety factors will allow. Only by working to capacity will the desired results be achieved. To build up a muscle, you must overload it. Lifting or running to capacity increases strength and endurance. This is known as the *overload principle*. There is fine line between working to capacity and demanding too much from a person, causing injury. It is the athletic trainer's, coach's, or strength and conditioning specialist's responsibility to help the athlete find this line.

9. **Duration.** The length of time a workout should last depends on the client's or athlete's level of fitness and the level of conditioning that is desired. For example, at least 30 minutes of aerobic work is necessary just to maintain one's fitness level. So, workouts should be no shorter than 30 minutes, not counting the warm-up and cooldown. However, if more than simple maintenance is desired, longer workouts should be scheduled, based on the individual's endurance. Keep in mind that a practice or exercise session that lasts longer than two hours may tire the participants mentally and physically, and cause an increase in injuries. A tired athlete is prone to more injuries. Initially, clients who are in extremely poor shape may not be able to complete even a 30-minute workout. Such clients or athletes should start slowly and gradually increase the length of the workouts.

10. **Balanced Strength.** Developing strength is a means of increasing greater endurance and power or speed. The strength training should be balanced. This means that when the muscles

in the front are worked, the muscles in the back should be worked, too. Some examples of balanced strength training include biceps/triceps, hamstrings/quadriceps, chest/back, and abdomen/low back. Try to vary the strength program as the year goes on. This can help keep the athletes excited about the program.

11. **Routine.** A daily routine of exercises should be established and defined for each phase of the program. Make sure each phase of the program works with the client's or athlete's schedule; if the workouts are not consistent, the program will fail.

12. **Modification.** The program must address any special needs the client or athlete has. This might include designing a program that can be done in a wheelchair, that won't aggravate existing back problems, or that emphasizes an athlete's special requirements, such as a strong arm for throwing.

13. **Fun.** The importance of working hard, playing hard, and enjoyment cannot be overemphasized. This is an important concept to daily living as well as a conditioning program. One way to increase the fun of a conditioning program is to work out with a friend.

14. **Relaxation.** Relaxation is an important aspect of good physical and mental health. A proper balance of work, leisure, and sleep promotes a healthy outlook on life and prepares the body to handle the physical and mental stresses of everyday life.

15. **Progression.** Make sure to add small amounts of work to each practice period. Remember that it takes anywhere from six to eight weeks for an athlete to attain a top level of physical conditioning and to physically adjust to the sport.

BASIC PRINCIPLES OF WEIGHT TRAINING

The goal of conditioning is to improve or maintain performance in terms of strength, endurance, and flexibility. When combined with flexibility and cardiovascular exercises, weight training is the most effective method of accomplishing these goals. The primary benefits of weight training are muscle strength and muscle endurance. Secondary benefits are **muscle tone**, **muscle mass**, **power**, and flexibility. Weight training is based on three basic principles: overload, variation, and specificity.

The Overload Principle

The **overload principle** is by far the most important concept when starting any weight lifting or weight training program. This principle involves overloading the body's muscular or cardiovascular systems by working them harder than normal activity requires (see Figure 7-1). If the overload principle is followed correctly, the muscle strength, endurance, and size will all increase without injury because the muscles will be overloaded in a controlled exercise activity.

Overload can be achieved using these methods:

1. Increase the amount of weight lifted.

2. Increase the number of repetitions in a **set**.

3. Increase the number of sets that are performed.

muscle tone
the shape of a muscle in its resting state.

muscle mass
the girth or size of the muscle.

power
the ability to apply force with speed.

overload principle
the application of greater than normal stress to a muscle, resulting in increased capacity to do work. Gradually the muscle will adapt to the increased demand, making it necessary to increase the stress again.

set

a group of repetitions.

4. Decrease the speed with which repetitions are performed.

5. Decrease the amount of time between sets.

The Variation Principle

variation principle

the alteration or modification of exercises to work an entire muscle or group of muscles and to combat boredom.

The **variation principle** refers to the modification or alteration of the type of exercise that is performed, as well as the intensity, speed, sequence, and duration of the exercises. Variation is important because it combats boredom and works the total muscle. To apply the variation principle, you can use the methods that are listed for applying the overload principle. In addition, change equipment, vary the order in which exercises are done, and change the body position as the exercises are done. For example, on a bench press, switch from a narrow grip in which the hands grasp the bar close together to a wide grip in which the hands are placed far apart. Or, when perform-

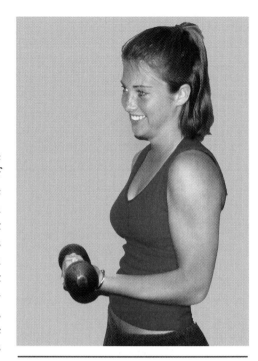

FIGURE 7-1 The overload requirement can be met in several ways, such as increasing the number of repetitions in a set.

ing lateral pulldowns, switch from a standard grip (palms facing forward) to a reverse grip (palms facing backward). Using a standard grip would emphasize the latissimus dorsi muscles; whereas using a reverse grip would emphasize the bicep muscles.

The Specificity Principle

specificity principle

the way in which an exercise relates to the activity for which performance enhancement is sought.

The **specificity principle** refers to the relationship between an exercise and the activity for which performance enhancement is sought. Exercises should be chosen based on the aspect of performance they enhance. For instance, those who participate in crew activities would be well-advised to use rowing machines as a part of their fitness routines, and athletes involved in throwing (e.g., baseball players, volleyball players, javelin throwers, football players, etc.) would benefit from exercises that strengthen the musculature of the rotator cuff. Specificity is important when improvement in a given activity is desired because an exercise that closely resembles the motion of the activity will improve one's ability more than an exercise that does not resemble the motion involved.

EXERCISING MUSCLES CORRECTLY

When starting clients or athletes with a weight training exercise, first consider their goals. Is the primary goal to gain muscle flexibility, tone, mass, endurance, or strength? In most cases all are desired results, but occasionally, one aspect may be the client's primary goal.

If the goal is flexibility, they will usually have a specific area of the body in mind, so the focus should be on **stretching** the muscle groups in that area of the body. When the goal is to tone the muscles, concentrate on performing as many repetitions as possible using relatively light weights. To gain muscle mass, heavy weights should be used with fewer repetitions. To increase endurance, concentrate on increasing the repetitions in each set, so instead of doing four sets of 10 reps, the athlete would do four sets of as many reps as tolerated before fatigue sets in, causing the loss of proper form. Strengthening will take place when muscle tone, mass, or endurance is increased. Therefore, when the goal is to strengthen the muscles, begin with the maximum amount of weight the client can comfortably lift 10 times without stopping (10 repetitions). When muscles are worked repeatedly, they become stronger and more toned.

Over time, your clients will find that the amount of weight being lifted no longer provides much **resistance** to their muscles, which are now stronger. This is the point at which it is appropriate to increase the amount of weight being lifted. Add a small amount of weight to the exercise, but decrease the number of repetitions (reps) performed in each set (e.g., begin again with 10 reps). The number of sets can remain the same, so if the client is accustomed to doing two sets of 20 reps, you might begin with increased weight for two sets of 10 reps. As the client's muscles become accustomed to the increased weight, more repetitions can be added to the sets.

To determine the proper amount of weight to add, you will have to consider the part of the body being strengthened. For example, for the small muscle groups, such as the biceps and triceps, 2-pound increments would be appropriate; and for the large muscle groups, such as the quadriceps, pectorals, and rhomboids, you would probably want to use 5-pound increments.

Don't forget the importance of strength balancing. As discussed in Chapter 3, balance means that what is done on the front or one side should also be done on the back or the other side. Therefore, to create balance of strength in the upper legs, if clients work the quadriceps for two sets of 10, they should also work the hamstrings for two sets of 10.

All weight exercises should be done following practice sessions—not before. Exercising following practice avoids injuries to the arm caused by muscles that are tired from exercising. If it is necessary to do the exercises prior to practice, the muscles should be allowed to rest for three hours before practice begins.

stretching

gently forcing the muscle to lengthen.

resistance

counterforce.

Safety Guidelines for Weight Training

The SCS needs to make sure that a client's weight training program is safe. Remind clients to use the following guidelines during every weight lifting session:

1. **Warm-Up/Cooldown.** As with any type of conditioning, it's important to warm up the large muscle groups for 5 to 10 minutes before proceeding to the exercise routine. Some warm-up activities include jumping rope, running in place, doing jumping jacks, and pedaling a stationary bike. A 5- to 10-minute cooldown will prevent the muscles from cramping by restretching the muscles following the exercise.

2. **Stretching.** All weight training sessions should be preceded by the stretching of the muscles to be worked.

3. **Spotting.** When using free weights, spotting is very important. A "spotter" is a person who protects the client by removing the weight from the client's grasp if the client loses control of the weight. Make sure to go over expectations with spotters before the start of an exercise set. Spotting is very important in the use of free weights; if a client is performing bench presses and is unable to complete the last repetition, the client may become trapped under the weight without a spotter there.

4. **Collars.** A collar (see Figure 7-2) is a device that secures the weights to the bar being lifted. When using free weights, make sure to use collars on the ends of the weight bars.

5. **Muscle Balance.** Make sure that the muscles are worked on the front side of the muscle group in the same way they are worked on the back side of the muscle group.

6. **Range of Motion (ROM).** Make sure your clients work the entire range of motion by achieving full flexion and extension of the muscle during each exercise.

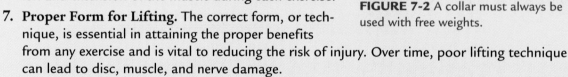

FIGURE 7-2 A collar must always be used with free weights.

7. **Proper Form for Lifting.** The correct form, or technique, is essential in attaining the proper benefits from any exercise and is vital to reducing the risk of injury. Over time, poor lifting technique can lead to disc, muscle, and nerve damage.

* All lifting is done in a slow and controlled manner. The **eccentric contraction** of bringing the weight down should take twice as long as it does to bring the weight up. For instance, when doing an arm curl, it should take about 2 seconds to go through the ROM on the way up during the **concentric contraction**, but it should take about 4 seconds to let the weight down during the eccentric contraction.

* To keep the natural curves of the back in proper alignment, a broad base of support, 1 to 4 feet in width, is maintained with the feet.

* To reduce the strain on the lower back and provide the proper leverage, the weight is kept close to the body.

* The resistance or weight should be tested before attempting to fully press or lift it. If it is too heavy, reduce the amount of weight before attempting to lift it again.

* Proper breathing helps facilitate the lift and is done by exhaling (breathing out) while performing the lift and inhaling (breathing in) when returning to the starting position of the exercise.

* Following the manufacturer's instructions for use and maintenance of all exercise equipment is extremely important. This helps ensure the user's safety and helps protect you from liability in the event an injury does occur.

* Using the momentum of a weight machine to assist with the next repetition should be avoided, as it interferes with obtaining the full benefits of the exercise. Bouncing the weight bar of either free or guided weights creates a similar momentum and also must be avoided. The bouncing of free weights may also cause injuries.

* Pausing before the completion of a repetition and holding the bar unevenly interferes with obtaining the full benefits of the exercise and should be avoided.

* As with all exercises, if the activity causes pain or increases pain, it should be stopped and the method reevaluated. Any pain that persists should be evaluated by a physician. Advise clients or athletes to stop the activity immediately if they feel dizzy or faint; experience pain in the chest, neck, or arm; or experience extreme shortness of breath. If symptoms persist or increase, contact the EMS.

FLEXIBILITY EXERCISES

Flexibility exercises (see Figure 7-3) are an important part of conditioning. Important on their own in terms of the range of motion they produce, they must also be performed regularly in conjunction with strength training, both before and after a workout. Performed prior to strengthening, these stretching exercises allow the muscles to work with less risk of injury. When performed after a workout, these stretches reduce the risk of muscle cramps and tightening.

To avoid injury and obtain maximum benefits, flexibility exercises should always be preceded by an appropriate warm-up period. Once the muscles are warmed up, they are stretched properly by filling the lungs with air just before the stretch and slowly releasing the air as the stretch is performed, easing and relaxing into the stretch as the air is exhaled. The stretch should produce moderate tension in the muscle but not cause pain. Stretches are held at moderate tension for 15 to

eccentric contraction
the lengthening of a muscle during contraction.

concentric contraction
the shortening of a muscle during contraction.

Flexibility Exercises for Target Areas

Body Part	Muscle Group	Stretch
Neck	Sternocleidomastoids	Lateral Neck Stretch
Chest	Pectorals	Chest Stretch
Shoulders	Deltoids	Anterior Deltoid Stretch
		Posterior Deltoid Stretch
Arms	Triceps	Triceps Stretch
	Wrist flexors	Wrist Stretch
Trunk/Hips	Low back muscles	Low Back Stretch (One Knee)
	Low back muscles	Low Back Stretch (Both Knees)
	Low to mid back muscles	Cat Stretch
	Hips/abdominals	Trunk Extension/Abdominals
	Low back and gluteals	Hip/Trunk Stretch
	Hip flexors	Hip Flexor Stretch
Groin	Adductors	Groin Stretch (Butterfly)
Legs	Hamstrings	Lying Hamstring Stretch
		Standing Hamstring Stretch
	Quadriceps	Standing Quadriceps Stretch
	Gastrocnemius/	Gastrocnemius Stretch
	soleus complex	Soleus Stretch

FIGURE 7-3 Suggested Flexibility Exercises and the Muscles They Stretch

30 seconds, inhaling and exhaling at a relaxed rate to obtain the full benefit of the stretch. Both sides of the body should be worked equally; stretch one side and then the other.

Lateral Neck Stretch (Figure 7-4)

Start Position: Instruct the client to stand up straight and place the palm of one hand on the top of the head with the fingers extending down the opposite side of the head. The other hand is placed behind the back.

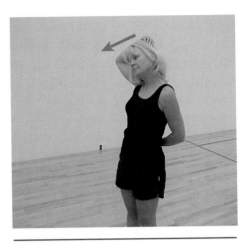

FIGURE 7-4 Lateral Neck Stretch

Stretch: The head is tilted laterally, in the direction of the upper hand, keeping the shoulders in line with each other. Resistance is created by gently pulling the head with the upper hand.

Chest Stretch (Figure 7-5)

Start Position: Instruct the client to stand facing the corner of a room at arm's distance away from the walls. The hands are placed flat against the walls at shoulder height, slightly in front of the body. One foot is placed in front of the other foot to provide support and balance during the stretch.

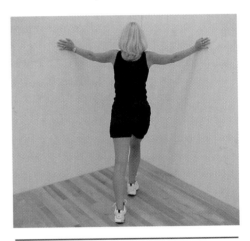

FIGURE 7-5 Chest Stretch

Stretch: The client leans into the corner, leading with the chest. The arms are kept straight as the client leans forward to stretch the chest muscles.

Anterior Deltoid Stretch (Figure 7-6)

Start Position: Instruct the client to stand with one side of the body a little closer than arm's reach to a wall. The inside hand is placed flat against the wall and behind the body as far as possible. The arm should be at shoulder level.

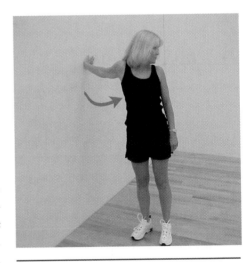

FIGURE 7-6 Anterior Deltoid Stretch

Stretch: Keeping the hand flat against the wall, the upper body is twisted away from the wall as far as possible without discomfort. Most of the twisting motion should come from the shoulder region.

Posterior Deltoid Stretch (Figure 7-7)

Start Position: Instruct the client to stand and extend one arm at shoulder level. The other hand is made into a fist and placed on the lateral aspect of the extended arm's elbow.

Stretch: The fist is used to pull the outstretched arm closer to the body, stretching the posterior deltoid.

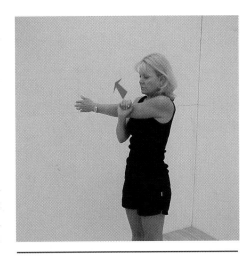

FIGURE 7-7 Posterior Deltoid Stretch

Triceps Stretch (Figure 7-8)

Start Position: Instruct the client to stand up straight and raise one arm up, bending the elbow to reach as far down the back as possible without discomfort. The opposite hand is placed on the elbow of the bent arm.

Stretch: The hand on the elbow is used to pull the elbow toward the back of the head until a stretch can be felt in the triceps, but not so far as to cause pain.

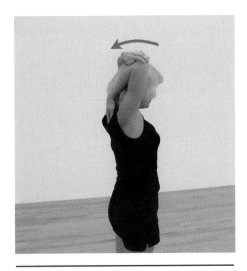

FIGURE 7-8 Triceps Stretch

Wrist Stretch (Figure 7-9)

Start Position: Instruct the client to bring both hands together in front of the chest, placing the fingers of one hand against the palm of the other hand.

Stretch: The client presses with the upper hand against the fingers in the palm, pushing them back toward the elbow. Resisting the pressure of the palm against the fingers should result in the stretching of the wrist tendons, but not so far as to cause pain. Hand positions should be switched to

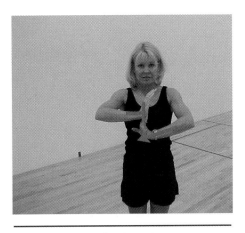

FIGURE 7-9 Wrist Stretch

achieve a balance in the flexibility of the wrists. This can also be reversed to stretch the wrist flexion.

Back Extension/Abdominals Stretch (Figure 7-10)

Start Position: Instruct the client to lie face-down on the floor or an exercise mat. The hands are then placed on the floor in line with the shoulders and used to raise the upper body off the floor.

Stretch: Keeping the pelvis as close to the floor as possible, the client pushes back with the arms, arching the back until a moderate stretch is felt in the abdomen, but not so far as to cause pain. The head and neck are kept straight.

Low Back Stretch (One Knee) (Figure 7-11)

Start Position: Instruct the client to lie in the supine position. One knee is then flexed, brought to the chest, and held with both hands. The other leg may remain extended, or it may be flexed at the knee with the foot flat on the floor.

Stretch: Keeping the back on the floor at all times, the client pulls the knee downward toward the chest, until a moderate stretch of the lower back and gluteal muscles is felt, but not so far as to cause pain.

Low Back Stretch (Both Knees) (Figure 7-12)

Start Position: Instruct the client to lie on the floor or on an exercise mat in the supine position. Both knees are then flexed, brought to the chest, and held with the hands.

Stretch: Keeping the back on the floor at all times, the client pulls the knees downward toward the chest, until a moderate

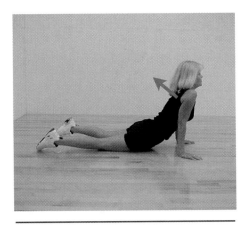

FIGURE 7-10 Back Extension/ Abdominals Stretch

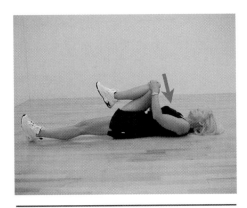

FIGURE 7-11 Low Back Stretch, One Knee to Chest

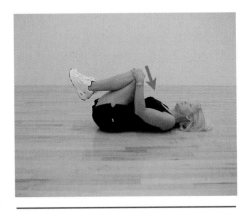

FIGURE 7-12 Low Back Stretch, Both Knees to Chest

stretch of the lower back and gluteal muscles is felt, but not so far as to cause pain.

Cat Stretch (Upper and Mid-Back) (Figures 7-13, 7-14)

Start Position: Instruct the client to get down on hands and knees, with the hands placed directly under the shoulders and the knees under the buttocks. The back is kept straight.

Stretch: This is a two-part stretch, requiring both an upward and a downward movement to obtain the full benefits. The client stretches the target area upward by simultaneously arching the back up, pulling the abdominals in, and tucking the chin toward the chest. The downward stretch consists of simultaneously allowing the back to sag, pushing the abdominal area toward the floor, and raising the head up.

Hip Flexor Stretch (Figure 7-15)

Start Position: Instruct the client to stand with feet apart, one placed in front of the body and one in back. The front leg is bent at the knee, and that foot is kept flat on the floor about 12 inches in front of the body. The back leg is extended behind the body as far as possible without discomfort. The arms are relaxed and either hang at the sides of the body or rest on the thigh of the forward leg.

Stretch: The client presses the hips forward and downward, bending the front knee and keeping the back leg as straight as possible. The back heel may come off the floor. The stretch should be felt in the front of the hip and in the quadriceps on the anterior thigh.

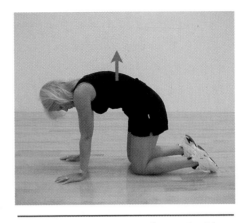
FIGURE 7-13 Cat Stretch, Up Position

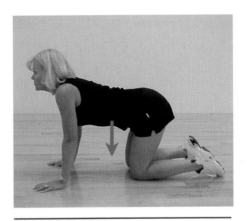
FIGURE 7-14 Cat Stretch, Down Position

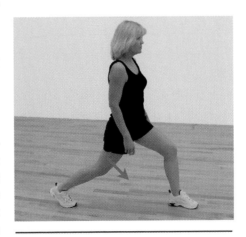
FIGURE 7-15 Hip Flexor Stretch

Hip/Trunk/Tensor Fasciae Latae (TFL) Stretch (Figure 7-16)

Start Position: Instruct the client to lie on the back with legs straight. One knee is flexed, brought toward the chest, and grasped with the opposite hand. The free arm is extended at a 90° angle to the body.

Stretch: The client crosses the knee over the body and presses the knee toward the floor until a moderate stretch is felt in the tensor fasciae latae on the lateral thigh. The lower back is kept in contact with the floor during the entire stretch.

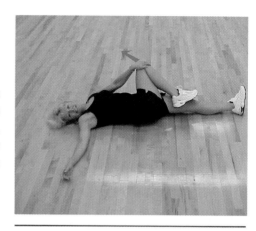

FIGURE 7-16 Hip/Trunk/TFL Stretch

Groin Stretch (Butterfly) (Figure 7-17)

Start Position: Instruct the client to sit on the floor or an exercise mat. The knees are flexed and the soles of the feet brought together at the midline of the body. The arms rest on the inner aspects of the legs, and the ankles are grasped.

Stretch: The client pushes the knees toward the floor until a moderate stretch is felt in the groin muscles. The client may gently press down against the legs with the elbows to increase the resistance of this stretch.

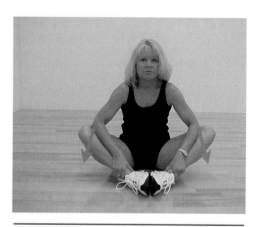

FIGURE 7-17 Groin Stretch, Butterfly

Lying Hamstring Stretch (Figure 7-18)

Start Position: Instruct the client to lie on the back with both knees flexed so the feet are flat on the floor. One leg is then straightened, and the toes of that foot are pointed toward the floor.

Stretch: The client raises the straight leg as far as possible, keeping it straight. The stretch should be felt in the hamstrings.

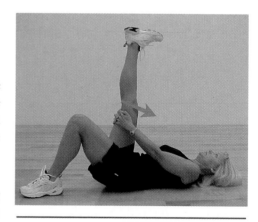

FIGURE 7-18 Lying Hamstring Stretch

To assist in the stretch, the client may interlock the fingers behind the straight leg and pull toward the chest.

Standing Hamstring Stretch (Figure 7-19)

Start Position: Instruct the client to stand and extend one foot in front of the body. The ball of the extended foot is placed on a platform, 4 to 8 inches high, and the heel is kept on the floor. The hands are placed on the hips to maintain balance through the stretch.

Stretch: The client leans forward from the hips, keeping the front leg straight, toe elevated, and heel on the floor, until a moderate stretch of the hamstring muscles is felt, but not so far as to cause pain. This can be done with or without toes elevated.

Standing Quadriceps Stretch (Figure 7-20)

Start Position: Instruct the client to stand at arm's distance away from a wall. One hand is placed flat against the wall at shoulder height, at a 90° angle to the side of the body. The knee of the leg closest to the wall is then flexed and the ball of that foot grasped with the opposite hand.

Stretch: The ball of the foot is pulled toward the buttocks until a moderate stretch of the quadriceps muscles is felt, but not so far as to cause pain.

Gastrocnemius Stretch (Figure 7-21)

Start Position: Instruct the client to stand facing a wall at arm's distance away from the wall. The hands are placed flat against the wall at shoulder height. One foot is placed in front of the other; the forward leg is bent at the knee and the rear leg is kept straight, with the heel on the floor.

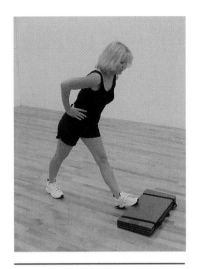

FIGURE 7-19 Standing Hamstring Stretch

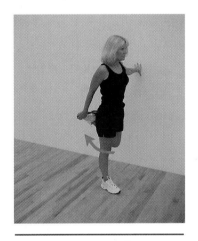

FIGURE 7-20 Standing Quadriceps Stretch

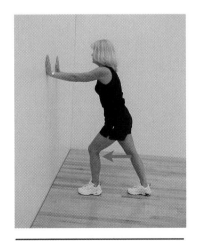

FIGURE 7-21 Gastrocnemius Stretch

Stretch: The client leans toward the wall, leading with the hips and flexing the arms as necessary. The heel of the rear foot is kept on the floor as the client leans forward to moderately stretch the gastrocnemius.

Soleus Stretch (Figure 7-22)

Start Position: Instruct the client to stand facing a wall at arm's distance away from the wall. The hands are placed flat against the wall at shoulder height. One foot is placed in front of the other with both knees bent and the feet flat on the floor.

Stretch: The client leans toward the wall, leading with the hips and flexing the arms as necessary. The heel of the rear foot is kept on the floor and the knee bent as the client leans forward to moderately stretch the soleus.

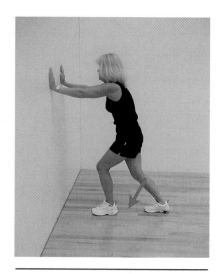

FIGURE 7-22 Soleus Stretch

STRENGTHENING EXERCISES

Muscles can be exercised in a variety of ways through different types of muscle contractions. The shortening of a muscle, accomplished through flexion, is called a concentric, or positive, contraction. The lengthening of the muscle is called an eccentric, or negative, contraction. Both types of contractions are essential to conditioning and can be produced in a variety of ways, using free weights, guided weights, or just the weight of the body, among other methods.

Isometric Exercises

> **isometric contraction**
>
> a muscle contraction with no motion that results in no change in the length of the muscle.

An **isometric contraction** results in no change in the length of the muscle; the muscle neither lengthens or shortens as it is contracted. This is done by applying pressure against a stable resistance, thereby increasing muscle tension, such as when a person pushes or pulls against an immovable object. For example, the rotator cuff can be strengthened isometrically by pressing the wrist and forearm against a wall through external rotation of the shoulder (Figure 7-23). Isometric exercises can help maintain and improve muscle strength and tone, but they can only build strength to a certain point because of their inability to work the muscle with an overload through the entire range of motion. Therefore, it is important to also include isotonic and isokinetic exercises in a strengthening program. Sometimes isometric exercises are only used

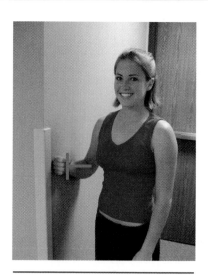

FIGURE 7-23 Isometric External Rotation, Shoulder

to test muscle strength—not to increase it. They are also useful in the early phases of physical rehabilitation because no range of motion is involved, limiting the amount of pain produced by the exercise.

When performing isometrics, it is important to work the whole muscle by varying the point of resistance during the muscle contractions. For example, in the rotator cuff exercise the point of resistance can be varied by shifting the position of the feet relative to the wall as well as the degree of shoulder rotation. This helps improve the range of motion for that muscle group.

The disadvantages of isometrics are their inability to work a muscle through the entire range of motion with movement. Reduced risk of injury due to the lack of a counter (opposing) force is the primary advantage of isometric exercises, but it is also helpful that no expensive equipment is required.

Isotonic Exercises

An **isotonic contraction** occurs when the muscle bears the same weight throughout the entire range of motion (see Figures 7-24 and 7-25). Isotonic exercises greatly improve joint mobility as well as muscle strength and tone. The muscle will shorten and lengthen as it goes through the contraction.

Disadvantages of isotonic exercises include the requirement of equipment, some of which is expensive, and the increased likelihood of injury if the exercises are done incorrectly, too much weight is applied, or spotting is done incorrectly. Advantages are that free weights, which are not terribly expensive, can be used in isotonic exercises. Furthermore, full jugs of water, sand-filled socks, or other similar homemade devices can be substituted for free weights to perform isotonic exercises without any expense at all. The use of free weights in isotonic exercises provides an additional benefit: they enhance **proprioception** by working the surrounding muscles more effectively than guided weights.

> **isotonic contraction**
>
> a muscle contraction produced by a constant external resistance.

> **proprioception**
>
> the ability to sense the location, position, orientation, and movement of the body and it parts.

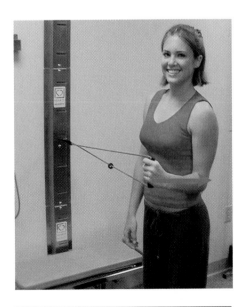

FIGURE 7-24 Isotonic External Rotation, Shoulder, Free Weights

FIGURE 7-25 Isotonic External Rotation, Shoulder, Pulley

Isokinetic Exercises

isokinetic contraction

a muscle contraction produced by a variable external resistance at a constant speed.

An **isokinetic contraction** occurs in the muscles when the speed of the exercise stays constant throughout the range of motion, while the resistance against the muscle varies according to the amount of force applied. This type of contraction will work the muscle to its full capacity through the entire range of motion (ROM).

Isokinetic exercises can be performed on equipment that provides hydraulic resistance or electronic resistance (see Figure 7-26). Both hydraulic and electronic resistance machines exercise muscles during concentric muscle contractions; some electronic resistance equipment can be adjusted to exercise muscles during either concentric contractions, eccentric contractions, or both. They are also used in strength testing concentricly, eccentricly, and isometricly. Eccentric contractions in the rotator cuff are important because they strengthen the muscles that decelerate the throwing action and cause the arm to stop.

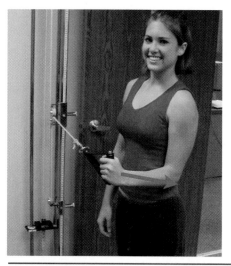

FIGURE 7-26 Isokinetic External Rotation, Shoulder, Isokinetic Machine

Another type of isokinetic exercise is called a **variable resistance** exercise. This is an exercise in which the client uses a guided weight machine or other equipment to vary the muscle resistance as the joint moves through its range of motion (see Figure 7-27). The variable resistance

variable resistance

a resistance exercise that varies through the range of motion.

equipment is designed to offer resistance that closely matches the strength curve of the exercised muscle through the range of motion. It has been shown that as a person goes through the ROM of a joint, certain muscle areas have more strength in them than other muscle areas because of the angles at which the joint may be flexing. Therefore, in order to overload every muscle area in the range of motion, the amount of weight must be varied as the range of motion changes. There is also the CAM system that delivers constant torque throughout the range of motion.

Isokinetic exercises have their drawbacks: the equipment required to do them is very expensive; there is an increased likelihood of injury if done incorrectly or if too much resistance is

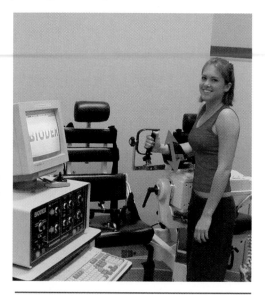

FIGURE 7-27 Isokinetic (Variable Resistance) External Rotation, Shoulder, Elastic Band

applied; and to get speeds fast enough to mirror sports activities is difficult, if not impossible. However, these exercises are great for maximum working of the muscle at every point along the range of motion.

Strengthening Exercises by Muscle Group

The following sections describe exercises that can be used to strengthen various muscle groups (see Figure 7-28). Many of these exercises can be done in a gym or using home equipment. Furthermore, variations of some of them can also be performed using nontraditional items such as surgical tubing and household items like bottles of water.

Strengthening Exercises for Target Areas

Body Part	Muscle Group	Exercise
Chest	Pectorals	Incline Bench Press
		Bench Press
		Chest Fly
Shoulders	Deltoids	Bent-Over Row
		Military Press
		Deltoid Raise
Arms	Triceps	Chair Dip
		Triceps Curl
	Biceps	Biceps Curl
Trunk/Hips	Latissimus dorsi	Lat Pulldown
	Rhomboids	Bent-Over Row
		Seated Row
	Trapezoids	Upright Row
	Abdominals	Sit-Up
		Internal & External Rotational Trunk Curls
	Low back	Trunk Extension
	Hips	Hip Adduction
		Hip Abduction
		Hip Flexion
		Hip Extension
		Squat
Legs	Quadriceps/gluteals	Leg Press
		Hack Squat
		Squat
	Hamstrings	Leg Curl
	Gastrocnemius/soleus	Heel Raise

FIGURE 7-28 Suggested Strengthening Exercises and the Muscles They Work

CHEST/PECTORALIS STRENGTHENING

The pectoral muscles are located in the upper thoracic region. These muscles are used in arm and shoulder movements such as pushing, pulling, and throwing, among others. For example, football offensive linemen rely on these muscles when blocking defensive opponents. To preserve the balance of strength, pectoral exercises should be accompanied by exercises that strengthen the back muscles—particularly the rhomboids.

Incline Bench Press—Free Weights

Start Position: Instruct the client to assume a comfortable position on the bench (Figure 7-29). The client grasps the bar with elbows flexed at approximately a 90° angle. The back is kept straight and flat against the back of the bench. The spotter assists the client in slowly pressing the bar off the stops; then the client assumes the entire weight and fully extends both arms.

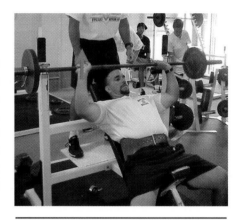

FIGURE 7-29 Incline Bench Press, Start Position with Spotter

Exercise: The client slowly lowers the bar to the chest. As soon as the bar touches the chest, the repetition is completed by pressing the bar back up to the start position, arms fully extended. The bar should be kept moving straight up and down as smoothly as possible, and it must not bounce off the client's chest to help in pushing the bar back up.

Bench Press—Free Weights

Start Position: Instruct the client to assume a comfortable position on the bench (Figure 7-30) and grasp the bars so that when the bar is lowered to the chest, both hands will be at about elbows' width apart, the upper and lower arms forming roughly a 90° angle. Be sure the client keeps the back flat against the back rest. The spotter assists the client in slowly raising the bar off of the stops, then the client assumes the entire weight and fully extends both arms.

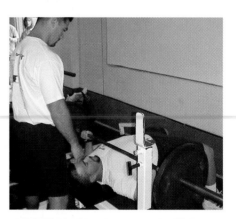

FIGURE 7-30 Bench Press, Start Position

Exercise: The client slowly lowers the bar to the chest. As soon as the bar touches the chest, the repetition is completed by pressing the bar back up to the start position, arms fully extended. The bar should be kept moving up and down as evenly as possible, and it must not bounce off the client's chest to help in pushing the bar back up.

Chest Fly—Guided Weights

Start Position: Instruct the client to sit on the bench, back straight and flat against the bench (Figure 7-31). The client then grasps the handles that provide the most comfortable position as well as proper form: the upper arms should form roughly a 90° angle with the side of the chest.

Exercise: The handles are pulled forward toward the middle of the chest through the machine's range of motion to achieve full flexion of the pectorals. The repetition is completed by returning to the start position, using the pectorals to resist the movement of the machine in an eccentric contraction.

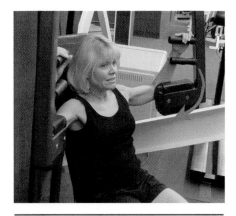

FIGURE 7-31 Chest Fly, Start Position

Incline Bench Press—Guided Weights with Variable Resistance

Start Position: Instruct the client to sit on the bench and grasp the handles. The bars should be about shoulder height, forming roughly a 90° angle between the upper arms and the forearms. The feet should be flat on the floor and the back flat against the back rest.

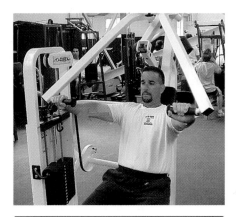

FIGURE 7-32 Incline Bench Press, Full Extension

Exercise: Using even and controlled motions, both handles are pressed out, away from the body through the machine's range of motion, until full extension is attained on both sides (Figure 7-32). The repetition is completed by returning the handles to the start position, using the pectorals to resist the movement of the machine. Since the right and left sides move independently of each other, proper form is maintained by keeping the handles in as straight a line as possible.

DELTOID STRENGTHENING

The deltoid is the large muscle covering the anterior, posterior, superior, and lateral shoulder, giving the joint its rounded appearance. Responsible for the types of overhead and swinging arm motions used in throwing, golfing, swimming, and tennis, this muscle also makes certain lifts possible—such as those performed in cheerleading and dance. When your clients are working on strengthening the deltoids, remind them that there are three aspects to the deltoid, and all three aspects must be strengthened. The military press exercises the entire deltoid, but the other exercises presented here strengthen only one aspect of the muscle: using the bench press or the incline bench will help to strengthen the anterior aspect of the deltoid; the deltoid raise will strengthen the lateral deltoid; and the bent-over row will help to strengthen the posterior deltoid. As an SCS or athletic trainer, you should make a conscious effort to make sure that the exercises for this muscle group are balanced. Clients with pain from a shoulder impingement should avoid deltoid exercises that extend the arm past 90° until the pain has subsided.

Bent-Over Row—Free Weights

Start Position: Instruct the client to stand behind the bar with feet flat on the floor about hip width apart. Bending approximately 20° at the hips and with the knees as necessary, the client then grasps the bar with the hands placed slightly more than shoulder width apart. The client then lifts the bar slightly so that the arms are fully extended and the bar is not touching the floor (Figure 7-33).

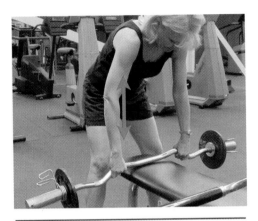

FIGURE 7-33 Bent-Over Row, Start Position

Exercise: The bar is pulled up toward the chest with the elbows pointing up. The repetition is completed by slowly lowering the bar back to the start position in a controlled motion. Note: You can also use dumbbells.

Military Press—Free Weights

Start Position: Instruct the client to sit on the bench, facing the weight bar. The bar is grasped at points that create 90° angles for both the elbows and shoulders.

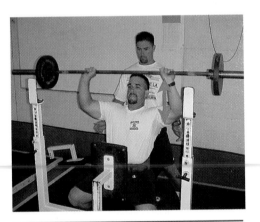

FIGURE 7-34 Military Press, Mid-Range Position

Exercise: With the spotter in position, the client lifts the bar off the stops and gently rests the bar across the chest. The client presses the bar as straight as possible above the head (Figure 7-34), until the arms are fully extended. The repetition is completed by slowly lowering the bar to the chest. The client must maintain complete control of the movements and avoid bouncing the bar off the chest. Bouncing the bar is poor form and may cause injury.

Military Press—Guided Weights

Start Position: Instruct the client to sit on the bench and grasp the handles (Figure 7-35). The bars should be about elbows' width apart and shoulder height, forming roughly a 90° angle between the upper arms and the forearms. The feet should be flat on the floor and the back flat against the back rest.

Exercise: Using even and controlled motions, both handles are pressed up, away from the body through the machine's range of motion, until full extension is attained on both sides. The repetition is completed by returning the handles to the start position, using the pectorals to resist the movement of the machine.

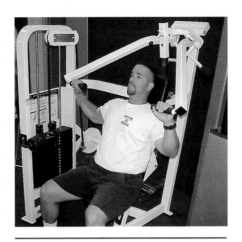

FIGURE 7-35 Deltoid Raise, Military Press, Start Position

Deltoid Raise—Guided Weights

Start Position: Instruct the client to sit at the machine and grasp the handles (Figure 7-36). The back should be flat against the back rest and the elbows should lie against the arm pads.

Exercise: The client raises the elbows up to, but not above, shoulder height. The repetition is completed by slowly returning the arms to the start position, using the lateral deltoid to resist the movement of the machine. Maximum benefits are obtained by squeezing the shoulder blades together during the raise.

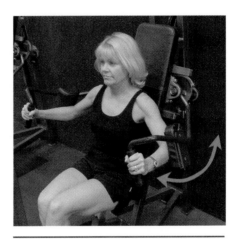

FIGURE 7-36 Deltoid Raise, Start Position

LATISSIMUS DORSI STRENGTHENING

The latissimus dorsi are large triangular muscles that fan across the upper back. These muscles assist in motions that pull the arms back. Swimmers, gymnasts, and others who rely on such arm movements will benefit from strong latissimus dorsi muscles.

Lat Pulldown—Guided Weights

Start Position: Instruct the client to sit on the bench facing the bar. The client grasps the bar slightly wider than elbows' width apart. The back is flat against the back pad.

Exercise: The client uses the latissimus dorsi to pull the bar through the machine's range of motion toward the abdomen (Figure 7-37). The bar, however, does not need to come into contact with the abdomen. The repetition is completed by returning to the start position using the latissimus dorsi to resist the movement of the bar.

RHOMBOID STRENGTHENING

The rhomboids are located in the back beneath the trapezius muscle layer. These muscles extend from the inner edge of the scapula to the spine and assist in pulling motions such as those used by rowers, swimmers, and wrestlers. For proper balance of strength, these exercises should be combined with pectoral strengthening.

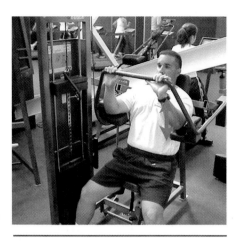

FIGURE 7-37 Lat Pulldown, Guided Weights, Mid-Range Position

Bent-Over Row— Free Weights

See the instructions for a bent-over row under "Deltoid Strengthening," earlier in this chapter.

Seated Row—Guided Weights

Start Position: Instruct the client to sit on the bench with the chest against the chest pad, facing the weight stack. The client grasps the handles and keeps the feet flat on the floor.

Exercise: Contracting the muscles of the upper back and retracting the shoulder blades, the client pulls the bars back so they are about even with the chest (Figure 7-38). The repetition is completed by returning the bars to the start position, using the rhomboids to resist the movement of the machine.

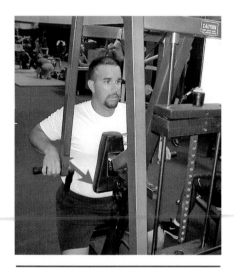

FIGURE 7-38 Rhomboids, Guided Weights, Full Flexion of Muscle

TRICEPS STRENGTHENING

The triceps extend down the entire length of the posterior surface of the humerus in the upper arm. Used to extend the arm, they also keep the head of the humerus in the glenoid cavity. Athletes engaged in javelin, baseball, softball, karate, or other throwing activities should be encouraged to develop strong triceps muscles.

Chair Dip—Body Weight

Start Position: Instruct the client to sit on a chair and grasp the front of the seat with both hands. The legs are either extended away from the chair or slightly bent at the knees. Using the strength of the arms, the client lifts the body out of the chair and away from the seat until the buttocks are in front of the chair (Figure 7-39).

Exercise: The client slowly lowers the body toward the floor as far as possible, flexing the elbows and keeping the hips, back, and neck aligned perpendicular to the floor. After a pause at the bottom of the movement, the client pushes back up with the triceps until the arms are fully extended. The client should avoid locking the arms at the elbows.

Triceps Curl—Free Weights

Start Position: Instruct the client to grasp a dumbbell with one hand and place the other hand on a bench for support. The upper arm of the weighted hand is kept parallel to the torso, while the elbow is flexed 90° (Figure 7-40).

Exercise: Keeping the upper arm still, the triceps is contracted as the lower arm is pulled back to full extension in line with the upper arm. After a pause at the top of the curl (full extension), the client slowly returns the dumbbell to the start position under control.

Triceps Curl—Guided Weights

Start Position: Instruct the client to sit on the bench facing the handles. The client then places the elbows in the middle of the elbow pads and grasps the handles with palms facing each other.

Exercise: The client tightens the triceps muscles to curl the bar toward the shoulders through the machine's range of motion (Figure 7-41). After a pause at full extension, the repetition is completed by returning the bar to the start position, using the triceps to resist the movement of the machine.

BICEPS STRENGTHENING

The biceps muscle extends down the length of the anterior surface of the humerus. This muscle is used primarily

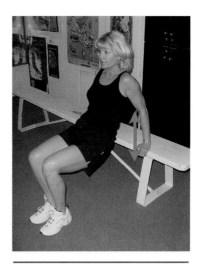

FIGURE 7-39 Chair Dip, Body Weight, Start Position

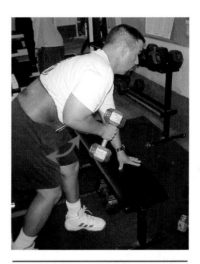

FIGURE 7-40 Triceps Curl, Free Weights, Start Position

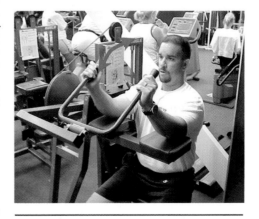

FIGURE 7-41 Triceps Curl, Guided Weights, Full Extension

in flexion of the arms. The biceps muscles assist in lifting and throwing motions such as those used in baseball, gymnastics, bowling, weight lifting, and racquet sports. When combined with triceps exercises, the following biceps exercises—and others like them—will produce balanced strength in the arm muscles and reduce the chance of injury.

Biceps Curl—Guided Weights

Start Position: Instruct the client to sit on the bench facing the handles. The client then places the elbows in the middle of the elbow pads and grasps the handles with palms facing the body.

Exercise: The client tightens the biceps muscles to curl the bar toward the shoulders through the machine's range of motion (Figure 7-42). After a pause at full flexion, the repetition is completed by returning the bar to the start position, using the biceps to resist the movement of the machine.

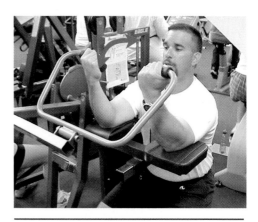

FIGURE 7-42 Biceps Curl, Guided Weights, Mid-Range Position

Biceps Curl—Free Weights (Dumbbell)

Start Position: Instruct the client to pick up a dumbbell and sit with both legs on one side of the bench. Bending from the hips, the client leans slightly forward and places the elbow of the weighted arm on the inner aspect of the thigh.

Exercise: Without moving the upper arm, the client contracts the biceps muscle to curl the dumbbell to approximately shoulder height (Figure 7-43). After a pause at the top of the curl, the repetition is completed by slowly lowering the dumbbell back to start position in a controlled motion, moving only the lower arm. The client should avoid bouncing the dumbbell to prevent injury.

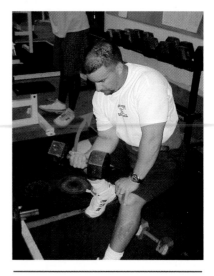

FIGURE 7-43 Biceps Curl, Free Weights (Dumbbell), Mid-Range Position

Biceps Curl—Free Weights (Curl Bar)

Start Position: Instruct the client to bend at the knees to grasp and lift the curl bar with both hands about shoulder width apart. After resuming a standing position, the feet are also placed about shoulder width apart to provide good balance. The bar is held in front of the thighs with the elbows fully extended.

Exercise: The client contracts the biceps muscles to curl the bar to approximately shoulder height (Figure 7-44). Touching the chest area with the bar or hands as a method of marking the top of the curl is optional. After a pause at the top of the curl, the bar is slowly lowered back to the start position, resisting the movement on the way down. Only the lower arms are moved during this exercise. There may be a tendency for clients to sway with the motion of the bar or bounce the bar off the thighs in an effort to get a little help to complete the next repetition. Swaying and bouncing are both poor form and should be avoided.

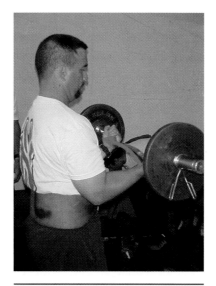

FIGURE 7-44 Biceps Curl, Free Weights (Curl Bar), Mid-Range Position

TRAPEZOID STRENGTHENING

The trapezius is the broad triangular muscle that extends from the mid-spine to the scapula, and across the upper back to parts of the neck and shoulder. It assists in shrugging and lifting motions. When lifting or carrying heavy loads, the stress felt in the neck is tension in the trapezius muscles. Weight lifters should be encouraged to develop strong trapezius muscles to increase performance and prevent injury.

Upright Row—Free Weights

Start Position: Instruct the client to stand in front of the bar with feet about shoulder width apart. The client bends over and grasps the bar in the middle and lifts the bar and rises back up to a standing position. Arms are fully extended and parallel to the body.

Exercise: The shoulders are raised and the bar is lifted evenly to about mid-chest level without touching the body (Figure 7-45). After a pause at the top of the lift, the repetition is completed by slowly returning the bar to the start position in a controlled manner.

TRUNK STRENGTHENING

The trunk muscles assist in almost every type of activity imaginable, so it is important to promote

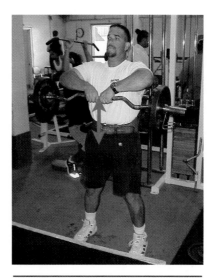

FIGURE 7-45 Upright Row, Free Weights, Full Flexion of Muscle

balance of strength by combining trunk extension, trunk flexion, and trunk rotation exercises in order to strengthen the back, abdomen, and oblique muscles (the muscles on the side of the trunk). Trunk flexion works the upper and lower abdominals; trunk extension strengthens the back; and internal and external rotational trunk curls strengthen the internal and external oblique abdominal muscles, located on the sides above the hip.

Sit-Up (Upper Abdominals/Trunk Flexion)

Start Position: Instruct the client to lie flat on the back with knees bent and feet flat on the floor, about shoulder width apart. Arms are folded across the chest or held at the sides of the head, and the chin should be tucked against the chest (Figure 7-46). A partner may hold the client's feet flat on the floor.

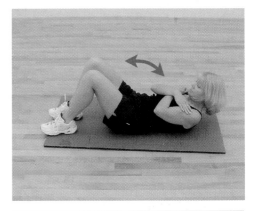

FIGURE 7-46 Sit-up, Start Position

Exercise: The client lifts the upper body away from the floor, curling toward the knees, until the elbows touch the thighs. The repetition is completed by slowly releasing the curl, contracting the abdominal muscles so the lower back comes in contact with the floor as the shoulders return to the start position.

Leg Curl (Lower Abdominals)

Start Position: Instruct the client to sit on the edge of a bench with the legs hanging over the edge. The hands are placed on the edge of the bench for support. The legs are extended, brought together, and raised about 4 inches above the level of the bench.

Exercise: The client bends the knees toward the chest as far as possible without discomfort (Figure 7-47). The repetition is completed by slowly releasing the curl, keeping the lower abdominal muscles contracted. The legs should be fully extended at the end of the curl and remain 4 inches above the level of the body.

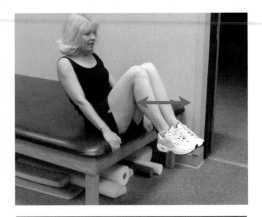

FIGURE 7-47 Leg Curl, Full Flexion

Internal and External Rotational Trunk Curls

Start Position: Instruct the client to lie on the back with knees bent approximately 90° and the feet flat on the floor. The arms are crossed on the chest and the chin is tilted toward the chest.

Exercise: The client contracts the abdominal muscles, rotates the upper body, and curls the upper body off the floor, one elbow curling to the opposite knee (i.e., right elbow touching the left knee) (Figure 7-48). After a pause at the top of the curl, in which the contraction is held, the client uncurls the body and returns to the start position. For this exercise, the client performs one complete set on one side of the body before switching to the other side.

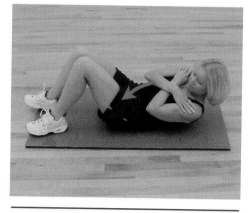

FIGURE 7-48 Trunk Curl, External Rotation, Left Oblique

Variations: The client may lift the legs off the floor and curl them toward the chest, with ankles crossed (Figure 7-49). Or the client may hold the legs straight out, but elevated above the floor. As the client rotates the body to the opposite knee, the client bends that knee and brings the elbow and the knee together (Figure 7-50). Both of these variations place greater emphasis on the obliques and lower abdomen muscles than if the feet are resting on the floor.

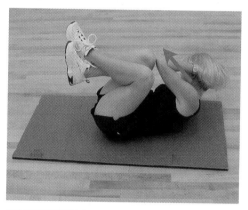

FIGURE 7-49 Trunk Curl, Legs Curled, External Rotation, Right Oblique

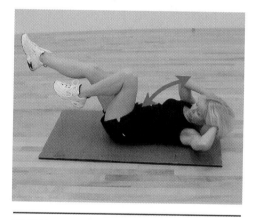

FIGURE 7-50 Trunk Curl, Legs Extended and Elevated, External Rotation, Left Oblique

Trunk Extension— Guided Weights

Start Position: Instruct the client to sit on the machine with the back against the weight pad. The arms are either placed across the chest or on the handle grips for support and balance. The feet are flat on the foot pad or the floor (Figure 7-51).

Exercise: Bending from the hips, the client pushes back against the pad through the machine's range of motion

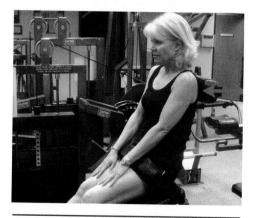

FIGURE 7-51 Trunk Extension, Guided Weights, Start Position

to full extension. The full extension is held for 2 seconds. The repetition is completed by slowly returning to the start position, using the muscles of the lower back to resist the weight of the machine. Note: Clients with bad backs should avoid this exercise or stay in pain-free ROM.

Trunk Extension— Body Weight

Start Position: Instruct the client to lie face-down on a bench, allowing the upper body to hang off the edge. A partner holds the client's legs on the bench to prevent the client from falling off. The clients hands are placed behind the head (Figure 7-52).

Exercise: The client extends the trunk upward, away from the floor, as far as possible and holds the position briefly. After a pause at full extension, the client slowly lowers the body to the start position.

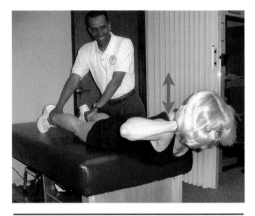

FIGURE 7-52 Trunk Extension, Body Weight, Start Position

HIP STRENGTHENING

A group of four exercises are used to achieve balance in the strength of the hip muscles. These exercises are adduction, abduction, flexion, and extension. The adduction and abduction exercises develop the groin and lateral thigh muscles used for sudden changes in lateral movements. The flexion and extension exercises develop the quadriceps, hamstrings, and gluteals used in forward and backward movements, such as running and cutting. Hip strengthening exercises are also used to help strengthen the groin muscles.

Hip Adduction— Guided Weights

Start Position: Instruct the client to stand on the foot board and face the machine with the legs to one side of the leg pad. Hands are placed on the handlebars to provide stability and balance. The leg closest to the leg pad is placed against the pad with the pad touching the medial portion of the thigh just above the knee.

Exercise: The client applies medial force with the weighted leg, pushing the weight across the body as far as possible without discomfort (Figure 7-53). After a pause at full adduction, the

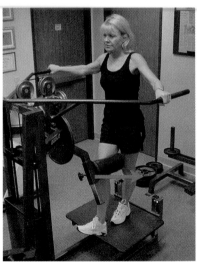

FIGURE 7-53 Hip Adduction, Guided Weights, Multi-Hip Machine

repetition is completed by slowly returning the leg to the start position, using the groin muscles to resist the weight of the machine.

Instruct the client to perform one complete set of this exercise before moving to the other side of the leg pad to work the opposite leg.

Hip Abduction—Guided Weights

Start Position: Instruct the client to stand on the foot board and face the machine with the legs to one side of the leg pad. Hands are placed on the handle bars to provide stability and balance. The leg nearest the leg pad is placed against the pad with the pad touching the lateral portion of the thigh just above the knee.

Exercise: The client applies lateral force with the weighted leg, pushing the weight away from the body as far as possible without discomfort (Figure 7-54). After a pause at full abduction, the repetition is completed by slowly returning the leg to the start position, using the lateral thigh muscles to resist the weight of the machine.

Instruct the client to perform one complete set of this exercise before moving to the other side of the leg pad to work the opposite leg.

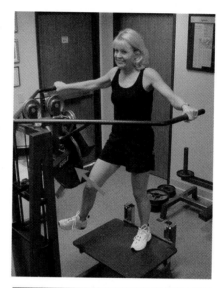

FIGURE 7-54 Hip Abduction, Guided Weights

Hip Flexion—Guided Weights

Start Position: Instruct the client to stand on the foot board, facing the leg pad. Hands are placed on the handlebars to provide stability and balance. The client places the leg closest to the rotating part of the machine under the leg pad so the anterior thigh rests against the pad.

Exercise: The client pushes the thigh forward and upward through the machine's range of motion (Figure 7-55). After a pause at full flexion, the client slowly returns to the start position, using the quadriceps to resist the weight of the machine.

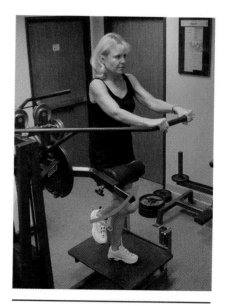

FIGURE 7-55 Hip Flexion, Guided Weights, Mid-Range Position

Hip Extension—Guided Weights

Start Position: Instruct the client to stand on the foot board in front of the leg pad. Hands are placed on the handlebars to provide stability and balance. The leg nearest the machine is flexed at the knee and the posterior thigh placed against the pad, just above the knee (Figure 7-56).

Exercise: The client pushes the leg backward through the machine's range of motion as far as possible without discomfort. After a pause at full extension, the repetition is completed by slowly returning the leg to the start position, using the gluteals to resist the weight of the machine.

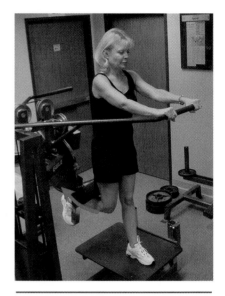

FIGURE 7-56 Hip Extension, Guided Weights

QUADRICEPS AND GLUTEAL STRENGTHENING

Located on the anterior aspect of the femur, the quadriceps assist in walking, running, jumping, skiing, skipping, and kicking. The gluteal muscles form the buttocks. Both the gluteals and the quadriceps are powerful muscles that assist in leg extension and are important muscles to exercise for sprinters, basketball players, weight lifters, and jumpers, among others.

Leg Press—Guided Weights

Start Position: Instruct the client to sit on the seat pad of the leg press machine with the back flat against the back rest and the hands grasping the handles. The feet are placed on the foot board, knees in line with toes, about hip width apart with toes pointed upward. The knees are flexed approximately 90°.

Exercise: The client presses against the foot board, extending the knees until the legs are straight (Figure 7-57). After a pause at full extension, the repetition is completed by slowly returning to the start position, using the quadriceps and gluteals to resist the weight of the machine.

Hack Squat Using the Leg Press—Free Weights

Start Position: Instruct the client to lie down on the bench and position the feet flat on the foot board about hip width apart, knees in line with toes. The position is adjusted to avoid

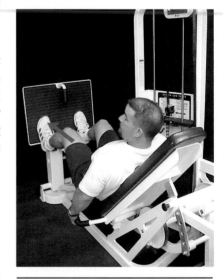

FIGURE 7-57 Leg Press, Guided Weights, Mid-Range Position

an angle of greater than 90° at the knees (Figure 7-58). The client grasps the handles for support and extends the legs fully, but without locking the knees.

Exercise: The client slowly lowers the weight by flexing the knees to an angle of no more than 90°. After a pause the weight is slowly raised back up to the start position in a controlled motion, moving only the legs. Bouncing the weight and using the momentum of the machine to complete the press are avoided to prevent injury and enhance the benefit of the exercise.

Squat—Free Weights

Start Position: Set the weight bar at a level slightly below the height of the client's shoulder. The bar must rest across the client's shoulders and back, not on the neck. With the spotter in place, instruct the client to step under the bar, grasp the bar at approximately shoulder width, and raise the head slightly. The client should look at a spot at or near the ceiling and stand with feet about shoulder width apart to give the best balance possible. Once in the proper position, the client stands straight up, lifting the bar off the stops of the apparatus and stepping back slightly to avoid coming in contact with the apparatus during the downward movement of the exercise.

Exercise: The client slowly bends from the waist as well as the knees to keep the bar traveling in a straight and controlled line toward the ground. After a pause with the knees at a maximum angle of 90°, the client completes the repetition by standing up straight in a slow and controlled manner using the quadriceps and gluteal muscles (Figure 7-59). The spotter must watch the client carefully and be ready to help if the weight begins to shift dangerously. To avoid injury, clients with knee problems should not flex the knees more than 90°.

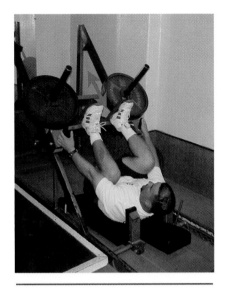

FIGURE 7-58 Hack Squat, Free Weights, Start Position

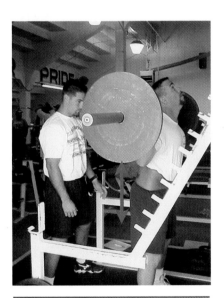

FIGURE 7-59 Squat, Free Weights, Finish Position

HAMSTRING STRENGTHENING

The hamstrings are located on the posterior aspect of the femur. Used primarily when flexing the leg, the hamstrings assist in activities such as running and climbing.

Overexerting tight or weak hamstring muscles may lead to injury and potentially lengthy rehabilitation; therefore, strengthening of the hamstrings is strongly recommended. Strong hamstrings also help prevent knee injuries.

Leg Curl—Guided Weights

Start Position: Instruct the client to lie face-down on the bench with knees just beyond the pad. The bar should touch the back portion of the lower leg at about ankle height. The hands are placed on the machine to maintain balance during the exercise (Figure 7-60).

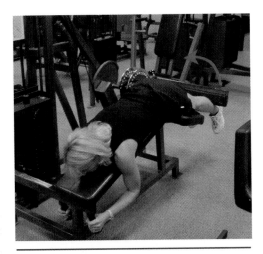

FIGURE 7-60 Leg Curl, Guided Weights, Start Position

Exercise: The client contracts the hamstrings and curls the lower legs up and toward the buttocks, keeping the hips on the machine. After a pause at full flexion, the client completes the repetition by slowly lowering the bar to the start position. To avoid injury, the client must not allow the momentum of the machine to extend the lower leg past straight, causing the knee to hyperextend.

GASTROCNEMIUS AND SOLEUS STRENGTHENING

The gastrocnemius and soleus complex is located on the posterior aspect of the tibia (the calf). The gastrocnemius muscle is located just beneath the surface of the skin and the soleus is beneath the gastrocnemius. This complex is primarily used in plantar flexion, but the gastrocnemius also assists in knee flexion. The gastrocnemius and soleus muscles are in constant use when the legs are in motion and, therefore, are important to running, jumping, and leaping abilities.

Heel Raise—Guided Weights

Start Position: Instruct the client to stand on the foot board, place the shoulder pads of the bars on the shoulders, and grasp the handles of the bars to maintain balance. Once comfortable and well-balanced, the client moves backward until the balls of the feet support the weight. The heels should hang below the foot plate of the machine.

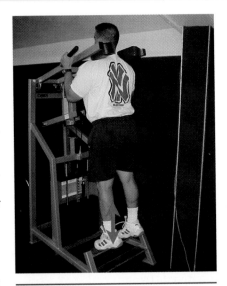

Exercise: The client contracts the calf muscles and presses on the balls of the feet to raise the heels above the level of the foot plate (Figure 7-61). Encourage the client to stretch

FIGURE 7-61 Heel Raise, Guided Weights

as high as possible to get maximum effect from this exercise. The client completes the repetition by slowly lowering the body until the heels are again below the level of the foot plate. Caution the client not to let the machine push him or her too low, which could result in injuries to the Achilles tendon and surrounding tissues.

Variation: The above exercise strengthens the gastrocnemius more than the soleus muscles. To place more emphasis on working the soleus, located anterior to the gastrocnemius, the client should perform the exercise with knees slightly flexed, rather than keeping the legs straight (Figure 7-62). Note: This can also be done with a barbell on the client's shoulders. The positioning would be the same as for the guided weights.

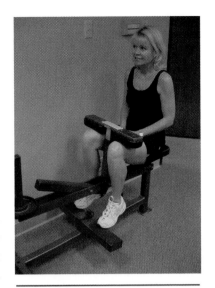

FIGURE 7-62 Heel Raise, Emphasizing Soleus Muscle, Guided Weights

CARDIOVASCULAR EXERCISES

Weight training results in the most visible aspect of physical fitness, increased muscle mass; but cardiovascular endurance is the most important aspect of physical fitness to one's health. The cardiovascular and respiratory systems transport oxygen and nutrients to the body's tissues for absorption, and carry carbon dioxide, a waste product, to the lungs for expulsion from the body. Cardiovascular exercises help build endurance in the heart and lungs, allowing people to do daily or athletic tasks without getting excessively tired. They also burn calories—an important consideration in weight loss and management programs. Cardiovascular exercises may also be performed at low intensity as part of the warm-up or cooldown phase in a weight training program.

The following cardiovascular fitness exercises can be used as part of an overall conditioning program. Some of the exercises do not require any equipment other than proper attire, making them economical as well as effective. As with all exercises, make sure to advise clients or athletes to stop the activity if they feel dizzy or faint; experience pain in the chest, neck, or arm; or experience extreme shortness of breath. If symptoms persist or increase, contact the EMS.

Power Walking

Power walking (Figure 7-63) is a cardiovascular activity that nearly anyone can do. Many people enjoy this form of exercise because it can be done outdoors in fresh air where the scenery can be changed by altering the course of the walk. Alternatively, the exercise may be done indoors, in a climate-controlled environment, on a treadmill.

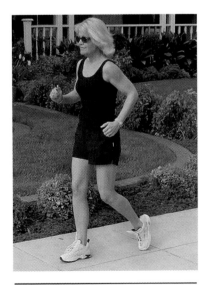

FIGURE 7-63 Power Walking

Clients should start with a short distance on flat ground and gradually increase the distance and intensity. To avoid injury, shoes worn while power walking should have a good arch support and the clothes worn should be appropriate for the climate. Advise clients who exercise outdoors to avoid wearing earphones, which can interfere with the ability to hear sounds that warn of impending dangers, such as cars.

Exercise: Instruct the client to walk swiftly, with the elbows held in at the sides and the hands relaxed. Pumping the arms increases the cardiovascular benefits of this exercise. The pace of the walk should allow the participants to carry on a conversation without getting out of breath.

Running and Jogging

Slightly more strenuous than power walking, running and jogging are cardiovascular activities that can be done by people of all ages and most fitness levels. As with all exercise programs, a doctor's approval should be obtained before beginning a running or jogging program. Individuals with knee, back, or other injuries may be cautioned against running or jogging because of the stress that is created on the joints; however, jogging and running may also be done in a pool where the buoyancy provided by the water greatly decreases the stress on the joints. Like power walking, running and jogging can be done outdoors, or it can be done indoors on a treadmill (Figure 7-64). As they would with any type of exercise, clients should ease into a running or jogging program and gradually increase the duration and intensity of the exercise.

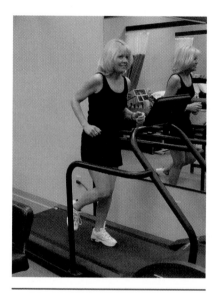

FIGURE 7-64 Running on a Treadmill

Exercise: Instruct the client to maintain proper form by holding the elbows in and moving smoothly rather than bouncing while running. To avoid injury to the joints, clients should avoid hard pounding of the ground with the feet. As with other cardiovascular exercises, the pace should allow the participants to carry on a conversation while exercising without getting short of breath.

Aerobics and Step Classes

Aerobics and step classes (Figure 7-65) are held by certified instructors at many gyms and health clubs. Many people enjoy them because they involve music and provide opportunity to share

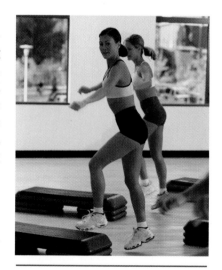

FIGURE 7-65 A Step Class (Courtesy of Photodisc)

the exertion and motivation with others. As with running and jogging, some people with certain injuries should not participate. All participants should start at a low-intensity level, or one that allows them to carry on a conversation while exercising, and work up.

Bicycling

Bicycling conditions the lower body as well as the cardiovascular system. Often an enjoyable activity, bicycling can be done outdoors on a regular bicycle, or indoors on a stationary bike (Figure 7-66). Regardless of the equipment used, the seat should be comfortable and adjusted so that the knees fully extend when the pedals are in the low position; excessive knee flexion resulting from a low seat may result in stress-related knee injuries. When off the seat, clients who use boys' bikes should make sure that both feet reach the ground to avoid injuries from the bar. As they would with any type of exercise equipment, clients should start slow when bicycling, gradually increasing in duration and intensity. Outdoor bicyclists should be cautioned to obey the rules of the road and wear protective equipment.

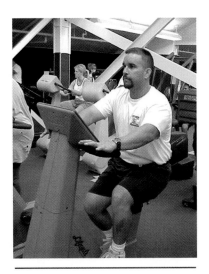

FIGURE 7-66 Stationary Bike

Start Position: Instruct the client to sit on the seat with the feet on the pedals and hands on the handlebars. The back is kept straight.

Exercise: On an outdoor bicycle, the hands are used to steer the bike as the feet work the pedals. Stationary bikes operate on the same principle, but do not require the use of handlebars as there is no need to steer; however, handlebar use is recommended for balance and stability.

Rowing Machines

Rowing machines (Figure 7-67) combine cardiovascular activity with upper-body strengthening exercises by simulating the motions used in rowing a boat. Individuals with back, knee, or shoulder problems should avoid these machines. Clients should start with a short workout at a low resistance and slowly increase in both intensity and duration.

Start Position: Instruct the client to sit on the seat and place the hands on the handlebars. Feet are placed in the stirrups or on the foot boards as available. The knees are flexed and the back is kept straight.

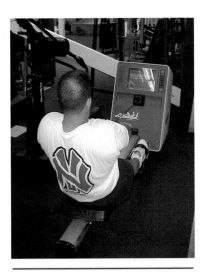

FIGURE 7-67 Rowing Machine

Exercise: The client pushes with the legs while simultaneously pulling with the arms, keeping the back straight. The client then slowly returns to start position in a controlled motion, using the quadriceps to resist the weight of the machine.

Ski Machines

By simulating the motions of cross-country skiing, ski machines (Figure 7-68) are great for total body conditioning; they provide upper- and lower-body workouts as well as cardiovascular benefits. For these machines in particular, the instructions vary for proper use. People with back problems may want to consult a sports medicine professional before using these machines, but those with knee problems may find that this type of machine does not aggravate their condition.

Start Position: Instruct the client to place the feet in the stirrups and hands on the handrails.

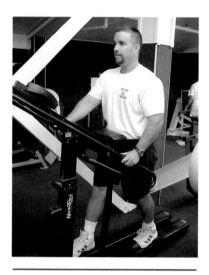

FIGURE 7-68 Ski Machine

Exercise: The arms glide up and down as the feet slide forward and backward. The arms and legs are moved in opposition (when the right arm moves up, the left leg moves back).

Stair Climbers

Like ski machines, stair climbers (Figure 7-69) provide a total body workout. By combining stepping and reaching motions, these machines work the upper and lower body as well as the cardiovascular system. Stair climbers may also be used for just a lower-body and cardiovascular workout by disabling the reaching features of the machine. Individuals with shoulder, knee, or back problems should avoid using these machines.

Start Position: Instruct the client to place the feet in the stirrups and hands on the handles.

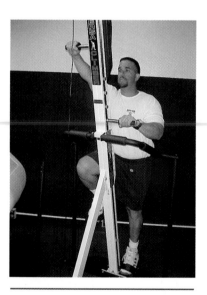

FIGURE 7-69 Stair Climber

Exercise: The right arm is extended as the right foot is raised, and then the left arm is extended as the left foot is raised, and so on. Or, the arms and legs may be moved in opposition.

Stair-Steppers

Stair-steppers (Figure 7-70) offer a variety of settings that make them appropriate for beginners as well as those who are highly conditioned.

Start Position: Instruct the client to step onto the foot boards and stand straight, facing the machine. One foot board will be in a low position and the other will be higher. The hands are placed on the handrails for balance, but caution the client that leaning on the handrails may result in carpal tunnel syndrome.

Exercise: The client shifts the weight to the foot on the high foot board and pushes the board down with that foot while simultaneously allowing the other foot and the low foot board rise. Then, again, the high foot board is pushed down as the low board rises. This motion is continually repeated throughout the course of the workout. Each workout is started at a slow pace. The speed is increased as endurance permits.

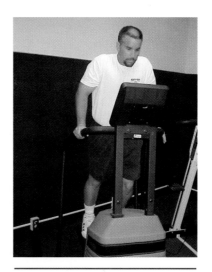

FIGURE 7-70 Stair Stepper

Elliptical Trainers

The elliptical trainer (Figure 7-71) is a piece of cardio equipment that provides a low-impact workout. Elliptical impact produces forces similar to those of walking, while treadmill running and pure running top the list in greatest amount of impact compared to other activities.

Start Position: On the elliptical as with all manufactured equipment, first check the manual and sports medicine professional for any start-up instructions or cautions. Elliptical trainers vary in that some have movable handlebars and other don't. To begin, have the client place both feet on the movable foot boards and hands on the rails or handlebars to establish balance. Then have the client push the appropriate controls and begin the exercise.

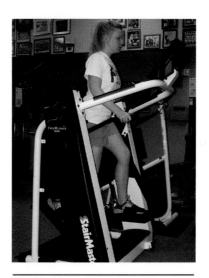

FIGURE 7-71 Elliptical Trainer

Exercise: With the feet moving in conjunction with the handlebars, have the client begin exercise. Ellipticals often have adjustments to increase resistance, increase the grade, and even reverse the direction of rotation. With the use of the upper body, clients have the ability to increase caloric output over the same time as others that don't work the upper body simultaneously. Remind clients to extend but not lock their knees while exercising.

Upper-Body Ergometers (UBEs)

The upper-body ergometer (UBE) (Figure 7-72) provides both upper-body strength and cardiovascular benefits. This machine is a good choice for people with lower-body limitations or temporary injuries who want to maintain or increase strength in the upper body.

Start Position: Instruct the client to sit on the UBE seat and place both hands on the handles. The feet are placed flat on the foot boards and the back is kept straight.

Exercise: The client rotates the arms forward and backward in the same manner that the feet work the pedals of a bicycle.

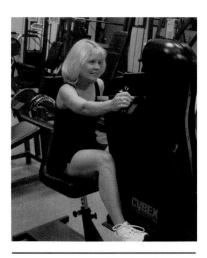

FIGURE 7-72 Upper-Body Ergometer

These flexibility, strengthening, and cardiovascular exercises—and exercises like them—are the tools an SCS or athletic trainer use to develop conditioning programs for clients and/or athletes. You will learn more about developing individual conditioning programs in Chapter 8. It is important to instruct clients or athletes in the proper ways of performing each exercise. Don't just assume they know how, and don't just hand someone a set of instructions. Always follow the manufacturer's guidelines for a given piece of equipment. The athletic trainer or strength and conditioning specialist is responsible for making sure clients and/or athletes know how to exercise properly. Demonstration is the best way to teach a new skill; show the client how to do it first, and then let the client try it while you watch. There are variations to practically every exercise, so keep an open mind about how they are done—but never compromise on safety!

THINKING IT THROUGH

Coach Churchill wanted to get together with his athletic trainer, Terri, to come up with a conditioning program the kids would follow through with. It had been a long football season and most came out uninjured, but the coach wanted to see if they could improve things even more.

Terri suggests first walking through the weight room and checking it out for safety. She has the coach make sure there are enough collars and belts and that the spacing between the stations is adequate. There's nothing worse than getting injured while trying to prevent injuries.

Second, Terri suggests comparing this season's injuries to those of previous seasons and national norms. Terri has all the injuries in a computer database, so it is easy to look for any increase in injuries over previous seasons and to compare to national norms. The coach had put a lot of work into the warm-up and cooldown phases of the training program this season, and it seemed to help, but the comparison Terri suggests would help them determine if the new warm-up drills had actually prevented any muscle strains. A reduced injury count is the best indication that a program is working.

Both the coach and Terri want to make sure that time wasn't wasted in the weight room. So they look closely at the duration and intensity of the program as well as the specialization and make some modifications, making sure that the duration is no longer than necessary and that the intensity of the exercises works the muscles to capacity. They also reassess the focus of the exercises, making sure the specialization is appropriate for each athlete. The ultimate goal is to make the kids stronger for the sports and positions they are playing.

What else could Coach Churchill and Terri look at in an attempt to improve the training program? How can they make the conditioning program interesting enough to the athletes to get them into the weight room to do their exercises? How can they track the effects of the changes they make to the program?

CHAPTER SUMMARY

Conditioning enhances the body's performance. A successful conditioning program must address muscular strength and endurance, flexibility, cardiovascular fitness, body composition, and individual special considerations. In addition, careful attention must be paid to the "Rules of Conditioning" to ensure the safety and success of the program.

Based on the principles of overload, variation, and specificity, weight training is an exercise method that helps improve an individual's fitness level by increasing muscular strength and endurance. Muscles can be exercised using isometric, isotonic, and isokinetic exercises. These exercises are performed in sets, using repetitions of each set, and using the resistance of weights and other muscles. It is important to emphasize the safety guidelines for weight training and other types of conditioning to clients and athletes.

Flexibility exercises increase range of motion. Although flexibility exercises can be performed on their own, they are also a vital aspect of weight training. When performed before and after a workout, flexibility exercises warm and gently stretch the muscles, reducing the risk of injury and cramping.

The heart and lungs can benefit from many different kinds of exercises. Cardiovascular exercise constitutes the most important aspect of developing and maintaining physical fitness. Such exercises also burn calories and help achieve a desired body composition. Advise clients or athletes to stop any exercise activity immediately if they feel dizzy, faint, or pain beyond that of a normal stretch. Furthermore, always instruct the client or athlete to follow the manufacturer's instructions for any type of fitness equipment used, and reinforce this advice by demonstrating the proper way to use it. The clients' safety and well-being are important; start their conditioning programs slowly, taking into consideration any special needs they may have such as back pain. As the clients become accustomed to the exercises, gradually increase the weight, duration, and/or intensity of the exercise to help them achieve their goals.

STUDENT ENRICHMENT ACTIVITIES

Complete the following exercises.

1. Put together two exercise programs: one for female basketball players' upper-extremity strengthening and one for males. Be inventive. Specify which days of the week they would do what. Make sure you include intensity, duration, capacity, warm-up, and balance strength in the programs.

2. Establish an exercise program for clients just starting out who want to strengthen their legs.

3. Explain the difference between isometric, isokinetic, and isotonic exercises, including when you would use them.

Write T for true, or F for false. Rewrite the false statements to make them true.

4.   T F   Isometric exercises are good to use during the final phases of the rehabilitation exercises.

5.   T F   During isotonic muscle exercises, the muscles contract but do not shorten and lengthen as they do in other muscle exercises.

6.   T F   Isokinetic exercises work the muscles to full capacity, through the entire range of motion.

7.   T F   A person should breathe out (exhale) while performing the weight lift.

8.   T F   The eccentric contraction of the muscle that brings the weight back down should take twice as long as it does to lift the weight up.

9.   T F   Always remind your clients to watch for signs of heart problems, such as pain or pressure in the left or mid-chest area.

10.   T F   The duration of each workout session should last for a minimum of 20 minutes.

11.   T F   The only body system ever affected when using the overload principle is the muscular system.

12.   T F   Stretching prior to working out reduces the chance of injury during the session.

13.   T F   When performing a soleus stretch, the rear leg needs to be kept straight.

14.   T F   A UBE machine uses the same motions as a bicycle, except that it is for the upper extremities.

Match the terms in Column A with the appropriate description in Column B.

Column A	Column B
15. isometric	**A.** uses a guided weight machine; the resistance varies as the exercised area goes through the range of motion
16. isotonic	**B.** muscle exercises using contraction and relaxation; contraction of a muscle against an immovable object
17. isokinetic	
18. concentric contraction	**C.** contraction of the muscle, using the same weight throughout the contraction
19. eccentric contraction	
20. muscle tone	**D.** the shape of a muscle at its resting state
21. muscle mass	**E.** muscle lengthens during contraction
22. variable resistance	**F.** muscle shortens during contraction
	G. the girth or size of the muscle
	H. the speed is controlled during the exercise so maximum contraction of the muscle through the full range of motion can be attained

Complete the following exercises.

23. Interview a local coach. Describe the way in which the "Rules of Conditioning" work into the team's conditioning program.

24. List all eight safety guidelines that the strength and conditioning specialist or athletic trainer needs to implement when using weight training exercises with athletes or clients. Briefly explain what each guideline means in terms of weight training safety.

25. Draw a layout for a home gym or fitness room. What equipment would the client need? Estimate the cost of that equipment.

26. Go evaluate your school's weight room and explain if they have the proper equipment to provide a balanced workout for the athletes. What would you add or delete from the weight room?

CHAPTER 8

Designing a Conditioning Program

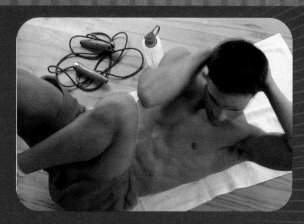

OBJECTIVES

After completing this chapter, you should be able to do the following:

1. Define and correctly spell each of the key terms.

2. Explain why it is important to keep each client's physical condition and medical history in mind at all times during the training program.

3. List the foundational elements of fitness program design.

4. List the structural elements of a fitness program.

5. Explain how duration, intensity, and frequency work together in the fitness program.

6. Discuss how to intensify a conditioning program using gradual steps.

7. Explain why it is important for clients to take responsibility for their own health.

KEY TERMS

* duration

* frequency

* intensity

* mode

* special populations

* target heart rate range

* target zone

INDIVIDUAL TRAINING PROGRAMS

Previous chapters have covered techniques for evaluating and assessing clients' physical conditioning and fitness. Now we take the next step and show how to create an appropriate conditioning program for a client.

Every client needs a physical conditioning and fitness program tailored to that client's own needs. With group instruction, such as teaching an aerobics class, remember to consider the purpose of the class and the needs of the group as a whole in deciding what to include in the program. More communication takes place between the client and the strength and conditioning specialist at the individual program level than in group instruction. So, although the same educational background is often required for either group or individual fitness instruction, the development of an individual training program is more time-consuming and requires more ongoing attention (see Figure 8-1). Individual clients require the undivided attention of their SCS, and their goals and fitness levels are in a constant state of change. This chapter will focus on individual training programs, as they are the programs that typically involve more-detailed information about the clients, their goals, and their current health status.

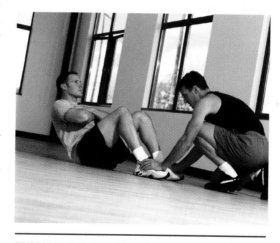

FIGURE 8-1 Outside of group instruction, clients need conditioning programs that are tailored to their individual needs.

KNOW YOUR CLIENT

Whether doing individual or group instruction, the SCS must always make sure that all clients or athletes have been cleared by a physician to begin a conditioning program. Be aware of any health problems a client may have (see Figure 8-2). Use the physical fitness assessment form in Chapter 5 to help decide which exercises clients are able to perform without risking their health, particularly if they have a history of heart problems. Make clients aware of additional symptoms, such as sudden dizziness, cold sweats, or fainting spells, that could be related to potentially undiscovered serious health problems. If clients experience any of these symptoms, refer them to their doctor before allowing them to continue with the program. The

American Heart Association and the American College of Sports Medicine both recommend that anyone 35 years or older who is starting a fitness program should receive a physical from a family doctor. It would be considered prudent to apply this rule to *all* clients, regardless of age, to help ensure clients' ability to participate in a safe and lasting program. Remember, *safety* is the first rule of conditioning, and a physician's clearance is the best way of ensuring that clients get off to a good start.

After reviewing a client's health history and addressing any restrictions made by the physician, begin planning the fitness program. Similar to designing and building a house, a fitness program must have a firm foundation, a solid structure, and room to grow. Remember to apply the remaining rules of conditioning presented in Chapter 7: warm-up/cooldown, progression, duration, intensity, capacity, balanced strength, motivation, specialization, routine, relaxation, fun, diet, and modification. These rules are links in a chain of fitness success. If one of the links becomes weak and breaks the chain, then the

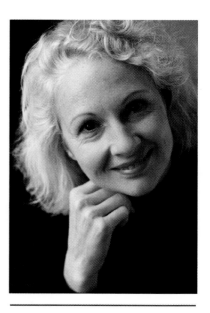

FIGURE 8-2 Talk to your client to confirm the client's physician's approval to begin a conditioning program. You will also need to learn what the client hopes to achieve with the program and how the client might like to do it.

client's ultimate goal of physical fitness may fail. Always consider how to put these rules of conditioning to use. The client's goals, motivation, time schedule, and existing habits and preferences will serve as the foundation of the program and will greatly affect its soundness and effectiveness.

Goals

As discussed in Chapter 3, a good fitness program is best begun by writing down what the client hopes to obtain from the program. These goals should be written as objective, measurable goals, rather than subjective goals (see Figure 8-3). For example, if a client is now at 20% body fat and would like to get down to 18% body fat, objectively evaluating the progress toward that goal by using skin calipers to measure the amount of body fat can greatly assist the client. Subjective data is harder to measure and evaluate. For instance, if the client feels tired and weak all day and would like to have more energy, assessing that client's progress toward that goal is subjective and therefore not measurable. This is because "tired and weak" is the way the client feels,

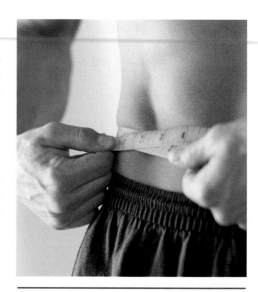

FIGURE 8-3 Your client's goals should be measurable; if he wants a flat stomach, a target waist size should be set.

and feelings, though valid, are not measurable. The goal records discussed in Chapter 3 are a great way to track a client's goals and will assist in planning the conditioning program.

Setting and achieving short-term and long-term goals is a good form of fitness management. For example, in a weight loss program, the long-term goal might be to lose a total of 20 pounds. But a realistic, short-term goal would be to lose 1 to 1½ pounds per week. Make sure that the goals are realistic and reachable, and that the goal setting does not take the fun out of the client's exercise program.

Goal setting provides benefits beyond communicating a desired outcome. Goals can and should be used to motivate the client throughout the course of the fitness program. If the client begins to lag a little in the pursuit of a goal, reminders of the end result help renew the incentive for continued effort. Goals are a great source of motivation. They are the psychological fuel that drives the effort being put forth. Although an individual's personal goals are probably the best source of motivation, the value of external motivation in the form of encouragement cannot be overstated. People need encouragement wherever and whenever they can get it. Be the clients' cheerleader as well as their fitness coach. Praise for a job well done, congratulations for meeting a short-term goal, and enthusiasm for even the smallest victory will do wonders for your clients' self-esteem and help spur them on to even greater achievements.

The client's goals should also be used to apply the specificity principle discussed in Chapter 7. These goals will help determine the types of exercises that are most appropriate. For instance, if the client is an administrative assistant who wants to ski, then the exercises should focus on strengthening the muscles of the lower extremities and enhancing cardiovascular fitness. If the client is an athlete who wants to increase the height of her high jump, then the exercises should be geared to condition the body in order to meet that goal. Use the sport specialization chart shown in Figure 8-4 as a guide in determining which areas of the body to focus on to boost an athlete's performance. For nonathletes, analysis of the demands placed on their bodies as a result of their daily activities will provide useful information for specializing their conditioning programs.

Setting achievable, meaningful goals is vital to the success of any conditioning program. The goals must be both important and realistic to the client; otherwise, there is no reason to put forth any effort. Specialization can help in the development of meaningful goals by focusing on the reason for the exercise.

Time Schedules

Help clients figure out ways they can work a conditioning program into their hectic daily lives, taking into consideration their preferences, habits, work schedules, family responsibilities, and other social and business activities (see Figure 8-5). For instance, some people find that exercising after work is best for them because it enables them to burn off some of the stresses that they may have built up during the workday. This way, when they go home after exercising, those workday stresses are behind them, and they can enjoy a more relaxed evening. Also, some people find that exercising decreases their appetite—a real bonus for cutting calories off the evening meal. However, other people notice that exercising in the evening makes it more difficult for them to get to sleep.

Sport Specialization

- foundation
- emphasize

	Pectorals	Deltoids	Rotator Cuff (SITS)	Latissimus dorsi	Rhomboids	Trapezoids	Triceps	Biceps	Back	Abdominals/Trunk Rotators	Hips	Quadriceps/Gluteals	Hamstrings	Gastrocnemius/Soleus	Cardiovascular
Baseball															
Field positions	•	•	•	•	•	•	•	•	•	•	•	•	•	•	•
Pitchers	•	•	•	•	•	•	•	•	•	•	•	•	•	•	•
Basketball															
Center	•	•	•	•	•	•	•	•	•	•	•	•	•	•	•
Forward	•	•	•	•	•	•	•	•	•	•	•	•	•	•	•
Guard	•	•	•	•	•	•	•	•	•	•	•	•	•	•	•
Diving	•	•	•	•	•	•	•	•	•	•	•	•	•	•	•
Field Hockey															
Field positions	•	•	•	•	•	•	•	•	•	•	•	•	•	•	•
Goalies	•	•	•	•	•	•	•	•	•	•	•	•	•	•	•
Football															
Linemen	•	•	•	•	•	•	•	•	•	•	•	•	•	•	•
Skill positions	•	•	•	•	•	•	•	•	•	•	•	•	•	•	•
Gymnastics															
Bars	•	•	•	•	•	•	•	•	•	•	•	•	•	•	•
Beam	•	•	•	•	•	•	•	•	•	•	•	•	•	•	•
Floor	•	•	•	•	•	•	•	•	•	•	•	•	•	•	•
Pommel horse	•	•	•	•	•	•	•	•	•	•	•	•	•	•	•
Rings	•	•	•	•	•	•	•	•	•	•	•	•	•	•	•
Vault	•	•	•	•	•	•	•	•	•	•	•	•	•	•	•
Ice Hockey															
Field positions	•	•	•	•	•	•	•	•	•	•	•	•	•	•	•
Goalies	•	•	•	•	•	•	•	•	•	•	•	•	•	•	•
Lacrosse	•	•	•	•	•	•	•	•	•	•	•	•	•	•	•

FIGURE 8-4 Sport Specializations

	Pectorals	Deltoids	Rotator Cuff (SITS)	Latissimus dorsi	Rhomboids	Trapezoids	Triceps	Biceps	Back	Abdominals/Trunk Rotators	Hips	Quadriceps/Gluteals	Hamstrings	Gastrocnemius/Soleus	Cardiovascular
Racquet Sports	•	•	•	•	•	•	•	•	•	•	•	•	•	•	•
Rodeo	•	•	•	•	•	•	•	•	•	•	•	•	•	•	•
Rowing/Crew	•	•	•	•	•	•	•	•	•	•	•	•	•	•	•
Skateboarding	•	•	•	•	•	•	•	•	•	•	•	•	•	•	•
Skiing															
Snow	•	•	•	•	•	•	•	•	•	•	•	•	•	•	•
Water	•	•	•	•	•	•	•	•	•	•	•	•	•	•	•
Soccer															
Field positions	•	•	•	•	•	•	•	•	•	•	•	•	•	•	•
Goalies	•	•	•	•	•	•	•	•	•	•	•	•	•	•	•
Softball															
Field positions	•	•	•	•	•	•	•	•	•	•	•	•	•	•	•
Pitchers	•	•	•	•	•	•	•	•	•	•	•	•	•	•	•
Swimming															
Distance	•	•	•	•	•	•	•	•	•	•	•	•	•	•	•
Sprinters	•	•	•	•	•	•	•	•	•	•	•	•	•	•	•
Track and Field															
Distance runners (cross-country)	•	•	•	•	•	•	•	•	•	•	•	•	•	•	•
Jumpers (high, long, and triple)	•	•	•	•	•	•	•	•	•	•	•	•	•	•	•
Mid distance	•	•	•	•	•	•	•	•	•	•	•	•	•	•	•
Sprinters	•	•	•	•	•	•	•	•	•	•	•	•	•	•	•
Throwers	•	•	•	•	•	•	•	•	•	•	•	•	•	•	•
Triathlon	•	•	•	•	•	•	•	•	•	•	•	•	•	•	•
Water Polo															
Field positions	•	•	•	•	•	•	•	•	•	•	•	•	•	•	•
Goalies	•	•	•	•	•	•	•	•	•	•	•	•	•	•	•
Weight Lifting	•	•	•	•	•	•	•	•	•	•	•	•	•	•	•
Wrestling	•	•	•	•	•	•	•	•	•	•	•	•	•	•	•

"Morning people" and those who have tight evening schedules will often choose the early morning hours for exercise. Many people have only pre-work time available to them, while others like the quiet solitude and easier availability of exercise facilities then. Also, morning exercise hours are often an easier time for clients to stick with their exercise plan. Studies have shown that morning exercisers adhere to their conditioning program better than evening exercisers do.

Lunchtime exercisers often have the advantage of working out or exercising with their working companions—another social factor that helps clients stick to their exercise goals. Although they may be limited in the amount of time they can spend exercising or in the ability to shower after the exercise, many people find that lunchtime exercise is very rewarding because they get a midday break that is both healthy and invigorating.

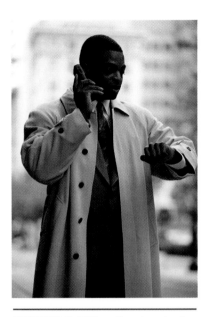

FIGURE 8-5 The client's schedule is always a factor in planning time for workouts.

Existing Habits and Preferences

An effective conditioning program must also work within the parameters of the client's existing habits and preferences (see Figure 8-6). If a client hates running, then a running program is not likely to provide motivation—a swimming program might be a better choice, but not if a client is afraid of the water or doesn't have access to a pool. Similarly, if a client likes to sleep late, a workout schedule that requires getting up at 5:30 in the morning isn't likely to be successful. The client must have a decent shot at following through with the program. Goals alone are not motivation enough. Other factors must also work in the client's favor in order to succeed. The job of the SCS is to stack the deck in the client's favor: Think of ways to make the program fun and inviting. Be innovative. Suggest to clients with long commutes to and from work that they avoid wasting time on the road by exercising at the office until rush hour is over. They can run up and down the stairs, jump on a mini trampoline, jump rope, or find other fun pieces of equipment that can be used to safely get them into shape. Clients who rely on public transit or a carpool for transportation can also put the time spent waiting for their ride to good use by exercising while they wait.

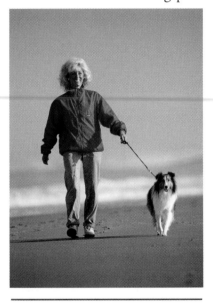

FIGURE 8-6 If your client walks her dog on a regular basis, you might suggest that she schedule her workout to follow the walk, allowing the walk to serve as her warm-up.

DESIGNING THE PROGRAM

With the client's goals, time schedule, habits, and personal preferences serving as the foundation of the program, it is time to begin to design the structure of the program. The structure consists of the mode, intensity, duration, frequency, special considerations, fun, and relaxation. In essence, these structural components *are* the program, but similar to building a house, a conditioning program must be built on a strong foundation and be able to expand to meet changing needs, or it will fail or become obsolete. In fact, to continue the analogy of constructing a house, the remaining rules of conditioning can be thought of as the hardware (the nuts, bolts, nails, and hinges) that holds the framework together.

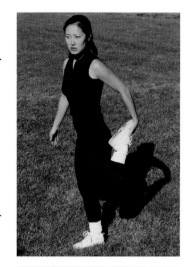

FIGURE 8-7 A proper warm-up and cooldown will help prevent injuries and muscle soreness resulting from exercise.

In helping clients to set goals, remember that they must build up their level of activity gradually, over a period of weeks. Do not set goals so high that clients push themselves and risk injury. Help them to build up to their **target zone** slowly, and show them how to warm up safely with stretching and 5 to 10 minutes of cardiovascular exercise before the workout and cool down slowly with 5 to 10 minutes of flexibility exercises afterward. Remind clients to listen to their body's early warning signs. For example, when a client has pain in the joints, it's possible the client may have pushed the body a little too hard, neglected the warm-up or cooldown phase, or possibly omitted both (see Figure 8-7). Fatigue is another signal that the body is not being cared for properly. Although it is natural to feel a little tired following a beneficial workout, poor nutrition and poor hydration can lead to unnecessary fatigue. As mentioned previously, a proper diet and sufficient water will provide important nutritional benefits by supplying the body with the fuel it needs to meet its new demands. Make sure to point this out to clients.

> **target zone**
> the desired level of fitness.

Mode

The **mode** refers to the type of exercises and equipment most appropriate for a client to perform to accomplish the fitness goals (see Figure 8-8). Mode is dictated by the client's goals, time schedule, habits and personal preferences, and access to equipment. For instance, one might choose swimming, hiking, kickboxing, aerobics, or basketball for a client whose primary goal is general or overall fitness. On the other hand, select specific strengthening exercises for a client who wants to improve strength in specific areas. If a client wants to play racquetball, but doesn't have a court readily accessible, then it won't work for the

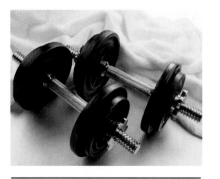

FIGURE 8-8 The equipment available to the client will help dictate the mode of exercise.

> **mode**
> the equipment and exercises used in an exercise program.

client to try to pursue playing racquetball every day on the way home from work. Or, if the client's goal is to ride in a bike race but she doesn't own a bike and hasn't been bicycling in years, then it would be best to begin slowly. First suggest that the client use the stationary bike in the gym to see how she responds to it, or suggest she purchase a used bicycle. Also make sure to assess the impact bicycling has on the client's physical health.

When clients exercise outdoors, they must take appropriate precautions for specific weather conditions they might encounter (see Chapter 19). On hot and/or humid days, they should try to exercise during the cooler parts of the day or try to find a place where they can exercise indoors. The cooler parts of the day are early morning or early evening—just after the sun has gone down. If there is a day or a week of high humidity, high heat, or both, people may have to decrease their exercise program until the weather cools a little. Clients should always drink plenty of fluids, particularly water, especially during hot or humid weather, and be aware of any kind of heat-related problems such as heat cramps, heat exhaustion, and heatstroke. Feelings of weakness or profuse sweating are symptoms of a heat and/or high humidity problem. Heatstroke is a medical emergency. If a client should experience heatstroke, cool off the person as fast as possible and activate emergency action procedures.

In very hot weather, clients will be more comfortable wearing light-colored, loose-fitting clothing. Sun-blocking lotions with a sun protection factor (SPF) of 35 or above should be worn on exposed parts of the body. In fact, the best first aid for sunburn is prevention. Caution clients to never wear a rubberized or plastic suit while exercising. This type of clothing can cause dangerously high body temperatures and may cause heat injury.

On cold days, it is better to wear several layers of clothing rather than to wear one heavy layer. This way, as a person goes through an exercise routine, layers can be removed as needed. Also, mittens, gloves, or even cotton socks should be used to protect the hands and keep them warm. Make sure to wear a hat during cold weather, since up to 40% of the body's heat is lost through the head and neck.

On rainy, icy, and snowy days, people who exercise outdoors need to be aware of the reduced visibility for themselves and for others around them, including drivers. Also, inclement weather reduces shoe traction on running routes, so remind clients to be extra careful during these weather conditions.

Intensity and Capacity

Intensity is the degree of effort required to complete a physical activity. The intensity affects the amount of stress placed on the body by the activity. If the work is too intense, muscle tissue is broken down and weakened, but if it is not intense enough, neither strength nor endurance increases. Intensity is usually measured by the heart rate in response to the amount of work involved (see Figure 8-9). A way to measure the intensity of a workout or exercise is to find out if a person's pulse count is within the **target heart rate range** appropriate for that person's age. The target heart rate range is 70 to 85% of

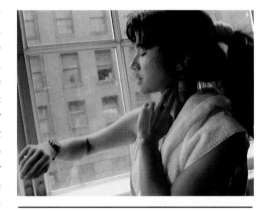

FIGURE 8-9 The pulse rate is used to measure the intensity of exercise.

"age predicted maximum heart rate," which is determined by subtracting the person's age from 220.

220 − (person's age) = age predicted maximum heart rate

age predicted maximum heart rate × .85 = target heart rate (upper range)

age predicted maximum heart rate × .70 = target heart rate (lower range)

Say, for example, that a man is 35 years old. One would determine his age predicted maximum heart rate by subtracting 35 from 220:

220 − 35 = 185

This person's age predicted maximum heart rate is 185 beats per minute. Then, to get the target heart rate range, simply multiply 185 by 70% for the low end of the range, and by 85% for the high end of the range.

185 × .70 = 129.5 (or 130 rounded off)

185 × .85 = 157.25 (or 157 rounded off)

target heart rate range = 130–157 bpm

A person's maximum heart rate can also be used to determine heart rate training zones. Exercising within each training zone will produce different results.

* Healthy zone (warm-up): 50 to 60% maximum heart rate

* Fitness zone (fat burning): 60 to 70% maximum heart rate

* Aerobic zone (endurance training): 70 to 80% maximum heart rate

* Anaerobic zone (performance training): 80 to 90% maximum heart rate

Capacity is a concept that is closely related to intensity. The intensity of the exercise must equal the client's capacity, or maximum capability, to produce the desired results. Capacity represents the threshold, or line, between productive exercise and overstressing a body system (see Figure 8-10). Strive to work a client to capacity, but do not exceed it. (See the overload principle in Chapter 7.)

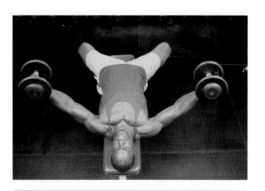

FIGURE 8-10 Working to capacity increases strength, power, and endurance.

capacity

maximum capability.

Duration

Duration refers to the length of time an activity is performed. It is easy to see why this aspect of structure is so important to a fitness program. Imagine that a 35-year-old man has chosen running as his mode of training. No matter how fast he runs, if he runs for only 5 minutes his body will not experience the overload necessary to build strength and endurance. Of course, some clients will have to start out with only 5 minutes of running and build up as their capacity increases, but if they never increase beyond that 5 minutes of work, they won't progress. In fact, at that rate, they won't even maintain their fitness level. Remember, it takes at least 30 minutes of aerobic work just to maintain one's fitness level.

duration

the length of time an activity is performed.

The American Heart Association has created guidelines for the development of training sessions that are designed to develop cardiovascular endurance. According to these guidelines, each training session should include the following:

1. A 5- to 10-minute warm-up and stretching session so that the heart and circulatory system are not taxed suddenly.

2. Sustained 20- to 30-minute exercise sessions in which the heart rate remains in the target zone.

3. A 5- to 10-minute cooldown session in which the intensity of the task is minimal. A cooldown is important because it allows blood to disperse throughout the body from the muscles where it has gone to support the activity. Otherwise, there is a chance the client may faint.

If clients are not able to keep their heart rate in the target zone for a 20- to 30-minute period of exercise, this is not considered a full workout. For example, let's say a client runs and uses the stair stepper and stationary bike three times a week for 20 to 30 minutes, keeping her heart rate in the target zone. Then, once a week, the client plays a recreational game of tennis in which her heart rate does not stay in the target zone for a full 20- to 30-minute period. The client cannot count the tennis activity as one of the regular fitness workouts for that week.

A final word about duration: balance of strength depends on working opposing muscles equally. This means that to be properly balanced in strength, the same time must be spent working the quads as the hamstrings, the biceps as the triceps, the pectorals as the upper back, and so on. The duration of the session must accommodate the time that it takes to strengthen all aspects of a given muscle or muscle group.

Frequency

frequency

the number of times an activity is performed within a specific time frame.

Frequency refers to the number of times something is done. Clients can maintain their current physical fitness level by doing regular workouts (training sessions that meet the American Heart Association's guidelines) three times per week. If the goal of a client's exercise program is anything other than maintaining the current fitness level, the client will have to increase the intensity, duration, or frequency of the exercises. For example, say that a client, Mike, is currently working out on a stationary bike three times a week for 30 minutes. To increase his fitness level, Mike will have to do one or more of the following:

1. Increase the frequency of the workouts by working out four times a week for 30 minutes.

2. Increase the duration of the workouts by increasing the exercise time to 35 minutes.

3. Increase the intensity of the workouts by increasing the resistance on the bike (changing to a higher gear).

Educating clients in the differences that intensity, duration, and frequency make in their fitness program will help them to achieve their goals efficiently and without confusion.

A routine or repeating schedule for exercise will help the client to make fitness a part of normal life and assure the frequency of the workouts. In fact, frequency hinges on routine. If exercise is viewed as anything but an important part of a consistent routine, it will be among the first things to be dropped when a schedule becomes hectic. In an effective fitness program, the workouts cannot be viewed as optional. Therefore, the program should provide options for different forms of exercise in order to keep the routine going when events occur that change the client's schedule. For example, if a client typically runs outside, this client can't just skip the workout when it snows; there needs to be a backup plan, such as running on a treadmill at the gym or jumping rope at home. Sometimes the client's own schedule will make a change necessary. If the client typically works out at the gym while the kids are in school, but one of the kids is sick at home, then the client must have some sort of contingency plan that allows staying with the routine of a workout at home. Likewise, businesspeople who travel must have a contingency plan; some hotels have gyms for guest use, or the client may take along elastic bands to do strengthening exercises in the hotel room.

Special Considerations

Certain populations require additional considerations in fitness program development. This is where the rule of modification becomes important. Programs for middle-aged or elderly clients, for example, must be approached differently and monitored even more closely than programs for younger individuals. Age often brings about certain ailments, such as heart disease. Furthermore, older clients may be more susceptible to injury because of past injuries such as a bad knee from high school football. Therefore, it is important to stay abreast of a client's health history and current status to avoid complications. In developing programs for this special population, begin by adding a maximum of three new exercises each session, avoiding the ones that cause pain. By adding only three exercises a session, you can track which ones do not agree with the client. As with other client populations, the lives of these clients will change, and sports medicine professionals will have to observe those changes and alter the individual conditioning programs accordingly.

Special populations also include individuals with special physical capabilities, such as professional athletes, or those with physical limitations, such as amputees, paraplegics, or individuals with back problems, to name a few (see Figure 8-11). Physical capabilities and limitations are determined by evaluating any history of injuries, operations, or other physical disabilities or chal-

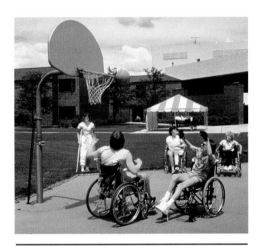

FIGURE 8-11 Individuals with physical limitations require special consideration in the development of a fitness program.

> **special populations**
>
> individuals with special physical capabilities or limitations that make adjustments necessary to a standard fitness program.

lenges; the resting heart rate; blood pressure; and overall fitness level (strength, flexibility, and endurance). For example, if the client has a history of asthma, that client's target zone goal may have to be changed accordingly. If a client has a history of back problems, there are certain activities, such as jogging, that this client should not do. Such clients should also avoid doing squats and dead lifts. Clients with back problems should be restricted to activities in which the feet stay on the ground and should avoid jumping and twisting to avoid distractions or separations of the discs followed by compression on a nerve.

The SCS can be creative in helping clients with physical health problems achieve fitness. For instance, if a client has had back surgery, that client may no longer be able to jog or run. Exercises such as swimming, biking, or using a stair climber can be used instead to achieve the client's goals. In the same manner, a client who is a professional athlete (and in top physical condition) will most likely need to start with a more aggressive training program in terms of strength, flexibility, and endurance than the average person would. So, the exercise plan will be based upon the physical health of client and will change from one to another.

Sometimes a program must be temporarily modified to meet an individual's changing needs. For example, when a client is recovering from an injury, the routine must be modified to retain as high a level of conditioning as possible, while allowing the injury to heal. Temporary modification of a training program may also be required for pregnant or fasting clients. Women who are pregnant should be guided by a physician in the development of their conditioning programs and should schedule check-ups on a regular basis to ensure that the exercise is providing the intended benefits to the client and the unborn child.

Clients who fast present a different type of challenge: While short fasts may not greatly affect a conditioning program, lengthy fasts can dramatically affect the body's energy reserves. For example, individuals who observe the Islam holy month of Ramadan do not eat or drink between the hours of sunrise and sunset during that month. Imagine sending an athlete out on a cross-country run in hot weather during such a fast! Without making the appropriate modifications to the program, the client may suffer needlessly.

Fun

From the client's standpoint, having fun while becoming fit is the most important component in the fitness program. If they do not find the fitness routine enjoyable physically, mentally, and socially, they will get bored and won't continue with the program. Realize that what clients might consider enjoyable when they start their physical fitness program may not still be fun after six months, let alone a year or five years later. As clients mature and change physically, mentally, and socially, so must their fitness routines change to reflect that important ingredient of fun—the component that keeps clients active and enthusiastic about their fitness program.

Also, the social factor of having fun in a fitness program should never be taken lightly (see Figure 8-12). For instance, many people need the companionship of a fitness partner in order to stay with their program. This fitness partner could be an individual, such as a friend or a spouse, or the fitness partners could be a group of people such as in a club or an aerobics class. Many times, the fitness companion may be a racquetball, tennis, or running partner. It's important, then, to plan clients' conditioning programs with an eye toward the amount of social interaction they need in order to have fun while getting fit and healthy.

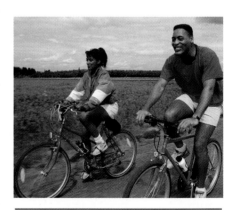

FIGURE 8-12 Working out with others can make the exercise more fun.

Schedule Time for Rest and Sleep

Relaxation is very important to good health. Though most people seek it, many cannot seem to achieve relaxation without a conscious effort. Relaxation takes time, so it is important to include it in a fitness schedule (see Figure 8-13). This means reserving adequate time for sleep and participating in activities that assist in inducing relaxation.

SAFELY INCREASING AND MAINTAINING FITNESS LEVELS

With the foundation and structure of the fitness program firmly established, the strength and conditioning specialist may help the client "move in" to this new lifestyle. However, clients will not be able to remain in the structure that has been designed for very long before modifications need to be made; plan for the modifications that will be necessary as the client's needs change. Follow-up testing will need to be done at appropriate intervals (every two weeks or so) to determine how the client's needs have changed. As the client's capacity increases, the frequency, duration, or intensity of the workouts must also be increased to further improve endurance.

Be sure to let clients know that strength training twice a week only *maintains existing strength*; it does not build it further. Remember, to *maintain cardiovascular health*, the workouts need to be done three times a week, and the sessions should involve at least 30 minutes of activity in the target heart rate range. The target heart rate range is the best guide for ensuring an appropriate intensity. Another useful guideline is to talk to clients as they exercise to see if they can talk comfortably while working out. If not, a client is working too hard.

Progression

The rule of progression dictates that small amounts of work be added to each practice period as capacity increases (see Figure 8-14). Getting into top physical condition doesn't happen overnight. It takes about two months of steady, progressive work to achieve optimum fitness. Though true, the "no pain, no gain" philosophy can be taken too far. If the body is pushed too far too fast, the risk of

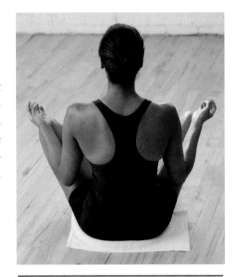

FIGURE 8-13 Meditation may be an effective relaxation technique for some clients.

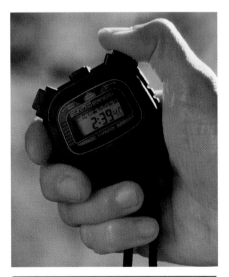

FIGURE 8-14 In a running program, clients can progress by increasing speed or distance.

injury is greatly increased and the work becomes counterproductive. The key to effective conditioning is slow and steady progression.

Variety

Year-round conditioning, known as periodization in athletic training, is important to everyone—not just to athletes. Training programs that vary by season keep athletes in good condition during their off-season, but nonathletes need variety too. Although conditioning programs for nonathletes are usually unaffected by seasons except for possible weather influences on outdoor activities, variety is still a vital aspect of their programs; it helps keep the participants interested.

Some people have found that if they do cardiovascular exercise on Mondays, Wednesdays, and Fridays and strength training on Tuesdays and Thursdays, it helps to break up their exercise routine. It also allows those muscles that have been worked hard an extended 48 hours to recover before clients work them out again.

When strengthening muscles, the muscles need time to recover after being exercised. Normally this time is around one day of rest before exercising that same group of muscles again. If the client exercises the same muscle groups for days at a time, the repeated stress to the muscle can result in breakdown, causing injury within the muscle rather than building it.

BASIC WALKING AND JOGGING PROGRAMS

Figures 8-15 and 8-16 are examples of basic conditioning programs that combine strength training with either walking or jogging for cardiovascular fitness. For many people, walking and jogging are great ways to burn calories and improve cardiovascular health because they offer the additional benefit of strengthening the lower extremities without the expense of weight equipment or a monthly membership fee to a gym. The primary advantage to the sample programs listed below is that they can each be done without the purchase of any equipment.

To begin a client or athlete on a walking or jogging program, first evaluate which would be more beneficial to that person: walking or jogging. For instance, if someone has bad knees, walking would be the best choice, because the repeated stress to the knee caused by jogging might aggravate that condition. Likewise, if an individual has not been exercising and is not in good condition, walking would again be the best choice because it creates less stress on the heart and lungs. On the other hand, someone who is in good condition to begin with, such as an athlete, would probably benefit more from a jogging program.

For someone who would prefer a jogging program to a walking program, but who must begin by walking because of a low fitness level, a transition must be made at an appropriate time. When walking becomes too easy or too boring, advise the client to phase in to the jogging program by alternating walking with jogging every other block. Remember to record the client's progress at each session, using progress reports or fitness assessment forms similar to those presented in earlier chapters of this book.

Regardless of the client's level of conditioning, always provide guidelines for performing the exercise to decrease the risk of injury and increase the benefits of the workout. For instance, in a walking program, the primary guidelines would be to wear comfortable shoes with an appropriate cushion and arch support; walk on a flat, even surface to avoid twisting an ankle; begin slowly (both in duration and

A Walking Program

Week #	Days	Warm-Up	Target Zone Exercise	Cooldown	Total Time
Week 1	M, W, F T, Th	Walk slowly 5 min. Walk slowly 5 min.	Walk briskly 5 min. Strengthen upper body: Push-ups, chair dips, and sit-ups: 1 set of each (5–10 repetitions).	Walk slowly 5 min. Walk slowly 5 min.	15 min.
Week 2	M, W, F T, Th	Walk slowly 5 min. Walk slowly 5 min.	Walk briskly 7 min. Strengthen upper body: Push-ups, chair dips, and sit-ups: 2 sets of each (5–10 repetitions).	Walk slowly 5 min. Walk slowly 5 min.	17 min.
Week 3	M, W, F T, Th	Walk slowly 5 min. Walk slowly 5 min.	Walk briskly 9 min. Strengthen upper body: Push-ups, chair dips, and sit-ups: 3 sets of each (5–10 repetitions).	Walk slowly 5 min. Walk slowly 5 min.	19 min.
Week 4	M, W, F T, Th	Walk slowly 5 min. Walk slowly 5 min.	Walk briskly 11 min. Strengthen upper body: Push-ups, chair dips, and sit-ups: 4 sets of each (5–10 repetitions).	Walk slowly 5 min. Walk slowly 5 min.	21 min.
Week 5	M, W, F T, Th	Walk slowly 5 min. Walk slowly 5 min.	Walk briskly 13 min. Strengthen upper body: Push-ups, chair dips, and sit-ups: 4 sets of each (5–10 repetitions).	Walk slowly 5 min. Walk slowly 5 min.	23 min.
Week 6	M, W, F T, Th	Walk slowly 5 min. Walk slowly 5 min.	Walk briskly 15 min. Strengthen upper body: Push-ups, chair dips, and sit-ups: 4 sets of each (5–10 repetitions).	Walk slowly 5 min. Walk slowly 5 min.	25 min.
Week 7	M, W, F T, Th	Walk slowly 5 min. Walk slowly 5 min.	Walk briskly 18 min. Strengthen upper body: Push-ups, chair dips, and sit-ups: 4 sets of each (5–10 repetitions).	Walk slowly 5 min. Walk slowly 5 min.	28 min.
Week 8	M, W, F T, Th	Walk slowly 5 min. Walk slowly 5 min.	Walk briskly 20 min. Strengthen upper body: Push-ups, chair dips, and sit-ups: 4 sets of each (5–10 repetitions).	Walk slowly 5 min. Walk slowly 5 min.	30 min.

Clients should check their pulse periodically to be sure that they are exercising within their target zone. As they get into better shape, they should try exercising within the upper range of the heart zone. As always, encourage them to explore fun ways of achieving their goals. At this point, the client may want to progress to a jogging program. Remember clients can increase time, speed of walk, and repetitions to keep at their target heart rate.

FIGURE 8-15 A Walking Program

A Jogging Program

Week #	Days	Warm-Up	Target Zone Exercise	Cooldown	Total Time
Week 1	M, W, F	Stretch 5 min.	Walk 10 min.	Walk slowly 3 min. Stretch 2 min. Walk slowly 5 min.	20 min.
	T, Th	Walk slowly 5 min.	Strengthen upper body: Push-ups, chair dips, and sit-ups: 1 set of each (5–10 repetitions).		
Week 2	M, W, F	Stretch 5 min. Walk 5 min.	Jog 1 min., Walk 5 min., Jog 1 min.	Walk slowly 3 min. Stretch 2 min. Walk slowly 5 min.	22 min.
	T, Th	Walk slowly 5 min.	Strengthen upper body: Push-ups, chair dips, and sit-ups: 2 sets of each (5–10 repetitions).		
Week 3	M, W, F	Stretch 5 min. Walk 5 min.	Jog 3 min., Walk 5 min., Jog 3 min.	Walk slowly 3 min. Stretch 2 min. Walk slowly 5 min.	26 min.
	T, Th	Walk slowly 5 min.	Strengthen upper body: Push-ups, chair dips, and sit-ups: 3 sets of each (5–10 repetitions).		
Week 4	M, W, F	Stretch 5 min. Walk 4 min.	Jog 5 min., Walk 4 min., Jog 5 min.	Walk slowly 3 min. Stretch 2 min. Walk slowly 5 min.	28 min.
	T, Th	Walk slowly 5 min.	Strengthen upper body: Push-ups, chair dips, and sit-ups: 4 sets of each (5–10 repetitions).		
Week 5	M, W, F	Stretch 5 min. Walk 4 min.	Jog 5 min., Walk 4 min., Jog 5 min.	Walk slowly 3 min. Stretch 2 min. Walk slowly 5 min.	28 min.
	T, Th	Walk slowly 5 min.	Strengthen upper body: Push-ups, chair dips, and sit-ups: 4 sets of each (5–10 repetitions).		
Week 6	M, W, F	Stretch 5 min. Walk 4 min.	Jog 6 min., Walk 4 min., Jog 6 min.	Walk slowly 3 min. Stretch 2 min. Walk slowly 5 min.	30 min.
	T, Th	Walk slowly 5 min.	Strengthen upper body: Push-ups, chair dips, and sit-ups: 4 sets of each (5–10 repetitions).		
Week 7	M, W, F	Stretch 5 min. Walk 4 min.	Jog 7 min., Walk 4 min., Jog 7 min.	Walk slowly 3 min. Stretch 2 min. Walk slowly 5 min.	32 min.
	T, Th	Walk slowly 5 min.	Strengthen upper body: Push-ups, chair dips, and sit-ups: 4 sets of each (5–10 repetitions).		
Week 8	M, W, F	Stretch 5 min. Walk 4 min.	Jog 8 min., Walk 4 min., Jog 8 min.	Walk slowly 3 min. Stretch 2 min. Walk slowly 5 min.	34 min.
	T, Th	Walk slowly 5 min.	Strengthen upper body: Push-ups, chair dips, and sit-ups: 4 sets of each (5–10 repetitions).		

Clients should check their pulse periodically to see if they are exercising within their target zone. As they become fit, clients can try exercising within the upper range of their target zone. Remind them that their goal is to continue to get the benefits they are seeking, while enjoying their exercise activity. Tell them that they should always listen to their body, and that they may want to build up to their goals less quickly, if needed. Remember clients can increase time, speed of jog, and repetitions to keep at their target heart rate.

FIGURE 8-16 A Jogging Program

speed), increasing the distance and speed gradually as the fitness level improves. For a jogging program, guidelines would include the same as those for walking, but would also include avoiding bouncing while jogging to avoid stress to the knees. Clients should also be told that while walking or jogging uphill increases the stress to the heart and lungs, walking or jogging downhill creates additional stress to the knees. The stresses of hills can be reduced by starting out with only small hills. Then once larger hills become appropriate, the downhill stress to the knees can be reduced by zig-zagging down the hill rather than going straight down.

Suggest that clients who exercise outdoors work out with a partner, especially in foul weather or in other situations that may be dangerous, such as exercising after dark. Clothing appropriate to both existing and anticipated weather conditions should be worn (see Figure 8-17). Earphones should not be worn, or at least not used at a high volume when walking or jogging outside. Loud music can mask the sounds of dangers such as moving cars or trains. When walking or jogging in unfamiliar areas, it may also be advisable to carry a cell phone. Keep in mind that many people will prefer to walk or jog outdoors, but for those who do not mind doing their workout indoors, treadmills can also be used to complete walking or jogging programs.

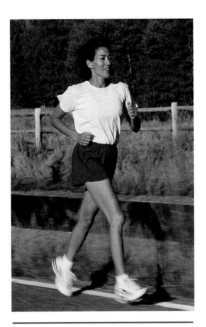

FIGURE 8-17 Running and power walking are great cardiovascular activities for people who want to exercise outdoors.

A SAMPLE INTRODUCTORY PROGRAM

The ability to understand and describe the elements of an effective conditioning program is important, but even more important is the ability to apply these concepts to meet the specific needs of each person. Therefore, an example of how these elements can assist in creating the outline and filling in the details of a conditioning program may be helpful. Consider the following individual and refer to Figures 8-18, 8-19, and 8-20.

Rafael Juarez is a 47-year-old stockbroker with a wife and two daughters. His work is fast-paced, requires a lot of his time, and causes considerable stress. Rafael really loves his job, but he is very dedicated to his family, too. He wants to spend as much time with them as possible. He also knows that the pace of his career could shorten his life if he doesn't stay in shape. Rafael is fortunate; he enjoys physical activity—especially racquetball—and works a game into his busy schedule whenever possible. But these sporadic bursts of exercise are not enough. He has realized that he needs a more structured program to get him into a little better shape and help him stay there.

His doctor has told him that he is good to go on a fitness program. However, since Rafael had back surgery six years ago, the doctor told him to avoid physical activities that cause him back or leg pain. His medical history has been checked and significant notations made on his Physical Fitness Assessment Form (Figures 8-18A and 8-18B). Remember, the medical history is *private,* not to be shared, and must be locked up where only the appropriate staff members have access.

Physical Fitness Assessment Form

Name _Rafael Juarez_   Date _9/22/XX_

Sex (M) F   Birthdate _10_ / _18_ / _XX_

Address _1111 Main Street_

City _Anytown_   State _TX_   Zip _99999_   E-mail _Rjuarez@work.net_

Phone (h) (_555_) _555-1111_   (w) (_555_) _555-2222_

Height _____   Weight _____   Target Weight _____

Medical Conditions Check all that apply

	Yes	No
1. Are you currently under a doctor's care for any reason?	☐	☑
2. Have you ever been hospitalized?	☑	☐
3. Have you ever had surgery?	☑	☐
4. Are you currently taking any medications or pills?	☐	☑
5. Do you have any allergies (medicines, bee stings, etc.)?	☐	☑
6. Have you ever been dizzy or fainted during or after exercise?	☐	☑
7. Have you ever had chest pain during or after exercise?	☐	☑
8. Have you ever had high blood pressure?	☐	☑
9. Have you ever been told that you have a heart murmur?	☐	☑
10. Have you ever had racing of your heart or skipped heartbeats?	☐	☑
11. Have you ever had a head injury?	☐	☑
12. Have you ever been knocked out or unconscious?	☐	☑
13. Have you ever had a seizure?	☐	☑
14. Have you ever had a stinger, burner, or pinched nerve?	☐	☑
15. Have you ever been dizzy or passed out in the heat?	☐	☑
16. Do you have trouble breathing during or after exercise?	☐	☑
17. Do you have any skin problems (itching, rashes, etc.)?	☐	☑
18. Have you had any problems with your eyes or vision?	☐	☑
19. Do you wear glasses or contacts or protective eye wear?	☐	☑

	Yes	No
20. Do you use any special equipment (splints, neck rolls, mouth guards, etc?)	☐	☑
21. Has anyone in your family died of heart problems or sudden death before age 50?	☐	☑
22. Do you have only one working organ of usually paired organs (only one eye, kidney, etc.)?	☐	☑
23. Have you ever sprained, broken, dislocated, or had repeated swelling or pain of any bones or joints?	☑	☐

Head ☐ Neck ☐ Chest ☐ Shoulder ☑ Back ☑
Hand ☐ Wrist ☐ Elbow ☐ Forearm ☐ Hip ☐
Thigh ☐ Knee ☑ Ankle ☐ Shin/Calf ☑ Foot ☐

	Yes	No
24. Are any of these bothering you currently?	☐	☑
25. Have you had any other medical problems? (asthma, mono, diabetes, etc.)	☐	☑
26. Have you had any medical problems or injuries since your last evaluation?	☐	☑
27. Any special instructions or precautions?	☑	☐

28. When was your last tetanus shot? _2 years ago_

Current medications

Additional notes

Age 47   Physician check every year – "all okay"

Back surgery 6 years ago for an entrapped sciatica nerve

Impingement of the G/H joint at times

Leg extension causes knee pain; Leg squats cause back pain;

Running up or down hills causes calf pain and foot numbness, but flat surfaces are no problem

Page 1/2

FIGURE 8-18A Physical Fitness Assessment Form, Page 1

Evaluation

Evaluation	Score			
	Week 1	Week 8	Week 20	Week 32
Muscular Endurance				
Bent-leg sit-ups (1 min)	22			
Push-ups (to fatigue)	14			
Bench jump/step (1 min)	25			
Flexibility				
Sit and reach (in.)	14"			
Back bend (in.)	16"			
Cardiovascular Endurance				
Recovery pulse (bpm)	112			
Body composition				
Triceps (mm)	9			
Biceps (mm)	9			
Subscapula (mm)	10			
Supra-iliac (mm)	14			
Total (mm)	42			
Total % body fat	22			

Work day starts at 6 a.m. and may lead to late evening; does not get a consistent lunch break.
Enjoys a physically active life when time permits
Plays racquetball once a week at a high level
Is not ready to give up sweets would rather work out harder

FIGURE 8-18B Physical Fitness Assessment Form, Page 2

NOTES

GOALS:

Wants body fat at around 18% — no higher than 20%
Not necessarily looking to gain strength, but doesn't want to lose strength
Wants to reduce and control leg pain resulting from back surgery
Wants to stay competitive in racquetball
Wants to be able to play with kids without suffering for a week afterward
Wants to reduce stress

TIME SCHEDULE:

Workouts have to be before work: from 4:25 to 5:30 a.m. This time doesn't break into the very important family time because the family is sleeping.

EXISTING HABITS AND PREFERENCES:

Likes desserts; doesn't want to give them up (note: schedule appointment with dietitian)
Likes racquetball

MODES:

Racquetball; Stair stepper; Treadmill (able to go 10 MPH); Guided Weights up to 10#'s; Rowing Machine; Seated Bench Press; Dumbbells (25 – 45#'s);

INTENSITY:

Monitor by keeping heart rate (HR) within target heart rate range (THRR). Increase gradually as capacity increases. Client has been advised to stop any exercise activity immediately if he feels dizzy, faint, or unusual pain.

DURATION:

Total workout time can be up to an hour. Since he tested average in CV fitness, CV exercises should keep HR within THRR for 20 minutes to start. Duration of strengthening exercises depends on muscles being worked. See program for details.

FREQUENCY:

3 days a week (M, W, F) Cardiovascular (CV) endurance and strengthening
2 days week (T, Th; or sometimes Sat. or Sun.) CV only

FIGURE 8-19 Fitness Program Notes

SPECIAL CONSIDERATIONS:

Need to keep the trunk strong and hamstrings flexible to control the leg pain resulting from his surgery. Avoid activities that cause undue pain to the back either at that moment or 1-2 days following the activity.

FUN:

Enjoys physical activity to begin with—especially racquetball. A morning workout program will give him time to think without interruptions and plan his day. It should also serve to gear him up for a fast-paced day.

REST & SLEEP:

The consistent exercise will help to burn off stress. We have also discussed the importance of adequate sleep and other forms of relaxation to his health.

PROGRESSION:

Will build gradually, primarily in intensity as his schedule keeps time pretty tight.

VARIETY:

Using the different modes will provide sufficient variety for a while. Will watch for signs that the routine is becoming old to him.

Rules of Conditioning Checklist:
✓ Safety: stayed within Dr's guidelines; advised client of safety cautions; will demonstrate proper use of all equipment.
✓ Motivation: see goals
✓ Specialization: Racquetball and general fitness
✓ Warm-up/Cooldown: see program
✓ Diet: likes dessert; schedule appointment with dietitian
✓ Intensity: see notes
✓ Capacity: starting slightly above existing levels as determined by fitness assessment to achieve overload; continue to monitor
✓ Duration: see notes
✓ Balanced Strength: see program
✓ Routine: see program
✓ Modification: no running or walking on slopes (see program)
✓ Fun: see notes
✓ Relaxation: see notes
✓ Progression: see notes

FIGURE 8-19 Fitness Program Notes *(Continued)*

THE PROGRAM

MONDAY, WEDNESDAY, FRIDAY (STRENGTHENING & CV)

Warm-up:
Stair stepper 15 minutes at a HR of 60-70% of THRR
Stretch hamstrings, gastrocnemius/soleus complex, and quadriceps (2 sets of 30 with a 30-second hold for each stretch)

CV Workout:
Treadmill 3 miles at 70-80% of THRR (no incline due to back pain)

Strengthening Exercises:
Biceps with dumbbell 2 sets of 12
Military press with dumbbells 2 sets of 12
Rowing machine 2 sets of 12
Triceps machine 2 sets of 12
Chest press machine 2 sets of 12
Guided weights for rotator cuff (Internal rotation 2 sets of 12; External rotation 2 sets of 12; Supraspinatus 2 sets of 12)

Cooldown:
Stretch hamstrings
Trunk exercises, including all four aspects of the abdominals (4 sets of 20; 1 set for each aspect) and core stabilization exercises

TUESDAY AND THURSDAY (CV ONLY)

Warm-up:
Stair stepper 15 minutes at a HR of 60-70% of THRR
Stretch hamstrings, gastrocnemius/soleus complex, and quadriceps (2 sets of 30 with a 30-second hold for each stretch)
On racquetball days, add chest, anterior deltoid, posterior deltoid, triceps, and wrist stretches

Workout:
1 hr of racquetball or do treadmill 4 miles at 70-80% of THRR (no incline due to back pain)

Cooldown:
Stretch hamstrings
Trunk exercises, including all four aspects of the abdominals (4 sets of 20; 1 set for each aspect) and core stabilization exercises

FIGURE 8-20 The Physical Fitness Program

TAKING RESPONSIBILITY FOR OUR HEALTH

Finally, in beginning a client on a new fitness program, one might want to emphasize certain points about the client's responsibilities in achieving and maintaining optimal health. The Surgeon General's January 2000 report *Healthy People 2010* (www .healthypeople.gov), dedicated to increasing the quality and years of healthy life and eliminating health problems for Americans, emphasizes the importance of individual responsibility for understanding and monitoring behavior in improving and maintaining health. The report indicates that the most significant factors of a healthy lifestyle can be achieved through personal habits. Consider the following facts:

* Engaging in regular moderate physical activity (30 minutes per day) increases muscle and bone strength; increases lean muscle and helps decrease body fat; aids in weight control; and enhances psychological well-being.

* Being overweight or obese substantially increases health risks of diabetes, heart disease and stroke, arthritis, breathing problems, a wide range of cancers, and sleep disturbance.

* Following the *Dietary Guidelines for Americans* (www.healthierus .gov/dietaryguidelines/) plays a critical role in health maintenance and disease prevention by reducing the occurrence of obesity and the risk of nutritionally related diseases (see Figure 8-21).

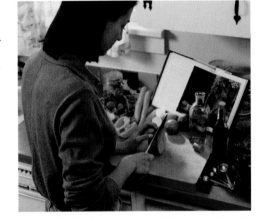

FIGURE 8-21 A healthy diet provides the body with needed nutrients and reduces the risk of obesity and various other health problems.

* Eliminating tobacco use of any kind adds 5 million years of potential life to Americans each year; significantly reduces risk of lung, mouth, throat, and organ cancer; and eliminates the risk of secondary-smoke disease for nonsmokers.

* Avoiding substance abuse including excessive alcohol consumption and illicit drug use eliminates the leading cause of death among Americans; reduces the risk of heart disease, cancer, pancreatitis, and liver disease; and offers the leading method of prevention for severe birth defects.

With this basic understanding, the following suggestions can be made to adults:

* Exercise regularly.

* Eat sensibly.

* Eliminate smoking.

* Control body weight.

* Limit alcohol consumption.

* Avoid drug use.

Exercise can make people feel better, look better, and sleep better. It can increase energy while reducing stress and tension. As if these benefits were not enough, exercise also can lead to increased productivity. Although it is up to each individual to be responsible for his or her own actions, an SCS or athletic trainer can help each individual stay on track.

THINKING IT THROUGH

The girls' soccer team at Encina High has a new coach who must develop a new in-season training program. This program must address the problems revealed by the new coach's analysis of last year's injury records.

PROBLEMS ENCOUNTERED LAST YEAR

High number of torn ACL (anterior cruciate ligament) of the knee
Sprained ankles
Loss of strength during the season (deconditioning)
Limited time (during the season it is very important to make sure that plenty of practice time remains to work on skills)

What goals should the new coach set to address last season's problems? What specific muscles should be targeted for conditioning and strengthening? What types of exercises could the team do to reach the desired goals? Should strengthening exercises precede or follow practice sessions, and why? How could the conditioning program be adapted for the indoors during inclement weather?

CHAPTER SUMMARY

When designing a fitness program for a client, it is important to keep in mind all of the elements that comprise the foundation, structure, and expansion capabilities of the program. The foundation is formed by the client's goals, time schedule, habits, and personal preferences. This is the part of the program that states *what* the exercises will accomplish, *why* they are being undertaken, and *when* they will be done. The foundation also addresses the personal characteristics of *who* the program is designed for. The structure consists of the mode, intensity, duration, frequency, special considerations, fun, and relaxation. Based on several of the rules of conditioning, the structure addresses the details of *how* and *where* the exercises are to be done. The program's expansion capabilities depend on progression and variety—two concepts that re-address *how,* and potentially *where,* the exercises are completed as the client moves toward a higher level of fitness.

Each of the above elements is vital to the success of a client's program. These elements, along with the remaining rules of conditioning (safety, motivation, specialization, warm-up/cooldown, diet, capacity, balanced strength, routine, and modification) will help outline and detail a safe, effective, and meaningful conditioning program for each client—one that is suited to the client's needs at that time. All of the rules should be considered essential, but safety is the rule that must override all others. Caution all clients that nothing is as important as their safety. Once they have been cleared by a physician to begin a conditioning program, make sure the clients know how to exercise safely: teach them how to monitor their heart rate; show them how to calculate their target heart rate range; and explain to them the importance of appropriate intensity in exercise. A safe and healthy client should be the ultimate goal and is the best guarantee of success in business.

STUDENT ENRICHMENT ACTIVITIES

Write T for true, or F for false. Rewrite the false statements to make them true.

1. T F Having fun, although important, is not a key element in becoming fit.

2. T F A person's idea of what is fun in a fitness program can change over time.

3. T F Most people would rather not be around others when doing fitness activities.

4. T F The mode is the method that is determined to be the best and most appropriate to accomplish fitness goals.

5. T F It's best for your clients to just exercise at any time of day that fits, depending upon how their day goes.

6. T F Studies show that those who exercise in the morning tend to stay with their exercise programs more often than those who exercise during the afternoon and evening hours.

7. T F To get a true cardiovascular benefit, the client must exercise at an appropriate intensity for a minimum of 20 minutes.

8. T F The intensity of exercise can be measured by monitoring the heart rate during exercise.

9. T F For a fitness program that involves muscle strengthening, the muscles need two days of rest before exercising them again.

10. T F According to the *Healthy People 2010* report, the most significant factors of a healthy lifestyle can be achieved through personal habits.

Match the terms in Column A with the appropriate description in Column B.

Column A	Column B
11. routine	A. individuals with special physical capabilities or limitations
12. target heart rate range	B. the length of time an activity is performed
13. special populations	C. a repeating schedule for exercise
14. intensity	D. the threshold between productive exercise and overstressing a body system
15. duration	E. the number of times an activity is performed within a specific time frame
16. frequency	F. nonmeasurable data, such as "felt more optimistic"
17. subjective	G. the degree of effort required to complete a physical activity
18. objective	H. used to assess intensity in exercise
19. capacity	I. exercises and equipment used to condition the body
20. mode	J. measurable data, such as "target rate sustained for 30 minutes"

Complete the following exercises.

21. Explain why it is important to keep the evaluation of each client's physical and medical history in mind at all times during the conditioning workouts and during the overall conditioning program.

22. Explain why it is important to have a written plan of objective goals for your clients.

23. What is your target heart rate range?

24. Choose another person and determine the person's target heart rate range.

25. Imagine you have a new client. What questions should you ask before developing a new fitness program?

CHAPTER 9

Emergency Preparedness and Assessment

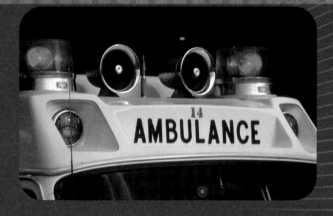

OBJECTIVES

After completing this chapter, you should be able to do the following:

1. Define and correctly spell each of the key terms.

2. Set up an Emergency Action Plan.

3. Identify the three body planes.

4. Describe the proper procedure for dealing with an unconscious athlete.

5. Perform primary and secondary surveys of injuries.

KEY TERMS

- active range of motion
- ashen
- assessment
- auscultate
- clammy
- coma
- cyanosis
- distended
- edema

- Emergency Action Plan
- emergency medical services (EMS)
- expiration
- HOPS
- inspiration
- isolated injury assessment
- log roll
- mechanism of injury

- mucus
- orientation
- paralysis
- passive range of motion
- PERL
- primary survey
- secondary survey
- stoma
- Trainer's Angel

EMERGENCIES ARE INEVITABLE

Injuries and other emergencies are an unavoidable aspect of sports. Imagine the following scenario:

> It is the end of the second quarter of the varsity football game, when you see a sweep around the right end. The defensive end holds his ground and makes the tackle after taking two head-on hits, one by the pulling guard and the other by the fullback. It's a great play, but the defensive end is a little slow getting up. Your instincts tell you to keep an eye on him as he goes back to the huddle. You can see that his balance is off and he is holding his head. At this point, you summon the coach to take the defensive end out so that you can evaluate him. As he approaches the sideline, you see that his eyes are glassy, and he has a vacant stare. It is time to remove the athlete from play and provide emergency care.

This is just one of the scenarios that a sports medicine professional may face. With this situation and many others, it is necessary to react quickly and confidently.

Certain information is required before the proper course of action can be determined. If the victim is conscious, much of this information can be gathered simply by talking to the patient, but information can be obtained in other ways as well. Accurate measurement of vital signs and careful observation of the patient are the keys to providing rapid and appropriate emergency care. Chapter 12 will describe how to accurately measure a patient's vital signs. This chapter will discuss the specific observational skills needed to perform both a primary and secondary survey on patients who are injured, as well as the procedures that must be followed to provide basic first aid to injured athletes.

THE IMPORTANCE OF GOOD OBSERVATIONAL SKILLS

assessment

evaluation of a patient's physical condition.

In order to provide the appropriate first aid to a patient, one must assess the extent of the person's injuries. Without this **assessment**, injuries that are not as obvious as others might go untreated, creating the potential for increased danger to the victim. To perform an accurate assessment of injured patients, learn to use a variety of observational skills, such as looking, listening, touching, and smelling.

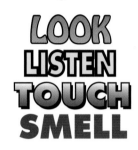

For example, deformities, swelling, discoloration, and the ability or inability to function can all be detected through visual observation of the patient. Red skin indicates a lack of oxygen or heatstroke, pale skin could indicate shock or heat exhaustion, and bluish skin is a signal that there may be an airway obstruction. Dark-skinned athletes who have a grayish cast around the nose or mouth may be in shock. These colors may also be observed on either the patient's fingernail beds or by gently pulling down the patient's lower lip. By listening to the patient, abnormal breathing sounds can be detected and the degree of pain can be assessed. By touching (palpating) the patient with the hands, one can determine swelling, skin temperature, and moisture. Cool and **clammy** skin may be a sign of shock, while hot and dry skin is a sign of heatstroke. Even the sense of smell can be used to detect certain conditions. For example, fruity smelling breath in an unconscious patient may indicate a diabetic coma.

clammy

moist.

PLAN FOR EMERGENCY ACTION

Emergency Action Plan

a written plan that describes procedures and roles that must be in place for emergency situations.

Establishing and implementing an **Emergency Action Plan** (Figures 9-1 and 9-2) is one of the most important duties an athletic trainer will perform. This plan is not something to just put on a board and perform when an emergency occurs. This is a written plan of emergency action procedures and roles that must be practiced during practice periods until everyone feels confident to perform the appropriate duties without confusion. Because certain gates normally open during the day may be locked at night, the plan must be practiced during both day and evening hours. This will prevent unwelcome surprises in the event of a nighttime or evening emergency. Make sure to record, and put on file, each date and time that the Emergency Action Plan is practiced.

Remember, the plan must work during after-school practices, evening practices, night and day games, at weekend events, and at events that are held off school premises, such as golf tournaments, cross-country races, and while traveling. Circumstances will change, such as gate closures, the ability to access fields in different locations on the athletic facilities, and the ability to carry cell phones. If phones are temporarily unavailable, such as in certain long-distance running events, have a teammate who is at a similar skill level assist in monitoring any of the athletes with known medical conditions. The athletic trainer will not be able to be everywhere at once, so prepare by delegating certain responsibilities to other members of the sports medicine team.

The Emergency Action Plan should also designate which person will take care of each emergency procedure (Figure 9-2). It is helpful to supply and practice

EMERGENCY ACTION PLAN
PROCEDURES

Organization_____

Sport _____ **Team** _____ **Year** _____

In the event of a medical emergency the on-duty physician, certified athletic trainer, or paramedic will administer immediate emergency aid to the injured person. If none of the above are present, then the head coach or designated first aider will assume responsibility.

The designated person will immediately initiate the Emergency Medical System (EMS). Please follow these procedures for a prompt and efficient response.

1. The designated care provider will remain with the injured athlete at all times.

2. Designated person use cell phone and dial 911 or other predetermined number.

    A. Identify self and exact location.

    B. State the nature of the injury. (Head/neck, fracture, loss of consciousness, or heat illness.)

    C. Instruct the emergency vehicle exactly where and how to reach activity area:
    - Street access
    - Entry gate
    - Building location
    - Building entry

    D. Stay on line until operator disconnects.

    E. Return to injury scene to be available for additional assistance.

3. Designated person meet the vehicle at the gate entrance. This person will have all necessary gate/door keys.

4. Designated person contact security for crowd control and other needs.

5. Designated person immediately call parents/guardian and advise them of circumstances, then call designated administrator and advise of circumstances.

6. Designated person document all information relating to injury and emergency response.

7. Designated person accompanies the injured athlete to the hospital and remains until parents/guardian or designated administrator arrives.

FIGURE 9-1 Procedures for the Emergency Action Plan

**EMERGENCY ACTION PLAN
DESIGNATED ROLES**

(Complete prior to activity/event.)

Name

1. _____ Attends to injured athlete, controls scene.

2. _____ Calls 911 or other predetermined number.

3. _____ Supervises team.

4. _____ Calls security and initiates crowd control.

5. _____ Meets paramedics at gate and guides to injured athlete.

6. _____ Gives emergency card to paramedics.

7. _____ Calls parents/guardian or alternate name on emergency card.

8. _____ Accompanies injured athlete to hospital.

PROCEDURES FOR CALLING 911

*This is to be filled out by the designated caller prior to the activity session,
and kept in his or her possession until the session is concluded.*

1. REMAIN CALM. This will aid the operator in receiving your information.

2. Dial 911. (Remember you may need to access an outside line first.)

3. My name is: _____

4. I need paramedics at: _____

5. My exact address is: _____
   The major cross streets are: _____ and _____, which
   is _____ blocks away.

6. There is an athlete with a _____ injury.
   The athlete's name is: _____

7. The athlete is located at: _____, which is on the
   _____ side of the facility.

8. I am calling from: _____ (phone number).

9. _____ will meet the ambulance/paramedics at: _____

10. Do not end the call until the operator hangs up first.

FIGURE 9-2 Designated Roles for the Emergency Action Plan

a script for making proper **emergency medical services (EMS)** telephone calls. For instance, prior to the event, someone must be designated to make sure that there is access to a phone and that the keys to any gates that may be needed are available. Someone also must be responsible for knowing how to access the athletic field so that the EMS unit can get to the injured athlete. During the event, one person can be designated to provide first aid to injured athletes, while a second person makes the emergency phone call. The person making the phone call must know the emergency phone number and any special number needed to get an outside line. Once in contact with EMS, the telephone person needs to tell EMS personnel what is wrong with the injured athlete. The written Emergency Action Plan should be placed above all telephones and carried with all cell phones, so that when an emergency does occur, the telephone person can read right through the plan.

When it is time to contact the EMS system, it is important to stay calm. The EMS authority will need the following information:

1. Any information on the severity of the injury.

2. What first aid is being provided.

3. The address and location of the injured athlete.

4. Where you will meet the EMS team.

Make sure to know the athletes; know their past injuries, any special medical conditions, and their tolerance to pain. This will help better understand the extent of any injuries that occur.

IMPLEMENTING EMERGENCY PROCEDURES

When approaching the injured athlete, make sure to move quickly and *do not panic*. Stay in charge of the situation until a more skilled health care provider arrives. For example, if a certified athletic trainer, emergency medical technician (EMT), paramedic, nurse, or a physician is available, step aside; however, stay available to help in any way possible. If no one else is around, proceed with the appropriate first aid until someone with higher qualifications arrives.

If the head athletic trainer is taking care of the injury, the athletic training student can make sure anyone who does not have anything directly to do with the injured athlete is kept away from the area.

> **emergency medical services (EMS)**
>
> mobile emergency health care providers.

NOTE:

It is recognized that gloves will not always be worn in all procedures. However, Universal Precautions require the use of gloves whenever blood or other body fluids are present. Because there is a greater chance of exposure to blood in contact sports, gloves are included in all procedures.

THE PRIMARY SURVEY

When in charge of administering first aid, immediately determine if the patient has a life-threatening condition by performing a systematic sideline evaluation. This is called the **primary survey**. Check a watch when approaching the patient (you may need to record the time if the patient is unconscious). The first thing to determine is level of consciousness. It is vital to immediately know if the patient is awake and alert, or unconscious. By introducing yourself and telling the patient why you are there, you are able to see how the patient can respond. Ask the patient how he or she is feeling: *"Hello, I'm John Smith. I'm an athletic trainer, and I'm here to help you. How are you feeling?"*

Does the patient respond? If so, are the answers appropriate to the question? Is the patient alert and oriented? If so, proceed to the secondary survey. If the patient is nonresponsive, begin the primary survey immediately. Remembering the primary survey is as easy as A-B-C.

* **A** = AIRWAY

* **B** = BREATHING

* **C** = CIRCULATION

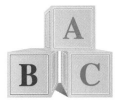

primary survey

an examination of the patient to determine the presence of any life-threatening emergencies; the initial assessment of airway, breathing, and circulation on a patient.

Airway

Is the airway open? If not, make an airway using the head-tilt, chin-lift maneuver (Figure 9-3; see also Chapter 13.) Always treat an unconscious patient as if there is a spinal injury. Therefore, in an unconscious patient use only this maneuver to open the airway. *Do not move the head or neck!* Spinal injuries and their symptoms are discussed in Chapter 15. Note: If blood or other body fluids are present, put on gloves before touching the patient.

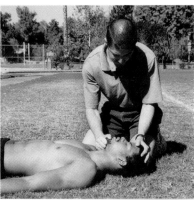

FIGURE 9-3 Head-Tilt, Chin-Lift Maneuver

If the Airway Is Not Clear

1. Wear gloves.

2. Grasp the mouth and *open the jaw* with the thumb and index finger.

3. Use the index finger to do a finger sweep (see Figure 9-4) to *remove any objects*. Note: This is done on a child or infant only if you can see the object!

4. *Make an airway using the head-tilt/chin-lift maneuver.*

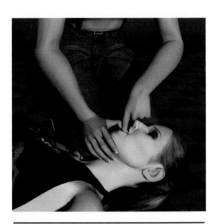

FIGURE 9-4 Finger Sweep

An injured football player's helmet must never be taken off if there is any chance of a neck injury. Taking the helmet off will jar the neck, and once the helmet is removed, the height of the shoulder pads will cause the head to hyperextend, creating the potential for increased damage to the spine. In an emergency, the airway of a player who is wearing a helmet with a face mask can be accessed by removing the face mask completely. This is done by cutting the face mask side attachments using the **Trainer's Angel**, FM extractor, or other face mask removal device that enables removal of the face mask within 30 seconds, while another rescuer stabilizes the head and neck. The helmet is left on the athlete. This procedure must be practiced with a CPR mannequin or with a friend under the supervision of a certified athletic trainer until it can be performed correctly. This is a skill that saves lives!

Trainer's Angel

a device made specifically to cut off the side tabs of the face mask to hinge it back or remove it.

NOTE:

If the removal of the face mask cannot be done easily within 30 seconds, the face mask and side attachments should be changed to other types so this can be done properly.

Breathing

Is the patient breathing? What is the rate of breathing? Look at the chest: is it moving (Figure 9-5)? Listen to the mouth for air movement (Figure 9-6). Feel for the presence of air. Again, is the patient breathing? Is it adequate? Place one ear near the patient's mouth and look toward the chest to evaluate the patient's respiration. From this position, one can hear the breath flow from the mouth, feel the breath on the ear, and watch the chest rise and fall as the patient breathes. If the athlete is face-down, this

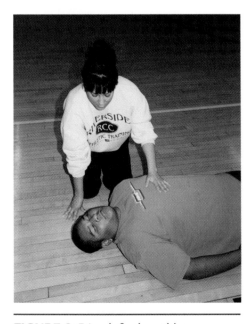

FIGURE 9-5 Look for breathing.

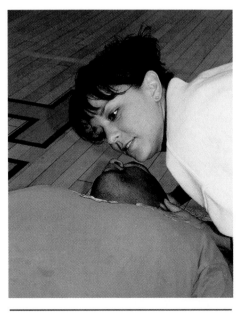

FIGURE 9-6 Listen and feel for breathing.

evaluation can be done by placing one hand near the mouth to feel for breath, and the other hand on the back to feel the rise and fall of the chest. Are the respirations noisy, labored, or gurgling? Gurgling respirations indicate fluid in the lungs.

FACE MASK REMOVAL USING THE TRAINER'S ANGEL

Materials Needed:

* Trainer's Angel
  or
* FM extractor (choose tool based on type of helmet)

1. **Procedural Step:** The athlete should be lying on the back. If necessary, gently log roll the athlete to achieve this position. Stabilize the head and neck.

   Reason: To avoid further injury to the athlete.

2. **Procedural Step:** Use the Trainer's Angel to cut the first clip in one of the following two ways:

   A. Position the blade on top of the clip and the notched end below the clip. This will involve a short downward cut through the clip.

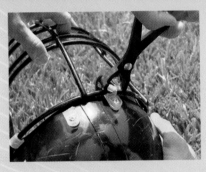

3. **Procedural Step:** Complete the cut by pressing the handles of the Trainer's Angel together.

   Reason: The clips must be cut to remove the face mask.

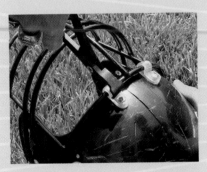

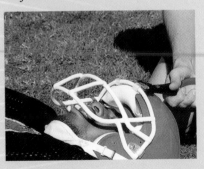

   B. Position the blade on one side of the clip and the notched end on the other side. This will involve a longer sideways cut through the clip.

   Reason: Either position will be suitable for cutting the clip.

4. **Procedural Step:** Cut the remaining clips in the same way.

   Reason: All of the clips must be cut before the face mask can be removed.

5. **Procedural Step:** Remove the face mask from the helmet.

   Reason: To gain access to the athlete's airway.

If the Patient Is Not Breathing

1. *Call for help.*

2. *Immediately correct any severe breathing problems.* (Clear the airway of any obstructions.)

3. *Begin rescue breathing.* (See Chapter 13.)

Circulation

Does the patient show signs of circulation? These signs are normal breathing, movement, coughing, or a carotid pulse.

If None of These Signs Are Present, Begin CPR

Assessment of the ABCs is known as the primary survey. It is done on all patients. If the patient is talking, it's obvious the patient is both breathing and has a pulse. If the patient is nonresponsive or in a **coma**, it is essential to do a primary survey immediately. Reassessment of the patient also is necessary at frequent intervals. A patient can be awake and responding one moment and unconscious the next. Always begin with the primary survey when approaching an unconscious patient.

> **coma**
>
> a state of unconsciousness or deep stupor.

If the athlete is face-down, but shows any of the signs of circulation and is breathing, there is no reason to turn the person over. However, if there are no signs of circulation or breathing and the patient is face-down, carefully **log roll** the victim to begin CPR. This procedure is detailed in Chapter 13. Remember, if the injured athlete is wearing a helmet with a face mask, *do not remove the helmet! Remove only the face mask to access the airway.* Do not give inhalants to an unconscious athlete. The athlete may have a neck injury, and inhalants may cause the athlete to jerk the head back, causing further damage to the neck.

> **log roll**
>
> the method used to turn a patient with a spinal injury, in which the patient is moved to the side in one motion.

Patients who are unconscious must *always* be treated as if they have a head or spine injury. Stabilize the patient's head and neck immediately with blankets or pillows and take all precautions. Monitor the patient's vital signs until the EMS arrives. Note the amount of time the patient was unconscious, and give the information to the EMS. If the patient regains consciousness, keep the patient calm while maintaining the head and body position until the EMS arrives.

THINKING IT THROUGH

It was the first game of the season and the team was playing at St. O'Leary High School. In the third quarter Germane, the starting defensive back, hit the running back head on, went down in a lump, and didn't move. Terry, one of the athletic training students, accompanied the head athletic trainer, Mr. Hill, out to the injured player, who was face-up. Mr. Hill checked his vital signs. The vitals were good, but Mr. Hill was concerned about Germane's neck. Mr. Hill stabilized Germane's neck while Terry used a Trainer's Angel to remove the face mask. If things took a turn for the worse, they would at least have unobstructed access to Germane's airway.

This was all very scary, but Terry knew what she had to do because they had practiced this very scenario many times and were ready for cases like this. They went to work without even thinking twice. As soon as Mr. Hill put his hands to the athlete's head, the athletic training students went about the jobs they were trained to do in situations like this: Terry stayed to assist Mr. Hill; Emily went to activate EMS and show them in; and Justin went to get Germane's insurance information.

The next day Germane was fine. He had been taken to the hospital for x-rays and further evaluation. All the athletic training students met with Mr. Hill and walked through what had happened the previous day. It was a great feeling to know that all the practicing they had done, which had seemed kind of boring at the time, was well worth it.

Why was it a good thing that the injured football player was face-up? Why is it important to have a plan for activating the EMS? What are the benefits of reviewing the plan of action before and after an emergency situation has taken place?

THE SECONDARY SURVEY

secondary survey

a head-to-toe physical assessment; an additional assessment of a patient to determine the existence of any injuries other than those found in the primary survey.

orientation

the ability to comprehend one's environment regarding time, place, situation, and identity of persons.

The **secondary survey** is a head-to-toe physical assessment that is done on patients to determine the extent of illness or injury. Some injuries and illnesses are obvious, but some are not so obvious. A head-to-toe assessment, or secondary survey, will help in locating all major injuries. Ideally, this should take about 2 minutes, but do not feel rushed. This survey will determine if the injured player will be allowed to leave the field independently, with assistance, or if an EMS squad is required. If it is determined the athlete will be lying on the field for any amount of time, a blanket should be placed around the patient. Make sure to stay calm and keep the athlete calm as well. Keep anyone who doesn't need to be there away from the immediate area. While examining the patient, ask questions about the injury or illness. Talking to the patient can relieve some of the anxiety and allow for the patient's **orientation** level to be checked at the same time.

The information obtained from the secondary survey must be used to evaluate whether the appropriate treatment can be provided to the athlete, or if the EMS should be called. Do not rush. Take all the time needed to make a good, thorough injury assessment and make the decision accordingly. Ideally, the patient should be lying down while being evaluated. In some cases, the patient may be allowed to sit up in a controlled environment while making the evaluation. If the athlete is more comfortable sitting up than lying down and is able to sit up without assistance, allow the athlete to sit while the assessment is done. Reassure the athlete at all times. Keep the athlete warm and continue to monitor all vital signs. Continue to ask how the athlete feels. Call the EMS using the Emergency Action Plan if unsure of how to proceed or if the situation requires a person with greater skills.

PERFORMING A SECONDARY SURVEY

Materials Needed:

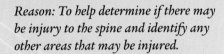

* gloves (if blood or other body fluids are present)

1. **Procedural Step:** Wash your hands if possible.

   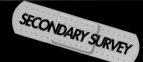

   Reason: Universal Precaution.

2. **Procedural Step:** Wear gloves if blood or any other body fluids are present.

   Reason: Universal Precaution.

3. **Procedural Step:** Explain the procedure to the patient using terms he or she will understand.

   Reason: To keep the patient calm and gather the information necessary for the patient to give informed consent.

4. **Procedural Step:** Beginning at the neck, handle the patient gently. Do not move the patient until you have deter-mined that there is no spinal injury.

   Reason: To avoid injuries to the patient's spine.

5. **Procedural Step:** Look for bleeding, swelling, or deformities.

   Reason: Presence indicates trauma.

6. **Procedural Step:** Determine the **mechanism of injury**. Did the patient hear or feel anything? Has the patient had any previous injuries or other problems with this area before? Did anyone else see what happened?

Reason: To help determine if there may be injury to the spine and identify any other areas that may be injured.

7. **Procedural Step:** While you are talking to the patient, obtain a history from the patient. Make sure you know the answers to any orientation questions you may ask the athlete. For example, you might ask, "What is your name?"; "What team do you play for?"; What is the score?"; and "What is the period?" Questions to ask to obtain a history might include: "How did the injury occur?"; "Where do you hurt?"; "Can you describe the pain?"; and "Do you have a headache or any ringing in your ears?"

   Reason: To check the patient's orientation and any possible retrograde amnesia.

8. **Procedural Step:** Does the patient have any pain in the neck? If so, assume there is a spinal injury.

   Reason: Pain may indicate injury.

9. **Procedural Step:** Look at the veins in the neck. Are they flat, **distended**, or bulging?

   Reason: When a person is lying down, the neck veins are normally slightly distended, stretched out, or inflated. A patient who is having problems with circulation may have neck veins that bulge.

(continues)

mechanism of injury

how the injury occurred.

distended

expanded or swollen.

PERFORMING A SECONDARY SURVEY (Continued)

10. Procedural Step: Is there any swelling in the neck?

Reason: Swelling can interfere with the airway.

stoma

surgically constructed opening in throat used for breathing.

11. Procedural Step: Look for a **stoma** in the throat.

Reason: A stoma is a permanent opening in the throat. The patient now breathes from this opening, rather than through the nose or mouth.

12. Procedural Step: Palpate (feel) the back of the neck for any deformity or tenderness.

Reason: Deformity or tenderness may indicate injury.

13. Procedural Step: Check the neck for a Medic-Alert tag.

Reason: These tags provide useful medical information when treating children, confused adults, or unconscious patients. (Note: you should already be aware of any medical conditions in the athletes you work with every day. This information should be on file as part of the athlete's medical history.)

14. Procedural Step: Gently palpate the entire scalp with both hands.

Reason: To search the entire scalp for bleeding, swelling, or deformity.

15. Procedural Step: Check the athlete for a possible concussion:

Ask the athlete to repeat a series of numbers forward and backward (e.g., 4-8-2-9).

Ask the athlete to recite the months of the year in reverse.

See if the athlete can remember three words (e.g., green, play, sports) and three objects (e.g., bench, ball, car) for 5 minutes.

Reason: A concussion may be a life-threatening injury.

16. Procedural Step: Feel for swelling by touching lightly all around the back of the head.

Reason: Lacerations may not be obvious on people with a lot of hair until the scalp is palpated.

17. Procedural Step: Palpate the face for tenderness or fractures.

Reason: A pain response pain may indicate an injury.

18. Procedural Step: Look at the patient's face for signs of symmetry (the equality of body parts). The parts should be equal in size, shape, and location.

Reason: Asymmetry may indicate an injury. For example, the eyes are symmetrical except when there is an injury. In this case, the injured eye may be swollen, or one pupil may appear to be a different size or shape than the other.

19. Procedural Step: Check the ears for any drainage.

Reason: Bloody drainage can indicate trauma. Clear drainage may be cerebrospinal fluid from a fractured skull.

20. Procedural Step: Look at the shape of the nose.

Reason: Deformity could indicate a fracture.

PERFORMING A SECONDARY SURVEY

21. Procedural Step: Check the nose for any fluid, drainage, or bleeding.

Reason: Clear drainage may be **mucus** *or cerebrospinal fluid.*

22. Procedural Step: Look in the mouth and check for any loose or missing teeth.

Reason: Teeth can block an airway if they get caught in the trachea. It may be possible to re-implant lost teeth if they are brought in with the patient.

23. Procedural Step: Look at the color of the lips and the inside of the mouth.

*Reason: A blue tinge to the lips (*cyanosis*) can indicate a lack of oxygen. This may indicate shock.*

24. Procedural Step: Check to see if there is any blood in the patient's mouth. If so, check to to see if the patient has bitten his or her tongue.

Reason: Blood in the patient's mouth not caused by biting the tongue may indicate a fractured rib.

25. Procedural Step: Check to see if the mouth is dry or if saliva is present.

Reason: Dry, cracked lips may indicate a fever, diabetic problem, or dehydration.

26. Procedural Step: Look at the eyes. Is the patient wearing contact lenses? If so, and if it is necessary to remove the lenses, place them in containers labeled with the patient's name, and make sure they are transported with the patient. Label one container *right eye lens* and one container *left eye lens.*

Reason: Contact lenses are personal property and must be accounted for. They can cause eye injury and can interfere with treatment.

27. Procedural Step: Look at the pupils by shining a penlight into each one.

Reason: Pupils that are constricted (small) can indicate a drug overdose or other medical problem. Normal pupils will react to light by becoming smaller (constricting). Pupils that do not react to light, or pupils that are dilated (large) can indicate a serious problem such as a head injury, drug abuse, etc. Unequal pupils can be a sign of head injury.

28. Procedural Step: When checking the pupils for reaction to light, make sure that an overhead light is not shining in the patient's face.

Reason: This may alter the results.

29. Procedural Step: Take the penlight from the side of the patient's face and shine directly into one eye and watch for a reaction. When done, repeat this procedure with the other eye.

*Reason: Pupils that are equal and react to light are normal (*PERL*).*

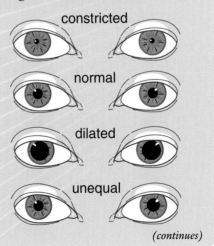

constricted

normal

dilated

unequal

(continues)

mucus
fluid secreted from the nose.

cyanosis
a bluish tint to the skin and mucous membranes caused by a decrease in oxygen.

PERL
the abbreviation for pupils equal and react to light.

ashen

a gray skin color seen in shock patients.

PERFORMING A SECONDARY SURVEY (Continued)

30. **Procedural Step:** While inspecting the head and face, check the skin. Is the skin warm and dry, hot, cold and clammy, **ashen**, or pale?

    Reason: Warm and dry is the normal skin condition. Hot skin can indicate fever or heatstroke. Cold skin can indicate shock or hypothermia.

31. **Procedural Step:** Is the skin diaphoretic (moist)?

    Reason: Wet skin can occur with fever, shock, heart attack, stroke, and diabetes.

32. **Procedural Step:** What is the color of the skin? Is it red, pale, or cyanotic (blue)? On patients with darker skin, check the nail beds or the inside bottom lip to determine the skin color.

    Reason: Color changes in the skin are indications of how well the blood is circulating and carrying oxygen to the tissues. Red skin can indicate heatstroke, high blood pressure, or carbon monoxide poisoning. Pale or ashen skin can mean insufficient circulation, shock, fright, bleeding, heat exhaustion, or insulin shock. Bluish skin or lips indicate the patient is not receiving enough oxygen and may have an obstructed airway.

33. **Procedural Step:** Check the chest for symmetry. Are both sides moving up and down with respirations?

    Reason: Normal breathing is quiet and effortless. Both sides of the chest should move with each breath. If only one side of the chest is moving, there may be a serious respiratory problem.

34. **Procedural Step:** If you suspect a problem with the chest area, look at the chest for scars, but respect the patient's privacy and maintain the patient's dignity. Do not expose the patient's chest unnecessarily.

    Reason: Scars may indicate previous surgery or injury.

35. **Procedural Step:** Look for any deformities, bruises, or contusions.

    Reason: Bruises and deformities can be caused by a fractured rib.

36. **Procedural Step:** Palpate the chest by feeling both sides of the chest. Watch the patient for signs of discomfort.

    Reason: Pain may indicate an injury.

37. **Procedural Step:** Feel the clavicles and ribs for tenderness, pain, or instability.

    Reason: Pain may indicate an injury.

38. **Procedural Step:** Listen to the breathing pattern. Is it regular or noisy? Is there a wheeze, rattle, or cough?

    Reason: There may be fluid in the lungs.

39. **Procedural Step:** If respirations are noisy or difficult, **auscultate** the chest with a stethoscope.

    Reason: To hear the chest sounds better.

40. **Procedural Step:** Listen to the front, back, left, and right sides of the chest, and compare the sounds heard during both **inspiration** and **expiration**. Listen in at least four places.

auscultate

to listen.

inspiration

inhalation; the act of breathing something into the lungs.

expiration

exhalation; the act of breathing out.

PERFORMING A SECONDARY SURVEY

Reason: To get an accurate assessment. If breath sounds are absent (or mostly absent) in one or both lobes, call the EMS and start artificial respiration immediately. (See Chapter 13.)

41. Procedural Step: Check the abdomen for scars, bruises, and distention.

Reason: Scars will alert you to any previous surgeries.

42. Procedural Step: Palpate the abdomen in all four quadrants (see illustration) for any tenderness, guarding (lying on side with knees flexed), pain, or rigidity.

Reason: A rigid or tender abdomen could be a sign of internal bleeding. Guarding is a nonverbal sign of pain.

43. Procedural Step: Start at the right upper quadrant and carefully palpate the entire abdomen in a clockwise direction.

Reason: To check the whole abdomen.

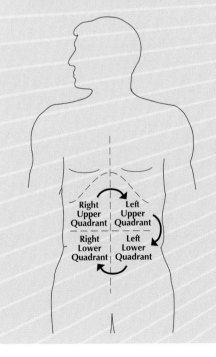

44. Procedural Step: Check to see if the patient appears to be in pain.

Reason: Facial grimace, abdomen clutching, and drawn up lower legs (guarding) are all signs of pain.

45. Procedural Step: Check for nausea or vomiting. What color is the vomitus and how much is there?

Reason: Bright red vomitus indicates bleeding. Yellow could be bile and may mean the liver has been injured. Dark red may indicate old blood in the stomach.

46. Procedural Step: Check the pelvis and look for signs of incontinence or bleeding.

Reason: Incontinence (loss of bladder or bowel control) may indicate a problem with the nervous system.

47. Procedural Step: Check for pain in the pelvic area.

Reason: Pain may indicate injury.

48. Procedural Step: Look at the lower extremities. Are there any deformities?

Reason: Deformity is one of the first signs of a fracture.

49. Procedural Step: Check to see how the legs are positioned. Palpate for the femoral pulse.

Reason: The femoral pulse is located in the groin on the inner side of the femur. A strong pulse indicates adequate circulation.

50. Procedural Step: Evaluate one leg at a time. Start with the upper thigh and palpate for any tenderness, swelling, or pain. Continue down the leg and feel the knee, lower leg,

(continues)

PERFORMING A SECONDARY SURVEY (Continued)

edema

swelling because of excess fluid in the tissues.

and foot. What is the skin temperature? Is the skin wet or dry?

Reason: To check for injuries and evaluate circulation.

51. **Procedural Step:** Compare the legs to each other.

    Reason: Deformities may indicate an injury.

52. **Procedural Step:** Check for sensation in both legs by brushing your fingers over them.

    Reason: To check for paralysis or other circulatory or neurologic problems.

53. **Procedural Step:** Check for movement in both legs. Without causing the athlete unnecessary pain, carefully check the range of motion (ROM) in each leg. First, have the patient demonstrate pain-free ROM without assistance. (Have the patient move the extremity in a manner that does not hurt.) Next, have the athlete move the extremity in the same direction against resistance by pushing against your hand. Finally, have the athlete demonstrate the ROM against resistance in the direction that causes pain, being careful not to cause further injury.

    Reason: To check for paralysis or other circulatory or neurologic problems.

54. **Procedural Step:** Check for pulses in the lower legs and feet. What color are the feet?

    Reason: A strong pulse indicates adequate circulation. Skin color also indicates the quality of circulation.

55. **Procedural Step:** Look for **edema**, especially in the ankles.

    Reason: Swollen ankles are signs of trauma, heart disease, and/or increased fluid.

56. **Procedural Step:** Ask the patient to move both feet. Can the patient feel and move both lower extremities?

    Reason: Indicates function of the nervous system.

57. **Procedural Step:** Check both arms as you did the legs. Look at the color of the skin and check for cuts or bruises.

    Reason: To check for injuries and evaluate circulation.

58. **Procedural Step:** Look for track marks (red marks over veins) or abscesses (localized collections of pus).

    Reason: May indicate IV substance abuse.

59. **Procedural Step:** Look for a Medic-Alert bracelet.

    Reason: This is a tag that provides information about known medical conditions or allergies.

60. **Procedural Step:** Feel for pulses at the brachial and radial arteries. The brachial pulse is located on the inside of the arm at the bend of the elbow. The radial pulse is located in the wrist on the thumb side.

    Reason: The strength of a pulse indicates the quality of circulation.

PERFORMING A SECONDARY SURVEY

61. Procedural Step: Ask the patient to move both hands, make a fist, or to squeeze your hands.

Reason: To assess the central nervous system.

62. Procedural Step: Check the strength of hand grips. They should be equal.

Reason: Weakness occurs in stroke victims and in patients with head or brachial plexus injuries.

63. Procedural Step: Depending on the patient's condition, you may need to log roll the patient to see the back. *Always* get help if there is any chance of a spinal injury.

Reason: To prevent injury to yourself and further injury to the patient.

64. Procedural Step: Look for bruises, scars, or wounds on the back.

Reason: To check for injuries.

65. Procedural Step: Palpate the thoracic, lumbar, and sacral areas for pain and tenderness.

Reason: Pain or tenderness may indicate an injury.

66. Procedural Step: Check to see if the athlete can run 40 yards and do five push-ups, five sit-ups, and five knee bends without headache or dizziness.

Reason: To assess the athlete's ability to return to play.

67. Procedural Step: Remove and dispose of your gloves if it was necessary to put them on.

Reason: Universal Precaution.

68. Procedural Step: Wash your hands.

Reason: Universal Precaution.

69. Procedural Step: Record your findings on the patient's chart.

Reason: To provide documentation.

If an injury is witnessed, an **isolated injury assessment** may be a more appropriate assessment than a secondary survey. This means that only the area of injury is evaluated. However, the secondary survey can help identify other signs and symptoms that may indicate further injury. One can never be overly cautious when assessing injuries. Remember that your job is to provide assistance to those with higher levels of medical training. If you begin to suspect that treatment of an injury is beyond your capabilities, activate the EMS.

HOPS

The key to injury assessment is to make sure that no injury is made worse by the process. All observations made and information gained in performing the assessment must be recorded and passed to the appropriate health care professionals to ensure effective continuity of care for the athlete. **HOPS** is an acronym for history, observation, palpation, and stress tests. The objective of the HOPS procedure is careful and

isolated injury assessment

a thorough examination of a specific part of the body to determine the extent of injury that may have occurred.

HOPS

a system of medical evaluation based on history, observation, palpation, and stress tests.

methodical injury assessment. It begins with the least invasive method of gathering information and slowly progresses to manipulation of the injury if appropriate. Therefore, the order in which these steps are taken is vital to safe assessment.

* History (based on subjective findings): How did the injury happen? When did it happen? Has this ever happened to the athlete before? What did the person hear or feel? Did anyone else see what happened?

* Observation (based on objective findings): Compare the uninvolved side to the involved side, always checking the uninvolved side first. Is there any swelling, deformity, numbness, discoloration, bleeding, or break in the skin? Look for any scars from previous surgeries, muscle atrophy, or loss of range of motion. Watch how the athlete leaves the field. Is the athlete limping? How quickly did the athlete get up? How is the athlete holding the injury? Did the athlete ask for assistance?

* Palpation: Ask the athlete to point to the area that hurts. Feel for deformities, spasms, pulses, breaks in the skin, and changes in temperature.

* Stress Tests: Check the **active range of motion**, then the **passive range of motion**, and finally perform resisted manual muscle testing. Additional special tests may also be needed. Some common special tests are discussed in the injuries sections of this chapter. If assessment or treatment of an injury is beyond your abilities, activate the EMS or refer the athlete to a physician as appropriate.

Asking about the injury provides information about the nature and location of the injury. Visually observing the injured area before feeling (palpating) it can avoid causing the athlete unnecessary pain and help determine the need for protective gloves before continuing with the assessment. Finally, performing palpation prior to stress testing can supply information to help prevent further injury. For example, in a compound fracture bone ends sometimes slip back beneath the skin, hiding the severity of the injury. By first asking questions, then looking at the injury, and then feeling for breaks in the skin, one can determine the possibility of such a fracture and avoid unnecessary movement of the injured body part that might lead to additional complications.

Body Planes and Directional Terms

When performing a secondary survey, it is important to keep in mind the terminology used in health care to describe different areas of the body. In the field of medicine, imaginary lines are used to separate the body into sections (see Figure 9-7). Because the results of the survey must be communicated to other emergency personnel, one of the most important aspects of accurate documentation and patient assessment involves the use of the appropriate anatomical terms.

The transverse plane refers to an imaginary, horizontal line that divides the body into a top half and a bottom half. The transverse plane also has two other directional terms associated with it. The first term, cranial, refers to body parts that are located near the head. The second term, caudal, refers to the body parts that are located near the lower back or sacral area.

---

active range of motion

AROM; movement of a joint through a range of motion produced by muscle contraction (i.e., without assistance).

passive range of motion

PROM; movement of a joint through a range of motion produced by an outside force (i.e., with assistance).

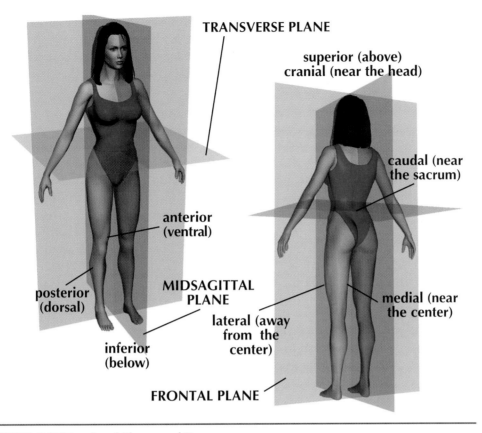

FIGURE 9-7 Directional Planes and Terms

Another directional plane that is used in the medical field is the midsagittal plane. This refers to the imaginary line that divides the human body exactly into right and left halves. This plane also has two other terms associated with the location of body areas: medial and lateral. Medial pertains to those parts located near the middle, or center, of the body. Lateral refers to those parts located near the outer sides of the body (away from the center).

The third and last directional plane used when referring to the location of body parts is the frontal, or coronal, plane. This plane uses an imaginary line to separate the body into a front and back section. The body parts located on the front are referred to as ventral, or anterior. Parts located on the back are referred to as dorsal, or posterior.

Body parts that are located above another are said to be superior to those located below. Body organs or parts that are located below others are inferior to those located above. For example, the thigh is inferior to the chest, but superior to the foot.

Other locational terms used extensively in the health care field are distal, proximal, external, and internal. Distal indicates that a body part lies distant to the original reference point (i.e., the radial pulse is distal to the upper arm). Proximal means the opposite of distal; the body part is close to the reference point. For example, in reference to the shoulder, the elbow is proximal and the wrist is distal. External generally refers to a location outside of or near the surface of the body.

For example, the ribs are said to be external to the heart because they surround the heart. Internal refers to a location that is inside the body. For example, the stomach is an internal organ. Internal wounds or incisions are said to be *deep* and external wounds are described as *superficial*. Make sure to understand these terms and use them correctly.

MOVEMENT OF THE ATHLETE

paralysis

loss of sensation and movement over an area of the body because of nerve damage.

Provide any necessary emergency first aid before moving the athlete. If the athlete shows any symptoms that indicate a head or spinal cord problem, such as **paralysis**, leave the athlete in the position produced by the incident (if breathing) and protect the head and neck until the EMS arrives. The one exception to this rule is if the spine-injured patient is not breathing. In this case, stabilize the spine, turn the patient carefully using the log roll procedure, and begin CPR while waiting for the EMS to arrive. (See Chapter 13.)

If the athlete has no symptoms that indicate a head or neck injury, the person may be assisted to a sitting position. Reevaluate the situation while the athlete is seated, checking for dizziness and evaluating the athlete's coherence. Bring the patient to a standing position, and recheck to make sure there is no change in signs or symptoms. This will give the athlete a chance to relax and confirm that dizziness or faintness is not a problem. If everything appears to be all right while the athlete is standing, assist the athlete back to the bench for a better assessment of the injury. If at any time the signs and symptoms change, help the patient lie down and call the EMS.

CHAPTER SUMMARY

Everything addressed in this chapter, as well as in other chapters in this book, will help in the preparation to provide quality care to athletes and patients. Practice these newly learned skills frequently. These skills must become second nature. When an emergency arises, there won't be time to refer to a book to look up what is supposed to be done. Do not ever guess at the correct way to approach an injury! Remember, people will be relying on your help. Take the time not only to learn this information, but also to understand why it is necessary to perform these tasks in a particular way. This will increase self-confidence and ability to competently take care of injuries when they happen—and they *do* happen!

Make sure that the entire sports medicine team is aware of the Emergency Action Plan and its importance. Practice this plan frequently, involving as many athletes and members of the sports medicine team as possible. Anticipate how conditions of the Emergency Action Plan might be affected during night or weekend use of the facilities.

STUDENT ENRICHMENT ACTIVITIES

Complete the following sentences.

1. The primary survey is an initial assessment of _____, _____, and _____.

2. The _____ _____ is a head-to-toe injury assessment.

3. HOPS is an acronym for _____, _____, _____, and _____ tests.

4. In an unconscious patient with a closed airway, the _____ maneuver should be used to open the airway.

5. After approaching a downed athlete and finding that he is unresponsive, you should begin the _____ _____ immediately.

6. The face mask of a potentially neck-injured football player can be removed safely using the _____ _____ or _____ _____.

Define the following terms.

7. distal

8. anterior

9. medial

10. posterior

11. superior

Write the letter of the correct answer.

12. Refers to a location outside of or near the surface of the body:

    A. distal.

    B. external.

    C. ventral.

    D. internal.

13. When you place an emergency phone call, the EMS will need all of the following information except:

    A. the first aid being provided.

    B. the exact location of the injured athlete.

    C. your address.

    D. where you will meet the EMS team.

14. If a patient is not breathing, the correct procedure is to:

    A. call for help, begin rescue breathing, and clear the airway.

    B. call for help, clear the airway, and begin rescue breathing.

C. begin rescue breathing, clear the airway, and call for help.

D. notify your supervisor.

15. If an athlete is face-down, is not breathing, and has no pulse, you must do this before beginning CPR:

A. perform a log roll.

B. attempt to revive the athlete with an inhalant.

C. remove the athlete from the field.

D. none of the above.

16. If you see an injury occur and the athlete is responsive, you will most likely:

A. perform a primary survey and secondary survey.

B. perform only a secondary survey.

C. perform only an isolated injury assessment.

D. perform an isolated injury assessment, followed up with a secondary survey if the athlete shows symptoms of additional injury during your assessment.

Complete the following exercises.

17. Establish a written Emergency Action Plan for every athletic team in your school or for a local school with athletic facilities.

18. Perform a "walk-through" of your Emergency Action Plan with a partner. What problems arose that you had not thought of before?

19. Using correct directional terminology, describe where the left foot is located.

20. Interview someone recovering from a sports-related injury. Have the person describe how the injury first felt when it occurred and then how it felt as the person left the field of play. Using the skills learned in this chapter, write out the steps of the Emergency Action Plan as you would have followed them with this patient. Include how you would have recognized the point at which you might have called EMS for help. What precautions would you have taken to keep this person's medical information confidential?

CHAPTER 10

Assembling the First Aid Kits and Equipment Bags

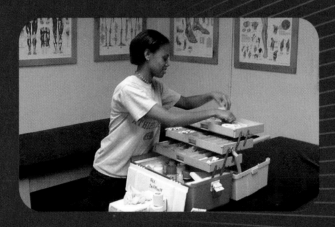

OBJECTIVES

After completing this chapter, you should be able to do the following:

1. Define and correctly spell each of the key terms.

2. Identify and describe the contents of each of the first aid kits described in this chapter.

3. List the forms that are a necessary part of the first aid kits.

4. Identify the items that are required in each type of equipment bag.

KEY TERMS

* athletic trainer's injury report
* basic first aid kit
* head injury and concussion information sheet

* injury report
* personal kit
* physician's kit
* physician's report

* treatment record

BASIC FIRST AID KITS

The proper materials can make anyone's job much easier. Athletic training is no exception. The supplies an athletic trainer uses for work are best kept in one or more organized kits. The number of kits necessary for the athletic trainer to maintain depends on the number of sports covered and the budget of the school or organization. This chapter describes the contents of a **basic first aid kit**, ways in which the basic first aid kit can be upgraded, additional upgrades for specific sports, and additional supplies that should be available for various sports.

> **basic first aid kit**
>
> a first aid kit appropriate for most sports activities.

It is the certified athletic trainer's responsibility to make sure that the first aid kits are properly stocked (see Figure 10-1), but an athletic training student can assist by making sure that all the necessary supplies are available in the kits. The athletic trainer will then double-check to confirm that the kits are properly equipped. A laminated checklist helps ensure that every item is present. The list should be readily available and easy to read because it is the only way of knowing if the kit is stocked and ready for every event or game.

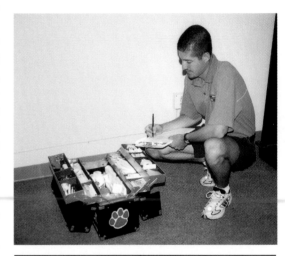

FIGURE 10-1 An athletic trainer makes sure his first aid kit contains the necessary items.

The Basic First Aid Kit

Below are suggested supplies and equipment for the daily basic first aid kit (see Figure 10-2) used to care for an athletic team. These supplies and equipment will vary depending on the sport, the number of athletes, and the time and distance away from the training room.

* Adhesive tape $1^{1}/2''$ (5 or more rolls)
* Analgesic/massage lotion

* Antibiotic cream
* Adhesive bandages in a variety of sizes and shapes

* Barriers: gloves, eye protection, and airways

* Blister kit (liquid bandage, felt, toe blister protectors)

* Butterfly strips, sterile strips

* Cotton swabs

* Disinfectant

* Disposable hazardous waste bags

* Elastic wraps (2″, 4″, and 6″) 2 each

* Heel and lace pads

* Liquid soap/hand wipes

* Lubricating ointment

* Mirror

* Mouth guards

* Nail clippers

* Non-sterile gauze pads (4″) 1 box (thicker for soaking up blood)

* Paper bag

* Pen/chalk/whiteboard marker

* Penlight

* Peroxide

* Pocket knife

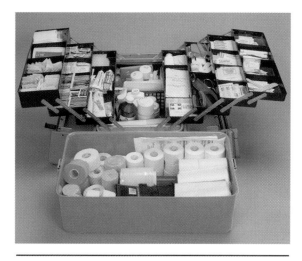

FIGURE 10-2 The Basic First Aid Kit

* Pre-wrap (2 or more rolls)

* Saline solution

* Spray adhesive

* Sterile gauze pads (4″) 1 box

* Tampons (can also be used as nose plugs for bleeding)

* Tape adherent spray

* Tape scissors

* Tongue depressors

* Triangular bandages

* Tweezers

Paperwork

* Emergency cards for athletes (emergency numbers, insurance information, parental release)

* Physician's reports (duplicate copies, one for your records, one to give)

* Athletic trainer's reports (duplicate copies, one for your records, one to give)

* Injury and treatment recording documents

* Emergency phone numbers: parents or guardians, coaches, administrators, physician, local EMS

* Laminated kit contents card (to ensure the kit is properly stocked)

The Forms

Paperwork is probably not the first thing that pops into one's mind when thinking of first aid. However, certain forms are an important part of a complete first aid kit and must be available at all practices and games. If forms are kept in the training room, they will not be available to you at away games. For this reason, these five forms should be kept as part of the first aid kit. In some cases a duplicate form may be needed to ensure everyone is properly informed.

* Injury reports

* Treatment records

* Athletic trainer's injury reports

* Physician's reports

* Head injury and concussion information sheets

injury report

a legal document containing information about the nature and treatment of injuries that is used in the evaluation of treatment procedures.

An **injury report** (Figure 10-3) and **treatment record** (Figure 10-4) should be used for every type of injury that occurs. These forms are very important because they document the injuries that have occurred and the treatments that have been provided. Injuries and treatments are recorded for three reasons:

1. The documentation may be used for legal purposes. For example, if an athlete is injured and the treatment that was provided is questioned, the reports will provide legal documentation that can help protect the team, school, coach, or athletic trainer from prosecution.

treatment record

a legal document used to track the course of care for an injured athlete and to evaluate various treatment methods.

2. The records help provide continuity of care by providing a means of communication between health care professionals. For example, the reports may be the only way an athletic trainer, who must remain at the athletic event, can communicate observations and first aid information to the physician who provides the next level of care at the hospital. Health care providers often do not have the opportunity for a face-to-face exchange of information.

3. The documents allow the athletic trainer to assess what the coach has been doing correctly and what needs to be improved. For example, if a coach does not have any athletes with back injuries, this indicates that the training practices have protected the athletes from unnecessary injuries. Likewise, if there is an abundance of back injuries, the coach may need to change some of the practice procedures.

athletic trainer's injury report

a report given to the coach explaining the nature of an athlete's injury or illness, treatment protocols, and suggestions for allowable activities.

The **athletic trainer's injury report** (Figure 10-5) explains, in writing, to the coach (and in a school setting, to the athlete's parents/guardian) the extent of an athlete's injuries. It also describes recommendations regarding the extent of activity that should be allowed and the course of treatment and/or therapy.

INJURY REPORT

Returning Athlete: ❏

Name: _____   School: _____

Address: _____

City/State/Zip: _____

Date of Birth: _____   Date of Injury: _____

Today's Date: _____   Position: _____

Sport: _____   Grade: _____

Level: V   JV   FR   COL   CLUB   REC   PRO   Home Phone: _____

Insurance: _____   Cell Phone: _____

Gender: M   F   E-mail address: _____

Do Not Write Below This Line

Gen. Structure: _____   **Onset:** Acute   Chronic

Spec. Structure: _____   Acute-recurring

Side: R   L   B   N/A   **Mechanism:** _____

Severity: 1 + 2 + 3   **Injury:** _____

Situation: OFF DEF N	**Game Outcome:** W L T N/A
Team Session:	
❏ Home Game _____ ❏ Away Game	❏ Weight Training _____ ❏ Conditioning
❏ Practice _____ ❏ Warm-Up	❏ Scrimmage _____ ❏ Recreation

Activity:

1. Batting	9. Defending	17. No Activity	25. Sliding
2. Being Blocked	10. Defensive Drill	18. Offensive Drill	26. Spike Volleyball
3. Being Tackled	11. Distance Running	19. Pitching	27. Sprinting
4. Blocking	12. Diving	20. Rebounding	28. Tackling Football
5. Bounding	13. General Sport	21. Running	29. Tackling Soccer
6. Catching	14. Jumping	22. Serve Tennis	30. Throwing
7. Conditioning	15. Kicking Football	23. Serve Volleyball	31. Unknown
8. Dance Activity	16. Kicking Soccer	24. Setting Screen	32. Weight Training

33. Other: _____

Notes: _____

_____

_____

FIGURE 10-3 An Injury Report

TREATMENT RECORD

Name: _____

Date: ____/____/____ Time: _____ (am/pm)

Age: _____ Sport: _____

Game/Practice/Other: _____

Injury site: _____ left/right

School: _____

Grade: 9 10 11 12

Position: _____

Home/Away: _____

Gender: male/female

Insurance Information on File as of _____

ICE
1. Ice Bag
2. Ice Massage
3. Ice Slush
4. Cold Whirlpool
5. Contrast

HEAT
6. Warm Whirlpool
7. Ultrasound
8. Phonophoresis
9. Moist Heat
10. Paraffin Bath
11. Iontophoresis

ELECTRICAL
12. Electrical Stim+
13. Electrical Stim-
14. E.M.S.
15. Interferential

OTHER TREATMENT
16. Compression
17. Phys. Med. -
    Stretch/Exercise
18. Phys. Med. - ROM
19. Pool Therapy

EXERCISES
20. Exercise -
    ISOM, ISOT, ECC
21. Flexibility
22. Proprio/Balance
23. C.V. Workout/Warm-Up
24. Rebounder
25. Slide Board
26. Body Blade
27. Surgical Tubing
28. Balance Board
29. Other _____

SERVICES
30. Tape/Wrap/Splint
31. Isokinetic Test
32. Injury Assessment
33. Home Program
34. Medication

REFERRAL INFORMATION
35. Family Pract. Ref.
36. Physical Therapy Ref.
37. Urgent Care Ref.
38. Other Phys. _____

STATUS OPTIONS
1. Full Go
2. Non-Contact
3. Light Participation
4. Alternative Exercises
5. Participate to Tolerance
6. Released

DATE	TREATMENT	STATUS	NOTES	TRAINER
1.				
2.				
3.				
4.				
5.				
6.				
7.				
8.				
9.				
10.				
11.				
12.				
13.				
14.				

FIGURE 10-4 A Treatment Record

ATHLETIC TRAINER'S INJURY REPORT

Name: _____   Date: _____

School: _____   Sport: _____

Athletic Trainer's Impression: _____

_____

_____

SEVERITY:	MILD		MODERATE		SEVERE
	1	+	2	+	3
EDEMA : 0	1	+	2	+	3

Treatment Recommendation:

_____ ice pack
20 min. on/1 hr. off
right after activity

_____ contrast baths
30 sec. cold/
2 min. warm x 20 min.

_____ whirlpool
hot/cold

_____ elevation

_____ crutches

_____ tape/pad/brace

_____ elastic wrap

_____ ice massage
7 min./3 x day

_____ moist heat
(hot shower, etc.)

Other Recommendations:

_____ come in for morning clinic

_____ full participation

_____ home exercise
program

_____ see family doctor

_____ participate to tolerance

_____ upper extremity
conditioning

_____ no activity until seen by doctor

_____ no contact

_____ lower extremity
conditioning

_____ coach evaluation of
athletic techniques

_____ follow up with high school
athletic trainer

Further Recommendations: _____

_____

_____

_____

Re-Evaluation Tentatively Set For: _____

FIGURE 10-5 An Athletic Trainer's Injury Report

PHYSICIAN'S REPORT

Patient: _____   Date: _____

Sport: _____   Athletic Trainer: _____

School: _____   Phone: _____

Physician: _____   Phone: _____

History: _____

_____

Physical Examination: _____

_____

_____

_____

Diagnosis: _____

_____

Medication: _____

Treatment Recommendation:

_____ ice pack
       20 min. on/1 hr. off

_____ elevation

_____ elastic wrap

_____ coach evaluation of
       athletic techniques

_____ upper extremity
       conditioning

_____ crutches

_____ ice massage – 7 min./3 x day

_____ follow up with high school
       athletic trainer

_____ lower extremity
       conditioning

_____ moist heat

_____ tape/pad/brace

_____ ROM exercises

Extent of Activity Recommended:

_____ Alternative Exercises

_____ Non-Contact

_____ Non-Contact Light

_____ No Activity Until Further Evaluation

_____ Participate to Tolerance

_____ Non-Contact Vigorous

_____ Full Contact

_____ Morning Clinic

_____ Call for Appointment
Family Practice/Orthopedic/
Physical Therapy

Further Recommendations: _____

_____

Re-Evaluation Tentatively Set For: _____

FIGURE 10-6 A Physician's Report

HEAD INJURY
AND CONCUSSION INFORMATION

Athlete:_____   Date of Injury: _____ Time: _____

Athletic Trainer/Physician: _____   Parent/Guardian: _____
Called/Follow Through:

Status: ❏ Released to Parent   ❏ EMS   ❏ Other

Recommendations: ❏ Observation Needed   ❏ ER   ❏ Follow up w/Physician

Your child has sustained a Head Injury/Concussion. Observation in the first 24 hours is vital to determine the possible severity. The following is to be used as a guide after a head injury has been sustained. If any of the following conditions occur, or if you feel your child needs further attention, contact your physician IMMEDIATELY or go to an emergency department at once, DAY or NIGHT. Look for the following:

Reduced Consciousness

Reduced consciousness is the main symptom to watch for — any decrease in consciousness is important. Some symptoms of reduced consciousness are noted below and should be assessed every 2-3 hours the first night.

Disorientation	Dizziness	Slurred or Incoherent Speech
Memory Loss	Lack of Coordination	Inability to Arouse or Awaken
Inability to Function	Vacant Stare	Poor Concentration
Delayed Verbal Response	Fainting	Lack of Awareness

Eye Changes
Pupils (the black part of the eye) are not equal.
Pupils fail to change in size when light is directed at them.

Personality Changes
Irritability • Anxiety or Depression • Confusion • Excessive Emotion

Persistent Headache
A headache is to be expected, but notice if it is long lasting or if it increases in severity.

Nausea and Vomiting
This is often from just the headache, but can be a sign of increased pressure in the head.

Dizziness or Ringing in the Ear
This might be accompanied by nausea and/or loss of balance.

Weakness of Limbs or Loss of Coordination
Even subtle changes should be reported.

Drainage of Blood or Clear Fluid from the Ears or Nose
Do not try to stop the flow. Note the color and type of fluid and
give this information to the appropriate medical personnel.

Convulsions / Seizures (Fits)
Try to prevent further injury to the patient while he or she is in the altered state.

Remember to awaken the patient every 2-3 hours to check for general mental clarity. Use no medications during the first 24 hours, including aspirin and aspirin substitutes (unless directed by a physician). After a head injury, the patient should start by taking small amounts of water or clear fluids and avoid excessive eating and drinking. **If you have any doubt, seek medical attention immediately.**

Athletic Trainer Phone: _____   Physician Phone: _____

Athletic Trainer Cell: _____

FIGURE 10-7 Instructions for Victims of Head Injuries

The **physician's report** (Figure 10-6) is sent with the injured athlete when going to the doctor. It is completed by the physician and returned after the athlete has been examined. Like the athletic trainer's report, the physician's report ensures that everyone understands the extent of the injury and what is expected from the athlete, the team, the athletic trainer, and the parents/guardian. This report also contains the physician's written instructions regarding the athlete's return to play.

Few forms are more important than the **head injury and concussion information sheet** (Figure 10-7). This is a set of instructions that must be given to the athlete or the athlete's parents/guardian when a head injury of any type is suspected. Because this form lists symptoms that may signal a more serious injury, it legally protects the athletic trainer in the event of a lawsuit by providing written precautions and instructions for proper care to the athlete and family. More important, the form protects the athlete from additional harm resulting from ignorance of complications that may arise in the hours following the head injury.

The Personal Kit

The **personal kit** (see Figure 10-8) is the first aid kit one has at all times during practices and games. At minimum, it consists of an airway, 4″ × 4″ sponge gauze, and gloves. It may also contain scissors, hydrogen peroxide, liquid soap, a flashlight, EpiPen, glucose, sterile saline, first aid cream, non-stick pads, and any other item particularly useful in treating athletes. Items may be added or removed depending on the sport, such as a face mask removal device for football and nose plugs for swimming. These items can be kept in a small zippered pouch worn around the waist. Keep the personal kit on hand at all times because life-threatening emergencies can occur when least expected—anytime and anywhere. Carrying the personal kit around the waist keeps one prepared for sudden emergencies.

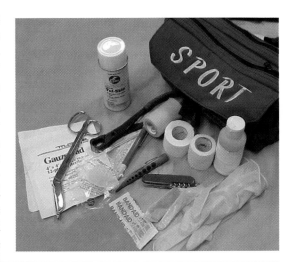

FIGURE 10-8 A Personal Kit

First Aid Kits for Transport Vehicles

A compact, ready-made first aid kit such as the one pictured in Figure 10-9 is good to have in any non-ambulance vehicle that may be used to transport athletes. At minimum, it should include cold compresses, bandages, gauze, tape, gloves, and a first aid manual.

Enhancing the Basic Kit

The following items can be used to upgrade personal kits. The size and type of the kit will also determine what is carried, but should not affect one's ability to provide the best care for the athletes.

---

physician's report

a report prepared by the physician that describes the extent of injury or illness, the course of treatment, and recommended activities. This report also provides the written authorization for the athlete's return to play, if applicable.

head injury and concussion information sheet

instructions for care given to an athlete or the athlete's parents/guardian when a head injury is suspected.

personal kit

the first aid kit that is kept with sports medicine professionals at all times and contains the most essential emergency supplies. This will vary with athletes' medical needs.

* Anti-fog and cleaner for glasses
* Antifungal spray for feet and other fungal areas
* Antiseptic towelettes
* Batteries (penlights, thermometer, etc.)
* Blood pressure cuff and stethoscope
* Cold spray (ethyl chloride)
* Contact lens case
* Ear plugs
* Elastic adhesive tape (various sizes, 1″, 2″, 3″) 2 each
* Extra-long elastic wraps (4″ and 6″) 2 each
* Eye patch
* Eyeglass repair kit
* Felt and foam of various thickness (foam open and closed cell)
* Flexible bandage wrap
* Gauze (non-sterile) several rolls
* Large assortment of adhesive bandages (knuckles, extra-large, etc.)
* Light key
* Lip protection
* Magnifying glass with or without light

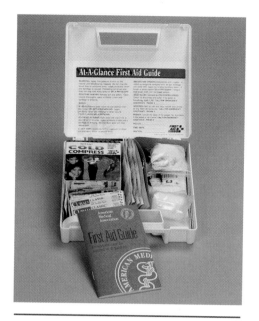

FIGURE 10-9 A Ready-Made First Aid Kit Suitable for a Transport Vehicle

* Plastic cups
* Razor blades
* Splint for fracture splinting
* Sewing kit
* Shoelaces (assorted sizes)
* Styptic pencil
* Suntan lotion
* Tape cutters (two each)
* Tape measure
* Thermometer (battery operated)
* Tweezers
* Water faucet key (various sizes)

Carrying Over-the-Counter Medications

Providing a single dose of a nonprescription medication to a high school athlete in most cases is prohibited. This must only be done under the directions of the team or family physician. At no time can anyone other than a legally licensed person lawfully prescribe or dispense prescription drugs.

Athlete-Specific Kit

This kit contains medications and items that athletes with preexisting illnesses may give to the athletic trainer to carry. The items must be accompanied with a note from the physician and family of the method, amount, and time they are to be dispensed.

* Asthma inhaler (possibly with a spacer)
* EpiPen (adrenaline/epinephrine)
* Glucose supplement

Additional Items

* Crutches to fit the sizes of the athletes

SPORT-SPECIFIC KIT UPGRADES

Basketball, Tennis, and Volleyball (Figure 10-10)

* Callous remover
* Cotton roll for making soft cast
* Elbow and knee pads
* Felt or foam horseshoes for ankle swelling
* Finger splints
* Glass cleaner and anti-fog for eyeglasses
* Glasses strap
* Heel and toe glides
* Lace-up ankle brace
* Powder
* Thermal sleeves (elbow, shoulder, and ankle)

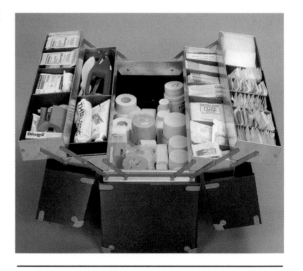

FIGURE 10-10 A Basketball, Tennis, and Volleyball Kit

Track and Cross-Country

* Calamine lotion (for poison oak and ivy)
* Callous remover
* Felt for arch supports (or ready-made supports)
* Heel cushions
* Sunscreen
* Toe glides
* Petroleum jelly

Baseball and Softball

* Elbow pads
* Extra-large telfa pads for abrasions
* Eye black (for eye glare)
* Flexible collodion
* Knee pads
* Stockinette (to hold gauze in place)
* Sunglass flip-ups
* Sunscreen
* Thermal sleeves (elbow, shoulder, and elbow-shoulder)

Football, Soccer, Lacrosse, IceHockey, and Rugby

* Callous remover
* Cervical collar
* Felt
* Foam padding
* Hard moldable rubber
* Knee brace (single and bilateral hinge)
* Mouth piece
* Neck collar
* Nose guard
* Packing foam
* Padded chin strap
* Protective cup
* Protective eye goggles
* Rib pads
* Shin guard
* Shoulder harness
* Trainer's Angel, FM extractor, or other face mask removal device (Figure 10-11)
* Wire bundle tie (substitute for shoe laces)

Gymnastics

* Grips (various types)
* Powder
* Wrist supports

The following kits will only be used where budget and qualified personnel are available. In most high school settings, these kits may not be practical. Although there might be individual items worth taking, examine the various kits/bags and evaluate each setting or situation separately (see Figure 10-12). These are meant to be guidelines.

Swimming, Diving, and Water Polo

* Razors
* Sunscreen
* Swimmer's eardrops
* Petroleum jelly
* Waterproof tape of various sizes

Wrestling

* Cervical collar
* Razors
* Tampons (for nosebleeds)

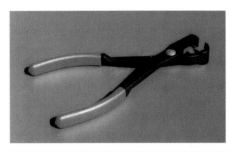

FIGURE 10-11 A Trainer's Angel, FM extractor, or other face mask removal device is useful when treating a football player with a potential spine injury. It prevents unnecessary movement of the spine by allowing removal of the face mask without removal of the helmet.

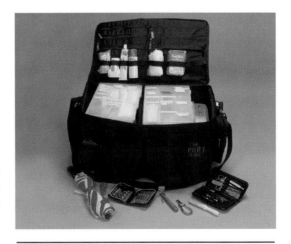

FIGURE 10-12 A soft-sided field kit. Note how the labeling of containers can make it easier to locate items quickly.

FOOTBALL FIELD KIT

Additional supplies and equipment may be needed for football. What is added will depend on the number of athletes and the available budget. The number of rolls of $1\frac{1}{2}''$ tape, pre-wrap, and heel and lace pads will depend on the number of athletes that will be taped. Always take extra supplies for unknown situations. There may be times a special pad needs to be constructed or a brace made available, so be ready for those moments.

* Adhesive foam $\frac{1}{8}''$
* Adhesive foam $\frac{1}{4}''$
* Airway
* Alcohol pads
* Assorted sizes of foam
* Athletic tape 1″, $1\frac{1}{2}''$
* Bag or pouch with assorted metal utensils (finger/toenail clippers, scissors, etc.)
* Betadine ointment
* Betadine pads
* Bioclusives 2″ × 3″ or 8″ × 10″
* Chalk and/or dry-erase pens and erasers
* Contact lens case
* Dacriose—eye wash w/cup
* Elastic wraps 2″, 4″, 6″
* Eye black
* Finger splints
* Flexi-wrap
* Foot powder
* Heel and lace pads
* Hydrogen peroxide
* Items for the weather (rain-suits, umbrellas, warm clothing, etc.)
* Knuckle bandages
* Latex gloves (large) 1 box

* Moleskin 2″
* Nasal sponges
* Non-adhesive pads 2″ × 3″
* Non-adhesive pads 3″ × 4″
* Non-sterile gauze 4″ × 4″
* Non-sterile gauze (roll)
* Nontear stretch tape 1″, 2″, 3″
* Orthoplast sheet
* Pre-wrap
* Taping-base adhesive
* Rosin/hand grip spray
* Safety pins
* Scissors/Trainer's Angel or other facemask removal tool
* Shark tape cutters
* Skin lube
* Sponge dressings 3″ × 4″
* Steri-Strips
* Sterile adhesive bandage strips (assorted)
* Sterile adhesive bandages—finger tip
* Sterile adhesive bandage strips 1″
* Sterile adhesive bandage strips—extra-large
* Sterile gauze 4″ × 4″
* Sterile gauze (roll)

* Sunscreen
* Super foam 12″ × 12″ (2 sheets)
* Tongue depressors

Bag One

* Elbow pads (1 pair of each size)
* Foam hip pads (1 set)
* Game jerseys (in appropriate numbers for various positions)
* Game pants (1 of each size)
* Hand pads (1 pair)
* Hip pads and tail pieces (2 sets)
* Jock straps (M, L, XL)
* Knee pads—regular, large, and youth (2 pair of each size)

* Lineman gloves (1 pair)
* Rib vests (M, L, XL)
* Socks (3 pair)
* Spider pads (2)
* Thigh pads—regular, large, and youth (2 pair of each size)
* Belts (1 of each size)

Bag Two

* Cowboy collars w/ backplates (regular and large)
* Helmets (M, L, XL)
* Shoulder Pads (44L, 68XL, QBL)

HELMET KIT

Although the athletic staff may be in charge of supplying these items (Figure 10-13), it is a good idea for the athletic trainer to know which items may be needed in case an item is lost or broken.

Top Shelf

* Air cast inflation tube (2)
* Air valves
* Chin strap snaps
* Cleats—with 3 keys (about 80, or enough to shoe about 5 pairs of shoes)
* Face mask posts
* Screwdrivers (Phillips and flathead)
* Screw-in snaps for helmet chin straps
* Screws
* "T" nut extractor

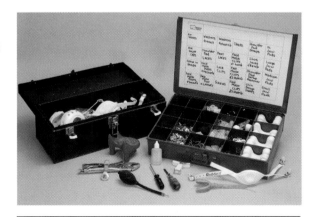

FIGURE 10-13 A Helmet Kit

* Valve stem grabber
* Washers
* Wrench

Bottom Shelf

* Hard chin straps (5)

* Helmet face mask fasteners bag

* Helmet pumps (3)

* Soft chin straps (5)

* Universal jaw pads (S, M, L, X, XX) (4 of each size)

SHOULDER PAD KIT

When building this kit, check the shoulder pads and all of the specialty pads first. Bring a supply of anything that can break or fall off.

Top Shelf

* Chalk (5 pieces) or white board markers

* Shoelaces—high and low-top (15 pairs)

* Shoulder pad lace fastener combos (10)

* Shoulder pad strap fasteners (15)

* Mouthpieces (15)

* Pant laces (10)

* Shoulder pad laces (10)

* Shoulder pad strap with fasteners (8)

* Uncut shoulder pad strap (1 roll)

Bottom Shelf

* Cups (5)

* Extra kicking tee (1)

FOOTBALL TAPE BAG

An athletic trainer should never run out of tape. Therefore, the tape bag (Figure 10–14) should be well stocked and have sufficient supplies for the number of athletes that may need treatment.

It is very important to rotate the tape in all of the kits. For example, if tape lies at the bottom of the kit for most of the season, it may become unusable. Also, once tape gets hot, it becomes harder to pull off of the roll, making it difficult to execute proper taping for the athletes.

Center Portion

* Assorted sterile adhesive bandage strips

* Athletic tape $1/2''$ (2 rolls)

* Athletic tape $1''$ (4 rolls)

* Athletic tape $1^{1}/2''$ (12 rolls)

* Athletic tape $2''$ (4 rolls)

* Elastic non-tear tape $1''$ (2 rolls)

* Elastic non-tear tape $2''$ (2 rolls)

* Elastic non-tear tape $3''$ (2 rolls)

* Elastic wraps

* Heel and lace pads

* Elastic tear tape $1^{1}/2''$ (4 rolls)

* Elastic tear tape 2″ (4 rolls)

* Elastic tear tape 3″ (4 rolls)

* Pre-wrap (4 rolls)

* Taping-base adhesive (1 large can for every 2 people who know how to tape)

Top Zipper

* Arch supports

* Foam cushion

* Plantar facia straps

* Skin lube

* Tongue depressors

* Turf toe straps

Front Pouch

* Flexi-wrap w/handle

* Scissors (1 pair)

* Tape cutters (6)

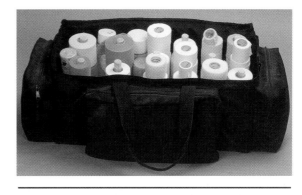

FIGURE 10-14 The contents of a football tape bag should be rotated regularly.

Right Pouch

* Biohazard bags

* Ice bags

Left Pouch

* Over-the-counter (OTC) medicines specifically prescribed to athletes

INJURY PAD BAG

One must be prepared for all types of injuries to the athletes—especially in contact sports. The injury pad bag (Figure 10-15) should contain supports, extra padding, and additional items to assist in the care of injuries.

Ankle Braces

* Right (1)

* Left (1)

Arm Slings

* Large (1)

* X-Large (1)

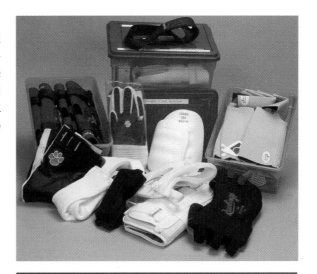

FIGURE 10-15 Contents of an Injury Pad Bag

Calf Sleeves

* Small (1)

* Medium (1)

* Large (1)

* X-Large (1)

Cervical Collars

* Hard (in appropriate sizes)

* Soft (in appropriate sizes)

Crutches

* Medium (1)

* Large (1)

* X-Large (1)

Elbow Sleeves

* Small (1)

* Medium (1)

* Large (1)

Groin Straps

* Small (1)

* Medium (1)

* Large (1)

* X-Large (1)

* XX-Large (1)

Hinged Knee Braces

* Medium (1)

* Large (1)

* X-Large (1)

* XX-Large (1)

Knee Immobilizers

* 18″ (1)

* 24″ (1)

Knee Sleeves

* Small (2)

* Medium (2)

* Large (2)

* X-Large (2)

* XX-Large (2)

Thigh Sleeves

* Small (2)

* Medium (2)

* Large (2)

* X-Large (2)

* XX-Large (2)

THE PHYSICIAN'S KIT

In the best of situations, the team physician would be either a family practitioner or an orthopedic surgeon who has had special training in sports medicine. This physician would be accessible during practice and come to all contact sports events.

In higher levels of sport competition, a physician may even come to practice, but that is rare. More commonly in high school competitions, a "game doctor" is available only for varsity football games. The game doctor may not have any specialty training and may not be familiar with the athletes or the sport. The doctor, could be a chiropractor or a podiatrist depending on league and state organizations' rules. The athletic trainer must be prepared to make the doctor aware of any preexisting injuries or illnesses the athletes may have and what the doctor might need to bring in the physician's kit.

Below are some items your team physician may want to carry in the **physician's kit** (Figure 10-16). The physician may also request additional items not listed below. Try to meet with the team physicians so that all can become familiar with the contents of each other's kits. This way everyone will be able to help each other in case of an emergency. Label the items clearly to identify them easily in an emergency.

physician's kit

items the team physician uses for advanced medical care and treatment the athletic trainer cannot provide.

Take nothing for granted. It is always best to be prepared. The physician's kit may include medications, sutures, syringes, and other items the athletic trainer is not trained or legally allowed to use. When not in use, this bag should be locked up.

Bottom Portion

* 0.9% sodium chloride (1 bag)
* Assorted elastic wraps
* Cast padding (4 rolls)
* Casting tape 3″ (4 rolls)
* IV set with 2 injection sites (1)
* Loose gloves
* Soft casting 3″ (4 rolls)
* Tourniquet

Middle Portion

* Non-adhering dressings 3″ × 3″ (5)
* Blank prescription pad (1)
* Blood pressure cuff
* Head injury/concussion forms (5)
* Hot temp cautery
* Note pad (1)
* Sterile gauze 4″ × 4″ (10)
* Sterile latex surgeon's gloves 7.5 (1 pair)
* Sterile latex surgeon's gloves 8 (1 pair)
* Stethoscope
* Stretch bandage 3″ (3 rolls)
* Suture removal set (1)
* Suture sets (2)
* Syringe (3 cc) w/22 G 1½ needle (3)
* Syringe 10 cc (2)

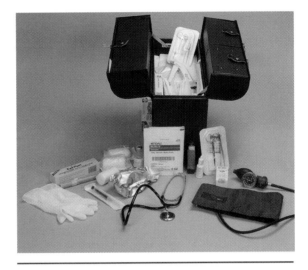

FIGURE 10-16 A Physician's Kit

Small Side Portion One

* 2% Lidocaine HCl, 50 ml (a numbing drug)
* Airway
* Cobalt blue diffuse light (ophthalmic)
* Eye pads (2)
* Flouri-strip (8)
* Nitrostat
* Ophthalmic ointment (Garamycin)
* Rx-OTIC ear drops
* Sterile eye irrigating solution (Dacriose)
* #11 surgical blade (1)
* Tetracain hydrochloride 0.5% dropperettes

Small Side Portion Two

* Aspirin
* Bacitracin zinc-polymyxin B sulfate ointment

* Cepastat
* Cold and sinus medicine
* EpiPen
* Ibuprofen
* Lidocaine HCl 2% and epinephrine 1:100,000
* Naprelan
* Skelaxin samples
* Tagamet HB
* Ventolin inhaler

Large Side Portion

* 4-0 Ethilon (2)
* 7-0 Ethilon (2)
* 25 G $^7/_8$ needle (3)
* 26 G $^1/_2$ needle (2)
* Alcohol prep pad (6)

* Angiocath 18 G $1^1/_4''$ 1.3 mm (1)
* Augmentin (5)
* Adhesive bandages (assorted)
* Benzoin applicator (4)
* High-impact spectacles
* Micropore 1" (2)
* Providone-iodine saturated swabsticks (2 packs of 3)
* Single-use scalpel #11
* Single-use scalpel #15
* Steri-Strips $^1/_4''$ (2)
* Steri-Strips $^1/_8''$ (3)
* Tongue blades
* Transpore 1" (1)
* Transpore $^1/_2''$ (1)

AWAY-GAME ITEMS

These are some examples of items needed when going to an away event. This information is based upon the approximate needs of a squad of 60 football athletes who are playing in a community or junior college setting during moderate weather. Items will vary depending on the size of the team, budget constraints, and weather conditions. Other factors that may affect this list include your knowledge regarding the proper use of certain items, the amount of space available to store the items, and supplies the home team might be able to provide. In fact, call the home team's athletic trainer prior to the event to find out what supplies may be available for the team and which ones should be brought along. Athletic trainers often make agreements among themselves as to what supplies will be made available by the home teams.

Coolers

* Coolers—2 six-gallon (locker rooms) (used to keep the athletes' drinks cool)
* Coolers—6 ten-gallon (sideline) (used to keep the athletes' drinks cool)
* Ice chests—2 (w/5 cases of drinks)
* Ice chests—2 (w/injury ice at sideline w/bags)

* Ice towels (in hot environments)
* Rapid-form immobilizer

Kits

* Apples (a healthy snack for the athletes on long bus rides prior to events)
* Biohazard and sharps containers

* Cleat cleaners (6)
  (Figure 10-17)
* Cups (4 sleeves)
* Folder for insurance papers
* Soft-sided bags
* Hose (short) (to fill coolers
  from a faucet)
* Injury pad bag (large, soft-
  sided bag)
* Sports chair
* Tape kit (soft-sided black)
* Towels (24)
* Trainer's kit

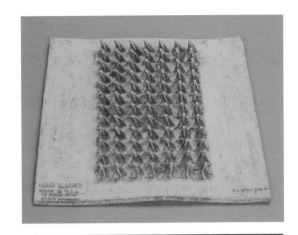

FIGURE 10-17 A Cleat Cleaner

* Water bottles (8 racks)

HOME- AND AWAY-GAME FIELD SETUP

These are examples of items needed during any football game, home or away. These suggestions are based upon the needs of a team of 60 to 70 athletes who are playing for a junior or community college.

Pre-Game

* Cleat cleaners (6—spread along
  sideline)
* Crutch box (have crutches in
  sizes appropriate for your athletes)
* Dry towels (24) (12 on benches
  each half)
* Equipment/athletic training
  supplies table (1) with:
    * Injury pad bag (large
      soft-sided)
    * Tape kit
    * Trainer's kit
* Ice chests filled with ice towels—
  in hot environments (2 chests
  with 12 towels in each)

* Sports chair
* Taping table (1 per athletic
  trainer)
* Treatment table (1) with:
    * Ice chests filled with bags
      of injury ice (2)
* Fracture splints
* Water tables (2) with:
    * Water (6 to 10 gallons)
    * Water bottles (8 racks)

Locker Room Setup

* Cooler—6 gallon (1 in each
  locker room)
* Drinking cups (4 sleeves; 2 in
  each locker room)

THINKING IT THROUGH

It was time to get ready for a road trip for a football game. Mr. Elton gave Bill the checklist and told him he was on his own to prepare the first aid kits and equipment bags. Bill was disappointed; he was hoping for a basketball game instead. This meant that he had to get everything ready for 80 football players. It was an afternoon game in the heat with no humidity. So that meant he had to pack water and ice—lots of it.

Mr. Elton also told Bill to call ahead to the game site, Southeastern State, and talk to Mrs. Doan, their head athletic trainer, to see what items would be available for his visiting team. Bill needed to know about access to water for pre-game and halftime. Mrs. Doan said an athletic training student and a physician would be available on the visitors' sideline and that she would supply a golf cart.

What else needs to be done to check the kits? How is calling ahead to see if any items are available for visitor use helpful? What are some of the differences in preparing first aid kits and equipment bags for a football game than for a basketball game?

CHAPTER SUMMARY

It is impossible to be too prepared for an emergency. For assembling first aid kits, the information in this chapter is extremely valuable. These lists can and should vary with the number and level of athletes. The keys to success in building kits are organization and resourcefulness. Many of the items on the lists are things that one might not normally anticipate, or are items that can be used for more than one purpose. Learn to anticipate the needs of the athletes and organize kits and bags according to need. There is no excuse for not having the proper supplies and equipment; running out of tape at an event or forgetting the coolers is *not* acceptable. It is the sports medicine professional's responsibility to be prepared!

Emergency forms are an essential part of the kits. The documentation provided by proper use of these forms covers everyone in the organization legally and provides the communication necessary for quality care. The information contained in the injury and treatment reports will help the sports medicine team understand and evaluate activities and their potential for injury. The athletic trainer's number-one priority is providing the medical attention necessary to maintain the health of the athletes.

STUDENT ENRICHMENT ACTIVITIES

Complete the following exercises.

1. Describe the items you will need for a basic first aid kit.

2. Imagine that you are an athletic trainer with a $3,000.00 budget for athletic supplies. Go to your local or online source for sports medicine supplies and get prices for the items on the list you created in Exercise 1. Then add up the total cost of the kit. See if your kit fits into your budget.

3. Write down at least three ways to bring funding into a school to provide the athletes with the needed supplies and equipment.

4. Describe how can you make sure that the athletes of visiting teams get the same quality of care as the athletes of the home team.

5. Describe how you can make sure that every person who is responsible for caring for injuries or who has access to your kit knows how to find the appropriate items.

Write T for true, or F for false. Rewrite the false statements to make them true.

6. T F The personal kit is carried with you only during games.

7. T F A Trainer's Angel is used to remove the face mask from a helmet.

8. T F The physician's kit may include items the athletic trainer is not trained or legally allowed to use.

9. T F Calling ahead to the home team's athletic trainer can help you know what supplies might be made available to you as the visiting team.

10. T F Food is never to be part of any of the kits.

Match the terms in Column A with the appropriate description in Column B.

Column A	Column B
11. athletic trainer's injury report	**A.** form that the injured athlete takes to the doctor's office for completion
12. physician's report	
13. head injury and concussion information sheet	**B.** set of instructions given to the athlete, or the athlete's parents/guardian, when a head injury is suspected or diagnosed
14. treatment record	**C.** provides documentation about the injury and its treatment
15. injury report	
	D. an injury report given to the coach by the athletic trainer explaining the nature of the athlete's injury or illness
	E. a legal document containing information about the nature and treatment of injuries used in the evaluation of treatment procedures

CHAPTER 11

Infection Control

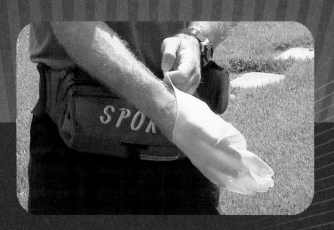

OBJECTIVES

After completing this chapter, you should be able to do the following:

1. Define and correctly spell each of the key terms.

2. Describe the six components of the infection cycle and methods of interrupting the cycle.

3. List the precautions for preventing puncture wounds from needles and other sharp objects.

4. Explain and demonstrate the proper procedure for putting on and taking off sterile gloves.

5. Name two serious illnesses clinical health personnel may contract from patients and explain how to prevent this from happening.

6. Demonstrate the procedure for proper handwashing.

7. Identify body secretions for which Universal Precautions must be used.

KEY TERMS

* AIDS
* aseptic
* clean technique

* hepatitis A
* hepatitis B
* pathogen

* sterile technique
* Universal Precautions

THE CHAIN OF INFECTION

Many sports involve skin-to-skin contact, and certain injuries can create breaks in the skin, placing both players and athletic trainers at risk of contracting a variety of infections. This is why it is very important for you to be aware of the *infection cycle*. Bacteria are single-celled microorganisms that can destroy blood cells. Bacterial infections are common complications of skin injuries. An athlete who has a bacterial skin infection may pass the infection to others via direct contact.

The infection cycle can be thought of as a chain of events (see Figure 11-1) that is given the opportunity to take place when a **pathogen**, or infectious agent, is present. There are six components of the infection cycle:

1. Pathogen: any disease-causing microorganism.

2. Reservoir Host: the individual in whom the infectious microorganisms reside. Humans or animals who do not show any outward signs or symptoms of the disease but who are still capable of transmitting the disease are known as carriers. In the world of athletics it is likely to encounter many carriers. Therefore, it is important to follow certain steps to prevent infection. These steps are known as *Universal Precautions* and will be discussed later in this chapter.

3. Portal of Exit: the pathogen's route of escape from the reservoir. Examples of portals of exit are breaks in the skin, saliva, reproductive secretions, and blood.

4. Route of Transmission: the method by which the pathogen gets from the reservoir to the new host. Transmission may occur through direct contact, air, insects, etc.

5. Portal of Entry: the route through which the pathogen enters its new host. The respiratory, gastrointestinal, urinary, and reproductive tracts, as well as breaks in the skin are common portals of entry.

6. Susceptible Host: the source, such as a human who accepts the pathogen, and depending on the degree of resistance, supports the pathogen's life and reproduction. Some examples of susceptible hosts include people who are malnourished, have suppressed immune systems, and who are in poor health.

It is essential to be aware of the various parts of the infection cycle and to take the appropriate steps to prevent infections from spreading. This will protect both sports medicine professionals and clients!

> **pathogen**
>
> a disease-causing microorganism.

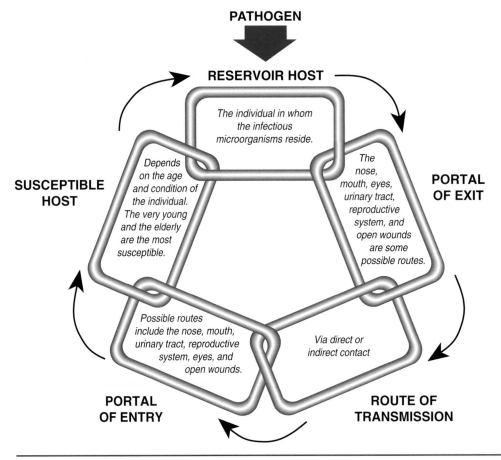

FIGURE 11-1 The Chain of Infection

BREAKING THE CHAIN OF INFECTION

The spread of disease can be stopped by removing any link in the chain of infection (see Figure 11-2). Links can be removed in the following ways:

1. Kill the bacteria before it enters the host (an organism that is invaded by a parasite and from which the parasite obtains its nutrition).

2. Change the environment in which the bacteria lives. If it needs moisture, the area should be kept clean and dry. If the bacteria requires a certain temperature, raise the temperature to kill the bacteria. This is why certain equipment items are sterilized. Sterilization is the complete destruction of all forms of microbial life.

The following steps can help prevent the spread of infection:

* Wash hands frequently. Correct handwashing technique is *the single most effective way to prevent the spread of communicable diseases*. Handwashing techniques are shown later in this chapter. For additional, printable handwashing facts and directions in English, Spanish, and other languages, visit www.dhfs.state.wi.us/communicable/factsheets/Handwashing.htm.

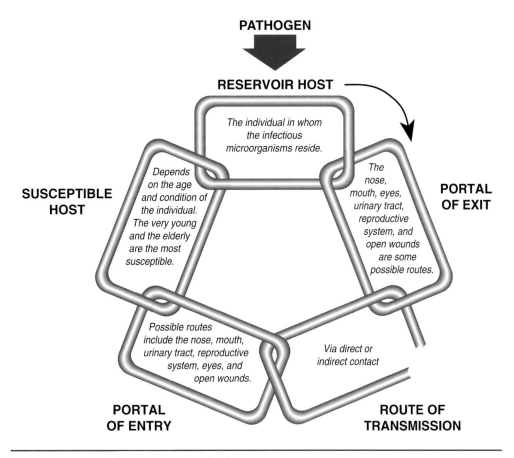

FIGURE 11-2 Breaking the Chain of Infection

* Wear gloves and other protective clothing (such as gowns, goggles, and masks) when the possibility of exposure to blood or other body fluids exists, and when working on patients who may be infectious.
* Keep immunizations up-to-date (especially hepatitis vaccinations).

CLEAN TECHNIQUE AND STERILE TECHNIQUE

It is vital that health care workers understand the importance of maintaining a clean, or **aseptic**, environment. Pathogens are everywhere, but they can be controlled or eliminated for a period of time by following certain procedures. Preventing the spread of pathogens is part of every health care worker's job.

Medical asepsis, also known as **clean technique**, refers to practices and procedures that are designed to ensure a clean environment by removing or destroying disease-causing microorganisms. In an outpatient physical therapy clinic, fitness center, or an athletic training room, the clinician will have the ultimate responsibility for most, if not all, of the cleaning. Even though the work environment may not be a part of the hospital setting, the standards for maintaining a clean environment may not be relaxed. Patients or clients deserve to be treated in an environment that is as free from potential sources of contamination as possible.

aseptic

sterile; preventing infection.

clean technique

the removal or destruction of infected material or organisms.

The first step in clean technique is proper and adequate handwashing. Other important factors in maintaining clean technique include wearing a clean uniform (if uniforms are required), remembering not to touch your face with your hands after working with a patient, and holding contaminated items away from the body. If a uniform is not required, make sure to be clean and well-groomed whenever providing patient or client care. Remember, the first impression patients will form will probably be based upon appearance. Personal attire must reflect the professional standards required by the work environment.

The highest level of protection for patients is surgical asepsis. Surgical asepsis, or **sterile technique**, is used whenever the skin is broken open, as in surgery or from a traumatic injury; when a normally sterile body cavity is entered; during the treatment of open wounds (i.e., dressing changes); and to decontaminate items between patients. Instruments and supplies used for putting in stitches or performing an operation are completely free from all microorganisms; they are sterile.

The Centers for Disease Control and Prevention (CDC) have established guidelines that, if followed, will minimize the risk of introducing disease-causing organisms to the health care provider and the patient. These guidelines will be described later in this chapter.

sterile technique

the procedure used by health care workers when performing or assisting with sterile procedures.

HANDWASHING—THE KEY TO CLEAN TECHNIQUE

Now that you are familiar with the concept of the infection cycle, it should be easy to understand how health care workers and patients contract illnesses in the health care environment. Staphylococci are bacteria that occur naturally on the skin and, therefore, are on hands. Research has shown the most effective method to reduce the risk of industrial illnesses and nosocomial infections is by frequent and correct handwashing. Health care workers are responsible for giving care to each patient with *clean* hands! This means that all patient contact must be preceded and followed by thorough handwashing. The procedure on the next page is the accepted method of handwashing to protect health care workers and patients from the spread of disease.

Proper handwashing will minimize the risk of spreading infection from one patient to another, from the health care worker to patients, and from patients to the health care worker. Handwashing must be done at the following times:

* When first arriving at work
* Before performing each medical procedure on a patient
* During a procedure if hands become contaminated
* Between each patient for whom medical care is provided
* After using the restroom
* After removing gloves
* Before eating

In short, handwashing is the key to successful clean technique.

HANDWASHING TECHNIQUE

Materials Needed:

* liquid soap
* dry paper towels

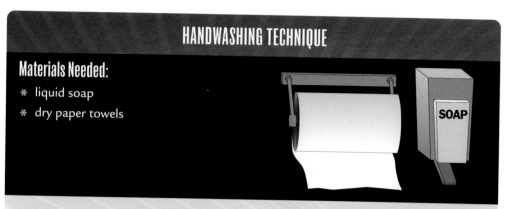

1. **Procedural Step:** Turn on the faucet. Adjust the temperature of the water to warm.

   Reason: To avoid burning yourself.

2. **Procedural Step:** Always wet your hands with the fingertips pointing down into, but not touching, the sink.

   Reason: Keeping your hands down keeps your forearms dry and prevents contaminated water on your forearms from running over your clean hands. (In most cases, your hands will be dirtier than your arms anyway, so concentrate on getting your hands clean.)

3. **Procedural Step:** Use a liberal amount of soap and rub the palms of your hands together several times.

   Reason: This friction will create a lather and help remove any unwanted viruses or bacteria from the skin surface.

4. **Procedural Step:** Put the palm of one hand over the back of the other hand and briskly rub them together.

   Reason: All parts of the hands are capable of carrying germs.

5. **Procedural Step:** Repeat step 4 using the opposite hands.

   Reason: To clean the other hand.

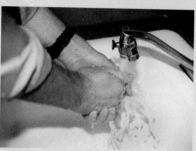

6. **Procedural Step:** Interlock the fingers of both hands and vigorously rub them together. You should scrub your hands for a total of two minutes.

   Reason: To remove harmful germs.

7. **Procedural Step:** Use an orange (cuticle) stick to clean under each nail. If a cuticle stick is not available, use a sterile brush.

   Reason: To remove germs from under the nails.

8. **Procedural Step:** Rinse all soapy lather from the wrists and hands, continuing to point the hands downward.

   Reason: To prevent contaminated water on your forearms from running over your clean hands.

9. **Procedural Step:** Leave the water running and dry all areas of the hands using a paper towel.

(continues)

HANDWASHING TECHNIQUE (Continued)

Reason: Paper towels are disposable and prevent the spread of germs.

10. **Procedural Step:** Dispose of the wet paper towel. Obtain another paper towel and, placing the paper towel on the faucet handles, turn off the water. Make sure the towel is dry.

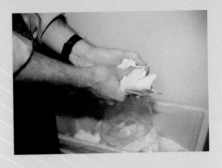

Reason: A wet paper towel allows microorganisms to pass through the towel and back onto your clean hands. The dry paper towel will shield your hands from germs on the faucet. The faucet and sink always are considered to be contaminated.

11. **Procedural Step:** Discard all debris and leave the sink and surrounding area clean, taking care not to recontaminate your hands.

Reason: The area must be ready for the next person who wants to wash.

USING GLOVES TO PROTECT YOURSELF AND OTHERS

Contact with or handling of blood or body fluids may be hazardous to health. Therefore, always protect yourself by wearing gloves whenever blood or body fluids are present, or if there is potential for them to be present (see Figure 11-3). Carry the gloves with you at all times when on duty. Injuries rarely occur near the first aid kits, so keep the most important supplies with you.

The procedure that follows is the correct procedure for donning sterile gloves when working in a clinical environment, such as when debriding a wound. This procedure protects both the caregiver and the patient from harmful pathogens. However, if blood or body fluids are present when you perform first aid, you will wear gloves primarily to protect yourself. In this case, you need not use the sterile procedure to don them. Just put them on and get to work.

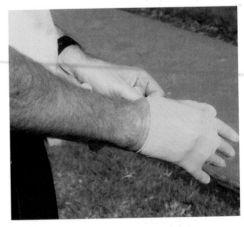

FIGURE 11-3 While working in the field, quickly put on gloves to protect yourself before providing first aid if blood or other body fluids are present. In a clinical setting, use the sterile technique.

DONNING STERILE GLOVES

Materials Needed:

* 1 pair sterile gloves

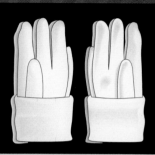

1. **Procedural Step:** Obtain a pair of sterile gloves in your hand size.

   Reason: For proper fit.

2. **Procedural Step:** Inspect the glove package for signs of contamination: water spots, moisture, tears, or rips.

   Reason: The gloves must be sterile.

3. **Procedural Step:** Remove all jewelry and scrub your hands.

   Reason: Universal Precaution. This reduces the number of normal bacteria on the skin.

4. **Procedural Step:** Dry your hands well.

   Reason: Moisture increases bacterial growth.

5. **Procedural Step:** Peel open the sterile package and lay the inner package on a flat, clean, dry surface so the end nearest you shows the word "cuff."

   Reason: This will allow you to don them properly.

6. **Procedural Step:** Open the inner wrapper like a book with right glove on the right, touching only the folded edge of the wrapper.

   Reason: A 1-inch border around the wrapper of the inner package is considered to be contaminated. The inside of the package is sterile.

7. **Procedural Step:** With the non-dominant hand pick up the glove touching only the inside of the cuff. (You will glove your dominant hand first.)

   Reason: The inside of the glove will be next to the skin. This area is not sterile.

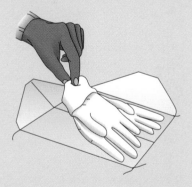

8. **Procedural Step:** Keeping your hands above your waist, step back from the table or tray. Hold your hands away from your body and

(continues)

DONNING STERILE GLOVES (Continued)

slide your dominant hand into the sterile glove. Leave the cuff folded for now.

Reason: To avoid contamination.

9. **Procedural Step:** Pick up the second glove with the gloved hand by slipping the fingers of the gloved hand under the cuff.

Reason: Sterile surfaces can only touch other sterile areas.

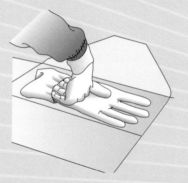

10. **Procedural Step:** Slide your second hand into the glove, keeping the gloved thumb extended (like a hitchhiker) to avoid touching your skin. Avoid touching anything else while you do this.

Reason: To avoid contamination.

11. **Procedural Step:** Move the glove up the hand and slide the fingers into position.

Reason: To secure the glove properly.

12. **Procedural Step:** Unroll the cuff of the first glove, touching only the

outside of the glove. Do not touch your bare arm with the sterile fingers of the glove.

Reason: To avoid contamination.

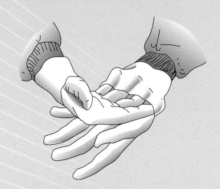

13. **Procedural Step:** Unroll the cuff of the second glove, touching only the outside of the glove. Do not touch your bare arm with the sterile fingers of the glove.

Reason: To avoid contamination.

14. **Procedural Step:** Interlock your fingers to adjust the gloves, but do not adjust the gloves below the heels of your hands.

Reason: To obtain a snug fit and to avoid contamination.

15. **Procedural Step:** Keep your hands above your waist and do not touch anything outside the sterile field. Ask for assistance if needed.

Reason: To avoid contamination.

Regardless of the environment is which you work, you will *always* need to remove your contaminated gloves correctly and dispose of them properly.

REMOVING CONTAMINATED GLOVES

Materials Needed:

* a trash can lined with a red biohazard bag

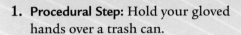

1. **Procedural Step:** Hold your gloved hands over a trash can.

   Reason: You will throw away your used gloves.

2. **Procedural Step:** Without touching the bare skin of your forearm, grasp the contaminated (or outside) area of the dominant glove cuff (approximately 1 to 2 inches from the top) with your gloved nondominant hand.

   Reason: To avoid contamination.

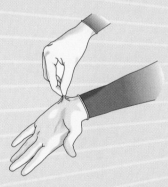

3. **Procedural Step:** Pull off the glove. It will now be inside out. Do not snap gloves when removing them.

   Reason: Microorganisms on the gloves could become airborne.

4. **Procedural Step:** Discard the glove directly into the trash container.

   Reason: Gloves cannot be reused.

5. **Procedural Step:** Place the bare fingertips of the dominant hand inside the other glove and grasp it near the top. Don't let your bare hand touch the contaminated portion of the glove.

   Reason: To avoid contamination.

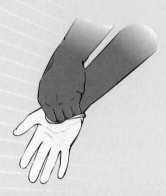

6. **Procedural Step:** Pull off the second glove. It also will be inside out. Discard it in the trash can lined with a red biohazard bag.
   NOTE: Never dispose of a biohazard bag into regular trash.

   Reason: Gloves cannot be reused. They are considered hazardous waste, and therefore must be disposed of in the proper manner.

7. **Procedural Step:** Wash your hands thoroughly before touching anything.

   Reason: Universal Precaution.

REMOVING BLOOD-STAINED CLOTHING

Sometimes blood stains clothing. When this happens, the clothing should be removed as soon as possible to avoid potential contamination from it. The stained clothing should be held away from the body if at all possible until either the blood or the clothing can be removed. Hydrogen peroxide and other blood-removal products are often used to remove blood from jerseys and other uniforms. A bloody shirt may be removed by rolling it up to conceal the bloody area, and then carefully pulling it off over the head, avoiding contact with the head. If these blood and shirt removal methods fail, the clothing may need to be cut from the body to reduce the risk of contamination.

The rule of thumb is that if the blood stain is removed, the athlete may return to play in that piece of clothing. However, it is important to note that removal of the red stain doesn't guarantee removal of the contaminants. The final decision is ultimately up to the officials.

AVOIDING CONTAMINATED SHARPS

A serious risk associated with providing clinical patient care is the possibility of receiving a puncture wound from a needle or other sharp object. In the field of health care there is a significant risk of contracting either hepatitis B or acquired immune deficiency syndrome (AIDS) from contaminated body fluid and blood.

All needles, scalpel blades, and other sharp objects should be disposed of in the proper puncture-resistant container. During orientation, try to learn the locations of all the sharps containers (Figure 11-4). Although the colors of these containers may vary, most of them will be either red or beige. Follow the manufacturer's instructions for the proper filling, sealing, and disposal of this container.

The following guidelines are suggested for reducing the risk of puncture wounds from contaminated needles or other sharp objects.

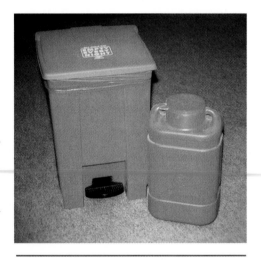

FIGURE 11-4 Proper disposal of sharp instruments will help protect you and others from accidental punctures.

1. Never recap, bend, or manually remove a dirty needle.

2. Always deposit the entire syringe and needle or sharp object in the puncture-resistant container.

3. Immediately clean any puncture wound with alcohol and betadine and cover the wound. Report the incident to a supervisor or instructor.

4. Never carry needles or sharps from one location to another with the tips pointing toward other people or yourself. *Point them toward the floor.*

Most needle sticks occur from carelessness. Always be aware of the location of needles or sharps as well as the location of surrounding people. Wear gloves and other protective wear. *Take all precautions*, and do not allow yourself, the patient, or a fellow worker to become a victim of a needle stick!

THE RISKS—HEPATITIS AND AIDS

There are several risks to the health care provider while providing care to patients. Using clean technique and making a conscious effort to reduce the risk of contamination for both the employee and the patient or athlete will help reduce the chances of contracting a very serious illness.

Two important diseases that can pose a significant risk to the employee are hepatitis and acquired immune deficiency syndrome, or **AIDS**. Hepatitis is a disease that results in inflammation of the liver. *Hepat-* means pertaining to the liver, *-itis* means inflammation of.

Many different agents can cause hepatitis. This disease may be caused by a virus, bacteria, or a variety of physical or chemical agents. There are several types of hepatitis, but the two most common types that can be contracted from patients and transmitted (transferred) to another are hepatitis A and hepatitis B. **Hepatitis A** is caused by a virus. It is the most common form of the disease occurring in children and young adults. Spread of the illness can occur through the fecal-oral route by failing to wash hands properly after using the restroom. This is important to the clinical health care worker providing direct patient care. Diligent and thorough handwashing *can* protect the health care worker. **Hepatitis B** is caused by a virus too; however, this form of the disease is spread through blood, blood products, semen, vaginal secretions, and saliva. Clinical health care workers in contact with blood *must* wear gloves and practice careful and frequent handwashing! Cover any breaks in the skin with a dressing *before* any patient contact occurs. If the dressing becomes wet, contaminated, or soiled, remove it, wash your hands, and apply a new dressing. Hepatitis can become a chronic, and sometimes fatal, illness. It is recommended that all first aid providers have hepatitis vaccines, especially providers in high contact sports (wrestling, football, etc.).

Acquired immune deficiency syndrome, or AIDS, is a fatal disease that, unfortunately, has become widespread. There is no cure for AIDS. This is a disease that is transmitted through blood and sexual contact. The illness is caused by a virus that attacks the immune system (blood cells that work together to fight off infections and disease). An immune system that does not function properly makes a person susceptible to many different kinds of infections, called opportunistic infections. For example, certain types of cancer and pneumonia are two of the most common disease processes that can be caused by opportunistic infections. Aids is a fatal illness, and no one is completely protected from the virus!

AIDS is recognized as a worldwide disease, and people from all ages and racial backgrounds can be infected. Take every precaution available to protect yourself from infection and to keep from transmitting the illness to patients or other health care providers.

One of the most controversial issues concerning this disease deals with patient confidentiality. According to current laws, it is *not* mandatory to inform health care providers if a patient is infected with the AIDS virus, known as the

---

AIDS

acquired immune deficiency syndrome; a viral disease caused by the human immunodeficiency virus (HIV), which destroys the immune system and renders the patient susceptible to other infections. It is contracted through blood and other body fluids, and is incurable.

hepatitis A

inflammation of the liver caused by a virus and spread by the fecal-oral route either from poor handwashing or contaminated food.

hepatitis B

inflammation of the liver caused by a virus and spread through contact with infected blood and body fluids. It is the most common form contracted by health care workers.

human immunodeficiency virus, or HIV. People who are infected with the virus may remain asymptomatic (not show any outward signs of the disease) for many years; therefore, health care workers should protect themselves as if every patient has the illness.

The CDC has devised protective measures for health care personnel. The CDC recommends that, because of the difficulty and inconsistency in identifying all patients infected with the AIDS virus, the following precautions be used for *all* patients. It is possible for patients to be HIV positive (carry the AIDS virus), yet show no symptoms. However, despite the fact that no symptoms are present, it is still possible for them to transmit the virus. For your own protection follow these guidelines, known as **Universal Precautions**, *exactly* as recommended if the possibility of direct contact with blood and/or body secretions exists.

Universal Precautions

guidelines developed by the Centers for Disease Control and Prevention (CDC) for protecting health care workers from exposure to blood-borne pathogens in body secretions.

1. *Wear gloves* whenever contact with blood, body secretions, or broken skin may occur. Do not re-use gloves!

2. *Wear protective eyewear and a mask* during any procedures that may expose you to splattering blood or other body fluids.

3. *Wear disposable gowns* if blood or body fluids may splatter.

4. *Thoroughly wash your hands* and other skin surfaces immediately following contamination.

5. *Avoid giving direct mouth-to-mouth resuscitation*; instead, use the mouth-to-mask method, resuscitator bags, and other available equipment. Keep an airway nearby when working in a health care environment.

6. *Avoid direct patient contact* if you have open wounds or other skin conditions.

7. *Wash your hands* after each patient contact and after removing gloves.

8. *Carefully and properly dispose of all sharp objects (needles, scalpel blades, etc.) in appropriate puncture-resistant containers.* Do not recap, bend, break, or manually remove needles! If stuck by a used needle, clean the area with Betadine, fill out the necessary forms to notify supervisors of the needle stick, and get a blood test for hepatitis and AIDS.

The Centers for Disease Control and Prevention have recommended these Universal Precautions to protect both health care workers and patients from contracting hepatitis B or AIDS. These guidelines and recommendations are not intended to make patient care time-consuming or difficult; they are intended to provide a safe, healthy environment for everyone concerned.

Body secretions for which Universal Precautions are appropriate include: urine, sputum, fecal material, wound drainage, semen, vaginal secretions, tissues, synovial fluid (fluid around a joint), cerebrospinal fluid (fluid around the brain and spinal cord), pleural fluid (fluid from the lung), peritoneal fluid (fluid from the abdominal cavity), pericardial fluid (fluid from around the heart), and amniotic fluid (fluid from the sac containing the growing fetus in the uterus). The CDC maintains that the risk of health care providers' contracting the hepatitis B virus or the AIDS virus from these secretions is not as high as the risk associated with blood and sexual secretions; however, the risk does exist! Recognizing common health hazards and infectious diseases can be difficult—especially because viruses and bacteria cannot be seen with the naked eye. Being aware of the potential hazards and risks and following the Universal Precautions established by the CDC as well as the recommendations of your facility, can greatly reduce your exposure to potentially fatal diseases.

THINKING IT THROUGH

Shanica was assigned to work a weekend wrestling tournament with Mr. Babcock, the head athletic trainer. Mr. Babcock requires that all his athletic training students be certified in CPR and first aid and have their hepatitis shots.

During the first match of the tournament Isaac, one of Mr. Babcock's wrestlers, got a bloody nose. The officials stopped the match for a blood time out.

What are some of the dangers associated with blood-borne pathogens? What should Mr. Babcock do to stop the nose bleed? What precautions should both Mr. Babcock and Shanica take? Under what conditions would Isaac be able to continue in the match?

CHAPTER SUMMARY

Pathogens are everywhere; therefore, the possibility of infection always exists. Understand how the chain of infection works, and what steps should be taken to help prevent the spread of disease. Universal Precautions have been recommended by the CDC for everyone's protection. These precautions can help protect you and others from serious health risks such as hepatitis and AIDS. Whenever in doubt about the potential for the transmission of disease, use Universal Precautions! Consistent and proper use of protective items, such as gloves and goggles, will help reduce the transmission of infectious diseases.

The most important step to help prevent the spread of pathogens is to wash your hands frequently and systematically. Proper and frequent handwashing helps to protect both the caregiver and the patient from potential infection. Remember, an ounce of prevention is worth a pound of cure.

STUDENT ENRICHMENT ACTIVITIES

Complete the following sentences.

1. _____ are single-cell microorganisms that can destroy blood cells.

2. Those who are capable of transmitting disease but who do not show any symptoms are known as _____.

3. Never recap, _____, or manually remove a dirty needle.

4. Photocopy and label the parts of the infection cycle.

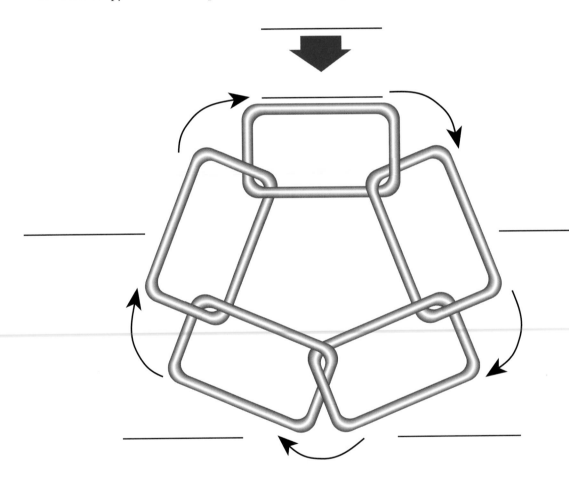

Define the following terms.

5. sterile technique

6. hepatitis A

7. hepatitis B

8. AIDS

9. Universal Precautions

Demonstrate the following techniques.

10. Practice the procedure for handwashing and have your instructor sign off when you have demonstrated the correct procedure.

11. Practice putting on gloves and have your instructor sign off when you have demonstrated the correct procedure.

12. Practice the removal of contaminated gloves and have your instructor sign off when you have demonstrated the correct procedure.

Complete the following exercises.

13. Look in your athletic trainer's kit. List what is in there for working with blood.

14. What would you need in a health club setting to prepare for blood?

CHAPTER 12

Vital Signs Assessment

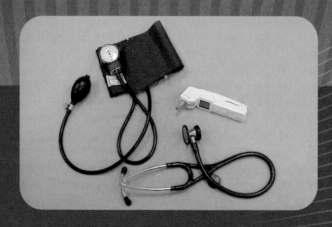

OBJECTIVES

After completing this chapter, you should be able to do the following:

1. Define and correctly spell each of the key terms.

2. Accurately measure and record the four vital signs.

3. Accurately measure and record a person's height and weight.

4. Identify several abnormal respiratory patterns.

5. Recognize the signs of shock.

KEY TERMS

* blood pressure
* core temperature
* homeostasis
* pulse
* respiration
* vital signs

THE VITAL SIGNS

The human body is an amazing system. As human beings, one of the abilities we possess is the ability to maintain a relatively constant internal environment by compensating for changes that occur in either the internal or external environment. This complex balancing act is achieved through the adaptation of various body systems to changes that occur. The process of maintaining this balance, known as **homeostasis**, is constant. Areas of the brain monitor conditions in the body at all times. When certain changes are detected, a response from the appropriate body system is stimulated. For example, if a low oxygen level is detected, the rate of breathing will increase until the amount of oxygen necessary for proper body function is achieved. Other homeostatic mechanisms include the regulation of body temperature and blood pressure.

> **homeostasis**
>
> a state of equilibrium within the body maintained through the adaptation of body systems to changes in either the internal or external environment.

The body systems function optimally within a relatively narrow range of conditions. This is why homeostasis is so important. When illness or injury occurs, the body's ability to maintain homeostasis can be impaired. Therefore, as a health care worker, it is essential to understand the signs of normal and abnormal body functions. **Vital signs** are used to assess the conditions of the various body systems, particularly the respiratory and circulatory systems. These signs will change as the body reacts to an injury or illness. The four basic vital signs are the pulse, respiration, blood pressure, and temperature. It is important to become skilled in the procedures for obtaining each of these vital signs. It is equally important to be able to communicate findings to a supervisor and others accurately by recording the results on the proper forms, using the correct terminology and abbreviations.

> **vital signs**
>
> assessments of pulse, respiration, blood pressure, and temperature; body functions essential to life.

> **NOTE:**
>
> During routine care, gloves are not usually worn unless there will be exposure to blood or other body fluids, or to broken skin, including open lesions. When in doubt, put on appropriate protective wear.

PULSE

The blood vessels expand and contract every time the heart beats. The blood flows through the vessels, and waves of blood cause a rhythmic throbbing in the arteries. This throbbing can best be felt by placing the fingertips over one of the large arteries that lie close to the skin and next to a bone. Veins are the blood vessels that carry blood from the body to the heart; arteries are the vessels that carry blood away from the heart to the rest of the body. This is why a pulse can only be felt in an artery.

pulse

a vital sign; a quantitative measurement of the heartbeat using the fingers to palpate an artery or a stethoscope to listen to the heartbeat.

The **pulse** reflects the condition of the patient's circulatory system and cardiac function. Therefore, changes in the pulse indicate a change in the patient's status. For example, a rapid but weak pulse may indicate shock, bleeding, diabetic coma, or heat exhaustion, while a rapid and strong pulse may indicate heatstroke, severe fright, or hypertension. A patient with a strong and slow pulse may have experienced a skull fracture or a stroke. The absence of a pulse indicates cardiac arrest or death. (See Chapters 17, 19, and 20 for more information on shock, heat exhaustion, and diabetic coma.)

Taking a pulse requires accurate counting and sensitivity to rhythms and quality. Pulse rates vary with the size of the patient, physical condition, and age, and are recorded in terms of beats per minute (bpm). The normal pulse rate for an adult is 60 to 100 beats per minute, with the average heart rate being 70 to 80. Rates higher than 100 are known as tachycardia, and rates below 60 are called bradycardia. In a trained athlete, the resting pulse will be lower (50–60 bpm) because the heart muscle receives more exercise. In this case, the lower pulse is not bradycardia, but rather a normal pulse rate for someone who is in good cardiovascular health. Exercise allows the heart to become stronger and more efficient, sending more oxygenated blood through the body with each beat.

The rhythm of the pulse is described as *regular* or *irregular*. Quality refers to the strength of the pulse, and is noted as *weak, strong*, thready (weak and rapid), or bounding (unusually full and strong). When noting the pulse on a medical or designated form, be sure to indicate the rate, the regularity of the rhythm, and the strength or quality.

The pulse can be felt in many places on the body, but one of the most common locations for obtaining the heart rate is near the radius, one of the bones in the wrist. This pulse is known as the radial pulse. Another common pulse site is the carotid pulse, located on the carotid artery in the neck. In an emergency the pulse rate should be recorded and the information given to a more qualified health care provider at the earliest opportunity. If a pulse is not detected, the EMS should be activated, and cardiopulmonary resuscitation (CPR) must be started immediately. (See Chapter 13.)

MEASURING A RADIAL PULSE

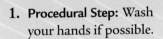

Materials Needed:

* a digital watch or analog watch with a second hand
* gloves (if blood or other body fluids are present)

1. **Procedural Step:** Wash your hands if possible.

   Reason: Universal Precaution.

2. **Procedural Step:** Put on gloves if there is any blood or other body fluid present.

   Reason: Universal Precaution.

3. **Procedural Step:** If in a clinical setting, identify the patient or client by asking the person for the first and last name. Repeat the full name back to the patient.

   Reason: To make sure you are working with the correct person.

4. **Procedural Step:** Have the patient sit, stand, or lie down, according to

MEASURING A RADIAL PULSE

the medical condition. If the patient has recently changed position, wait a few minutes before taking the pulse.

Reason: This allows the heart rate to adjust to the patient's shift in position.

5. **Procedural Step:** Tell the patient what you are going to do using terms the patient can understand.

Reason: This keeps the patient calm and provides the patient with necessary information to give informed consent.

6. **Procedural Step:** Place the palm of the hand downward. If the patient is lying down, rest the patient's forearm across the chest.

Reason: This position will help you count the patient's respirations, when you get to that assessment, without the patient being aware that breaths are being counted. Such awareness may alter the result.

7. **Procedural Step:** Place the pads of your first two fingers directly over the radial artery. Apply slight pressure.

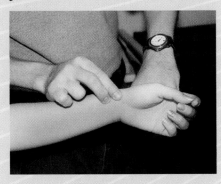

Reason: The fingertips are sensitive and can feel the pulse, located on the inside of the wrist on the thumb side.

8. **Procedural Step:** Feel for the pulsations as the heart beats. Don't push too hard.

Reason: You could stop the blood flow and stop the pulse.

9. **Procedural Step:** Look at the second hand on your watch and begin counting. Ideally, the pulse should be counted for 1 full minute; however, if the pulse is regular it is acceptable to count for 30 seconds and multiply the number by 2.

Reason: This will give you the beats per minute quickly. The pulse rate is charted as the beats per minute.

10. **Procedural Step:** If the rhythm is irregular, then count it for a full minute.

Reason: It is possible to miss some heartbeats by not counting an irregular pulse for a full minute.

11. **Procedural Step:** When measuring a pulse rate, note the *rhythm* and *quality* of the beat as well.

Reason: Rhythm refers to whether the pulse is regular (doesn't change) or irregular (speeds up and/or slows down). Quality refers to the strength of the pulse. A weak, thready pulse may indicate shock, while a full bounding (strong) pulse could indicate high blood pressure.

12. **Procedural Step:** Remove and discard your gloves.

Reason: Universal Precaution.

13. **Procedural Step:** Wash your hands before providing care to another patient.

Reason: Universal Precaution.

(continues)

MEASURING A RADIAL PULSE (Continued)

14. Procedural Step: Record the rate, rhythm, and quality of the pulse in the designated place on the proper form.

Reason: To provide documentation.

15. Procedural Step: Immediately report any abnormalities to your supervisor or contact the EMS.

Reason: An abnormality may indicate a health problem.

Chart it like this: *P = 80, R/S* (regular & strong) or *P = 116, irreg/thready* (irregular, thready)

NOTE: Although the radial artery is the most common place for measuring the pulse rate, a pulse can be measured anywhere the pulsations of an artery can be felt.

MEASURING A CAROTID PULSE

Materials needed:

* a digital watch or analog watch with a second hand
* gloves (if blood or other body fluids are present)

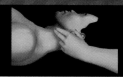

1. Procedural Step: Wash your hands if possible.

Reason: Universal Precaution.

2. Procedural Step: Put on gloves if there is any blood or other body fluid present.

Reason: Universal Precaution.

3. Procedural Step: If in an inpatient setting, identify the patient or client by asking the person for the first and last name. Repeat the full name back to the patient.

Reason: To make sure you are working with the correct person.

4. Procedural Step: Tell the patient what you are

doing in terms the patient can understand.

Reason: This keeps the patient calm.

5. Procedural Step: Check the carotid artery on one side and then the other side. The carotid pulse is used to check for a pulse when cardiac arrest is suspected. Pressing on both carotid arteries at the same time could decrease the blood supply to the brain.

Reason: The carotid pulse is the closest point to the heart that can be easily detected without a stethoscope. It can still be felt when a patient may only have fainted. There will be no pulse on a patient in cardiac arrest. Patients who have experienced a stroke may have a carotid pulse on only one side.

MEASURING A CAROTID PULSE

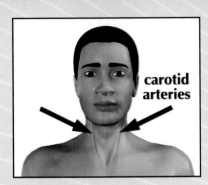

carotid arteries

6. Procedural Step: Use the pads of your first two fingers, and place them directly over one side of the front of the patient's neck. Check both the right and the left pulse for 5 to 10 seconds. If no pulse is felt, then begin cardiac compressions.

Reason: This is how the carotid pulse is measured.

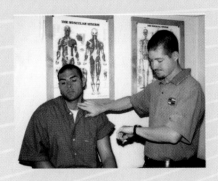

7. Procedural Step: Remove and discard your gloves.

Reason: Universal Precaution.

8. Procedural Step: Wash your hands before providing care to another patient.

Reason: Universal Precaution.

9. Procedural Step: Record your findings on the patient's chart.

Reason: To provide documentation.

10. Procedural Step: Immediately report any abnormalities to your supervisor or contact the EMS.

Reason: An abnormality may indicate a health problem.

Chart it like this: *P = 62.*

NOTE: This pulse is generally used in emergency situations and for self-monitoring of the pulse during cardiovascular exercise, rather than for patient monitoring. Therefore, rhythm and quality are not usually noted for a carotid pulse.

There are many other places in the human body where the pulse may be felt (see Figure 12-1). Some of the more common pulse sites are listed below:

* The temporal artery: This artery is located on the face in front of the ear. Since this pulse may be difficult to locate, it is generally not used for a pulse rate.

* The brachial artery: This artery is found on the inside of the arm at the crease near the elbow. The pulse that is palpated at this location is used primarily for a blood pressure check.

* The femoral artery: Found in the right and left groin, this pulse is often used to check for circulation in the legs.

* The popliteal artery: This pulse is located behind the knee and, like the femoral artery, may be used to check for circulation in the legs.

* The dorsalis pedis: This pulse is located on top of the foot and is used primarily to check for circulation in the feet.

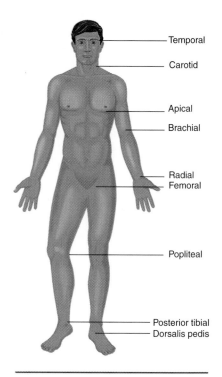

Temporal
Carotid
Apical
Brachial
Radial
Femoral
Popliteal
Posterior tibial
Dorsalis pedis

FIGURE 12-1 Pulse Sites

RESPIRATION

Breathing, or **respiration**, is the process of bringing oxygen into the body where it can be utilized by the cells, and expelling carbon dioxide, which is eliminated as a waste product from the cells. This process is controlled by the brain and regulated by the changing carbon dioxide levels in the bloodstream. To allow air to enter and exit the body, the ribs, chest muscles, and diaphragm move spontaneously in response to messages from the brain.

Respiration provides the cells of the body with the energy required to perform their specific functions. This energy is obtained when food is metabolized (chemically altered) at the cellular level. The conversion of food to energy requires oxygen. Respiration provides this oxygen to each of the cells, via the bloodstream. When more energy is required by the muscle cells, such as during exercise, the rate of respiration increases. The normal rate of breathing can also be altered by excitement, drugs, and a number of disease processes (e.g., diabetes, kidney abnormalities, and heart and lung diseases). In addition, pain, fever, and trauma may also affect the breathing process. If breathing patterns are altered and the body is deprived of oxygen, serious damage can occur to the vital organs. The absence of respiration indicates a blocked airway or death.

A single respiration consists of one inspiration and one expiration. Use the following general guidelines for the normal rates of respiration:

* Age 15 and older: 15 to 20 breaths per minute

* A well-trained athlete: 6 to 8 breaths per minute

Although respiration is mostly spontaneous, voluntary muscles may also be used to breathe. When a person focuses on breathing, the rate of respiration is often altered. Therefore, to prevent a patient from inadvertently altering the true rate, try to conceal the fact that respirations are being counted. For example, respiration can be measured without a person's knowledge by observing and counting breaths after taking the pulse.

In addition to measuring respirations, it is also important to observe the patterns of the respirations. Respiratory patterns are defined as follows:

* Abdominal: respirations using primarily the abdominal muscles while the chest is mostly still

* Apnea: the cessation of breathing; may be temporary or permanent

* Bradypnea: breathing that is abnormally slow

* Cheyne-Stokes respiration: a grossly irregular breathing pattern composed of intermittent periods of apnea lasting from 10 to 60 seconds followed by periods of fast and slow breathing

* Decreased: very little air movement in the lungs

* Dyspnea: difficult or painful breathing; shortness of breath

* Hyperpnea or tachypnea: breathing that is faster or deeper than that which is produced during normal activity. Also known as hyperventilation

* Kussmaul's breathing: deep, gasping respirations; *air hunger*

* Labored breathing: difficult breathing that uses shoulder muscles, neck muscles, and abdominal muscles

The volume of air that is exchanged with each respiration can be determined by placing one hand on the patient's chest and feeling the chest rise and fall. The volume of respirations can be described as deep or shallow (restricted). When respirations are deep, the patient takes long, deep breaths. A prolonged inspiration might indicate an upper airway obstruction, or a prolonged expiration could indicate chronic obstructive pulmonary disease (COPD), like asthma, bronchitis, or emphysema. If the breathing is shallow, shock may be indicated. Irregular breathing or gasping may indicate cardiac involvement. Under normal circumstances breathing (respiration) is quiet and effortless. Noisy respirations indicate an obstruction in the air passages.

Patients who are having difficulty breathing usually will sit up and lean forward in an effort to breathe easier. The first signs of oxygen deprivation are mental confusion and restlessness. A person who is experiencing these symptoms must be seen immediately by the physician.

MEASURING RESPIRATION

Materials Needed:

* a digital watch or analog watch with a second hand
* gloves (if blood or other body fluids are present)

1. **Procedural Step:** Measure the respiration after obtaining the patient's pulse.

   Reason: To prevent the patient from knowing when breaths are being counted.

2. **Procedural Step:** Wash your hands if possible.

   Reason: Universal Precaution.

   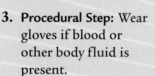

3. **Procedural Step:** Wear gloves if blood or other body fluid is present.

   Reason: Universal Precaution.

4. **Procedural Step:** If in an inpatient setting, identify the patient or client by asking the person for the first and last name. Repeat the full name back to the patient.

   Reason: To make sure you are working with the correct person.

5. **Procedural Step:** Do not tell the patient when you will be monitoring the respiratory rate.

   Reason: This could alter the results.

6. **Procedural Step:** If you measured the radial pulse, keep the patient's arm across the chest and count one inspiration and one expiration as one breath.

   Reason: Having the patient's arm in this position will make it easier to detect the rise and fall of the patient's chest.

7. **Procedural Step:** Count the rate for 30 seconds and multiply that number by 2. This final value will be the number of breaths per minute (i.e., if you count eight full respirations in 30 seconds, multiply $8 \times 2 = 16$ breaths per minute).

   Reason: Respiration is documented as the breaths per minute.

8. **Procedural Step:** Remove and discard your gloves if it was necessary to put them on.

   Reason: Universal Precaution.

9. **Procedural Step:** Wash your hands.

   Reason: Universal Precaution.

10. **Procedural Step:** Record the results on the patient's chart.

    Reason: To provide documentation.

11. **Procedural Step:** Report any difficulty in breathing to your supervisor or activate the EMS and note it on the patient's chart.

    Reason: Difficulty in breathing indicates a health problem.

    Chart it like this: *R = 16, labored*

BLOOD PRESSURE

Blood pressure is a measurement of the pressure of the blood exerted against the walls of the arteries. This pressure is recorded as two measurements: systolic and diastolic. The systolic pressure is the top number in a blood pressure reading. It reflects the blood pressure when the heart contracts. The diastolic pressure reflects the blood pressure when the heart is at rest and is recorded as the bottom number of a blood pressure measurement. For example, if a person has a systolic pressure of 120 and a diastolic pressure of 80, the blood pressure would be recorded as 120/80.

The blood pressure is affected by a number of factors, such as the amount of blood and other fluids that are present in the body, the condition of the arteries, and the force of the heartbeat. These factors, in turn, can be affected by many other considerations. Age, exercise, obesity, food, pain, stress, stimulants, steroids, and some medications can cause the blood pressure to increase; whereas weight loss, fasting, depression, and blood loss can lower the blood pressure. Gender and heredity can also influence a person's blood pressure. For example, pre-menopausal women tend to have blood pressure measurements that are approximately 10 mm Hg lower than men. Similarly, a person's chances of having low blood pressure or high blood pressure increase if one or both parents suffered from the condition.

Although blood pressure increases during exercise, an exercise program helps to lower blood pressure overall. The heart beats (or works) as fast as it needs to in order to get blood, oxygen, and nutrients to the entire body. A strong, healthy heart that pumps efficiently allows blood to circulate throughout the body at a lower pressure than a heart that is in poor condition and has to work harder to perform the same function. This is why trained athletes tend to have lower blood pressure than average people. Physical training increases the heart's pumping efficiency and improves the health of the peripheral vascular system.

The blood pressure measurement is a source of valuable information for the health care provider. Specific abnormalities in blood pressure are indications of various health problems. If a positive result is obtained, meaning that the blood pressure is either too high or too low, experienced medical assistance should be sought immediately.

Positive test results:

1. A systolic value below 100 mm Hg or above 139 mm Hg

2. A diastolic value below 65 mm Hg or above 89 mm Hg

Implications:

1. Low blood pressure (hypotension) may indicate shock, dehydration, or internal injury. Possible causes might be heart failure, heat exhaustion or heatstroke, diabetes, or liver disease.

2. High blood pressure (hypertension) can be a dangerous precursor to cardiac problems and strokes. High blood pressure can exert extreme pressure on blood vessels, including the vascular regions of the brain. Possible causes might be obesity, lack of physical activity, too much salt in diet, and stress.

blood pressure
the pressure exerted by the circulating blood against the walls of the arteries.

In emergency situations, blood pressure should be measured as soon as possible, and the information should be given to EMS personnel when they arrive. If the blood pressure cannot be obtained, activate the EMS or find someone who can take a proper reading.

To measure a person's blood pressure, a sphygmomanometer (blood pressure cuff) and a stethoscope will be needed. To get an accurate reading, the width of the sphygmomanometer should cover approximately three-fourths of the patient's upper arm. If the cuff is too narrow, a false high reading can be obtained, and a cuff that is too wide can produce a false low reading (see Figure 12-2).

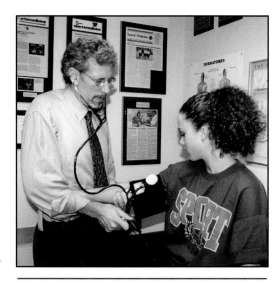

FIGURE 12-2 The width of the blood pressure cuff can affect the accuracy of the measurement. Make sure the sphygmomanometer is the proper size for the patient.

AUSCULTATING A BLOOD PRESSURE

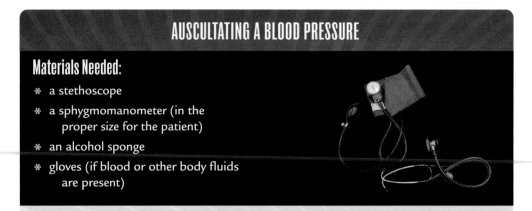

Materials Needed:

* a stethoscope
* a sphygmomanometer (in the proper size for the patient)
* an alcohol sponge
* gloves (if blood or other body fluids are present)

1. **Procedural Step:** Wash your hands and assemble the equipment.

   Reason: Universal Precaution.

2. **Procedural Step:** Put on gloves if there is any blood or other body fluid present.

   Reason: Universal Precaution.

3. **Procedural Step:** If in an inpatient setting, identify the patient or client by asking the person for the first and last name. Repeat the full name back to the patient.

   Reason: To make sure you are working with the correct person.

4. **Procedural Step:** Explain the procedure using terms the patient can understand.

AUSCULTATING A BLOOD PRESSURE

Reason: This keeps the patient calm and provides the information necessary for the patient to give informed consent.

5. **Procedural Step:** Have the patient sit or lie down. Roll the patient's sleeve about 6 inches above the elbow. If the sleeve is too tight, remove the arm from the sleeve. Extend the arm, palm up, at heart level.

   Reason: A sleeve that is too tight may compress the brachial artery and distort the results. If the arm is above heart level, the reading may be incorrectly low.

6. **Procedural Step:** Palpate the brachial artery on the inner aspect of the elbow. Then place the blood pressure cuff smoothly and securely around the patient's arm about 2 inches above the bend in the elbow. Be sure the middle of the cloth-enclosed cuff is directly over the brachial artery on the inner aspect of the upper arm. If the cuff has an arrow to indicate right or left arm, the arrow should be placed over the brachial artery.

   Reason: The cuff should be tight enough to stay on, but not so tight as to be constricting. It should be high enough so that the stethoscope will not touch the cuff and cause extraneous sounds. By placing the center of the bladder of the cuff over the brachial artery you assure that the pressure is applied equally over the artery.

7. **Procedural Step:** Place the earpieces of the stethoscope in your ears with the tips pointing slightly forward. Avoid letting the tubes rub together.

Reason: The forward position of the earpieces will make it easier to hear because they will be following the direction of the ear canal. The tubes should be hanging freely so extraneous sounds won't be heard.

8. **Procedural Step:** Palpate the pulse at the brachial artery. Place the diaphragm of the stethoscope firmly over the point of maximal impulse (PMI).

   Reason: Proper placement of the diaphragm will help you hear the sounds of the blood pressure.

9. **Procedural Step:** Hold the diaphragm in place with your non-dominant hand, close the control valve, and quickly squeeze the bulb with your dominant hand until you can no longer hear the pulse.

   Reason: The range of 20 to 30 mm Hg is sufficient to be sure you have pumped the cuff high enough to accurately hear the systolic pressure. Inflating the rubber bladder in the cuff stops the flow of blood in the artery. The cuff is inflated quickly and smoothly to avoid congestion in the blood vessels.

10. **Procedural Step:** Slowly and steadily open the control valve at a rate of approximately 2 to 3 mm Hg per heartbeat. This will release the air in the cuff. Listen for the first clear, tapping sound. This is the systolic pressure. Notice the reading on the calibrated scale.

    Reason: The systolic blood pressure represents the pressure against the walls of the arteries when the ventricles of the heart contract and blood surges through the aorta and pulmonary arteries.

(continues)

AUSCULTATING A BLOOD PRESSURE (Continued)

11. Procedural Step: Continue to steadily deflate the cuff until the last sound is heard. This is the diastolic pressure.

Reason: The diastolic pressure refers to the point at which there is the least pressure in the arteries and occurs when the heart relaxes (diastole) before the next contraction (systole).

12. Procedural Step: Quickly release the rest of the air from the cuff and remove the cuff from the patient's arm.

Reason: If left inflated, it will prevent circulation to the hand and arm.

13. Procedural Step: Report any abnormalities to your supervisor or activate the EMS. Immediately record the measurements obtained as a fraction, noting the time, arm used (right or left), and the patient's position (lying, sitting, or standing).

Reason: Abnormalities may indicate a health problem. Charting immediately will ensure accuracy.

14. Procedural Step: If you have trouble obtaining a reading on one arm, take a reading on the opposite arm and report the problem on the chart.

Reason: An abnormality may indicate a problem with one of the arteries.

15. Procedural Step: Clean the earpieces and the diaphragm of the stethoscope with an alcohol sponge.

Reason: The equipment will be ready for use the next time.

16. Procedural Step: Remove your gloves and discard if it was necessary to put them on.

Reason: Universal Precaution.

17. Procedural Step: Wash your hands before giving care to another patient.

Reason: Universal Precaution.

Chart the blood pressure like this, indicating which arm was used and whether the patient was sitting or lying down: *BP = 160/90 RA, sitting* meaning the blood pressure was 160 mm Hg systolic and 90 mm Hg diastolic, and the reading was taken on the right arm with the patient in a sitting position.

NOTE: When listening for the diastolic pressure, you will notice a change in the quality of the sounds before they completely disappear. Some physicians consider this first diastolic sound to be the diastolic blood pressure. If you are asked to record this sound, chart it as follows: *B/P 180/100/90*. This would mean that the first sound you heard was 180 (systolic blood pressure), a change or muffled sound was noted at 100 (first diastolic sound), and the last sound you heard was at 90 (final diastolic pressure).

THINKING IT THROUGH

At Valley Community College the beginning of soccer season signals the need for every player to have a physical exam. It typically takes the entire athletic training staff all morning to perform the necessary physicals, and this year promised to be no different.

On the date set for the physicals Ms. Morgan, the head athletic trainer, set up a different station for each vital sign. She then assigned athletic training students to each station. Steve was assigned to take blood pressures, and he was doing a good job of it. Ms. Morgan was getting the same pressures as he was nine out of 10 times.

One of Steve's friends, Rudy, was in line to have his blood pressure taken. To Steve's surprise, Rudy's blood pressure was 170 over 92. Steve did not know how to tell a friend that his blood pressure would jeopardize his chance to play soccer. So, Ms. Morgan and Steve sat down with Rudy to discuss his unusually high blood pressure. Rudy assured them that he had a condition called "White Coat Syndrome," in which he gets nervous when someone takes his blood pressure. He promised to have his family physician check him out and forward the results to the school's athletic department.

Why is it important for an athletic trainer to check the athletic training student's work periodically? How elevated is Rudy's blood pressure when compared to the normal range? Is it acceptable to have a family physician perform the physical and forward the results instead of having it performed by the athletic training staff?

TEMPERATURE

The body's **core temperature** must remain within a relatively narrow range in order for the body's various systems to function efficiently. The body's temperature is regulated by an area in the brain known as the hypothalamus. This important group of cells monitors the temperature of the blood and stimulates a response to compensate for any changes in temperature that occur. For example, heat is normally produced as we burn calories obtained from the food we eat. If this fails to produce enough heat, the hypothalamus will compensate for the lack of heat by sending a message (via the nerves) to the muscles to create heat by shivering. The hypothalamus also causes the blood vessels in the skin to constrict so that the body's heat can be retained. Similarly, if the body generates too much heat, the sweat glands are stimulated, and the blood vessels are dilated to promote the loss of heat.

Normal body temperature is 98.6° Fahrenheit (37° Celsius). Oral temperature reading is the preferred method for obtaining a patient's temperature. However, for those who work in the field, it is often more practical to take a temperature reading of the tympanic membrane (the membrane that covers the eardrum) using a digital

core temperature

the internal body temperature.

ear thermometer called a tympanic thermometer. The tympanic membrane shares the same blood supply as the hypothalamus, the portion of the brain that controls the body's temperature. The temperature reading obtained from the tympanic membrane is actually the temperature of the blood flowing through the tympanic membrane. The thermometer's speculum is inserted into the patient's ear next to the tympanic membrane. Within seconds, the thermometer provides a read-out of the patient's temperature. *Be careful not to insert the probe too far—this can injure the tympanic membrane!*

There are two temperature scales that are used to assess a patient's temperature: Fahrenheit and Celsius. Proper measurement of the body's core temperature can help identify changes in the patient's condition. The following pages describe the correct procedures for taking a patient's temperature using tympanic and oral thermometers.

MEASURING A TYMPANIC TEMPERATURE USING A TYMPANIC THERMOMETER

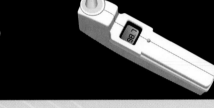

Materials Needed:
* a tympanic thermometer (electronic)
* a disposable thermometer cover
* gloves (if blood or other body fluids are present)

1. **Procedural Step:** Wash your hands.

   Reason: Universal Precaution.

2. **Procedural Step:** Put on gloves if any blood or other body fluid is present.

   Reason: Universal Precaution.

3. **Procedural Step:** If in an inpatient setting, identify the patient or client by asking the person for the first and last name. Repeat the full name back to the patient.

   Reason: To make sure you are working with the correct person.

4. **Procedural Step:** Explain the procedure using terms the patient can understand.

Reason: This reassures the patient and provides information necessary for the patient to give informed consent.

5. **Procedural Step:** Remove the thermometer from your kit.

   Reason: The device is portable.

6. **Procedural Step:** Place the disposable cover over the ear speculum.

   Reason: Clean technique.

7. **Procedural Step:** Have the patient turn the head to one side. If the patient is a child, gently turn the head to one side and hold it in place.

   Reason: This makes the ear easily accessible.

8. **Procedural Step:** Place the speculum in either ear canal for 5 seconds. It only has to cover the opening!

MEASURING A TYMPANIC TEMPERATURE USING A TYMPANIC THERMOMETER

Reason: This measures the temperature of the tympanic membrane.

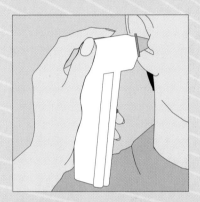

9. **Procedural Step:** Press the scan button, and release it when the temperature is flashing on the display screen.

   Reason: The signal indicates the thermometer is ready to be read. It usually takes about 2 seconds.

10. **Procedural Step:** Remove the thermometer from the patient's ear.

    Reason: The temperature has been obtained.

11. **Procedural Step:** Read the thermometer and discard the disposable cover.

    Reason: Universal Precaution.

12. **Procedural Step:** Remove and discard your gloves if it was necessary to wear them.

    Reason: Universal Precaution.

13. **Procedural Step:** Wash your hands.

    Reason: Universal Precaution.

14. **Procedural Step:** Return the thermometer to your kit.

    Reason: It will be ready for use the next time.

15. **Procedural Step:** Chart the temperature.

    Reason: To provide documentation. 98.6°F is normal.

    Chart it like this: $T = 98^4$ or $T = 98.4$.

MEASURING AN ORAL TEMPERATURE USING A DIGITAL THERMOMETER

Materials Needed:
* a digital thermometer
* a disposable thermometer cover
* gloves (if blood or other body fluids are present)

1. **Procedural Step:** Wash your hands if possible.

   Reason: Universal Precaution.

2. **Procedural Step:** Put on gloves if blood or other body fluids are present.

   Reason: Universal Precaution.

(continues)

MEASURING AN ORAL TEMPERATURE USING A DIGITAL THERMOMETER (Continued)

3. Procedural Step: If in an inpatient setting, identify the patient or client by asking the person for the first and last name. Repeat the full name back to the patient.

Reason: To make sure you are working with the correct person.

4. Procedural Step: Explain the procedure using terms the patient can understand.

Reason: This keeps the patient calm and provides information the patient needs to give informed consent.

5. Procedural Step: Remove the thermometer from your kit and place a disposable cover over the probe.

Reason: To avoid contamination.

6. Procedural Step: Have the patient discard anything in the mouth.

Reason: It may affect the temperature reading.

7. Procedural Step: Ask if the patient has had anything by mouth within the last 15 minutes. If so, wait 15 minutes more.

Reason: It may affect the temperature reading.

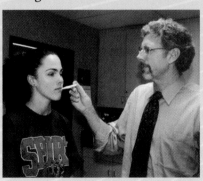

8. Procedural Step: Wait for the *ready* signal to be displayed on the thermometer.

Reason: This means the thermometer is ready for use.

9. Procedural Step: Place the probe in the patient's mouth under the tongue. Have the patient close the lips.

Reason: This area is close to a rich blood supply.

10. Procedural Step: At the sound or flashing light, remove the probe from the patient's mouth.

Reason: The signal indicates the thermometer is ready to read.

11. Procedural Step: Without touching the portion of the cover that was in the patient's mouth, dispose of the cover.

Reason: This allows removal of the probe cover without touching it and prevents alteration of the thermometer reading.

12. Procedural Step: Remove and discard your gloves if it was necessary to put them on.

Reason: Universal Precaution.

13. Procedural Step: Wash your hands.

Reason: Universal Precaution.

14. Procedural Step: Read the display. Record the temperature on the patient's chart.

Reason: To provide documentation.

MEASURING AN ORAL TEMPERATURE USING A DIGITAL THERMOMETER

15. Procedural Step: Return the thermometer to the kit.

Reason: The equipment will be ready for the next use.

16. Procedural Step: Immediately report any abnormalities to your supervisor or contact the EMS.

Reason: This may indicate a health problem. A normal oral temperature is 98.6°F.

Chart it like this: $T = 98^6$ or $T = 98.6$.

WEIGHT AND HEIGHT

Most people want to achieve a certain weight so that they will look and feel attractive. But there are health reasons for maintaining a particular weight, too. Excess weight or fat can contribute to a variety of health risks. Some of these risks are listed below:

* Increased risk of cardiovascular disease because of additional stress on the heart, and heightened risk of hypertension and atherosclerosis

* Decreased life expectancy

* Impeded circulation in the legs

* Increased risk of diabetes

* Increased stress on muscles and joints supporting the extra weight

Since weight is such an important factor in maintaining good health, a person's height and weight are almost always measured in the course of a physical examination. The following pages contain the proper procedures for measuring weight and height.

MEASURING THE WEIGHT OF AN ADULT

Materials Needed:
* a scale with a measuring device

1. Procedural Step: If in an inpatient setting, identify the patient or client by asking the person for the first and last name. Repeat the full name back to the patient.

Reason: To make sure you are working with the correct person.

(continues)

MEASURING THE WEIGHT OF AN ADULT (Continued)

2. **Procedural Step:** Ask if the patient knows his or her weight.

   Reason: This will assist you in setting the weight on the scale in the general area; it also avoids embarrassment if you misjudge the patient at a too-heavy weight.

3. **Procedural Step:** Ask the patient to remove any heavy outer wear such as coats and sweaters. The shoes may be removed too.

   Reason: Clothing and footwear can add 3 to 6 pounds.

4. **Procedural Step:** Make sure both the weights on the scale are pushed completely to the left, at the *zero* position. The scale must be on a flat, balanced surface.

   Reason: To prevent an inaccurate reading.

5. **Procedural Step:** If the patient is barefoot (as may be the case in an inpatient setting), place a paper on the scale to stand on.

   Reason: Clean technique.

6. **Procedural Step:** Inform the patient the scale may move and assist the patient onto the scale by gently taking an arm for extra support.

   Reason: To prevent the patient from falling.

7. **Procedural Step:** Always be ready to physically assist the patient. Constantly watch for any unsteadiness.

   Reason: To prevent a fall if the patient loses balance.

8. **Procedural Step:** Instruct the patient to stand still, with arms at sides. The patient should not hold on to any part of the scale or you.

Reason: If the patient touches you, the scale, or anything else, some of the weight will be displaced, causing an inaccurate reading.

9. **Procedural Step:** The bottom weight on the scale marks increments of 50 pounds. Slide this weight to the mark (50, 100, 150, or 200) that is closest to, but not over, the patient's stated weight. Make sure the weight rests securely in the incremental groove on the register.

   Reason: Unless this bottom weight is properly set, your measurement may be off by several pounds.

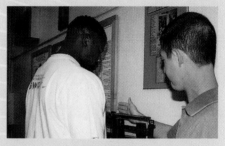

10. **Procedural Step:** Gradually move the upper weight, which indicates individual pounds, across the upper register until the pointer on the right end of the set of registers rests in the center of the metal frame. The registers should not touch the sides of the frame.

    Reason: When the set of registers balances in the center of the metal frame, the scale is set to the patient's correct weight.

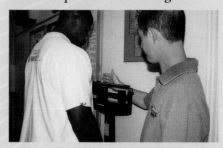

MEASURING THE WEIGHT OF AN ADULT

11. Procedural Step: Assist the patient from the scale.

Reason: To prevent the patient from falling.

12. Procedural Step: Return the weights to the *zero* setting.

Reason: To prepare the scale for the next patient.

13. Procedural Step: Record the patient's weight in pounds.

Reason: To provide documentation.

14. Procedural Step: Remove and discard the paper if it was necessary to place one on the scale.

Reason: Clean technique.

Chart it like this: *9:00 a.m. 150 lbs.*

MEASURING THE HEIGHT OF AN ADULT

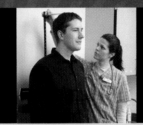

Materials Needed:

* a scale with a measuring device

1. Procedural Step: If in an inpatient setting, identify the patient or client by asking the person for the first and last name. Repeat the full name back to the patient.

Reason: To make sure you are working with the correct person.

2. Procedural Step: Have the patient remove shoes and step on the scale, facing away from it.

Reason: To obtain the most accurate measurement. Shoes can substantially alter a person's height reading.

3. Procedural Step: With the hinged arm in the lowered position, raise the height bar above the patient's head.

Reason: To prevent the arm from injuring the patient.

4. Procedural Step: Instruct the patient to look straight ahead.

Reason: This will keep the top of the head level.

5. Procedural Step: Extend the hinged arm and gently slide the measuring bar down until it rests lightly on the patient's head.

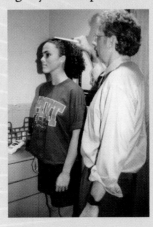

(continues)

MEASURING THE HEIGHT OF AN ADULT (Continued)

Reason: If done too quickly, the patient may be injured.

6. **Procedural Step:** Read the last digit or fraction of a digit that is visible on the moveable portion of the bar, just above the stationary portion.

read here in inches

Reason: This is the patient's height.

7. **Procedural Step:** Record the patient's height in inches. If the patient wants to know the height in feet, remember that 12 inches = 1 foot. Therefore, a person with a height of 72 inches is 6 feet tall.

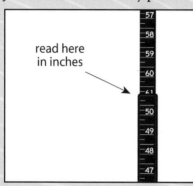

Reason: To provide documentation.

Chart it like this: *9:00 a.m. 60 ¾ ins.*

CHAPTER SUMMARY

One of the most valuable skills a health care provider can learn is how to measure a patient's vital signs properly. The four basic vital signs include the pulse, respiratory rate, blood pressure, and temperature. There are specific procedures for obtaining accurate measurements of each of these vital signs. Anyone who wants to work in the field of sports medicine must know what these procedures are and be able to perform them quickly and accurately. In addition to being able to obtain accurate measurements, one must be able to use this information to detect changes in the patient's health status. Understanding the factors that can affect each vital sign also will help ensure the quality of care provided to each patient and client.

It is not enough for a health care provider to simply measure and record vital signs; the key to quality care is communication. Many times the sports medicine professional will be the first to arrive at the scene of an injury and will be responsible for passing information to the EMS, physicians, and family members. The importance of good communication in providing high quality health care cannot be overemphasized! This means every sports medicine professional must carefully observe the patient's signs and symptoms, initiate appropriate emergency action, record all vital patient information, and report all the necessary patient information to the appropriate people (i.e., EMS personnel, the patient's physician, and the patient's family).

STUDENT ENRICHMENT ACTIVITIES

Complete the following sentences.

1. The body's temperature is regulated by an area in the brain called the _____.

2. _____ is the process of bringing oxygen into the body and expelling carbon dioxide.

3. A single respiration consists of one _____ and one _____.

4. Blood pressure is measured with a _____ and a _____.

5. When recording a blood pressure reading, the top number is the _____ pressure and the bottom number is the _____ pressure.

Define the following terms.

6. vital signs

7. bradycardia

8. dyspnea

9. bradypnea

10. apnea

11. hyperpnea

Complete the following exercise.

12. Copy this chart on a sheet of paper or into a computer file you name "vitals." Practice taking the vital signs of five classmates, and record your findings in your chart.

NAME	BP	P	R	T
1.				
2.				
3.				
4.				
5.				

CHAPTER 13

Basic Life Support

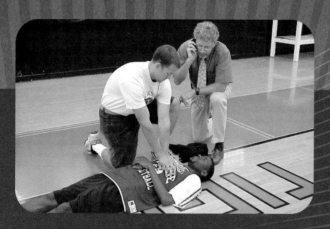

OBJECTIVES

After completing this chapter, you should be able to do the following:

1. Define and correctly spell each of the key terms.
2. Name and describe the steps involved in CPR.
3. Explain the importance of early access to AED.
4. Demonstrate the obstructed airway maneuver.
5. Explain and demonstrate the three-person log roll.

KEY TERMS

* automated external defibrillator (AED)
* cardiac arrest
* cardiopulmonary resuscitation (CPR)

* chest compressions
* full arrest
* head-tilt, chin-lift maneuver
* obstructed airway maneuver
* sudden cardiac arrest

INTRODUCTION TO LIFESAVING PROCEDURES

Basic life support involves the prompt recognition of breathing difficulties and/or cardiac arrest and emergency treatment for them. This chapter introduces you to the skills needed to clear an obstructive airway, perform CPR, and use an AED. This in no way should take the place of the proper training and certification needed to be prepared for a lifesaving event.

It is imperative to have an Emergency Action Plan (see Chapter 9) for every event, athletic site, and possible known situation. This plan must be written and practiced, and each practice must be recorded. This must be ongoing. With proper training comes confidence and experience, and with that comes the ability to save lives.

> **NOTE:**
>
> Remember, wear gloves and other protective devices (such as goggles, face masks, etc.) whenever there is potential for exposure to blood or other body fluids. If you are not wearing them at the time of the incident (sudden hemorrhage, vomiting, etc.), don them immediately.

CARDIOPULMONARY RESUSCITATION

Cardiopulmonary resuscitation (CPR) is a procedure that combines rescue breathing, which supplies oxygen to the lungs, and chest compressions, which circulates blood throughout the body. When performed correctly, CPR can maintain life in a victim of cardiac or respiratory arrest while emergency personnel gather to provide advanced life support. Because CPR has proven to be effective in restoring a pulse and respirations, it is done whenever the heart and lungs stop working.

The absence of a heartbeat is called **cardiac arrest**. When both respirations and pulse cease, the patient experiences clinical death. However, the body cells have a residual oxygen supply and can survive a short time without new oxygen. After 4 to 6 minutes without a pulse or respirations, the brain does

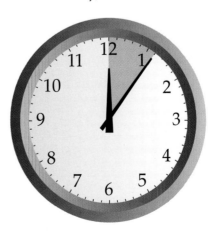

cardiopulmonary resuscitation (CPR)

a lifesaving procedure involving artificial ventilation and chest compressions that is done for cardiac arrest.

cardiac arrest

asystole; the absence of a heartbeat.

not receive the oxygen that is vital to all the body organs, and the brain cells begin to die. When the brain cells die, it is called biological death. The period between clinical and biological death is very short. If a person recognizes the **full arrest** and immediately begins CPR, the patient can be saved from biological death. The key is *immediate recognition* of cardiac arrest and *immediate response* with CPR.

full arrest

respiratory and cardiac arrest.

SUDDEN CARDIAC ARREST

Surviving **sudden cardiac arrest** is often dependent on how fast a patient is defibrillated. For each minute a patient is in arrest, the chance of survival decreases by about 10%. Very few people are successfully resuscitated after 10 minutes.

sudden cardiac arrest

a sudden stopping of the heartbeat, which may cause death.

Chain of Survival

The chain of survival consists of four links: early access to EMS (emergency medical services), early CPR (cardiopulmonary resuscitation), early defibrillation, and early advanced care. Any weak link in the chain will reduce a patient's chances of survival.

Several steps in advanced preparation are key in ensuring the first aid provider (*rescuer*) is not in danger before providing CPR for a patient in cardiac arrest. Most important, the emergency situation itself can be dangerous, so when approaching an unknown emergency, maintain distance and call for help.

SETUP

The acronym SETUP can be a useful tool to remember personal safety.

* <u>S</u>top. Pause for a moment and look for any obvious hazards.

* <u>E</u>nvironment. Account for any environmental barriers or dangers.

* <u>T</u>raffic. Be extremely careful when providing first aid near a roadway.

* <u>U</u>nknown hazards. Be aware of unknown hazards that were not initially apparent. The rescuer may have to retreat from the scene.

* <u>P</u>rotect yourself and the patient. The use of gloves and breathing barriers is important, because infectious diseases can be transmitted through open cuts or sores of the skin and the mucous membranes of the mouth, nose, and eyes.

Assess Responsiveness

* Introduce yourself. Introduce yourself to the patient and inform the person that you are trained in first aid. Do this even if the person seems unresponsive. The patient may be able to respond. Ask if the person needs help (see Figure 13-1).

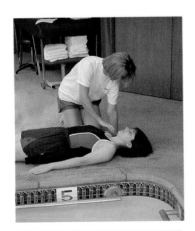

FIGURE 13-1 Determine Unresponsiveness

* Tap and shout. Tap the patient on the clavicle and ask if the person is okay. If there is no response, immediately access emergency medical services (EMS). If there are bystanders, have them call for EMS and then meet the EMS and bring them to the scene. If there is no one there, the rescuer must call the EMS before proceeding.

Check Airway—Head-Tilt, Chin-Lift

To perform the **head-tilt, chin-lift maneuver**, position one hand on the patient's forehead, while placing the fingertips of the other hand under the bony part of the chin to open the airway. Apply firm, backward pressure on the patient's forehead while lifting the chin upward. This should tilt the head backward and move the jaw forward (see Figure 13-2). If this does not establish an airway the first time, try it again. Once the airway is open, keep one hand on the forehead to maintain the airway.

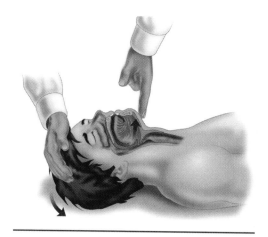

FIGURE 13-2 Head-Tilt, Chin-Lift Maneuver

> **head-tilt, chin-lift maneuver**
>
> a procedure for opening a blocked airway in which a patient's head is titled back and the chin is lifted.

* Inspect the patient's mouth. If there are any visible foreign materials in the mouth, remove them.

Assess Breathing

Place one ear next to the patient's mouth, look to see if the chest rises and falls, listen for any sounds of breathing, and feel for exhaled air. This check should proceed for no longer than 10 seconds. If the patient is breathing, maintain airway and scan for signs of serious bleeding. Assess the patient's skin color and temperature for signs of shock. To assess darker-skinned patients, examine their lips or finger tips. If breathing is absent, begin cardiopulmonary resuscitation (CPR).

> **NOTE:**
>
> If the patient is face-down and does not have respiration or other signs of circulation, you will need to log roll the patient to begin CPR or rescue breathing. Patients who need CPR or rescue breathing are not left face-down—even if you suspect a spinal injury. As you perform the log roll, make sure that proper care is taken to protect the spine.

Ventilations

To begin ventilations, place a shield over the patient's mouth; take a normal breath, then press your mouth against the shield to create an airtight feel (see Figure 13-3). If the patient is not breathing, provide two rescue breaths. Each breath should be one second long and have sufficient volume to create a visible rise in the patient's chest. Then, remove your mouth and allow the patient to completely exhale while taking a fresh breath to provide the second ventilation.

Signs of Circulation

To determine the difference between respiratory arrest and cardiac arrest, you will need to effectively assess for an obvious sign of circulation. This is done primarily by checking for a pulse in the neck, the carotid pulse (see Chapter 12). Because this is a relatively complex skill, do not use it if you have limited training and experience. (Although checking a pulse is no longer taught to the layperson, the present guidelines do continue to recommend that trained healthcare professionals check for a pulse, in addition to looking for signs of circulation, before doing chest compressions on an unconscious victim.)

Signs of circulation indicate the presence of adequate blood flow through the patient's circulatory system. These signs include normal breathing, patient movement, and most important, a clearly obvious carotid pulse.

While maintaining the head tilt, find the pulse next to the bony structure of the neck (trachea). Place two fingers on top of the neck and slide them toward yourself in the groove, compressing the fingers (see Figure 13-4). This groove contains the carotid artery where the pulse will be felt. Take no longer than 10 seconds to assess for adequate signs of circulation. If there is no pulse or if you are unsure if the pulse is present, consider it to be absent.

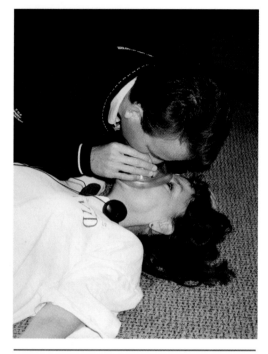

FIGURE 13-3 Mouth-to-Mask Emergency Resuscitation

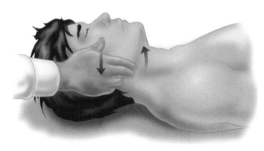

FIGURE 13-4 Hand Placement to Check for Carotid Pulse

Circulation—Chest Compressions

For **chest compressions**, the patient must be on the back on a flat, firm surface. The rescuer should place the heels of the hands on the center of the sternum. At the same time, place the other hand on top of the first while interlacing the fingers to maintain this position (see Figure 13-5). The rescuer should be as close to the patient as possible. The rescuer's body should be positioned up and over so that the shoulders are directly above the hands. The elbow and

---

chest compressions

controlled and repeated application of pressure to the sternum of a victim of cardiac arrest to keep the supply of oxygen moving throughout the body.

shoulders should be locked; then begin compressions at a depth of 1½ to 2 inches at a rate of 30 compression to two ventilations. The rate of compressions should be about 100 times per minute. Remember to allow the chest to fully expand to a normal position between compressions. The compressions should always be deep and fast.

Early defibrillation by a trained first aid provider prior to the arrival of EMS is the most successful treatment for sudden cardiac arrest. Remember, for every minute a patient is in arrest, the chance of survival decreases by about 10%.

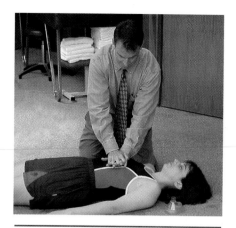

FIGURE 13-5 Chest Compressions

> **NOTE:**
>
> All athletic trainers must be certified in CPR! This applies to athletic training students as well.

AUTOMATED EXTERNAL DEFIBRILLATOR (AED)

Historically, defibrillation has been provided by EMS personnel. EMS response time from collapse to defibrillation is often longer than 10 minutes and in most cases too late. With the **automated external defibrillator (AED)** the trained rescuer has the ability to provide defibrillation much earlier than EMS. AEDs are small, portable devices that can accurately identify whether defibrillation is needed. The AED analyzes the heart rhythm, advises the rescuer when the shock is indicated, and provides the necessary shock to the patient through electrode pads adhered to the patient's chest. When an AED is accessible and a program is in place for using it, it can dramatically improve survival rates, up to 50%.

automated external defibrillator (AED)

small, portable device that can accurately identify need, analyze rhythm, alert the rescuer, and provide the necessary shock through electrode pads adhered to the victim's chest.

Basic AED Operation[*]

The AED is simple and safe to use; even the complex analysis and decision to deliver a shock is made by the AED. The rescuer simply has to attach the device and push a button to deliver a shock when it is indicated by the AED.

The four basic steps in operation of an AED are:

1. Turn the AED on.

2. Attach the electrode pads to the patient.

3. Allow the AED to automatically analyze the patient's heart rhythm.

[*]Copyrighted material owned by MEDIC FIRST AID International, Inc. is reproduced herein with permission.

4. Get all others to step away from the patient when indicated by the AED, and press the button to deliver the shock.

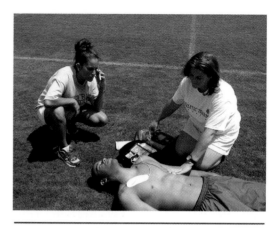

FIGURE 13-6 Placement of AED Pads

The AED should be positioned next to the rescuer and near the patient's head. Open the case, turn the power on, and follow the verbal instruction from the AED. Once the AED is available, stop CPR and attach the AED to the patient. Do this by exposing the chest and preparing it for the AED (also know as "bare and prepare"). Depending on the device, it may be necessary to plug the pads into the AED.

If the patient's chest is wet, it must be dried. The rescuer must peel the backing off the pads one at a time and place them on the patient's chest in the correct spot. To assist in this process, the AED pads have pictures to show the proper placement (see Figure 13-6).

* The first pad should be placed below the patient's right clavicle and beside the sternum. The rescuer should make sure the pad adheres to the skin by pressing it flat.

* The second pad should be placed lower on the patient's right side, over the ribs, and a few inches below the armpit. Once again, make sure the pad is pressed on firmly.

Once it is fully connected, the AED will automatically analyze the patient's heart rhythm. Do not move the patient, or the analysis may be interrupted. At this point the AED will verbally make an alert to shock or not to shock. If it says to shock, it will begin to charge automatically. Make sure no one is touching the patient; warn everyone by stating out loud, "Stand clear." Most AEDs will have the rescuer push the shock button to deliver the shock.

After the defibrillation shock, CPR should be started immediately. Once started, the rescuer should not stop CPR unless instructed by the AED, directed to do so by an EMS provider, or the patient clearly moves. The AED may direct the first aid provider to deliver additional shocks to the patient. The rescuer must continue to follow all voice instructions given by the AED.

Once EMS arrives, the rescuer should provide a brief summary of what happened, including the condition of the patient when found, how long the patient was down, and what care was provided.

FOREIGN BODY AIRWAY OBSTRUCTIONS

An unconscious person can have an obstructed airway because of the position of the airway. For example, the tongue or epiglottis can block the air passage in certain positions. Making an airway using the head-tilt, chin-lift maneuver can correct this problem.

A foreign body obstruction or choking emergency can occur in a conscious or unconscious person. Choking results from a partial or complete airway obstruction. If there only is a partial obstruction, the victim will be able to cough and exchange some air. In this case, encourage the victim to cough and do not interfere. If the airway is completely obstructed, the victim won't be able to cough, speak, or breathe. Usually the victim's hands grasp the neck. This is the universal sign for choking.

To perform the **obstructed airway maneuver**, ask the victim if he is choking. If the victim can talk, cough, or breathe, he is not choking. If the victim indicates that he is choking, perform the obstructed airway maneuver (Figure 13-7). This maneuver is performed with the rescuer standing behind the conscious victim. Wrap your hands around the victim's waist and make a fist with one hand. Place the thumb side of the fist against the victim's abdomen directly above the navel but below the xiphoid process, the bony tip of the sternum. Grasp the fist with your other hand, and with a quick upward thrust, attempt to knock the wind out of the person to remove the obstruction. This is done in sets of five repetitions until the obstruction is removed or the victim becomes unconscious.

If the victim becomes unconscious, lay him in a supine position and kneel astride the victim's thighs. Place the heel of one hand against the victim's abdomen above the navel but below the xiphoid process. Place your other hand on top of the first hand and deliver upward abdominal thrusts five times. Open the victim's mouth and do a finger sweep as described in Chapter 9. Remove the object if you can find it.

If the victim is pregnant or obese, an alternate chest thrust can be used. Stand behind the victim, place your arms under the victim's armpits, and encircle the chest. Place the thumb side of your fist in the middle of the victim's chest, grab your other hand, and with a quick backward thrust, attempt to knock the wind out of the person to remove the obstruction. Do this in sets of five repetitions until the obstruction is removed or the victim becomes unconscious.

The procedures for CPR and rescue breathing in infants and children are essentially the same as with adults except for a few modifications because of the size of the individual. Because the focus of this book is on treating adult injuries, the procedures for children and infants are not discussed here. However, it is important to know there are some important differences in the procedures when the victim is a child or an infant.

FIGURE 13-7 The Obstructed Airway Maneuver

obstructed airway maneuver

quick upward thrust performed against a patient's abdomen while standing behind a patient to remove an obstruction and open free passage of air from the mouth or nose to the lungs.

THE LOG ROLL

The log roll is a procedure that is used to turn over a patient who is lying face-down without causing additional injury to the spine.

> ***WARNING!*** Improper lifting and moving is a leading cause of back injury. Do not practice this move if you have a history of back problems. Practice of emergency moves may aggravate previous back injuries. Careful attention must be given to proper lifting and moving techniques at all times. When possible, use your legs, not your back, and keep your weight as close to the patient's body as possible. Although it is not always possible, try to avoid twisting, sustained or intense exertion, and awkward or extreme postures.

A single rescuer can accomplish the log roll. However, the more rescuers that are available, the safer the log roll is for the patient. A log roll procedure for three rescuers (R1, R2, and R3) is described below. The procedure is based on a scenario where there is no spine board, no evidence of a spine injury, and the patient is not breathing. In this situation, the patient must be turned as carefully as possible while ensuring minimal if any movement of the spine. Once the patient is turned, the rescuer will be able to access the airway.

PERFORMING A THREE-PERSON LOG ROLL

1. **Procedural Step:**

   R1: Kneel above the patient's head. Stabilize the head. Position your hands in anticipation of rotation. (This means to place your hands to the side of the patient's head in the position that they will be after the patient has been rolled. Then, keeping your hands in that position, rotate them and gently grasp the patient's head. See photo in step 2 for final hand placement.)

   R2: Kneel at the patient's waist. Straighten the patient's arms and legs, extending the arm nearest to you over the patient's head, next to the ear. (Note: if the arm appears to be injured, or if moving it causes the athlete additional pain, do not extend the arm.) Place the patient's other hand, palm-in, next to the patient's torso.

   R3: Kneel at the patient's knees.

   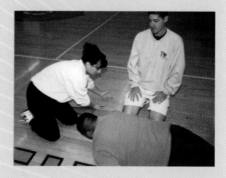

2. **Procedural Step:**

   R2: Grasp the patient at the shoulder and the elbow.

PERFORMING A THREE-PERSON LOG ROLL

R3: Grasp the patient at the hip and the ankle.

(Notice how R1's hands are positioned in anticipation of rotating the patient's head as described in step 1.)

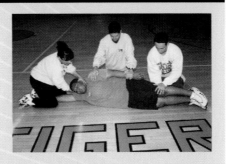

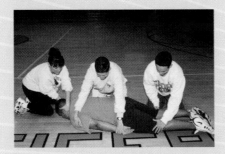

3. **Procedural Step:**

   R1: Signal to begin log roll. For example, say "Roll on three. One, two, three."

   R2 and R3: Slowly roll the patient toward you, in the opposite direction from which the head was facing if the patient is not face-down.

4. **Procedural Step:**

   R1: Maintain stabilization in line with the patient's rotating torso.

   R1, R2, and R3: Continue the log roll until the patient is face-up.

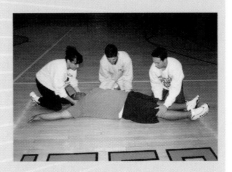

Based on information provided by EMP International, Inc. Eugene, OR. Used with permission.

THINKING IT THROUGH

Today at basketball practice, Mike Mathews got low-bridged while shooting a lay-up. Raphael was in charge because the head athletic trainer, Lisa, as usual, was overseeing wrestling practice and couldn't be in both places at once.

Mike was hit hard. When Raphael, the athletic training student, got out on the court, Mike's eyes were rolling back into his head and he was having trouble breathing. Raphael did a quick assessment, checking Mike's pulse and breathing. Raphael could feel a strong pulse, but Mike's breathing was labored. Raphael started the

Emergency Action Plan by telling the equipment person to call for EMS first, and then to call Lisa on the radio to inform her of the situation.

Raphael put on his gloves and took out the airway that he always carried with him. As he did this, he started to run the procedure for CPR through his head. He checked Mike's vitals again, using two fingers on the chin to assure a good airway, and placed his ear close to Mike's mouth to hear him breathe. Raphael kept talking to Mike to reassure him that everything was going to be fine. Meanwhile, Raphael was preparing himself to administer CPR if necessary. It seemed to take forever, but Lisa and the EMS finally arrived and took over while Raphael filled them in on the details as to what had happened and the care he had provided up to that point.

Lisa and Raphael told the coaches to clear Mike's teammates away from him and to stay out of the way of the paramedics. When the paramedics finally took Mike away, Raphael sat down with Lisa and everyone involved and wrote down exactly what happened. Raphael then spent some time talking with Lisa about what happened and gearing down from the event.

Why did Raphael put on gloves to treat the injured player? Why is it important to check vital signs periodically? What are some ways to instill confidence in the injured player that he is going to be fine in what must feel like a dire situation? Why does the athletic training student need some time to wind down after a situation like this?

CHAPTER SUMMARY

Although this chapter on basic life support is in no way intended as replacement for CPR training and certification, it does offer an excellent overview and introduction to one of the most important skills a person can possess. The ability to recognize and respond to life-threatening signs and symptoms may be most useful when least expected. This skill is not only essential to sports medicine but also in everyday life, at home, on the athletic field, at the park, in the grocery store, etc.

All members of the sports medicine team should practice techniques for opening an airway—the head-tilt, chin-lift maneuver and the obstructed airway—until these techniques can be performed confidently without hesitation.

Take care to protect your patient and yourself during any repositioning that might be necessary. When log rolling an unresponsive athlete into a supine position for rescue efforts, maintaining the patient's axial (spinal) alignment will help prevent complications and further injury. It is important not to let the weight of the patient's head cause extreme flexing of the neck; this is particularly important with unconscious patients. Protect yourself by bending your knees when you lift, utilizing all available assistants during repositioning, and trying to avoid awkward bending or twisting whenever possible.

STUDENT ENRICHMENT ACTIVITIES

Complete the following sentences.

1. CPR stands for _____ _____.

2. _____ _____ occurs when the heart has stopped beating.

3. For one-rescuer CPR, the chest should be compressed _____ times for every _____ rescue breaths (ventilations).

4. For CPR to be most effective, the patient must be _____ and on a _____ surface.

5. When respiration stops, the body loses its means of obtaining _____.

Complete the following exercises.

6. Copy and number the following CPR steps in the correct procedural order from 1 to 7.

   Begin chest compressions.

   Assess circulation.

   Open airway.

   Call for help.

   Determine unresponsiveness.

   Assess breathing.

   Begin ventilations.

7. Research locally available CPR classes. Make up a poster or flyer with sign-up information on three of them.

CHAPTER 14

Injuries to the Tissues

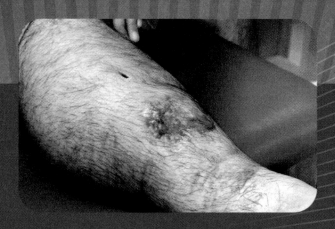

OBJECTIVES

After completing this chapter, you should be able to do the following:

1. Define and correctly spell each of the key terms.

2. Name and explain the function of at least four cellular components.

3. Name and describe the four different types of tissue groups.

4. List the main components of a body system.

5. Describe several types of joints in the body and their category.

6. Identify and discuss soft tissue injuries.

7. Discuss the different symptoms of sprains, strains, dislocations, and fractures.

KEY TERMS

* abrasion
* anaphylactic shock
* anatomy
* articulation
* avulsion
* blister
* bursitis
* callus
* cardiac muscle
* cell
* contusion
* crepitation
* dislocation

* ecchymosis
* fracture
* hematoma
* incision
* joint laxity
* laceration
* ligament
* myositis ossificans
* organ
* paresthesia
* physiology
* PRICE procedure
* puncture wound

* skeletal or striated muscle
* smooth or visceral muscle
* splint
* sprain
* strain
* subluxation
* synovitis
* systemic reaction
* tendon
* tendonitis
* tissue

INJURIES ARE INEVITABLE

A wide variety of injuries can occur during sports and physical fitness activity. Some of the more common injuries involve the tissues. These injuries include cuts and abrasions, contusions, muscle strains, ligament sprains, inflammation of the tendons, joint dislocations, fractures, and injuries to specific organs. Furthermore, because sports and exercise often involve repetitive body motions, athletes are also especially prone to overuse injuries of the limbs and joints. Athletic trainers must be able to recognize different types of injuries, distinguish between levels of injury severity, and apply appropriate first aid and ongoing treatment to an injured person. When providing treatment, make sure to address the cause of the symptoms; don't just treat the symptoms. If symptoms do not improve after continued treatment, discuss other possible causes of such symptoms with the athlete and the coach, and explore methods of eliminating these potential causes.

> **NOTE:**
>
> Initial findings regarding any injury should always be relayed to the physician who will handle the case. Information that is obtained at the scene of the injury is very valuable!

To work in sports medicine, one must have a basic understanding of the structure of the human body, namely, how the various structures make it possible for us to move and function in so many different ways. Therefore, in this chapter and those that follow, information regarding basic **anatomy** and **physiology** is provided along with the discussions of common injuries, their treatment, and their prevention. For example, before we can discuss tissue injuries, we must first understand what tissues are and what functions they perform.

Tissues are a group of specialized cells and their cell products. There are four main categories of human tissue: epithelial tissue, connective tissue, nerve tissue, and muscle tissue. The cells in a particular category of tissue are specialized to perform a certain function. For example, the cells in muscle tissue are specialized to contract.

Just as cells combine to form a particular type of tissue, two or more tissues that combine to perform a specific function form an **organ**. The lungs, heart, stomach, and liver are examples of organs, or viscera. When organs and other body structures combine to perform a common function, they form a body system, such as the circulatory system, the respiratory system, the nervous system, the muscular system, and the skeletal system (see Figure 14-1). The circulatory, respiratory, and nervous systems will be discussed in detail in later chapters.

anatomy

the study of the structure of the body (how the body is put together).

physiology

the study of the function of the body (how the body works).

organ

a structure within the body made up of tissues that allow it to perform a particular function.

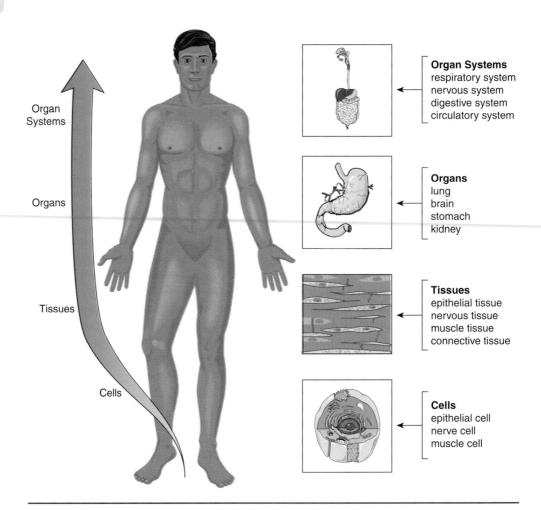

Organ Systems
respiratory system
nervous system
digestive system
circulatory system

Organs
lung
brain
stomach
kidney

Tissues
epithelial tissue
nervous tissue
muscle tissue
connective tissue

Cells
epithelial cell
nerve cell
muscle cell

Organ Systems

Organs

Tissues

Cells

FIGURE 14-1 From Cell to System

CELLS AND TISSUES

Cells

The **cell** is the basic structural and functional unit of all living organisms; it is the smallest structure capable of performing all the activities vital to life (Figure 14-2). Cells and the tissues they form allow the body to perform the functions that are vital to life, such as breathing, eliminating waste products, and maintaining homeostasis.

Cells are made up of a jelly-like material known as cytoplasm (protoplasm). Cytoplasm is made of water, carbon, hydrogen, calcium, nitrogen, oxygen, phosphorus, food particles, pigment, and tiny structures called organelles. Mitochondria are organelles that release energy and are responsible for the chemical reactions that occur within the cell. Enzymes are contained within the mitochondria and influence the amount of energy released during these chemical reactions. Enzymes increase the speed of the reaction without changing themselves. At the center of the cell is the nucleus, which controls the metabolism, growth, and reproduction of the cell. Chromosomes are found within the nucleus of the cell and contain the genes. The physical and mental characteristics of an individual are determined by the genes found within the chromosomes of the cells.

The semipermeable outer covering of the cell is called the cell membrane. This covering plays an important role in maintaining the body's homeostasis by allowing only certain substances to enter and/or exit the cell. The cell membrane detects changes within the cell and its surrounding environment and allows only

cell

the basic unit of life.

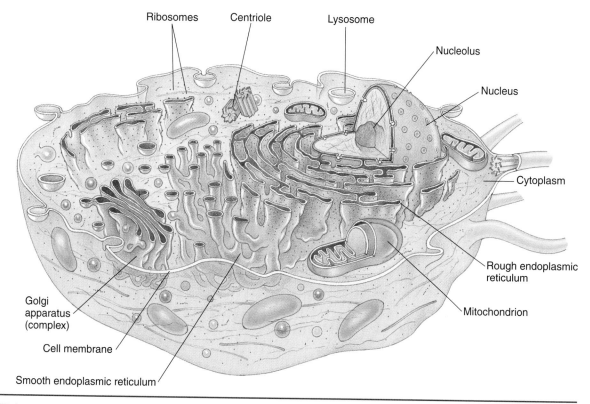

FIGURE 14-2 The Parts of the Human Cell

the substances that benefit the cell to remain inside. The substances that are not needed are allowed to leave the cell.

Cells reproduce through a process known as cell division. Within the human reproductive organs, this division is called meiosis. This type of cell division is specific for the ovaries and testes only, and creates cells that contain half the number of chromosomes that nonreproductive cells contain. This type of division is necessary for proper fertilization and reproduction. Cell division that occurs elsewhere in the body, such as skin cells producing more skin cells, is called mitosis. Cells of the same type divide and form tissues.

Tissues

tissue

a collection of similar cells and their intercellular substances that work together to perform a particular function.

Tissues are composed of similar cells that are specialized to perform a particular function. Tissue fluid (interstitial fluid) occupies the tiny spaces between the cells of the body. This tissue fluid is composed primarily of water, but it also contains sodium, potassium, and other substances that are vital to the proper functioning of the body. If there is not enough tissue fluid, the body is dehydrated. Signs and symptoms may include dry mucous membranes, thirst, and weakness. But, if too much tissue fluid is present, edema (swelling) occurs, and the patient is said to have fluid overload. Either of these conditions can impair the functioning of the body's systems.

There are four main categories of tissue in the human body: epithelial tissue, connective tissue, nerve tissue, and muscle tissue. Epithelial tissue is the main tissue of the skin. It lines the cavities of the body and the principal tubes and passageways that lead to the outside. Epithelial tissue helps protect the internal organs and assists in regulating the body temperature. It also forms the glands that produce hormones responsible for regulating various body functions. Injuries common to this type of tissue are usually traumatic, including abrasions, laceration punctures, and avulsions. Tissues may also be affected by infection, inflammation, and disease.

Connective tissue provides the framework for most organs. It supports and connects other tissues and parts. There are two types of connective tissue: *soft* and *hard*. Adipose, or fatty tissue, is soft connective tissue that stores fat. This fat serves as a food reserve, insulator, and energy source. Adipose tissue also forms fibrous connective tissue that supports the joints of the body and helps connect certain structures. For example, tendons are fibrous connective tissue that connect muscles to the bone, and ligaments are fibrous connective tissue that connect bone to bone. Bone and cartilage are made of hard connective tissue. Bone (osseous tissue) is the tissue that comprises the skeletal system. Cartilage is a dense, elastic, connective tissue. It is found in the moveable joints of the body, such as the knee and between the spinal discs, where it acts as a shock absorber by distributing the forces that are applied to the joint. Cartilage also creates the contour of the nose and the ears, and is found in the larynx (voice box).

Nerve tissue is the third type of tissue. It serves as the pathway for communication from the central nervous system (i.e., the brain, spinal cord, and the nerves) to the muscles, organs, and various systems in the periphery. Nerve tissue is composed of neurons, which are special cells that carry commands and information between the brain and the rest of the body. Minor injuries such as contusions can cause short-term damage to the nerves, temporarily impairing sensations and movement. But if a nerve is crushed or severed, long-term disability such as paralysis can result.

Muscle tissue has tiny muscle fibers that are able to contract, allowing the muscles to produce movement and power. There are three types of muscle tissue: **skeletal or striated muscle**, which attaches to the bones and permits movement; **cardiac muscle**, which causes the heart to contract; and **smooth or visceral muscle**, which is found principally in the organs. Each of these types of muscle tissue will be discussed in more detail later in this chapter.

CONTROLLING BLEEDING

Since the body does not have an excess supply of blood, all bleeding must be controlled. Remember to always wear gloves when dealing with blood or other body fluids. Profuse bleeding, or a hemorrhage, is a serious life-threatening condition that can lead to shock. Bleeding can be either internal or external. Internal bleeding often is the result of blunt trauma or a medical condition (i.e., ulcers, ectopic pregnancy).

External bleeding can occur from capillaries, veins, or arteries. Capillary bleeding is the most common type of external bleeding and occurs with most injuries. Applying a sterile pad and compression will usually control the capillary bleeding found in minor cuts, scratches, and abrasions. If a vein is punctured or severed by a cutting instrument, the dark maroon blood will flow steadily. The amount of blood loss depends on the size of the vein.

To control venous bleeding, a sterile compress is placed over the wound and a gloved hand applies direct pressure to the site (Figure 14-3). It takes normal blood 4 to 6 minutes to clot, so pressure should be applied for at least 6 minutes. If a person has a bleeding condition such as hemophilia or takes blood thinning medication (e.g., Coumadin, heparin, or aspirin), the pressure will have to be continually applied until the patient is seen by the doctor. If the first compress becomes saturated with blood, apply another over the top of it and reinforce it.

Arterial bleeding is caused by a punctured or severed artery. Arterial blood is

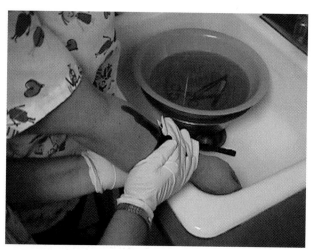

FIGURE 14-3 Apply direct pressure to control bleeding.

bright red and pulsates (spurts) because it is under pressure. These are more serious injuries, and the bleeding must be controlled to prevent shock. Direct pressure is the best method for controlling arterial bleeding.

Elevating the injured part also can help control bleeding. However, there are some circumstances in which the extremity should *not* be moved, such as with a fracture or spinal injury. Therefore, most, but not all, injuries will be elevated.

skeletal or striated muscle

voluntary muscles that can be consciously controlled, unlike involuntary muscles that work whether the body is conscious or unconscious.

cardiac muscle

the muscle of the heart, adapted to continued rhythmic contraction.

smooth or visceral muscle

muscle tissue that contracts without voluntary control; contracts slowly and sustained over a longer time; found in internal organs and blood vessels.

If direct pressure with elevation is not successful, use indirect pressure, or pressure points. To apply indirect pressure, locate the pressure point directly above the injury and apply pressure to that artery until the pulsation in the artery stops or the bleeding from the wound is controlled. Pressure points exist at the following arteries (see Figure 14-4):

* The temporal artery, located in front of the ear

* The carotid artery, located to the side of the Adam's apple just below the jaw bone

* The subclavian artery, located deep in the hollow near the collarbone

* The brachial artery, located on the inner side of the upper arm, about 3 inches below the armpit

* The ulnar artery, located in the forearm

* The radial artery, located in the forearm

* The iliac artery, located in the groin

* The femoral artery, located in the leg

* The popliteal artery, located behind the knee

* The dorsalis pedis artery, located on top of the foot at the bend in the ankle

Ice is the next method of controlling the flow of blood. The ice, because it is cold, causes vasoconstriction and slows the flow of blood (see Figure 14-5). Place a paper towel or a cloth between the skin and the ice.

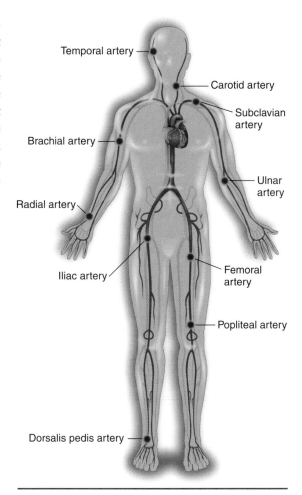

FIGURE 14-4 If bleeding cannot be controlled through direct pressure, apply indirect pressure.

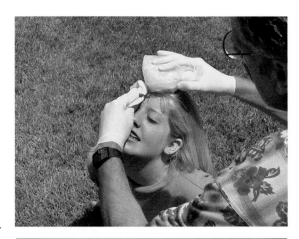

FIGURE 14-5 Ice can slow the loss of blood if direct pressure, elevation, and indirect pressure are unsuccessful.

GENERAL PRINCIPLES OF WOUND CARE

It is helpful to keep all the materials necessary for wound care in a personal kit. While these items can be kept in a basic kit, keep the following supplies nearby at all times as minor wounds occur frequently in sports: gloves; 4" × 4" gauze sponge (to soak up blood); sterile saline; nonsticking pads (to cover the wound); and antiseptic first aid cream. Soap and water should also be kept handy in order to thoroughly clean wounds.

The following principles should be applied when treating any type of wound.

* *Always wear gloves when handling wounds.*

* Control any bleeding.

* Prevent infection.

* Cleanse the wound.

* Immobilize the injured part.

* Apply ice (except for snakebite).

* Handle the wound gently.

* Have a physician rule out infections such as methicillin resistant staphylococcus aureus (MRSA).

A clean wound will heal quickly, but a dirty wound will become infected and can cause multiple complications; therefore, the wound must be cleaned. Some of the patient's clothing may need to be removed to gain access to the wound. If this is the case, remember to always do this in an appropriate manner, exercising discretion at all times. If the abrasion is painful or deep and a physician is present, the doctor may order some anesthetic jelly to be applied before cleansing it. Dirt may be ground into the wound, so a thorough cleansing is essential. Asphalt ground into the skin can cause a permanent tattooing of the skin if it is not removed.

Wounds must be cleansed before a dressing is applied. Scrub the wound with a surgical scrub brush for 5 to 10 minutes using gloves and sterile technique to decrease the chance of infection. Start from directly over the wound, and scrub the area in a circle working away from the wound. Rinse with sterile water or saline. The doctor will irrigate (wash out) the wound with sterile saline again later. Dry the area with a dry, sterile towel and cover the wound with additional dry, sterile towels. Make sure the patient has a current tetanus immunization. If the patient's immunization has lapsed, alert the nurse or physician.

DRESSINGS AND BANDAGES

Dressings and bandages prevent infection to open wounds, promote healing, and offer comfort to the patient. Use a great deal of care in putting on the dressing and bandage. The dressing must cover the wound and be constructed to stay in place until the dressing can be changed and the wound evaluated. A great deal of creativity is allowed in designing a dressing that will fit the area of injury and accommodate the needs of the patient. Dressings must be sturdy enough to stay in place throughout the day's activities and absorbent enough to soak up blood and drainage. Dressings protect the wound, so padding is needed to cover tender areas.

Some dressings apply pressure to help control bleeding. Stretchy rolled bandages are designed to be used for pressure dressings such as these. Design a dressing covering the entire wound area that is both comfortable and neat.

Dressings are materials applied directly on the wound. Bandages are the material used to hold the dressing in place. There is usually drainage from the wound, so the first dressing that is applied should be of sterile, soft, nonstick material and be able to conform to the shape of the wound. It is important that these dressings not stick to the wound because the skin can take longer to heal if it sticks to the dressing when the dressing is changed. Some examples of this type of dressing include Vaseline gauze, telfa, adaptic, and xeroform gauze.

The second layer of dressing should be of absorbent material and large enough to cover the wound. Dressings should not be any bigger than necessary. This layer protects the wound and absorbs the drainage. Examples of material suitable for this layer of dressing include 4 × 4s, fluffs, ABD pads, 5 × 9s, tube gauze, sanitary pads, oval eye pads, occlusive plastic wrap or foil, and adhesive bandages.

The outer layer is the bandage that holds the dressing in place. It should conform to the wound and be stretchable enough to allow for any swelling to occur yet snug enough to hold the dressing in place without interfering with circulation. Examples of appropriate bandages include roller gauze, Kerlix, Kling, rolled stockinette, and stretchy rolled bandages.

The bandage is secured to the skin with tape. Choose a tape that is best suited for the patient's skin and the type of dressing used. Tape can be adhesive, cloth, paper, or hypoallergenic. Paper tape is used on the face and other sensitive skin surfaces. It may be necessary to shave hairy skin before applying adhesive tape. Another method to secure the dressing in place is with a stretchy net dressing. This type of dressing, called stockinette, is especially suitable for head dressings and burns.

There are as many different ways to apply a bandage as kinds of material from which to choose. Here are some guidelines.

* Always remove rings, watches, or bracelets from the patient if dressing a hand or wrist. If the hand swells, these items can interfere with normal circulation. Put the ring on the other hand or give it to the patient or a family member. Be sure to document what was done with the patient's belongings.

* Try to leave the fingers and toes exposed so circulation and sensation can be checked.

* Use sterile material.

* Control any bleeding.

* Open the dressing package using sterile technique, and touch only the corners, *not* the part that goes directly over the wound.

* Cover the entire wound.

* Apply the bandage snugly, but not too tightly.

* The bandage should not be too loose or it may slip.

* Secure all loose ends with tape or tuck them inside the bandage.

* Put the bandage on in the position in which it is to remain. Do not try to bend a bandaged joint.

* Ask the patient how the dressing feels. If it is uncomfortable, rearrange it.

* Stay within Occupational Safety and Health Administration (OSHA) guidelines. (See www.osha.gov.)

Patients should be given instructions for wound care. These instructions will probably come from the physician, but the athletic trainer should follow up to make sure the patient understands what to do.

* Keep the dressing clean and dry; the dressing may need to be changed daily.

* If the dressing soaks through, reinforce it with another gauze pad.

* If it gets wet, remove the dressing and replace it or return to the doctor.

* Watch the circulation in the injured extremity. Call the doctor if the extremity becomes numb, tingly, pale, blue, or cold, or if the athlete experiences severe pain with motion.

* Watch for the following signs of infection: redness, swelling, increased pain, a red streak up the arm or leg, foul-smelling drainage, or an elevation in temperature.

* If sutures were required, the patient will be instructed to return for removal of the sutures in 5 to 14 days.

* Protect yourself. OSHA requires employers to make available to their employees who are exposed to blood or other bodily fluids a vaccine to prevent the hepatitis B virus (HBV) at no cost.

SUPERFICIAL INJURIES TO THE SOFT TISSUES

Soft tissue injuries (wounds) involve damage to one or more of the tissues surrounding the bones and joints. Soft tissue injuries can involve the skin, fascia, cartilage, muscles, tendons, ligaments, veins, or arteries. These injuries can occur alone or they may accompany a fracture or blunt trauma.

Wounds are either *open* or *closed*. A closed wound does not break the skin, unlike open wounds, which involve a break in the skin or mucous membranes. All open wounds require at least first aid treatment. Even minor cuts and scrapes should be treated to prevent a serious infection. The goals for treating open wounds are to control bleeding and prevent infection.

Abrasions

Abrasions are caused by sliding or skidding on pavement, concrete, dirt, or sand. They result from running, skating, softball, baseball, football, volleyball, and other activities that cause people to fall. Abrasions can be quite large and painful. However, bleeding usually is not a problem in treating these injuries as the wounds are not deep, but because the ground is dirty, the possibility of infection is great (see Figure 14-6).

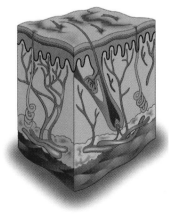

abrasion

an open wound, road burn, or rug burn in which the outer layer of skin has been scraped off.

FIGURE 14-6 An Abrasion

Immediate Treatment: The first aid for an abrasion is to wash the area with antibacterial soap and debride the wound with a soft scrub brush. Then flush the area with water or sterile saline. Apply a petroleum-based first aid cream to the abrasion to keep the area moist and to prevent a scab from forming. Dress the wound by applying a non-adhesive sterile pad over the ointment. Taping and wrapping procedures for simple abrasions are described in Chapter 21.

Follow-up Treatment: Change the sterile pad every day. For the next few days up to a week, watch the area of or around the abrasion for signs of infection such as redness, drainage, excessive warmth, or swelling. Red streaks extending from a wound indicate blood poisoning. Send the athlete to a physician if any of these symptoms occurs. Always use barriers such as latex or rubber gloves when dealing with blood or other body fluids.

Prevention: Abrasions can be prevented, or at least minimized, by wearing clothes that cover the skin as much as possible. Covering the skin reduces the chance of direct exposure to rough surfaces.

Lacerations

laceration

a jagged tear in the flesh.

Lacerations are wounds caused by a tearing motion, resulting in wound edges that are jagged. These wounds can be minor or very deep, and they can involve other tissues (Figure 14-7). Deep wounds may have associated nerve, blood vessel, muscle, tendon, ligament, and bone damage and usually will be repaired in an operating room.

Immediate Treatment: For first aid, clean the laceration with soap and water or sterile saline, and then apply sterile compression dressing to stop the bleeding. Use barriers such as latex or rubber gloves when dealing with blood or other body fluids. The procedure for repairing small lacerations is found in Chapter 21. If the size and depth of the wound indicates stitches are needed, send the athlete to a physician for further evaluation. Stitches are necessary when the edges of the laceration will not close, when the wound is deep, or the laceration is 1 to 1½ inches long. In addition to stitches, the athlete may need to receive a tetanus injection.

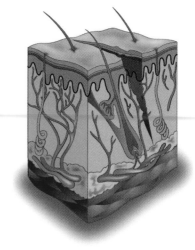

FIGURE 14-7 A Laceration

Follow-up Treatment: If a physician is involved, make sure doctors' orders are followed. Monitor the wound for redness, heat, swelling, red streaks, or drainage. Send the athlete to a physician if any of these symptoms occur.

Prevention: Protective clothing and appropriate padding should be worn by athletes whenever possible. Pay special attention to areas of the body that have high potential for contact injuries in the sport being played.

Puncture Wounds

A **puncture wound** results when a pointed object directly pierces soft tissue (Figure 14-8). This type of wound is often the most susceptible to infection; be aware of the possibility of tetanus infection. Sometimes the penetrating object remains embedded in the skin. Foreign bodies embedded in tissue require the attention of a physician. A history of the location, the method of entry, and type of puncturing object are helpful items of information.

People can become impaled by sharp objects like arrows, darts, and screwdrivers. When someone is impaled, the object is still in the body and partially sticking out.

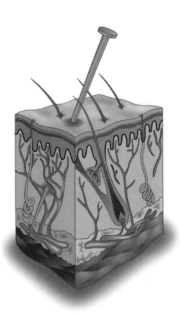

FIGURE 14-8 A Puncture Wound

puncture wound

a soft tissue injury caused by the penetration of a sharp object.

Immediate Treatment: The immediate treatment for a victim of impalement is to stabilize the object in place and then evaluate the patient for further injuries. To stabilize the object, tape it securely in place with very minimal movement. Be very careful and move the victim as little as possible. *Protruding objects are left in place and should not be removed until the patient is evaluated by the physician.*

To treat minor puncture wounds, clean the wound with soap and water or sterile saline, and then cover it with sterile gauze. Always use barriers such as latex gloves when dealing with blood and other body fluids. Send the patient to a physician for evaluation and, if needed, a tetanus injection.

Wood splinters also require special attention. Wood splinter wounds should *not* be soaked, because the water will cause the wood to decompose. Some woods, like cedar and redwood, can cause serious tissue reactions and must be dealt with immediately. Special pointed splinter forceps are used to remove the object, and efforts are made to prevent squeezing and pressure to surrounding tissue. Splinters under the fingernail may require partial removal of the fingernail by a physician in order to remove the splinter.

Follow-up Treatment: A patient with a puncture wound must be evaluated daily for signs and symptoms of infection or blood poisoning. Change the dressing daily.

Prevention: Make sure the event area (field, court, etc.) is free from nails and other sharp objects. Protective clothing also should be worn by the athletes.

Incisions

Sharp, knife-like objects can cause cuts called **incisions**. These usually are clean cuts, but they can be very deep, and other tissues may be involved (Figure 14-9). A deep incision can cut muscles, tendons, ligaments, veins, arteries, and nerves. Incisions often occur on hard, bony areas that are poorly padded.

incision

a clean, straight, knife-like cut.

Immediate Treatment: For first aid, clean the area with soap and water or sterile saline. Swab the edges of the wound with tape adherent and allow it to dry. Then pull the edges of the wound together using Steri-Strips. If the incision bleeds or the athlete has not had a tetanus injection in the last 10 years, send the patient to a physician for further evaluation and possibly sutures and a tetanus injection. Always use barriers such as latex or rubber gloves when dealing with blood or other body fluids.

Follow-up Treatment: Change the dressing daily. As with other soft tissue injuries, monitor the wound for signs of infection or blood poisoning. Send the athlete to a physician if evidence of any of these symptoms is noted.

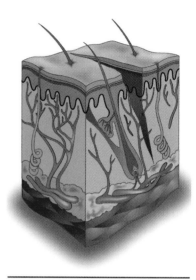

FIGURE 14-9 An Incision

Prevention: Make sure the event area is free from sharp objects. Protective clothing also should be worn by the athletes.

Avulsions

> **avulsion**
>
> a painful soft tissue injury in which a flap of tissue is torn loose or pulled off completely.

An **avulsion** is a loss of tissue. If the tissue still is attached it is called a flap avulsion (Figure 14-10).

Immediate Treatment: The first aid for an avulsion is to clean the area and use compression with a sterile dressing to stop the bleeding. Use barriers when dealing with blood or body fluids. Cover the area and send the athlete to a physician for further care.

  If a large flap of tissue has been torn away, efforts should be made to locate it, because some tissue can be reattached. Place the avulsed tissue in a gauze wrap that has been moistened with normal saline and sealed in a plastic bag to prevent destruction of the tissue. The bag should be placed on ice. The area of avulsion should be protected with a moist saline dressing.

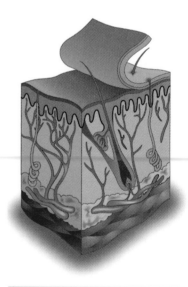

FIGURE 14-10 An Avulsion

Follow-up Treatment: Change the dressing daily and watch for signs and symptoms of infection or blood poisoning.

Prevention: Protect the body areas with the highest potential for contact, based upon the sport that is being played (e.g., protect the shins of soccer players).

Calluses

A **callus** is a reaction in which the skin becomes thickened due to a high friction area or intermittent pressure (Figure 14-11). A callus can occur when something, such as a shoe that doesn't fit properly, rubs against a bony protrusion.

Immediate Treatment: The treatment for calluses is to use a pumice stone on the calluses to file off the thick skin and to stop the problem that is causing the friction.

Follow-up Treatment: Monitor the callused area to see if the steps taken to reduce the friction are working. If the callus becomes hard or begins to crack, apply lotion to soften the area.

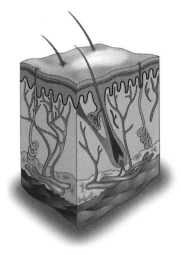

callus

a thickened, usually painless, area of skin caused by friction or pressure.

FIGURE 14-11 A Callus

Prevention: To prevent calluses, a lubricant may be put on the area of pressure. To reduce friction on the feet, make sure that shoes fit properly and that there is break-in period before shoes are used for regular activity. In addition, the athlete can wear two pairs of socks with powder. Thin pads or topical applications that mimic the protection of skin may also be used to reduce friction.

Blisters

A **blister** is a build-up of fluid that collects under the skin in response to friction (Figure 14-12).

Immediate Treatment: To treat a blister, clean the area and place a donut pad around the blister to disperse the pressure to the area. Taping and wrapping procedures for blisters can be found in Chapter 20. If the blister is large or if it might be infected, send the athlete to a physician for evaluation.

Follow-up Treatment: Try to eliminate the source of friction (see prevention below). Monitor the affected area for signs of infection or blood poisoning. Send the athlete to a physician if there is evidence of any of these symptoms.

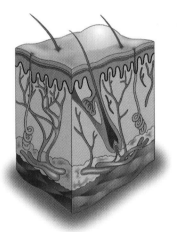

blister

a bubble-like collection of fluid beneath or within the epidermis of the skin.

FIGURE 14-12 A Blister

Prevention: As with calluses, the prevention of blisters requires the removal of the source of friction. Talcum powder may be used to reduce moisture and help prevent friction. Other methods of reducing friction include applying petroleum jelly or skin-like pads or topical applications to the area of friction. To prevent blisters on the feet, shoes should fit properly and two pairs of clean, dry socks can be worn. New shoes should not be worn for long periods until they are broken in.

Bites and Stings

Bites and stings occur from insects, reptiles, animals, and even humans. They can result in puncture wounds, lacerations, or avulsions. Athletes have been known to accidentally bite their own tongues or lips as the result of a fall. Mosquitoes, spiders, scorpions, ticks, chiggers, wasps, bees, and ants are all insects known to bite or sting humans. Insect bites can be rather serious, as some spiders are poisonous and ticks and other insects can carry a number of infectious diseases and transmit the disease to man from a bite.

Snakebites can be deadly if the bite is from a poisonous snake. The most common types of poisonous snakes in the United States are rattlesnakes, cottonmouths, water moccasins, copperheads, and coral snakes. Sometimes the snake is taken to the hospital with the patient to help with identification of the snake. Do not, however, put yourself (or allow others to put themselves) in any danger by attempting to capture a live snake! The symptoms of a snake bite include fang marks, swelling, **paresthesia** (numbness), **ecchymosis**, and pain.

Animals can be infected with rabies, a potentially fatal disease of the nervous system. If the bite is from a domestic animal, information about the animal's rabies immunization must be obtained. If the bite is from a wild animal, and the animal can be captured, it will be examined by an animal control officer. If the animal is unavailable, it will be assumed the animal had rabies, and a rabies treatment will be given to the victim in an effort to prevent the disease.

Immediate Treatment: Bites must be cleansed thoroughly, and any bleeding must be controlled. Bites from anything other than a mosquito should be evaluated by a physician. Mosquito bites can be treated with first aid cream to help reduce the itching. Caution the patient not to scratch the bite as this will delay the healing process and may lead to infection. If an athlete receives a bite that cannot be identified, or if the patient shows signs or symptoms that indicate any kind of **systemic reaction** to the bite, get the victim to an emergency room or the family physician immediately. Animal bites are reported to the animal control officer.

Many people are allergic to bees and wasps. For those who are allergic, a sting from one of these insects can cause an immediate reaction which could lead to **anaphylactic shock**, requiring resuscitation and IV medications. If the stinger is still attached, remove it with a massaging motion using a wooden tongue depressor. Do not squeeze or apply pressure to the area. There are many commercial bee sting kits on the market. Those in charge of a sport that puts the athletes at an increased risk of a sting (e.g., cross-country) should carry a bee sting kit. Understand how to use the kit before an emergency occurs.

If any bite may have come from a poisonous spider or snake, activate the EMS and watch for signs of allergic reaction to the venom. The patient history is very important in the treatment of poisonous bites because the patient may have seen the snake or spider. Attention is given to the ABCs of emergency care. If the venom is in the person's circulation, a systemic reaction will occur and may result in respiratory arrest, cardiac arrest, or both. Watch for the signs and symptoms of shock, and prepare the patient for rapid transport for treatment by a physician. If the reaction is local, attention is paid to the site of the bite. The area of the bite must be immobilized, and efforts must be made to calm the patient and localize the toxins. A constricting band may be applied close to the wound. This is done to prevent the venom from entering the circulation. With a constricting band in place, a distal

paresthesia

an abnormal sensation of the skin, such as numbness, tingling, prickling, or burning, with no apparent cause.

ecchymosis

ruptured blood vessels in the subcutaneous tissue, noticeable by a purple discoloration of the skin.

systemic reaction

a reaction that involves the whole body rather than just a part of it.

anaphylactic shock

a severe, sometimes fatal allergic reaction that causes a sharp drop in blood pressure and breathing difficulties.

pulse should be present. *Ice is never applied to a snakebite wound.* Ice constricts the blood vessels and slows the healing process.

Bites of the tongue or lips may be deep and can bleed profusely. To treat these types of wounds, make sure the airway is clear, control the bleeding, and send the patient to a physician. Bites from humans, if they are acts of assault, should be reported to the police. Because many types of bacteria live in saliva, human bites are serious wounds.

Follow-up Treatment: Check the affected area daily for signs and symptoms of infection or blood poisoning.

Prevention: First, in areas where mosquitoes are a problem, make sure the athletes use an insect repellent that will help prevent mosquito bites from occurring. Second, try to have the athletes stay away from areas in which the risk of animal or insect encounters is high.

Skin Infections and Other Dermatological Conditions

The skin can be affected by a wide variety of medical conditions, including tinea pedis (athlete's foot), tinea corporis (ringworm), herpes, papillomavirus (warts), and impetigo.

There are many other types of skin infections, but these are among the most common. If an unfamiliar skin condition is encountered, play it safe and send the affected individual to a physician.

Tinea corporis is a dermatophyte infection. Dermatophytes are fungi that produce a well-defined, itchy, red patch of skin bordered by a scaly red ring, giving rise to the nickname ringworm (Figure 14-13). Ringworm is contagious; the rash will spread on both the infected individual and to other individuals as a result of contact. These fungi and yeasts are the cause of most fungal infections, including tinea.

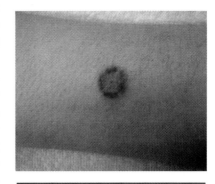

FIGURE 14-13 Tinea corporis (ringworm) is a fungal infection of the skin on the body.

Tinea pedis is a fungus that generally occurs between the toes and on the bottoms of the feet (Figure 14-14). It is caused by heat, moisture, and failure to change socks. It can also be contracted from a shower floor. Signs and symptoms include a red rash and extreme itchiness in the affected area. The rash is characterized by small pimples that contain a yellow serum which will leak out when the rash is scratched. Severe cases are indicated by a red, white, and gray scaling of the affected area.

Herpes is a viral infection that most commonly affects the face, trunk, and genitalia. It is characterized by blisters, inflamed skin, and pain. Sometimes the blisters form crusty yellow scabs,

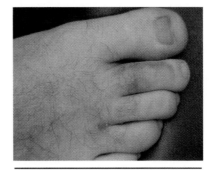

FIGURE 14-14 Tinea pedis (athlete's foot) can usually be treated with an over-the-counter medication.

while fever is another possible symptom. Herpes is a highly contagious infection that is a disqualifying condition for athletes in contact sports. When treated properly, the condition clears up two weeks following beginning treatment.

The papilloma virus causes raised, flesh-colored lesions with small dark spots on the affected areas of the body. Warts affecting the feet are the most common for athletes and are called plantar warts. The infection is contagious, particularly to some individuals who seem to be more susceptible than others. Warts should be protected with a donut pad to disperse pressure until they are treated by a physician. Do not attempt to treat a wart.

Impetigo is a bacterial infection contracted through contact. It is characterized by redness, itching, soreness, and yellow pustules. It tends to develop on areas of the body subject to high friction. This highly contagious infection is also a disqualifying condition for athletes in contact sports. It responds rapidly to proper treatment by a physician.

Immediate Treatment: To avoid spreading the condition, athletes and others with any of these disorders should be cautioned not to scratch or touch the rash. Make sure athletes don't share towels or use common whirlpools. Athlete's foot can be treated with an over-the-counter medication for athlete's foot. If the rash does not clear up within a week, send the patient to a doctor for treatment. For the rest of the described conditions, cover the affected area with a nonstick pad and send the patient to a physician for treatment. Athletes with herpes or impetigo are not allowed to return to play in contact sports until authorized by the physician.

Follow-up Treatment: To prevent the spread of infection, clean and disinfect any surfaces (shower floors, mats, etc.) and equipment the athlete may have touched. Make sure all potentially affected clothing is either disinfected or discarded (Note: uniforms are almost never discarded). When the athlete returns, monitor the affected area daily and send the patient back to the physician if the area fails to improve or if symptoms get worse.

Prevention: The bacteria and viruses that cause these skin conditions like warm, moist, and dark environments. So, to prevent these conditions from occurring, athletes should practice good hygiene by keeping their skin clean and dry and using their own sideline towels rather than sharing them with other athletes. A moisture-absorbing powder may be used to help keep the feet dry. Disinfect surfaces and equipment on a routine basis. Equipment that requires disinfection includes wrestling mats, knee pads, shoulder pads, elbow pads, and any other items that come in contact with the skin.

Hematomas

hematoma

a blood-filled swollen area; a goose-egg mass caused by bleeding under the tissues.

A **hematoma** is a closed wound. There is usually considerable damage to the soft tissues surrounding the area, including the muscles, blood vessels, and skin. Bruising also may occur. The discoloration of the skin is caused by the ruptured capillaries bleeding into the tissues. A blood blister is a type of hematoma in which blood pools in the superficial layers of the skin. Blood blisters are caused by friction.

Immediate Treatment: Ice, compression, and elevation (ICE). When applying ice to a wound, ice should be kept in place for 20 minutes, followed by an hour during which the ice is taken off. Repeat this cycle for a 24- to 72-hour period during waking hours, or until the swelling subsides. Always check back with the athlete/patient to make sure he or she is okay. Monitor the patient's vital signs, and if the condition worsens, contact the EMS.

Follow-up Treatment: Make sure the patient is seen by a physician. Sometimes hematomas are accompanied by other injuries, such as internal bleeding, that require treatment by physician.

Prevention: Make sure all objects near the field of play are padded so that athletes are protected in case they hit the objects.

Contusions

A **contusion** is a bruise received from a sudden traumatic blow to the body, causing bleeding in the tissue that later leads to discoloration at the injury site (Figure 14-15). The severity of the contusion is directly related to the amount of soft tissue crushed and the amount of force applied to the tissue. These injuries are quite common with sports-related activities; therefore, it is recommended that athletes wear protective gear to decrease the possibility of injury. Contusions commonly affect the quadriceps of basketball players and football running backs; however, it is important to note that contusions may occur to any part of the body.

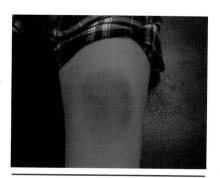

FIGURE 14-15 A Contusion

> **contusion**
>
> a soft tissue injury caused by seepage of blood into tissue; a bruise.

A person with a mild contusion will experience point tenderness and local pain at the injury site. Limbs with mild contusions retain normal range of motion. Mild contusions on the legs generally do not cause the person to walk with a limp. Most signs and symptoms of a mild contusion will lessen in a short time. A moderate contusion will also cause swelling at the point of injury. A limb with a moderate contusion may have a decrease in its range of motion, and the patient may walk with an abnormal gait if the injury is to the leg. A severe contusion will feature marked tenderness and increased swelling. It will cause a severe decrease in range of motion and inability to maneuver. A person with a severe contusion to the leg will be unable to walk without a limp.

Immediate Treatment: Contusions should be treated with ice, compression, and elevation (ICE). Use the icing procedure described in the treatment of hematomas. Apply the compression first by applying an elastic cloth wrap around the injury, which keeps blood from flowing into the injury. The compression material should be left on both during and after the ice application in order to decrease the swelling. The ice should be applied for 20 minutes to constrict the blood vessels, and then the ice is removed for one hour. The ice can be held in place with plastic wrap, which will also help keep the compression wrap dry. If possible, and if the possibility of a fracture does not exist, the injured area should be elevated higher than the heart during treatment periods until the swelling has subsided. This will reduce swelling and decrease the pain.

If a contusion occurs, ice the area *immediately* with the muscle flexed. For example, to flex a contused quadricep, the knee should be kept in flexion during the icing period. However, a contused bicep should be kept extended by extending the elbow. After the 20-minute ice treatment is removed, the athlete should do range-of-motion exercises. A stationary bike can be used for a quad contusion to work on range of motion (ROM). If the athlete cannot walk without limping, provide the athlete with crutches. Monitor the girth (the distance around) of the involved extremity and compare it to the girth of the uninvolved extremity. For example, on a quadricep contusion, measure the girth of the quadricep approximately 4 to 6 inches from the superior aspect (top) of the patella, making sure that the point of measurement includes the area of the contusion (Figure 14-16). A cloth measuring tape is necessary for accurate measurement. Measure this same area on the uninvolved quadricep. By taking these measurements and recording them, any changes in swelling can be detected.

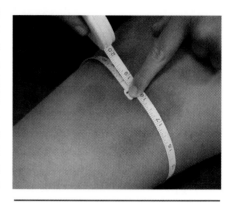

FIGURE 14-16 Measure the girth of the injured area and the same area on the uninvolved limb to monitor the degree of swelling associated with the contusion.

Follow-up Treatment: Continue the treatment schedule (ice for 20 minutes; off for an hour while protecting the skin) and elevation during waking hours until the swelling has subsided. Mild stretching through pain-free range of motion also is encouraged. Isometric exercises can be used to maintain strength during rehabilitation. As with all other injuries, if the injury does not seem to be healing, or if unsure of how to proceed, send the patient to a physician.

Once the area has started to heal, the athlete may return to play. To protect the area from additional injury, cut a donut-shaped pad out of closed-cell foam and place it over the injured area to distribute the force of potential blows away from the injured tissue (see Figure 14-17). Cover the donut pad with a hard plastic pad, and hold both pads in place with a neoprene sleeve or elastic wrap, which will provide warmth and compression to the injured area. The protective padding should conform to the appropriate rule book guidelines and should also be checked by the game officials to make sure the athlete's injury padding conforms to legal specifications. If the injured athlete is playing in an event, game officials will also check to be sure that the injured player will not cause further harm to the injury and that the athlete's padding will not harm other players, should they come in contact with it.

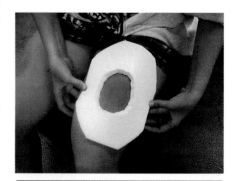

FIGURE 14-17 A donut-shaped pad can help distribute the force of a new blow to a healing contusion.

Prevention: Athletes who are vulnerable to receiving direct hits in certain areas from other players should be covered with protective pads, such as thigh pads, so that any hits will be dispersed over a broader area of the body (see Figure 14-18). In football, for example, the running backs or other players who have large thighs will need a larger pair of quadriceps pads than will other athletes who have smaller thighs and require standard-size quad pads. Athletes who wear thigh pads should wear tight practice and game pants so that the quad pads don't slide off to one side while they are running or are playing in hip flexion positions. Although having larger players wear larger protective pads seems logical, it is a preventive measure that is often overlooked.

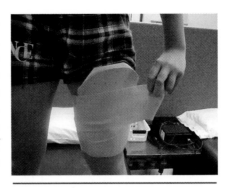

FIGURE 14-18 An elastic wrap helps keep the protective pads in place and provides comfort while the injury heals.

THE MUSCULAR SYSTEM

The human body is composed of over 600 muscles that help us move in different ways. Muscles are made up of bundles of tiny contractile muscle fibers, which are held together by connective tissue. These highly conductive muscle fibers initiate movement when they are stimulated by nerve endings. This stimulation causes the muscle fibers to become short and thick (contract) causing movement of the organs and parts of the body.

There are many types of movement, and different muscles are capable of causing different types of movement (see Figure 14-19). Rotation is the turning, or

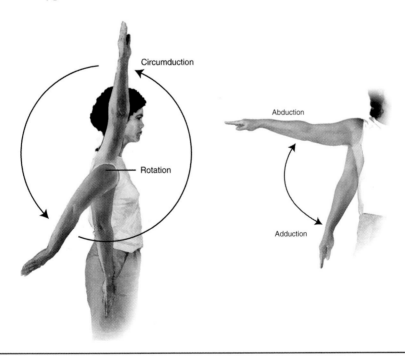

FIGURE 14-19 Types of Movement

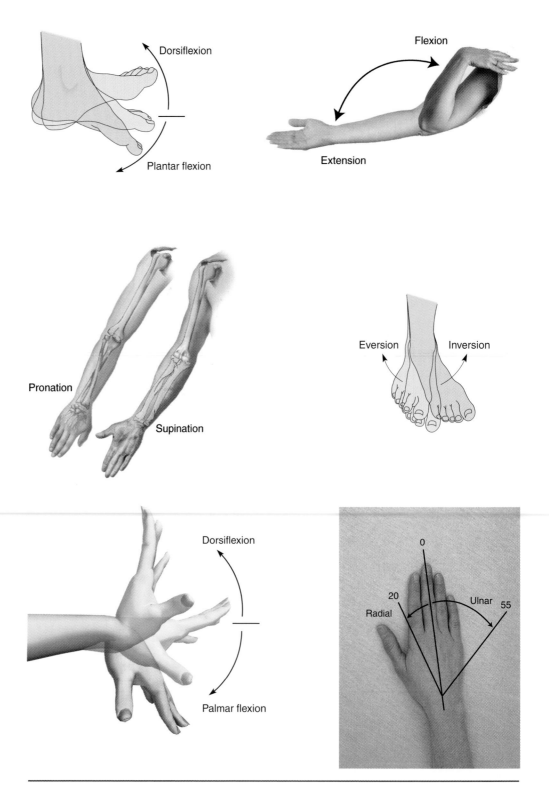

FIGURE 14-19 Types of Movement *(Continued)*

circular motion, of a body part on its axis. The movement of a body part toward the middle of the body is called adduction; and the opposite motion, the movement of a body part away from the middle of the body, is called abduction. Extension is the movement that results in an increased angle between two bones, or straightening of a body part; and the movement that results in a decreased angle between two bones, or bending a body part, is known as flexion.

Plantar flexion is the downward movement of the foot, and palmar flexion is the bending forward of the wrist so as to create a decreased angle between the palm and the inner surface of the forearm. Dorsiflexion is the movement of a joint toward the dorsal aspect. This means that dorsiflexion of the foot is movement in which the foot flexes upward, toward the top of the foot, and dorsiflexion of the hand indicates movement in which the hand is bent backward at the wrist. Eversion means turning outward, and inversion is turning inward or inside out. The muscular system performs hundreds of movements daily; many times without a person consciously thinking about them!

As discussed in the section on tissues, there are three different types of muscle tissue (see Figure 14-20). The first is called cardiac muscle. This type of muscle fiber makes up the walls of the heart. Cardiac muscle is involuntary; that is, the brain controls it automatically. The heart continues to beat and pump blood to the lungs and throughout the body without a person having to think about it.

The second type of muscle fiber found in the body is known as smooth or visceral muscle and is found throughout the body in the internal organs. Visceral muscle is found in the respiratory and digestive tracts, in the blood vessels, and in the eyes. Smooth muscles are made up of long and circular fibers. This special arrangement allows for wavelike movement, called peristalsis, to occur throughout the digestive tract, or alimentary canal. Like the cardiac muscle, this type of muscle is involuntary.

The third kind of muscle is known as skeletal or striated muscle. These muscles are attached to the bones and produce movement upon command from the brain. There are two points of attachment: the point of origin and the point of insertion. The point of origin is the end where movement does not occur. The point of insertion is the end where movement occurs. Skeletal muscles are attached to bones

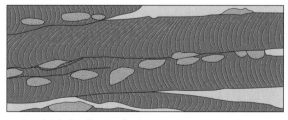

Striated (skeletal) muscle tissue

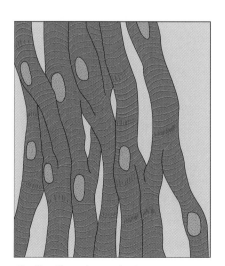

Cardiac (heart) muscle tissue

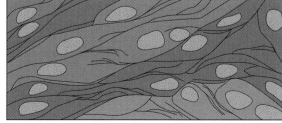

Visceral (smooth) muscle tissue

FIGURE 14-20 Types of Muscle

by tendons, a very strong, fibrous connective tissue that acts as an anchor. An example of a tendon that secures a muscle to a bone is the Achilles tendon. This tendon is located at the lower portion of the calf, on the gastrocnemius muscle, and secures that muscle to the calcaneus, or heel bone. Some muscles are attached to other body parts or other muscles by fascia. Fascia are fibrous membranes that cover, support, and separate muscle. For example, lumbodorsal fascia surround and protect the deep muscles of the back. Fascia also connect the skin to underlying tissues.

Muscles remain partially contracted at all times. This is true even when the muscles are at rest. This partial state of contraction is known as muscle tone. Proper muscle tone means that the muscles are ready for action. When muscles are not used over a period of time, they lose their tone. This is known as atrophy, and occurs with paralysis and other conditions. When atrophy exists for an extended time, a joint may become damaged and remain in a flexed position. This condition is known as a contracture. If this occurs, the patient is unable to extend those muscles or move those joints.

Muscles throughout the body are different sizes and shapes and contribute to the body's contour or form. For example, the muscles of the trunk are long, broad, flat, and expanded. So too is the trunk of the body. In contrast, the muscles of the extremities are long and round, as are the extremities themselves. The major muscles of the body are shown in Figure 14-21.

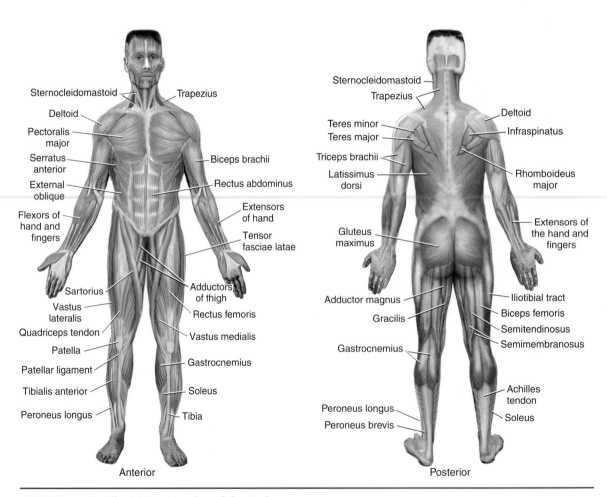

FIGURE 14-21 The Major Muscles of the Body

INJURIES TO THE MUSCLE TISSUES

Muscle Strain

A **strain** is an overstretching or tearing of the muscles and/or adjacent tissues such as the fascia or tendon. Most muscle strains occur where the tendon meets the muscle and commonly affect the hamstring or quadricep groups.

Mild strains are often caused by muscle spasms. A person with a mild strain will experience local pain with contraction that decreases with stretching, some decrease in range of motion, point tenderness, mild loss of function, and possible muscle spasms. A moderate strain will be more painful than a mild strain when the muscle is contracted and/or stretched. A snap or a tearing sound is sometimes heard by the patient when a moderate strain occurs, and delayed discoloration of the tissues may also occur (see Figure 14-22). There will be point tenderness, moderate swelling, moderate to severe loss of function, and possible muscle spasms. The patient also will experience a decrease in range of motion. A severe strain is a rupture of the tendon or muscle tissue. There will be a decrease or increase in range of motion, severe loss of function, possible muscle spasms, and a defect in the muscle that is palpable. If pain is present with a severe strain, there will be no change in the degree of pain when the muscle is contracted or stretched, because the muscle is completely torn (see Figure 14-23).

Immediate Treatment: First aid for a mild strain is to use the ICE technique (apply ice using the icing procedure, compress the injured area with an elastic wrap, and elevate it above the heart).

strain

a pulled muscle.

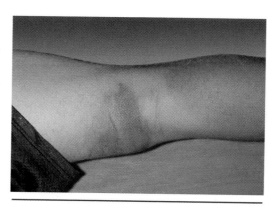

FIGURE 14-22 Residual bleeding and delayed discoloration will accompany a moderate or severe strain or muscle tear, such as with this hamstring strain.

Strain Classifications

Sign/Symptom	1st Degree	2nd Degree	3rd Degree
muscle damage	mild tearing	moderate tearing	complete tear
pain w/contraction	mild	moderate to severe	none to mild
pain w/stretching	yes	yes	no
muscle spasm	possible	possible	possible
loss of function	mild	moderate to severe	severe
ROM	decreased	decreased	decreased or increased
edema	mild	moderate	moderate to severe
palpable defect	none	none	yes

FIGURE 14-23 Strain Classifications

For the most part, the immediate treatment for a moderate strain is the same as for a mild strain. In addition, observe the amount of initial swelling to the injury to establish a baseline guide for gauging how well the injury is responding to treatment.

Treatment for a severe strain requires ice, compression, and elevation as do the other types of strains. In addition, immobilize the affected area, make the athlete as comfortable as possible, and activate the Emergency Action Plan. The athlete may require surgery to repair the damage and may be unable to return to play for as long as one month to one year.

Follow-up Treatment: Perform static stretching to maintain range of motion by lengthening the muscle to the point of tightness or pain—then hold that position for 15 seconds. Repeat this procedure at least three times a day, stretching the muscle morning, noon, and evening. Rest the area for one to five days. The injured person can return to regular activity when able to run forward, backward, and in a "figure-8" without limping, and has been evaluated by the athletic trainer. Also, the athlete might want to see a physician to rule out fractures or other complications.

When treating a moderate strain, monitor the amount of swelling—whether it decreases, increases, or remains the same and whether the pain increases or won't go away. Further, note whether the injured area is getting smaller, which can be caused by muscle atrophy.

To evaluate the degree of swelling a strain has produced, compare the injured area with the uninjured area by measuring the girth (the distance around) of the involved and uninvolved extremities. If the injury is to a leg or foot, the athlete may need to be put on crutches until able to walk without a limp. If unsure about treatment, have the patient see a physician.

Prevention: Teach athletes strengthening and flexibility exercises for the areas of the body that are vulnerable to injury, depending on the sport being played. Appropriate taping or bracing of vulnerable body parts will provide additional protection. Protect the athletes by checking the event area for possible hidden dangers such as holes on the field, water on the court, etc.

Myositis Ossificans

myositis ossificans

a condition in which bone forms in and replaces muscle tissue as a result of trauma.

Myositis ossificans is a condition in which calcium is produced within the muscle after a blow (see Figure 14-24). Pain is the primary symptom. Sometimes an immovable mass can be palpated in the muscle. It will be visible on X-rays three to four weeks post-injury.

Immediate Treatment: Send the athlete to a physician for further evaluation, and protect the affected area with a donut pad. Measure the girth of the affected area to establish a baseline for future evaluations. If the injured

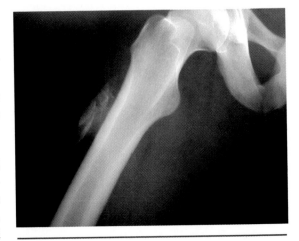

FIGURE 14-24 Myositis ossificans affecting the femur and the surrounding soft tissue.

area involves an extremity, measure the same area on the uninvolved extremity for additional comparison information. Record these measurements.

Follow-up Treatment: Keep a donut-shaped closed-cell pad around the area to displace any pressure on the point of pain. Keep ROM by having the person ride a stationary bike.

Prevention: Make sure that athletes are wearing proper padding to protect them from blows.

Tendonitis

Repeated stress to the tendons often results in microtearing of the tendon sheath resulting in inflammation of the tendon, a condition known as **tendonitis**. Sports that use repetitive motions such as swimming, baseball, water polo, and football (some positions), as well as throwing and jumping sports, carry increased risk of tendonitis. Tendonitis may also be caused by improper body mechanics or poor conditioning. Symptoms include general soreness and point tenderness, with or without motion and possible mild swelling.

> **tendonitis**
>
> inflammation of a tendon.

Immediate Treatment: Ice the area as soon as symptoms develop, using the ICE procedure. In severe cases, resting the injured area is also recommended. In some cases, protective braces may help ease the pain and speed the healing of the injury. A neoprene compression sleeve may also be helpful.

Follow-up Treatment: Massage the area with ice for 7 to 10 minutes, four times a day. If the injury does not improve within one to two weeks, the athlete should see a physician. Anti-inflammatory medicine or additional treatment, such as ultrasound therapy, may be prescribed by the physician.

Prevention: Ice applied to high-stress areas after practices and games can help prevent tendonitis. Proper conditioning (warm-up, pre-season and off-season) and good sport-specific body mechanics can also help prevent injury. Consult with the coaching staff regarding proper use of mechanics for the sport. Bring to their attention different ways that proper mechanics can prevent injuries.

THE JOINTS

Joints, or **articulations**, allow movement according to their range of motion. There are three categories of joints:

> **articulation**
>
> a joint; the point at which two or more bones meet.

1. Fibrous: (immovable) includes the bones of the cranium, or skull
2. Cartilaginous: (slightly moveable) includes the vertebra in the spine
3. Synovial: (freely moveable) includes the elbow, knee, fingers, etc.

Mobile joints are the most frequently injured joints and are grouped according to the way in which they work. For example, pivot joints allow rotation on a single axis, and hinge joints allow the adjoining parts to flex (bend) and extend (straighten). Some joints, like the knee, may have more than one component. The knee is a hinge joint, which glides anteriorly and posteriorly. It is also capable of internal and external rotation. See Figure 14-25 for examples of the different motion groups for joints.

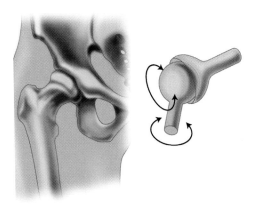

Ball & socket A round end of one bone fits into a cup-like end of another bone, allowing a wide range of movement. The shoulder and the hip are examples of ball and socket joints.

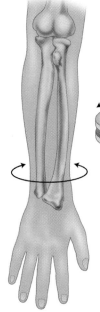

Pivot A projection fits through a ring made up of bone and ligament, allowing only pivoting movement. The first and second cervical vertebrae are pivot joints. A pivot joint in the wrist permits the palm of the hand to turn upward or downward.

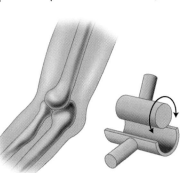

Hinge A joint in which the two surfaces are molded together closely, allowing a wide range of flexion and extension along a single plane. The elbow and the knee are hinge joints.

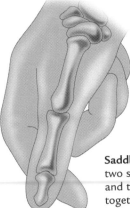

Saddle A joint in which two surfaces, one convex and the other concave, fit together. A saddle joint can be found in the thumb.

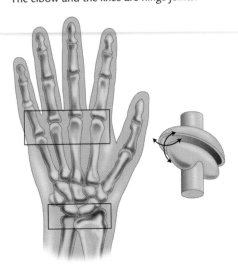

Condyloid (ellipsoid) A round or oval end of a bone fits into an oval cavity, allowing all types of movement except pivoting. One of the wrist joints is a condyloid joint. This type of joint can also be found in the metacarpals.

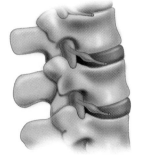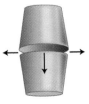

Gliding Two facing bone surfaces meet, allowing only gliding movements. Motion is limited by surrounding tissues and ligaments. The wrist and the ankles as well as the vertebrae in the spine contain gliding joints.

FIGURE 14-25 Motion Groups for Synovial Joints

Special bands of white connective tissue help hold bones together at the joint. These connective tissues that connect bone to bone are called **ligaments**. **Tendons** are fibrous connective tissues that attach muscle to bones. The joint is enclosed in a protective capsule that contains synovial fluid. This fluid is colorless and contains mineral salts, fat, and other substances. It acts as a shock absorber and cushions both ends of the bone so that they do not irritate each other. There are other structures that protect the bones, too. A bursa is a sac full of synovial fluid that reduces friction between tendons, bones, ligaments, and other structures. A meniscus is a cartilaginous disc surrounded with fluid that also reduces friction during movement and adds stability.

INJURIES TO THE JOINTS

Ligament or Capsular Sprains

Excessive force applied to soft tissues will cause injury. Three types of force can damage soft tissues: compression, tension, and sheer. *Compression* is a force that, with enough energy, crushes the tissue. Soft tissue can withstand some compressing force; however, if the force is excessive and not absorbed, a contusion will occur. *Tension* is a force that pulls and stretches tissue. *Shear* is a force that moves against the parallel organization of collagen fibers. Tendons and ligaments are designed to effectively withstand tension forces, but do not resist sheer or compression forces well. Excessive tension or sheer forces cause injuries such as ligament or capsular sprains or muscle strains with varying degrees of severity.

A **sprain** is the overstretching and/or tearing of ligaments or other connective tissues caused by traumatic twisting of a joint (see Figure 14-26). A sprain may also involve the articulating capsule or the synovial membrane. In general, symptoms of a sprain include deformity, **crepitation**, point tenderness, and immediate swelling. If, while examining a sprain, indications are found that a fracture has occurred, send the injured athlete to a physician.

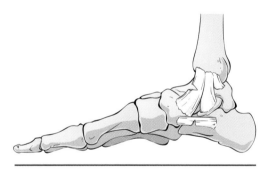

FIGURE 14-26 A Sprain

Sprains vary in degrees of intensity (see Figure 14-27). A first-degree or mild sprain will consist of minor tearing of the ligament and/or articulating capsule, with symptoms such as mild point tenderness and mild loss of strength. There should be no **joint laxity**, and no decrease in range of motion (ROM). The lost strength will return after a short time.

A second-degree or moderate sprain is a partial tearing of the ligament- and/or articulating capsule and is indicated by marked swelling, tenderness, decreased range of motion, and moderate loss of function of the injured area. When stressed for evaluation, a moderately sprained joint will exhibit some laxity when compared to the uninvolved side, indicating instability. The laxity will have an "endpoint." The endpoint is the point at which the natural tightness of the ligaments and tissue resists pressure, an actual endpoint that prevents further intrusion into the area.

A third-degree or severe sprain is a complete tearing of the ligaments and/or articulating capsule. There will be a complete loss of function in the injured area,

ligament

a band of white, fibrous, connective tissue that helps hold bone to bone.

tendon

fibrous connective tissue around a joint that connects muscle to bone.

sprain

a stretching or tearing of the ligaments, characterized by the inability to move, deformity, and pain.

crepitation

a crackling or grating sound heard upon movement of a damaged bone or joint.

joint laxity

joint play; motions occurring between the ends of two or more bones that form a joint as it moves through its range of motion.

Sprain Classifications

Sign/Symptom	1st Degree	2nd Degree	3rd Degree
ligament damage	mild tearing	moderate tearing	complete tear
point tenderness	yes	yes	yes
loss of function	mild	moderate to severe	severe w/instability
ROM	not affected	decreased	decreased or increased
edema	mild	moderate	moderate to severe
stress test results	no laxity	some laxity w/endpoint	increased laxity w/no endpoint

FIGURE 14-27 Sprain Classifications

abnormal motion, and possible deformity. Local tenderness and swelling will also be present. When stressing the ligaments for evaluation, an opening of the joint that appears to have no endpoint will be found. While applying stress to a joint injury, if it seems the injured ligaments are offering no resistance, then there is no endpoint—no resistance by the ligaments to the pressure being applied—and a third-degree or severe sprain is indicated.

Always compare the involved (injured) side with the uninvolved side. When doing this, check the uninvolved side first. This provides information about what type of appearance and movement to look for in the injured side. Knowing what to look for is important because there will be only one opportunity to check the involved side—the athlete won't let the examiner do it again. It will hurt!

Immediate Treatment: When giving first aid to someone with a sprain, use the five steps of the **PRICE procedure**:

> **PRICE procedure**
>
> systemic steps taken to mitigate or minimize injury: protect, rest, ice, compress, and elevate.

* Protect: The first step is to avoid further injury. For example, if the athlete suffers a sprained ankle on the field, have the athlete avoid putting pressure on the injury while walking off of the field. To accomplish this, have two or more people support the athlete or have the athlete use crutches.

* Rest: Rest the injured area.

* Ice: Use the icing procedure. Ice the surrounding tissues immediately for 20 minutes, followed by an hour during which the ice is off. Repeat this cycle for a 24- to 72-hour period during waking hours, or until the swelling subsides. For comfort, place a cloth or towel between the ice and skin.

* Compress: Compress the sprained area with an elastic wrap.

* Elevate: Elevate the injured area above the level of the heart.

Taping and wrapping procedures for foot and ankle ligament sprains can be found in Chapter 21.

Follow-up Treatment: Isometric strengthening should be done to maintain strength as the injury heals. Flexibility exercises should also be performed within the athlete's pain-free ROM. Once tissues have recovered, strengthening should increase to isotonic exercises. Braces can add external support to damaged ligaments while the injury heals (see Figure 14-28). There are many different kinds of braces: neoprene adds warmth; plastic and metal provide stability; and cloth or athletic tape can add additional stability and hold everything together.

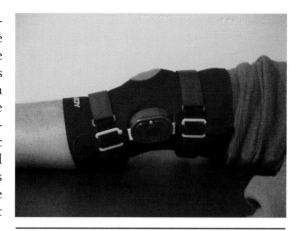

FIGURE 14-28 Braces can add support to damaged ligaments while they heal.

Prevention: Check the event area for possible hidden dangers such as holes on the field, water on the court, etc. Also, instruct the athletes in the appropriate strengthening exercises for the areas of the body that are vulnerable to injury, depending on the sport being played. Appropriate taping or bracing of vulnerable body parts can provide additional protection (see Chapter 21).

Dislocations and Subluxations

A **dislocation** is an injury resulting from a force that causes a joint to go beyond its normal anatomical limits. A subluxation is a partial dislocation. Usually, a person can identify that a **subluxation** has occurred because often the injured person will state that at the time of the injury, the joint "felt as though it slipped out and then went back in." The signs and symptoms of shoulder dislocation include point tenderness, loss of strength, complete loss of motion, swelling, and deformity. Almost always there will be damage to the joint capsule and ligaments. These symptoms can be detected by comparing the injured shoulder to the uninjured one. Signs and symptoms of a subluxation include dead arm weakness (the inability to lift the arm) and pain.

dislocation

the separation of a joint and malposition of an extremity.

subluxation

a partial dislocation.

Immediate Treatment: Check the area below the injury for a pulse and sensation. If either the pulse or sensation seem to be impaired, call the EMS immediately. While waiting for the EMS or if pulse and sensation seem normal, splint the injury in the most comfortable position possible. Recheck the area below the injury for pulse and sensation to make sure that nothing has been made worse by the movement and splinting. Apply ice using the proper procedure. If the weight of the ice causes the athlete more pain, reduce the amount of ice being applied. If the pulse and sensation below the injury seem normal, but there is any uncertainty about the situation, call for EMS. In all cases, have the athlete see a physician. Sometimes, a dislocated joint may "pop" back into position. If this happens, the urgency to see a physician is not as great, but still needed. Do not attempt to relocate (reduce) the dislocated joint.

Follow-up Treatment: Have the athlete perform flexibility and strengthening exercises to increase range of motion and strength in the affected body part. Start with isometrics, then move to isotonic lifting.

Prevention: Shoulder braces will decrease external rotation and abduction of the shoulder girdle (a common point of dislocation). Elbow and knee braces can help protect the elbows and knees from becoming dislocated. Strengthening exercises that work the musculature on all sides of the joint should also be performed by the athletes. Working the muscles on all sides of the joint helps prevent an imbalance in muscle strength that could lead to injury.

Synovitis and Bursitis

bursitis

inflammation of a bursa.

synovitis

inflammation of the synovial membrane in a joint, characterized by pain, swelling, localized tension, and increased pain with movement.

Patients with synovitis or bursitis typically have a history of repeated movement or overuse, such as repeatedly throwing overhand in baseball, or repeatedly doing an overhead serve in tennis. Both disorders can also be caused from direct trauma. **Bursitis** is inflammation of a bursa, located between two bony prominences and/or a muscle or tendon. For example, in the shoulder the bursa will become inflamed between the head of the humerus and the acromial arch. **Synovitis**, the inflammation of a synovial membrane, in the shoulder will cause pain when moving the arm in abduction or rotation. Both disorders may cause crepitation and increased pain when resistance is applied.

Immediate Treatment: If no swelling is present, treatment for overuse injuries includes the use of deep-heating modalities such as moist heat packs. If swelling is present, use the ICE (ice, compression, and elevation) or PRICE technique, depending on the pain with movement and the severity of the injury. Use the proper icing procedure whenever ice is applied for anything other than controlling bleeding or snakebite.

Follow-up Treatment: After the swelling subsides, use moist heat treatments. Careful, static stretching to preserve range of motion also is important when an athlete suffers from bursitis or synovitis—it is crucial that the athlete does not lose the range of motion that remains. For example, to maintain range of motion in the shoulder, have the athlete perform rotator cuff strengthening exercises in a pain-free range of motion (see Chapter 7). If pain increases or persists for over a week, send the patient to a physician.

Prevention: Educate the athletes in the proper use of body mechanics. Improper use of the body's muscles will cause unnecessary stress to the joint and/or overuse of the joint.

THE SKELETAL SYSTEM

The skeletal system provides a framework of support for the soft tissues of the body and protects the internal organs from damage. Each of the 206 bones that form the human skeleton affects our movement in some way. The skeletal system performs five specific functions:

1. Provides support for the muscles, fat, and soft tissues
2. Protects the internal organs

3. Provides leverage for lifting and movement through the attachment of muscles
4. Produces blood cells
5. Stores the majority of the body's calcium supply

Bones (osseous tissue), which are composed primarily of calcium and phosphorous, are classified into five groups. Long bones are bones in which the length is greater than the width, such as the femur, humerus, tibia, and radius. Short bones are blocky bones that are closely joined and those in which there is no relationship between their length and width, such as the wrist (carpals) and ankle (tarsal) bones. Flat bones are bones that are composed of two relatively parallel plates of compact bone that are separated by a layer of spongy bone, such as the scapula (shoulder) and skull. Irregular bones are bones of complex shape and structure, such as the facial bones and vertebrae. Sesamoid bones are small bones found within various tendons, such as the patella.

The long bones have four basic parts (Figure 14-29). The long shaft is known as the diaphysis, and at each of its ends is an epiphysis. The medullary canal is the cavity in the diaphysis that is filled with yellow marrow (fat cells). The endosteum is the lining of the medullary canal that keeps the yellow marrow intact.

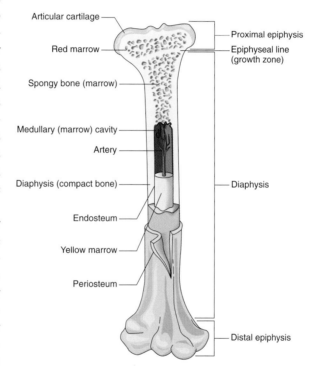

Articular cartilage

Red marrow

Spongy bone (marrow)

Medullary (marrow) cavity

Artery

Diaphysis (compact bone)

Endosteum

Yellow marrow

Periosteum

Proximal epiphysis

Epiphyseal line (growth zone)

Diaphysis

Distal epiphysis

FIGURE 14-29 The Parts of the Bone

The outside layer of every bone is called the periosteum. The specialized cells in this layer promote bone growth (ossification), nutrition, and repair.

Some bones contain red bone marrow, which is responsible for producing erythrocytes (red blood cells) and some leukocytes (white blood cells). The bones that contain red bone marrow are the ribs, sternum (breastbone), vertebrae (spinal bones), scapula (shoulder), and the proximal ends of the femur (thigh bone) and humerus (upper arm bone). These bones contribute greatly to the body's ability to heal by producing red bone marrow, which produces red and white blood cells.

The skeletal system is divided into two sections: the axial skeleton and the appendicular skeleton (see Figure 14-30). The axial skeleton is the main trunk of the body and includes the skull, spinal column, ribs, and sternum. The appendicular skeleton is formed from the extremities (arms and legs), shoulder girdle, and pelvic girdle.

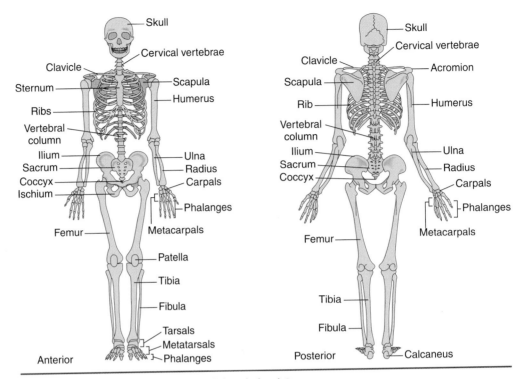

FIGURE 14-30 The Major Bones of the Skeletal System

INJURIES TO THE SKELETAL SYSTEM

Fractures

A **fracture** is a partial or complete break in the continuity of a bone. Although athletes are not the only people who are prone to fractures, those who participate in certain sports have a higher risk than others of breaking a bone: skiers break legs, wrestlers break wrists, and skateboarders break arms. These injuries can result from any one of a variety of forces including direct impact, compression, torsion, or indirect impact. Fractures may also be caused by disease processes, such as cancer; repeated stressful motions, such as running; or sudden muscle contraction, such as seizures. The following are signs and symptoms of a fracture:

* Pain at the site of the injury
* Deformity
* Edema (swelling) at the injury site
* Ecchymosis (bruising)
* Grating or crepitation
* Immobility
* Numbness or tingling
* Pale or cold skin due to impaired circulation

Be alert to the possibility of damage to the tissues surrounding the area of the break. Be gentle in handling the patient and do not move the injured area while

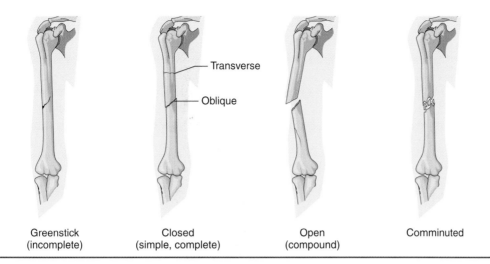

Greenstick (incomplete) Closed (simple, complete) Open (compound) Comminuted

FIGURE 14-31 Some Common Types of Fractures

checking for sensation or feeling; it is vital not to make the injury worse by impairing the circulation or causing nerve damage.

Bones can fracture in a variety of ways, sometimes causing additional injury as they break (see Figure 14-31). A fracture that does not break the skin is called a closed fracture. An open fracture, or compound fracture, occurs when the bone protrudes through the skin, leaving an open wound such as a laceration. Not all compound fractures are obvious; sometimes the ends of the fractured bone settle back under the skin, making it look as if the wound is only superficial. Anyone with an open wound resulting from any type of sudden force or impact should be checked for the signs and symptoms of a fracture. Be aware of the potential hazard of secondary puncture wounds that may result from sharp bones protruding through the patient's skin.

An avulsion fracture is commonly found when a person sprains an ankle or another joint in the body where a ligament attaches to the bone. During the injury, a fragment of bone is torn away at the point of attachment of a tendon, ligament, or muscle. Basketball players often are prone to this type of fracture.

A stress fracture can be caused by repeated stress over a period of time as compared to an acute fracture caused from one specific injury. Stress fractures, or fatigue fractures, result from repeated wear and tear on the bones of body parts that have great demands placed on them, such as the tibia or fibula in the legs of marathon runners. A bone scan may be needed to diagnose this type of fracture; stress fractures are so small they may not show up on a regular x-ray until the healing and calcification process has begun. The best indication that a stress fracture has occurred will be the athlete's persistent complaints of pain in an area of repeated stress.

A greenstick fracture is an incomplete break in a long bone shaft in which the bone is also partially bent. This fracture, which occurs in children and adolescents because of their soft bone tissue, earned its name because of its similarity to the way in which a green twig breaks.

An impacted fracture is a break in which one bone fragment becomes embedded in the interior of another bone fragment. Athletes who participate in rodeo and contact sports are more likely to receive impacted fractures than athletes in other sports.

A longitudinal fracture is a break in which the bone splits or cracks lengthwise, typically caused by impact such as a hard landing after a jump. Thus, long jumpers may receive such fractures.

An oblique fracture is an oblique or diagonal break that occurs when one end of a bone receives a torsion while the other end remains fixed.

A spiral fracture is a break in a bone that has an S-shaped, or helical, separation. Basketball players are among those most prone to this type of fracture in the event the foot is firmly planted while the upper body twists violently to maintain control of the ball.

A transverse fracture is a break that occurs across the bone shaft at a right angle to the long axis of the bone; usually the result of direct blows, such as those received in contact sports.

A comminuted fracture is a break having three or more fragments at the fracture site. Again, players of contact sports are most likely to experience a comminuted fracture.

A blowout fracture is a break in the floor of the orbital socket resulting from a direct blow to the eye. Athletes participating in baseball, lacrosse, racquetball, and squash are especially vulnerable to this injury.

Immediate Treatment: In the event of a compound fracture, a sterile dressing is applied over the wound and bleeding is controlled using a pressure point. Direct pressure must be applied with care to control bleeding when a fracture is suspected. The pressure will cause the patient more pain and may even cause additional bone displacement, making the fracture worse. As with any occurrence of bleeding, it is important to protect yourself and others from coming in contact with possibly infectious blood by wearing gloves.

For any fracture, put the person in the most comfortable position possible, and call for the EMS. While waiting for the EMS to arrive, restrict the athlete's movement of an extremity with a **splint**. This can decrease much of the pain and help prevent additional injury to the patient. Splints should be applied so that they extend above and below the fracture site. Magazines, boards, and Sam® splints can all be used to splint the injury, and can be held in place with an elastic wrap. Sam® splints are especially useful in providing support as they mold to the shape of the fractured area. To decrease swelling, elevate the involved extremity and apply ice using the icing procedure to the injury site. Keep the athlete as quiet as possible and avoid any unnecessary movement of the injured area. The procedures for taping and wrapping avulsion or incomplete fractures can be found in Chapter 21.

Avoid elevating an injured limb if it would involve movement of a fractured joint, if there is a possible spine injury, or if it causes the patient additional pain. For instance, do not elevate a fractured arm if there is a possibility the shoulder is also fractured. But, if there is a suspected fracture of the elbow and the shoulder is uninvolved, the arm can be elevated at the shoulder—just keep the bones of the elbow from moving with respect to each other. The physician will cast the involved site.

Continue to monitor the athlete's vital signs while awaiting the EMS. Monitor the quality of the blood circulation below the injured area by checking the distal pulse (the pulse directly below the fracture) frequently. The distal pulse tells whether circulation is present below the area of injury. An additional assessment for circulation involves checking the temperature and color of the skin: cool or pale skin indicates decreased circulation.

splint

a rigid device that holds parts of the body together and limits motion.

Follow-up Treatment: An x-ray will be necessary to determine the nature and extent of a fracture. Make sure the physician's recommendations for continued care are followed. Make sure the cast stays dry and continue to monitor the patient's circulation. Watch for signs of swelling and infection. If any of these symptoms occur, send the patient back to the physician immediately.

Prevention: Watch for potential sources of injury on and around the field of play. Alert the athletes to the presence of any holes or other hazards.

THINKING IT THROUGH

Mike Meredith has been the city high-hurdle champion ever since he was a freshman—quite a feat to say the least. His ultimate goal was to place a dime on each hurdle and come so close that he could knock them off without slowing down or knocking over a hurdle. With this drill there was always the chance of hitting one and falling down, but the drill increased his speed. Mike was lucky: he had never had a hard fall—until today.

Tired from a long day at school and staying out late the night before, Mike didn't concentrate very hard. He had done this drill a hundred times; in fact, he thought he could do it in his sleep. His final drill was a time trial. The coach set off the cadence: Ready . . . set . . . go.

For some reason the starting blocks weren't secured very well, and they slipped slightly, slowing Mike's start and putting him behind on his first hurdle. This didn't bother him; he knew how to catch up. He buried his head down and went for it. Coming up to the sixth hurdle he was way behind and hit the hurdle hard, sliding across the all-weather track. Lying on his side, Mike looked like he was in a lot of pain. Tammy, the athletic training student, was ready. She went right over to Mike and began first aid.

What should Tammy do for Mike's abrasions? What should she have in her fanny pack to protect herself from coming into contact with blood? What are some things Tammy should watch the wound for over the next few days?

CHAPTER SUMMARY

Injury to tissues may cause bleeding, inflammation, and/or swelling. While minor injuries to the skin may cause only short-term damage and pain; injuries to the deeper tissues, such as crushed or severed nerves, may cause long-term disability, such as paralysis. Care must always be taken to carefully assess the degree of damage and to administer the appropriate first aid. Above all, anyone providing treatment to an injured athlete must be extremely careful to avoid making an injury worse through improper treatment.

Controlling bleeding and preventing infection are the most important considerations in treating injuries to the tissues. Direct pressure and indirect pressure are the two primary methods of controlling bleeding. Ice can also be effective in slowing the flow of blood. Remember to wear gloves when treating any injuries involving blood or other body fluids, and keep the site of the injury as clean as possible through proper cleansing and dressing of the wound.

The muscular system provides strength and helps control movement. Different muscles are capable of causing different types of movement. There are three types of muscle tissue: cardiac, visceral, and striated. Cardiac and visceral muscles are involuntary muscles. Striated muscles, or skeletal muscles, are attached to bones and produce movement upon command from the brain. As with injuries to nerve tissue, the severity of the injury has a direct impact on the degree of damage and the length of the recovery process. During recovery, efforts must be made to preserve the range of motion of the affected muscles.

The skeletal system provides the framework for the body and protects the internal organs. Some of the bones contain red bone marrow, which contributes to the body's ability to heal by producing blood cells. Bones attach to each other by ligaments and form joints, which allow various body parts to move. The most common sports injuries to affect bones are fractures. The obvious signs of a fracture are pain, immobility, and deformity, but others symptoms include swelling, bruising, numbness, crepitation, and impaired circulation. Wounds resulting from compound fractures must be covered with a sterile dressing, and precautions must be taken to avoid contact with blood products and the possibility of puncture from protruding bones. Do not attempt to reposition deformities that result from fractures—this is a job for the physician.

STUDENT ENRICHMENT ACTIVITIES

Complete the following exercises.

1. What type of movement is involved when your arm moves away from your body?

2. What kind of joint is in your elbow?

3. Explain why a stress fracture is sometimes missed in a standard x-ray.

4. Describe the technique and purpose of applying ice to a sprain.

5. List three key elements of follow-up treatment for fractures.

6. List the poisonous insects and snakes that inhabit the area in which your team practices and plays.

7. What attaches bone to bone?

8. What attaches bones to muscles?

Define the following terms.

9. cell

10. semipermeable

11. edema

12. adipose

13. vertebrae

14. meniscus

15. atrophy

Write T for true, or F for false. Rewrite the false statement to make them true.

16. T F A compound fracture is easily identified by bone protruding through the skin.

17. T F Pulse and sensation must be rechecked after splinting a dislocation or subluxation.

18. T F An oblique fracture is typically the result of a twisting motion.

19. T F The sports medicine professional should attempt to reposition severely deformed fractures to reduce the patient's pain.

20. T F In some cases, ice and elevation may be used to treat swelling resulting from fractures.

Describe the type of activities that might result in the following types of fractures.

21. longitudinal fracture

22. spiral fracture

23. stress fracture

24. blow-out fracture

25. transverse fracture

26. As an athletic trainer, how would you prepare for some of the above fractures? What would you carry in your kit?

Photocopy and label the following diagrams.

27. The Major Bones of the Skeletal System

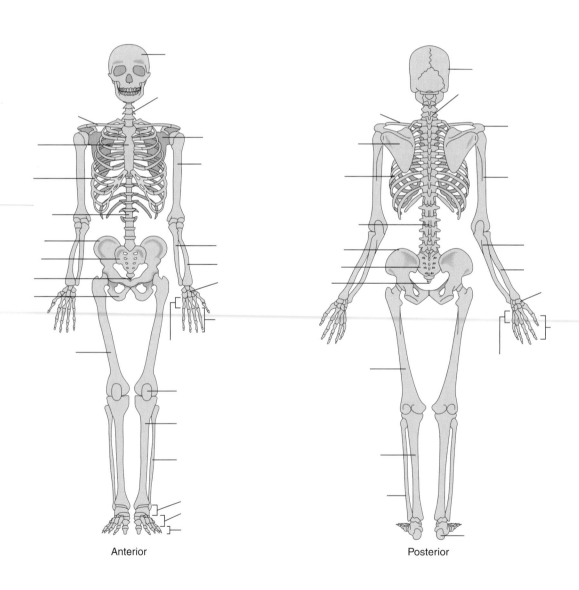

Anterior   Posterior

28. The Major Muscles of the Body

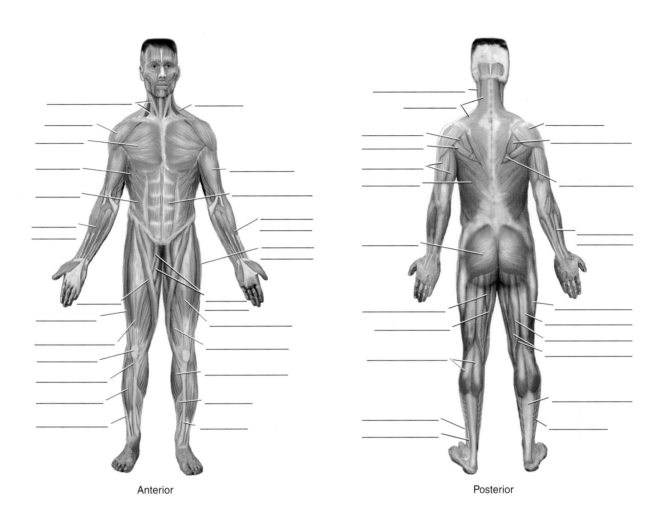

Anterior

Posterior

CHAPTER 15

Injuries to the Head and Spine

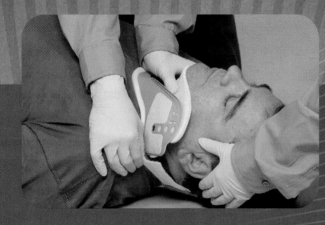

OBJECTIVES

After completing this chapter, you should be able to do the following:

1. Define and correctly spell each of the key terms.

2. List and explain the major parts and functions of the brain.

3. Explain some common injuries to the head and describe their initial treatment guidelines.

4. Describe the symptoms of three common facial injuries and explain their treatments.

5. Briefly describe the composition of the spine.

6. Explain the purpose of the nervous system.

7. Discuss how to treat injuries to the head and spine.

KEY TERMS

* central nervous system (CNS)
* concussion
* contact sports
* disc
* epistaxis
* hemorrhage
* posttraumatic amnesia
* radiating pain
* referred pain
* second-impact syndrome
* vertebrae

INTRODUCTION

Any injury to the head or spine is a serious matter. For instance, if a person receives an injury to the head, it can cause a brain **hemorrhage** (bleeding in the brain or its surrounding tissues). Trauma to the head, such as that which may occur in contact sports, can fracture the skull and may even send fragments of the skull into the brain. Injuries to the brain may cause swelling (edema) and are serious medical emergencies. Spinal injuries are serious matters, too. Because the spinal cord serves as the communication pathway between the brain and the rest of the body, injuries to the spine can be life-threatening. Spinal injuries can also result in paralysis.

Sports that carry a higher risk of neck injury include gymnastics, ice hockey, basketball, football, rodeo, diving, and extreme sports. In general, head and neck injuries can be prevented by maintaining the flexibility and strength of the neck musculature in all motions. Properly fitted protective gear, such as shoulder pads, helmets, and face masks, is also very important in preventing head and spine injuries, as is adherence to the safety rules of the game being played. For instance, one important rule in football forbids players to dive into other players head first in order to tackle them. Most of the neck injuries that occur in football result from breaking this rule.

hemorrhage

the severe, abnormal internal or external discharge of blood.

THE HEAD: AN OVERVIEW

What is commonly known as the head is comprised of the skull and the face. The skull is made up of the bones of the cranium, together with the facial bones and teeth. The head contains several of the special sensory organs such as the eyes, ears, nose, and mouth (sight, sound, smell, and taste). Facial muscles, the vertebral column, and the cerebral meninges all are attached to the bones of the cranium and face.

The skull consists of the cranium, the face, and the teeth. The cranium consists of eight bones: one occipital, two parietal, one frontal, two temporal, one sphenoid, and one ethmoid. Housed within the cranium (in the cranial cavity) are the brain and the primary neural tissues of the **central nervous system (CNS)** that send vital nerve impulses to and from the brain (see Figure 15-1).

The anterior portion of the head is the face. Extending from the forehead to the chin (excluding the ear area), this small, complex area contains a number of bones and intricate arterial-venous systems. There are 14 facial bones: one mandible; two maxillae; two zygomatic; two nasal bones; two lacrimal bones; one vomer (includes the superior nasal concha); two palatine; and two inferior nasal conchae

central nervous system (CNS)

the body system composed of the brain and the spinal cord.

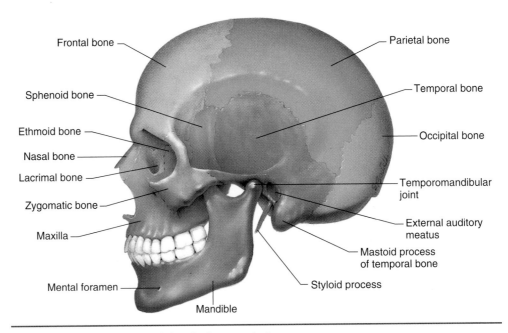

FIGURE 15-1 The Bones of the Skull, Lateral View

(see Figure 15-2). Blood is carried to both sides of the face by pairs of arteries that branch off from the external carotid artery: the maxillary, facial, and superficial temporal arteries. Blood is then carried away from the face by the exterior and interior jugular veins. Also known as the maxillo-facial region, the face includes two orifices (openings) in its bony structure: the mouth and the nasal cavity. Thus, in addi-

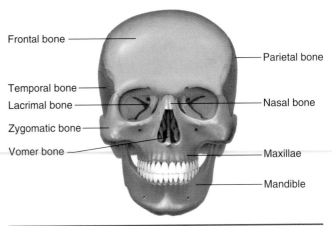

FIGURE 15-2 The Bones of the Skull, Anterior View

tion to containing the first parts of the nervous system, the skull also houses the beginnings of the respiratory and the digestive systems.

Between the cranium and the face are the orbital cavities, which house the eyes. These cavities, like the cranial cavity and the nasal cavity, are open spaces that are surrounded by bone. The hard, bony surfaces of such cavities provide a degree of protection for the delicate tissues they contain.

The skull also contains other types of open spaces. For instance, the foramen magnum, which is located in the occipital bone, creates a hole through which the brain stem passes before becoming the spinal cord. The paranasal sinuses, another type of open space in the skull found in several of the skull bones, are hollow or air-filled spaces found in the maxillae as well as in the sphenoid, frontal, and ethmoid

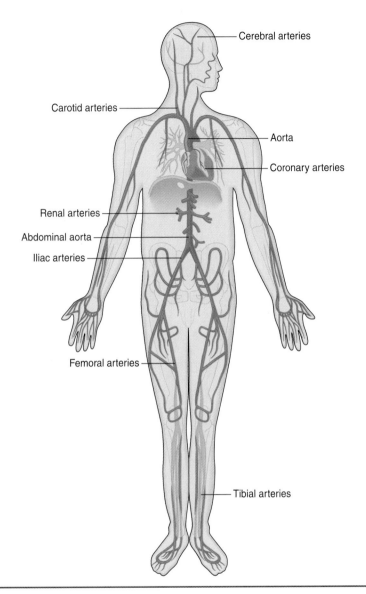

Cerebral arteries

Carotid arteries

Aorta

Coronary arteries

Renal arteries

Abdominal aorta

Iliac arteries

Femoral arteries

Tibial arteries

FIGURE 15-3 The Arteries

bones. Within the temporal bones, still another type of open space contains the middle and inner ear structures.

Except for the mandible, the bones of the skull articulate with one another via immovable joints called sutures. The temporomandibular joints, which are freely movable, join the mandible with the temporal bones.

The skull is supported by the vertebral column on the atlas (the first cervical vertebra). The atlas is a ring-shaped bone that articulates, or joins, superiorly with the occipital bone and inferiorly with the axis (the second vertebra). These joints and the muscles that surround them allow the head to turn and nod. Nodding of the head is made possible by the articulation of the atlas and the occipital bone, and turning of the head is an ability created by the articulation of the atlas and the axis.

The face and head are nourished through the body's blood supply by specific veins and arteries. Typically the name of each artery (see Figure 15-3) corresponds to a vein with the same, or at least very similar, name. The main artery of the body is the aorta. The aorta branches off of the left ventricle of the heart to direct the blood flow throughout the body. The first part of the aorta is called the ascending aorta and contains the aortic arch. Branching off the ascending aorta and its arch are two arteries called the carotid arteries. There is a right and a left carotid artery. Each branch ascends the right and left lateral aspects of the neck, respectively, and further subdivides into the internal and external carotid arteries. These arteries are the main blood supply to the neck and head. The location of the external carotid artery is important to remember as the site where the pulse is palpated to determine whether or not CPR is required. Arteries transport the blood away from the heart, bringing newly oxygenated blood and nutrients to the areas they serve. Wherever a pulse is palpated, an artery exists.

The veins are named in the same fashion as the arteries. Veins carry blood back to the heart and lungs so the waste products can then be excreted from the body and the blood re-oxygenated for the cells. Because of the abundant blood supply to the head and face, open wounds to these areas tend to produce what can appear to be a large amount of bleeding.

The Nervous System

One of the most complex and fascinating systems of the human body is the nervous system. Its main components are the brain, cranial nerves, spinal cord, spinal nerves, and peripheral nerves. A highly organized and intricate system, its main function is to coordinate and regulate the body's many responses to internal and/or external environmental changes. The nervous system also determines the body's response to stimuli. A stimulant is anything that produces a temporary increase in the functional activity or efficiency of an organism.

The basic structural unit of the nervous system is the nerve cell, or neuron. Neurons differ from common cells in their design and specific function. A neuron has a cell body that contains a nucleus, several dendrites (cytoplasmic branches off the cell body that transmit impulses to the body of the cell), and an axon (a branch off of the cell body that conducts impulses away from the body of the cell). The main function of the neuron is to cause the body to react to its environment.

Two types of neurons exist in different areas of the body (see Figure 15-4). Sensory neurons, or afferent neurons, are found in the skin and in the sensory organs. These neurons transmit messages, or impulses, from the sensory organs and the skin to the brain and spinal cord. The second kind of neuron is the motor, or efferent, neuron. Motor neurons originate in the brain or spinal cord and carry impulses to the muscles and glands of the body, enabling the body to react to its environment. For example, if a person touches a hot surface, the sensory neurons will detect heat, and the motor neurons will cause the body to remove the hand away from the heat source. Mixed nerves, as the name implies, are a combination of sensory and motor neurons.

A nerve is a combination of several identical nerve fibers located outside the brain or spinal cord. Nerves originate in a specific nerve center, either the brain or the spinal cord, and infiltrate other organs as well as the muscles and skin, conveying impulses from one part of the body to another.

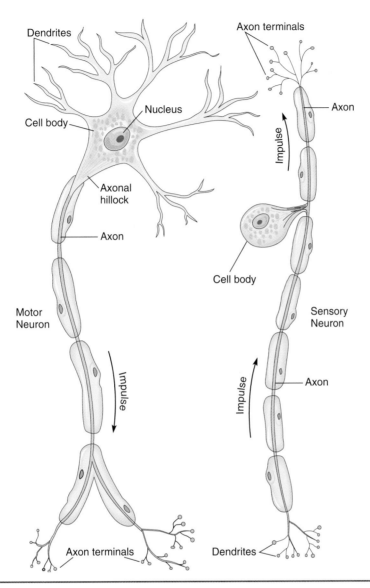

FIGURE 15-4 The Neurons

The Central Nervous System

There are two main divisions within the nervous system: the central nervous system (CNS) and the peripheral nervous system (PNS).

The central nervous system consists of the brain and the spinal cord (see Figure 15-5). The brain is located within the skull and performs numerous functions, primarily controlling and coordinating the body's activities. In order to perform at its highest potential, the brain requires an ample supply of oxygen and dextrose, a form of sugar.

The brain is surrounded by a protective barrier of membranes called meninges (see Figure 15-6). There are three layers of meninges: the outer layer, called the dura mater, is thick and strong; the middle layer, called the arachnoid

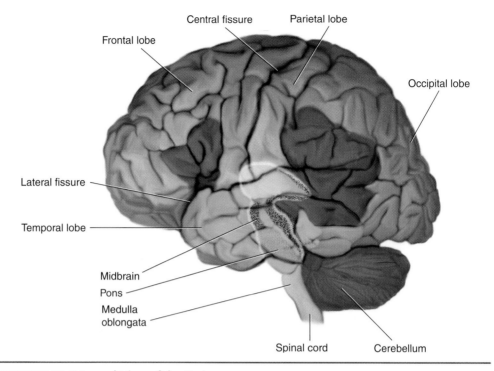

FIGURE 15-5 Lateral View of the Brain

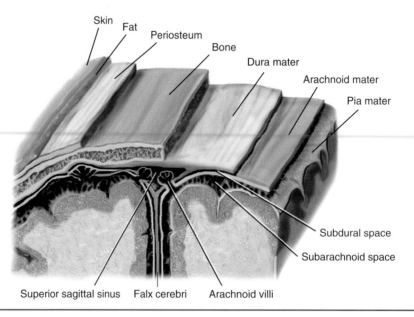

FIGURE 15-6 Meninges and Related Structures

membrane, is very delicate and resembles a spider's web; and the inner layer, called the pia mater, is directly connected to the brain and the spinal cord. The pia mater contains many blood vessels that provide nourishment to both structures. Between each of these layers is a space. The space between the dura mater and the skull is the epidural space; the subdural space is between the dura mater and the arachnoid membrane; and the subarachnoid space is between the arachnoid layer and the pia mater.

Contained within the brain are four hollow spaces, called ventricles, that connect to each other and the subarachnoid space. The ventricles constantly produce cerebrospinal fluid (CSF)—a clear, colorless, watery fluid that flows through and protects the brain and the spinal cord by acting as a shock absorber. Cerebrospinal fluid provides nourishment to and removes different waste products from the brain and spinal cord. Eventually, CSF becomes absorbed by the veins of the dura mater.

The brain contains many specialized areas. However, for the purposes of this book, only the larger sections will be addressed.

The cerebrum controls willful actions; interprets sensory messages gained from sound, sight, smell, touch, and taste; and governs thought and speech. The cerebrum is the largest part of the brain. Taking up most of the cranial cavity, it is separated into two halves and made up of two layers: gray matter, the outer layer; and white matter, the inner layer.

The cerebellum is responsible for muscle coordination and tone and for maintaining balance and posture. It is located below the cerebrum in the posterior cranial cavity.

The midbrain is located below the cerebrum and above the brain stem. It is responsible for conducting impulses throughout the brain and for conducting certain visual and auditory reflexes.

The pons is located within the brain stem, below the cerebrum. It acts mainly as a bridge between two or more sections of the brain and is responsible for conducting certain impulses throughout the brain and for some reflexive actions, such as chewing and salivation.

The medulla oblongata is located at the base of the brain stem and protrudes slightly over the spinal cord. It controls involuntary actions such as respiration, heartbeat, blood pressure, swallowing, and coughing.

The spinal cord is attached to the medulla oblongata and continues down to the first or second lumbar vertebrae of the back. It is protected by the vertebrae, cerebrospinal fluid, and meninges. The spinal cord's two major functions are to conduct impulses through afferent and efferent nerves, and to connect the body parts to the brain.

The Peripheral Nervous System

The peripheral nervous system is outside the central nervous system and is responsible for gathering information and carrying the response signals to and from the CNS. It is composed of the nerves located outside the brain and spinal cord. The peripheral nervous system is subdivided into the somatic nervous system and the autonomic nervous system.

The somatic nervous system is the part of the peripheral nervous system that controls skeletal muscles responsible for voluntary movement. There are 12 pairs of cranial nerves within the brain. Each pair is responsible for one or more functions, such as sight, taste, hearing, smell, and facial responses, such as smiling. The spinal cord contains 31 pairs of specialized nerves called spinal nerves.

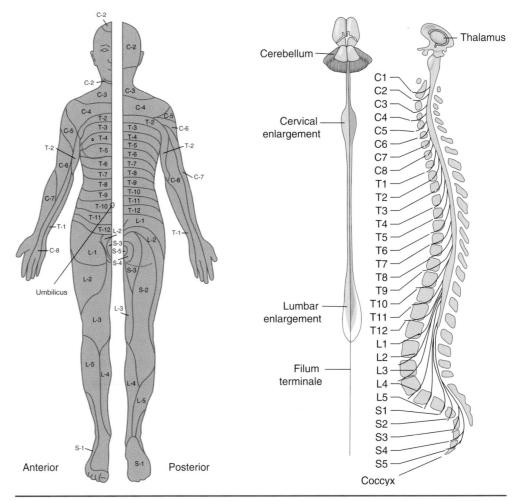

FIGURE 15-7 Areas of Skin Innervation and Associated Nerves

The axons and dendrites of these cranial and spinal nerves extend into the outer parts of the body. These cranial nerves, spinal nerves, and their axons and dendrites make up the somatic (pertaining to the body) nervous system (see Figure 15-7). The right side of the brain controls the left side of the body and vice versa. When the spinal cord sustains injury, the degree of damage depends on where the spinal cord was injured.

The autonomic nervous system regulates the balance between the involuntary functions of the body and causes the body to react in emergency situations (see Figure 15-8). This system also is separated into two divisions that maintain homeostasis within the body: the sympathetic nervous system and the parasympathetic nervous system.

The sympathetic nervous system controls many involuntary activities of the glands, organs, and other parts of the body. It prepares the body for a "fight-or-flight" response to an emergency situation by increasing the respiratory and heart rate, raising the blood pressure, and slowing the digestive processes. The parasympathetic nervous system, which has the opposite effect on the body, complements the activities of the sympathetic nervous system. It acts as a brake by slowing the heart and respiratory rates, lowering blood pressure, and increasing the activity of the digestive system. These two systems work together to keep the body's involuntary responses to stimuli in balance.

TREATING A DOWNED ATHLETE: A REVIEW

Head and spine injuries require immediate attention. As discussed in Chapter 9, if the athlete is down and unconscious, always treat the athlete as if he or she has a possible head or spine injury. As with any injury in which the player is down, start the athlete's injury assessment by doing a primary survey (see Chapter 9). Also, when approaching the downed athlete, note the time in case the athlete is unconscious. The total time of unconsciousness will need to be noted on the injury assessment. If there is a second person available, have that person keep nonessential personnel away from the athlete. Establishing control of the environment will aid in concentrating on the

Parasympathetic Nervous System		Sympathetic Nervous System
constricts pupils		dilates pupils
stimulates salivation		inhibits salivation
slows heart rate		accelerates heart rate
constricts bronchi	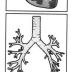	dilates bronchi
stimulates gastric juice production		inhibits gastric juice production
no action		stimulates release of epinephrine and norepinephrine
accelerates digestive process and relaxes the rectum		inhibits dgestive process and contracts the rectum
contracts bladder muscles		relaxes bladder muscles

FIGURE 15-8 The Autonomic Nervous System

assessment and will help keep the athlete from panicking. Record all findings during the history and evaluation.

Remember, any face mask must be removed to perform CPR. However, do not take off the helmet, because this might injure the player further. Removal of the face mask can be done using the Trainer's Angel or another tool to cut all clips of the helmet (procedure is explained in Chapter 9). Then lift the mask off. Cutting off the face mask and turning the athlete from face-down to face-up should be practiced to the point that the rescuer is very comfortable doing either maneuver in an emergency.

If the athlete is not breathing or there is no pulse, call for EMS (emergency medical services) and begin CPR. Continue CPR until the EMS arrives. If the athlete is face-down, has no pulse, and is not breathing, carefully turn the athlete using the log roll method, making sure the head, neck, and body rotate as a unit as shown in Chapter 13. Once the athlete is on the back, CPR can be administered.

> ### NOTE:
>
> If the athlete is face-down but is breathing and has a pulse, stabilize the head and neck and leave the athlete in that position. Call the EMS. Continue to monitor the vital signs. If the athlete's pulse or respiration stops, log roll the athlete, and then begin CPR.

If the athlete is breathing and has a pulse but is unconscious, continue the evaluation by first trying to revive the athlete. Gently try to get the athlete's attention, calling the athlete's name as you speak. Do not try to wake the athlete by shaking—this might cause further injury. As soon as possible, have someone call EMS. While waiting for EMS, continue to check all vital signs and attempt to revive the athlete. Get a history of what happened from officials or anyone else who saw the event.

If the athlete regains consciousness, note the total time that the athlete was unconscious. This information will be useful in the present and future treatment of the injured athlete.

While maintaining the athlete's body and head in a stable position until EMS arrives, continue with the secondary survey and assure the athlete that everything possible is being done to avoid further injury.

Obtain a history of events from the athlete; this information can be used to check mental orientation. Make sure you know the answers to any questions you ask the athlete.

Start with simple questions such as:

* What is your name and the name of your school?

* Do you know where you are?

* Do you remember what happened?

* Do you have a headache or ringing in your ears?

* Does your neck hurt? Do you have pain or numbness anywhere?

* Give the person four numbers to repeat (4, 8, 2, 6) immediately and again in 5 minutes while continuing to check for any signs of impaired consciousness.

Calm the athlete if necessary and check the eyes for a glassy look or vacant stare. Check the pupils for reaction to light; normal pupils will react to light by constricting. If the pupils are equal in size, ask the athlete if he or she has any blurred or double vision. If the pupils are unequal, it may or may not be a sign of a head injury; some people normally have unequal pupils. It is important to take the time to know the normal size of each athlete's pupils before injuries occur so it will be apparent if an injury has made one or both unusually large for that athlete. If the pupils seem abnormal, make sure these findings are relayed to the EMS and the physician.

Check to make sure the athlete is able to move hands, feet, and toes without help. Make sure the athlete has feeling in both legs and arms. Glide one hand over the athlete's neck to feel for any possible deformities or point tenderness. If at any time the athlete shows symptoms of a spinal cord injury (numbness anywhere below the neck, decreased strength, or decreased motion), stabilize the head and neck and call the EMS. Never put a pillow under the neck of a patient with a potential neck injury. Continue to protect the head and spine and monitor vital signs until the EMS arrives.

When evaluating the athlete, remember the steps of the secondary survey (see Chapter 9). Performing the entire secondary survey may or may not be necessary. For instance, if you see the injury occur, and the athlete is not complaining of any other concerns, the isolated injury assessment is the more logical choice. However, if while doing the assessment any signs or symptoms of additional injury are noticed, call the EMS and proceed with the step-by-step secondary survey. It is always better to be extra cautious than to risk oversight.

If the athlete has no symptoms of a spinal cord injury, the athlete is then permitted to sit up without assistance. Then reevaluate the situation, and check to see if the athlete is still coherent and not dizzy. Bring the athlete to a standing position and once again recheck to make sure the athlete is not dizzy and does not have any increase in signs or symptoms. Have the injured athlete walk to the side of the field or gym where the athlete can be reevaluated for any further problems. Statistics show that as many as 25% of those *with* spinal fractures are often able to walk under their own power and do *not* complain of any symptoms or show any signs of spinal cord injury. Always maintain a high index of suspicion based on the mechanism of injury. If allowing an athlete to walk off the field, continue monitoring until the athlete is released from the event.

Once the athlete is on the sidelines, check coordination by asking the athlete to stand on two feet with eyes closed (known as the Romberg test). Check to see if the athlete loses balance. Follow this with the tandem gait test by asking the athlete to walk a straight line as if on a rope (place the heel of one foot directly ahead of the toes of the other foot) for about 5 feet. Report any inability to complete these tests to the physician or EMS.

As with all injuries, make sure to document what occurred. In a school setting or working with minors, contact the parents or guardian with any concerns and make sure they receive the Head Injury and Concussion Information form discussed in Chapter 10.

INJURIES TO THE BRAIN

The brain regulates and coordinates the body's activities and is the primary organ of the nervous system. As such, it is responsible for receiving sensory impulses, interpreting sensations, and forming perceptions. These processes are what make thought, speech, action, emotion, memory, reason, and judgement possible. A network of nerves (the peripheral nervous system) that extends from the central nervous system to every part of the body serve as the information pathways along which the sensory impulses travel to and from the CNS. The brain then generates an appropriate motor response from the body, such as moving away from a source of perceived heat or responding to a question. (See the section about the nervous system earlier in this chapter.) Given this information, it should be easy to see why injuries that may involve the brain must be taken very seriously.

EVALUATING A HEAD INJURY

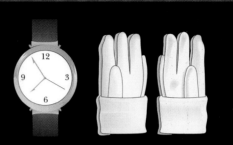

Materials Needed:

* a digital or analog watch with a second hand
* gloves (if blood or other body fluids are present)

1. **Procedural Step:** Wash your hands if possible.

   Reason: Universal Precaution.

2. **Procedural Step:** Put on gloves if there is any blood or other body fluid present.

   Reason: Universal Precaution.

3. **Procedural Step:** Check the time on your watch as you approach the athlete.

   Reason: If the athlete is unconscious, you will need to keep track of how long unconsciousness lasts.

4. **Procedural Step:** Perform the primary survey (check the ABCs) (see Chapter 9). Activate the EMS and begin CPR if needed (see Chapter 13).

   Reason: To make sure the victim is breathing and has a pulse, and to check for consciousness.

5. **Procedural Step:** If the athlete is conscious and shows no signs of a spinal injury, evaluate the athlete for the following symptoms of a concussion: headache, dizziness, lack of awareness of surroundings, and nausea (with or without vomiting).

   Reason: To start the evaluation for a concussion and rule out spinal injury, knowing both of these can be fatal.

6. **Procedural Step:** If the athlete shows one or more of the above symptoms, ask the athlete to do the following tests:

   Repeat a series of numbers (e.g., 4-8-2-9).

   Recite the months of the year in reverse.

   Remember three words (e.g., green, play, sports) and three objects (e.g., bench, ball, car) for five minutes.

   Do a Romberg test, followed by a tandem gait test.

   Increase activity by having the athlete run 40 yards, do five push-ups, five sit-ups, and five knee bends without headache or dizziness.

   Reason: Loss of memory and/or the inability to understand and follow instructions may indicate a brain injury.

7. **Procedural Step:** If the athlete is unable to perform any of the above activities, the athlete should be excluded from play. See Chapter 22 for more return-to-play guidelines.

   Reason: If the athlete is allowed to play, the injury could become worse.

EVALUATING A HEAD INJURY

8. Procedural Step: Recheck the athlete in 5 minutes. If the athlete passed all the tests in step 6 and passes them again after 5 minutes, the athlete may return to play after 15 minutes if monitored closely. If the athlete fails the tests at any time, call the EMS.

Reason: Head injuries can be fatal.

9. Procedural Step: Remove and dispose of your gloves if it was necessary to put them on.

Reason: Universal Precaution.

10. Procedural Step: Wash your hands.

Reason: Universal Precaution.

11. Procedural Step: Record all steps you have taken and provide a copy of that information to the physician or the EMS if they become involved.

Reason: To provide continuity of care.

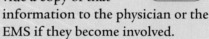

Continuous blood flow to the brain is necessary in order to provide all of the brain cells with oxygen and dextrose. An interruption in the blood flow to any part of the brain may result in a brain injury. Any type of brain injury can result in an accumulation of waste products such as carbon dioxide and lactic acid, which can cause the brain to swell. As the brain swells, there is increased pressure within the skull. Increased intracranial pressure may also result from an accumulation of excessive blood or excessive production of cerebrospinal fluid. Swelling of the brain tissue can reduce the blood supply to the brain, leading to further complications including permanent brain damage or death.

Concussions

Cerebral **concussions** occur frequently in sports; in football alone, over 250,000 concussions occur each year. They are caused most frequently by direct blows to the head; however, sudden jerks of the head and neck can also produce concussions. A cerebral concussion causes immediate symptoms—headache, dizziness, nausea, and symptoms of disorientation and confusion resulting from swelling at the point of contact. The injury causes a temporary stoppage in the blood supply to the brain. The injured person should be examined very carefully immediately after the injury has occurred.

Concussions can be aggravated by a condition known as **second-impact syndrome (SIS)**. This syndrome results when an athlete with a concussion returns to play before the signs and symptoms are resolved and receives another jarring blow. The shock from the second blow can lead to more serious complications and may be fatal.

At times, the sports medicine professional may not have the benefit of knowing that an athlete has received a head injury; he or she may not be present when the injury occured and the athlete may not want to or even be able to admit that something is wrong. For this reason, learn to recognize the following post-concussive symptoms.

---

concussion

injury to the brain or spinal cord, accompanied by loss of neural function, resulting from a blow to the head or a fall.

second-impact syndrome (SIS)

a second concussion received before the signs and symptoms of the first concussion have been resolved: a life-threatening emergency.

* Any loss of consciousness

* Persistent low-grade headache

* Light-headedness

* Poor concentration

* **Posttraumatic amnesia**, either retrograde amnesia (no memory of some of the time immediately before the injury) or anterograde amnesia (no memory of being injured or of the time immediately following the injury)

* Sleepiness

* Loss of coordination

* Slurred or incoherent speech

* Irritability

* Anxiety

* Depression

* Ringing in the ears (tinnitus)

* Vacant stare

* Disorientation

* Nausea and/or vomiting

* Pupils not reacting evenly to light or unresponsive

posttraumatic amnesia

loss of memory for events immediately before or following a trauma.

These can be severe, life-threatening symptoms. Even if only one of these symptoms is present, the victim may have a concussion. Make sure all interested parties (athlete's family, the coach, other team members, etc.) are made aware of the above symptoms. Because concussions can be life-threatening, they are categorized according to severity. Guidelines for concussion severity have been created by several organizations and authors, such as the Colorado Medical Society, Robert Cantu, M.D., and the American Academy of Neurology. The guidelines shown in Figure 15-9 are based on information derived from these sources.

Concussion Severity Reference Guide

Concussion Grade	Cantu Grading System (2001 Revision)[*]
Grade 1 (mild)	* No loss of consciousness (LOC) * Either posttraumatic amnesia (PTA) or post-concussion signs and symptoms that clear in less than 30 minutes
Grade 2 (moderate)	* LOC lasting less than 1 minute and PTA *or* * Post-concussion signs or symptoms lasting longer than 30 minutes but less than 24 hours
Grade 3 (severe)	* LOC lasting more than 1 minute *or* * PTA lasting longer than 24 hours *or* * Post-concussion signs or symptoms lasting longer than 7 days

[*]Cantu, R.C. "Posttraumatic retrograde and anterograde amnesia: Pathophysiology and implications in grading and safe return to play." *Journal of Athletic Training.* 2001; 36(3): 244–248. This grading system modifies the original Cantu grading system proposed in Cantu, R.C. "Guidelines for return to contact sports after a cerebral concussion." *Physician Sportsmed.* 1986; 14(10): 75–83.

FIGURE 15-9 Concussion Severity Reference Guide

Guidelines the Physician May Use

Concussion Grade	Number of Concussions Suffered	Cantu Guidelines (Revised)[*]
Grade 1 (mild)	First	* Return to play after 1 symptom-free week * End season if CT or MRI abnormal
Grade 1 (mild)	Second	* Return to play in 2 weeks after 1 symptom-free week
Grade 1 (mild)	Third	* End season * May return to play next season if no symptoms
Grade 2 (moderate)	First	* Return to play after 1 symptom-free week
Grade 2 (moderate)	Second	* May not return for minimum of 1 month * May return to play then if symptom-free for 1 week * Consider ending season
Grade 2 (moderate)	Third	* End season * May return to play next season if without symptoms
Grade 3 (severe)	First	* May not return to play for minimum of 1 month * May return to play then after 1 symptom-free week
Grade 3 (severe)	Second	* End season * May return to play next season if no symptoms

[*]Cantu, R.C. "Posttraumatic retrograde and anterograde amnesia: Pathophysiology and implications in grading and safe return to play." *Journal of Athletic Training.* 2001; 36(3): 244–248. This grading system modifies the original Cantu grading system proposed in Cantu, R.C. "Guidelines for return to contact sports after a cerebral concussion." *Physician Sportsmed.* 1986; 14(10): 75–83.

FIGURE 15-10 Guidelines the Physician May Use

Immediate Treatment: Athletes with any type of concussion must be removed from play. If an athlete has a Grade 1 concussion, an adult must accompany the athlete to the physicians (the athlete should not be allowed to drive). If the athlete is a minor, make sure the parents are notified of the injury. For a Grade 2 or Grade 3 concussion, activate the EMS. Monitor all vital signs while awaiting the EMS. Again, if the athlete is a minor, make sure the parents are notified of the injury (record this conversation in a note with the injury report). Use the Head Injury and Concussion Information form in Chapter 10 to inform the athlete and/or parents/guardian of the warning signs of possible complications.

Follow-up Treatment: Regardless of the injury's grade, do not allow the athlete to return to play until cleared (in writing) by a physician. Figure 15-10 shows guidelines for return to play that a physician might be expected to use, depending on the number and severity of concussions the athlete has received. See Chapter 22 for further information on return to play.

Prevention: Make sure athletes wear appropriate head protection and that it fits properly. Even a haircut can alter the way a helmet fits. Therefore, all head gear should be checked daily for proper fit. Sports requiring protective head gear include bicycling, baseball, wrestling, rodeo, football, and hockey. Mouthpieces may also help to reduce the shock of a blow to the head. In addition, exercises that increase neck strength and flexibility are recommended.

INJURIES TO THE EAR

The ear makes it possible for us to hear and maintain our balance, or equilibrium. It is divided into three sections: the outer ear, the middle ear, and the inner ear (see Figure 15-11). The outer ear, known as the auricle or pinna, is made of cartilage that projects from the head. The pinna leads into the external auditory canal and ends at the tympanic membrane (the eardrum).

The middle ear, or tympanic cavity, is between the tympanic membrane (eardrum) and the inner ear, and leads to the internal auditory canal, called the eustachian tube. This tube conducts sound to the inner ear by passing sound vibrations from the air outside to the fluid in the inner ear via a chain of three tiny bones called ossicles: the malleus, the incus, and the stapes. Air enters and leaves the middle ear through the eustachian tube. This tube is directly connected to the upper part of the throat, making the ear and throat susceptible to infection. The eustachian tube allows the air pressure in the middle ear to equal the air pressure entering the external auditory canal, keeping the air pressure on both sides of the tympanic membrane equal. When pressure is unequal, a popping sound can often be heard. The tympanic membrane and the ossicles are extremely delicate and may be injured by the violent movement of air waves (e.g., explosions, loud music, or shouting directly into the ear).

The inner ear is the most important and complex structure of the ear. The anterior of the inner ear contains the oval window and the cochlea, which holds the sensory receptors for hearing; and the posterior contains the vestibule and the

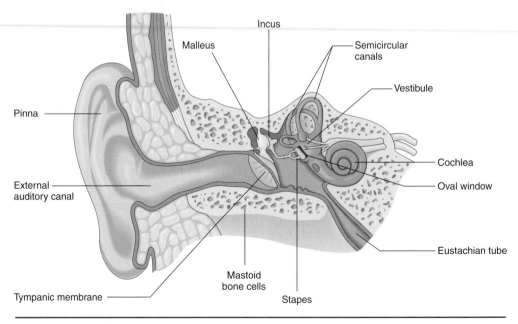

FIGURE 15-11 The Ear

semicircular canals, which include the receptors for equilibrium and the sense of position. These canals contain fluid that moves in response to head and body movements. The movement of the fluid is sensed by tiny hair cells that line the canals. These cells convey messages about the movements to the brain via nerve fibers, forming our sense of balance and equilibrium. Any forceful blow to the side of the head can affect one's balance as well as one's ability to hear.

In sports, injuries to the ear usually involve the external ear and can include any of the tissue injuries discussed in Chapter 14. To prevent tissue injuries to the ears, make sure the athletes wear proper head protection, including helmets and/or ear guards. Apply petroleum jelly or skin lube to the ears to prevent friction, and caution the athletes to remove all earrings prior to play.

> **NOTE:**
>
> Any time clear fluid or blood is present in the ears, send the athlete to a physician for further care or contact the EMS.

Cauliflower Ear

Hematoma auris (cauliflower ear) is the most common injury of the ear in sports activity. It is caused by extreme friction, or by repeated trauma to the ear as occurs in such sports as wrestling and boxing. The signs and symptoms include tearing of the cartilage in the external ear, which results in bleeding and fluid accumulation around the ear.

Immediate Treatment: For first aid, apply ice, use compression, and put a bandage on the ear. Send the athlete to a physician for further care. In the event that the injured person experiences dizziness or hearing loss immediately following the blow to the ear, send the person to a physician *at once* to avoid any permanent damage to the ear.

Follow-up Treatment: Because the ear is vulnerable to reinjury while it is healing, make sure the athlete wears proper head gear and/or ear guards during practice and play. Make sure the physician's orders are followed. Check the ear daily for signs and symptoms of infection.

Prevention: To prevent cauliflower ear, apply petroleum jelly to the ears to reduce friction, and make sure the athletes wear proper ear guards and other appropriate head gear (e.g., helmets) for protection.

Otitis Externa (Swimmer's Ear)

Otitis externa is an infection of the ear canal. It occurs when moisture is trapped in the external ear canal by an accumulation of ear wax, a foreign object, swelling, or some other blockage. This frequently affects swimmers, which is why it is often called "swimmer's ear." Symptoms include dizziness, pain, itching, discharge, and partial hearing loss.

Immediate Treatment: Dry the ear thoroughly, use the drops mentioned below, and send the athlete to a physician.

Follow-up Treatment: Make sure the physician's orders are followed.

Prevention: Advise athletes to dry the ears thoroughly and use ear drops containing a 3% boric acid and alcohol solution before and after swimming. They may also wear rubber or wax ear plugs to keep water out of the ear. Caution them to never stick objects, such as cotton swabs, in the ear, as this may force fluid farther into the ear. Cold temperatures and wind can aggravate the condition, so athletes should avoid ear exposure to such elements, especially if water is in the ears.

Rupture of the Tympanic Membrane

A rupture of the tympanic membrane is most likely to occur in contact sports, water polo, and diving. It can be ruptured as a result of a sudden change in pressure, such as that experienced by a diver, or from a fall or slap to an unprotected ear. The membrane can also be ruptured by an object that is inserted too far into the ear. Victims of this condition will complain of a loud pop, followed by pain, dizziness, hearing loss, nausea, and vomiting. Bleeding and tinnitus may also occur. The hole created by the rupture can be viewed using an otoscope.

Immediate Treatment: Send the patient to a physician as quickly as possible. It will usually heal spontaneously in about two weeks, but the physician will need to monitor the ear for infection and check for any additional injury. This injury requires removal from play in aquatic sports.

Follow-up Treatment: Monitor the area for signs of infection or any other concerns. Make sure the physician's orders are followed. Do not allow the athlete to return to play without written permission from the physician.

Prevention: Make sure the athletes wear ear protection in contact sports, especially wrestling, during both practice and games. Caution the athletes not to insert objects into the ears.

Foreign Bodies in the Ear

Rarely, foreign objects can enter and/or become trapped in an athlete's ear. For instance, it is possible for a bug to fly or crawl into the ear. Symptoms may include pain, itching, and potential hearing loss.

Immediate Treatment: Send the athlete to a physician for care. *Do not* stick anything into the ear as it could force the object further into the ear and potentially puncture the tympanic membrane.

Follow-up Treatment: Make sure the physician's orders are followed.

Prevention: Caution the athletes not to insert objects into the ears.

INJURIES TO THE EYE

The eye is a delicate and detailed organ. The eyeball is spherical in shape and is protected anteriorly by the skull bones and inferiorly by facial bones that form the eye socket, or orbit. The eyelid and eyelashes protect the anterior portion by helping to keep out foreign bodies such as dust, dirt, and pathogens.

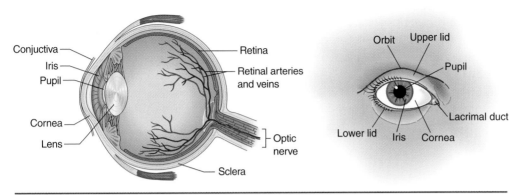

FIGURE 15-12 The Eye

The eye is made up of many different parts, each one playing a significant role in a person's ability to see (see Figure 15-12). The eyeball is surrounded by three layers of protective tissue. The outer layer, called the sclera, is made from firm, tough, connective tissue and is white in color. The middle layer, called the choroid coat, is a delicate network of connective tissue that contains many blood vessels. The inner layer, which is called the retina, contains the nerve receptors for vision and approximately ten different layers of nerve cells. Two kinds of nerve cells are contained within the retina: cones, which are used mainly for light vision; and rods, which are used when it is dark or dim.

There are several other important structures contained in the eye. The cornea is the clear front portion of the eye. The cornea is very sensitive to injury; visual problems can result if it becomes scarred. The main function of the cornea is to permit light rays to pass through to the retina, which allows the image to be relayed to the brain. Lacrimal glands located within the orbit constantly produce tears, which lubricate the eye and allow it to glide smoothly within the socket and under the eyelid. A clear, mucous membrane, called the conjunctiva, covers the inner eyelids and the front of the eyeball—except for the cornea. Both the lacrimal glands and the conjunctiva protect the eye.

A person's eye color is determined by the color of the iris. This muscular structure at the front of the eyeball allows the pupil to adjust its size, depending on the amount of light entering the eye. The pupil is the black circle in the middle of the iris. It constricts (becomes smaller) when bright light enters it and when focusing on something at close range. The pupil dilates (becomes larger) when the light is dim and when focusing on distant objects. Certain drugs, injuries to the head, eye surgeries, and neurological disorders also can affect pupil size. As light enters the iris, it passes through to the lens, which is located directly behind the iris. The lens then refracts, or bends, the light rays directly to the retina.

The shape of the eyeball is maintained by the aqueous humor and the vitreous humor. The aqueous humor is a clear, watery fluid found in the anterior and posterior chambers of the eye. It refracts light rays to the retina. The vitreous humor fills the entire cavity behind the lens and helps in light ray refraction.

Each eye has six extraocular muscles that coordinate eye movement. Five nerves also serve each eye: two sensory nerves and three motor nerves. Sensory nerves detect sensory information such as pain, temperature, and burning, while motor nerves transmit messages that result in movement.

In sports activity, the eyes are vulnerable to trauma from impact with fingers, elbows, and other objects. In fact, certain equipment involved in games such as racquetball, squash, badminton, tennis, baseball, and basketball are potential sources of injury to the eye. For instance, imagine the force at which a baseball or tennis ball might strike the eye. Blows to the eye can cause a variety of injuries ranging from the mild, such as a black eye, to the serious, such as a detached retina. Symptoms of injury to the eye include eye irritation, pain, discoloration, bleeding, tearing, and any vision disturbance, including double vision (diplopa).

Contusions

A blow to the eye may cause a contusion (bruise). If there is bleeding in the blood vessels around the eye or the temporal regions of the face, raccoon's eyes (black eyes) may occur (see Figure 15-13). Swelling may also result.

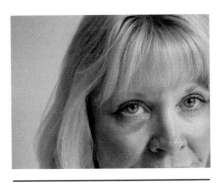

FIGURE 15-13 Black eyes are known as raccoon's eyes and can be caused by a fracture of the skull at the eyebrow.

Immediate Treatment: Ice the surrounding tissues immediately for 20 minutes, followed by an hour in which the ice is off. Repeat this cycle for a 24- to 72-hour period during waking hours, or until the swelling subsides. Raccoon's eyes can be a symptom of a fracture of the orbit, so, athletes who develop a black eye should be seen by a physician. In all cases, if the injury is not slight and easily resolved, it's best to have the injury looked at by a doctor. If the bleeding occurs in the anterior portion of the eye (a condition known as hyphema) or if there is double vision, the injury could be very serious, and the injured person should consult a physician immediately.

Follow-up Treatment: Monitor the wound to make sure the swelling decreases, and make sure the physician's orders are followed. Also check the patient for any additional signs or symptoms that may have occurred from the blow to the eye. If any of the signs or symptoms get worse, have the injured person go to a physician for further care.

contact sports

sports in which physical contact between players is expected during the normal course of play.

Prevention: Athletes and others who engage in high-risk **contact sports**, particularly sports that use high-velocity objects in play, (such as racquetball or squash) should wear face guards.

Corneal Abrasions or Lacerations

Sand, dirt, insects, or other airborne particles can fly into and scratch the corneal surface of the athlete's eye, causing a corneal abrasion or laceration. Such injuries can cause severe pain and watering of the eye and sometimes even a spasm of the muscle around it. Corneal abrasions and lacerations may also be caused by contact with another player's fingers.

Immediate Treatment: Do not allow the athlete to rub the eye. Patch the eye and send the athlete to the physician. Ask the athlete to try turn the head to look in a different direction rather than to shift the eyes, because eye movement can cause additional irritation. If the athlete seems to have difficulty remembering to avoid eye movement, patch both eyes to reduce the potential for further injury to the affected eye.

Follow-up Treatment: Make sure the physician's orders are followed. If any of the signs or symptoms get worse, have the athlete contact the physician for further care. Remind the injured person of the importance of taking any prescribed medication.

Prevention: When the activity area is dry and windy, it is a good time to cover one's eyes. In sports such as motocross, eye goggles are recommend to prevent such eye problems.

Retinal Detachment

A blow to the eye can cause retinal detachment, which is the separation of the retina from the underlying epithelium. The detachment is painless; the patient will see flashes of light and have blurred vision. When it worsens, the patient will complain of a "curtain" or something similar covering the field of vision.

If the retina is detached, the symptoms may not be immediate, but over a period of days (sometimes much more) the injured person's vision will contain floating particles, vision distortion, and abrupt light changes.

Immediate Treatment: Patch the eye and send the patient immediately to the physician (ophthalmologist) for further care and diagnosis.

Follow-up Treatment: Make sure the physician's orders are followed. If any of the signs or symptoms get worse, have the injured person contact the physician for further care. Remind the injured person of the importance of taking any prescribed medication.

Prevention: Protective eye goggles should be worn in sports such as racquetball, squash, and other sports that carry risk of direct blows to the eye.

Foreign Bodies and Embedded Objects

During sports activity it is possible for foreign bodies such as dust particles to become embedded in the eye. Symptoms include pain, itching, tearing, and redness.

Immediate Treatment: Make sure that the athlete does not rub the eyes. Use an eyecup to flush the eyes with water. Also try to attract small particles out with the corner of a moistened cloth. If unable to draw out any of the particles, patch both the affected eye and the unaffected eye with sterile gauze and transport the athlete to the physician for further evaluation. Both eyes are patched to prevent further damage to the eye containing the particle; since both eyeballs move together, it is important to limit the movement of the unaffected eye so the damaged eye will not move with it.

Follow-up Treatment: Make sure the physician's orders are followed. Remind the athlete of any medication that needs to be taken and monitor the eye for signs of infection. If at any time the injury seems to worsen, contact the athlete's physician for further care.

Prevention: Eye protection such as goggles should be worn in dusty or dirty conditions—such as on baseball fields and tracks—and when the wind is blowing.

Fractures—Orbital Roof and Blowout

An orbital fracture is a fracture of the orbital roof of the eye, caused by a direct blow to the eye. A blowout fracture is a break in the floor of the orbital socket resulting from a direct blow to the eye. Symptoms for both of these fractures include swelling, hemorrhaging, and possible double vision (diplopia). There are also nerves around the area that can be involved.

Immediate Treatment: Control any bleeding using direct pressure, but in doing so, be careful not to cause unnecessary additional pain to the athlete. Patch the eye with sterile gauze and send the patient to the physician (ophthalmologist) for further care and diagnosis.

Follow-up Treatment: Make sure the physician's orders are followed. Remind the athlete of any medication that must be taken and monitor the wound for signs of infection. If at any time the injury seems to worsen, contact the athlete's physician for further care.

Prevention: Baseball, lacrosse, racquetball, and squash players are particularly vulnerable to fractures of the eye. Therefore, these athletes and any others who engage in activities involving objects that move at high speeds should wear protective goggles during play.

Conjunctivitis

Conjunctivitis is inflammation of the conjunctiva. Signs and symptoms include burning and itching around the eye and swollen eyelids. Occasionally, a yellow discharge is present as well.

Immediate Treatment: Acute conjunctivitis (pinkeye) can be highly contagious, so whenever contact is made with infected eyes be sure to wear gloves and wash your hands. Regardless of the type of conjunctivitis, send the athlete to a physician for further care and diagnosis. Caution the patient not to touch the eyes to avoid the potential of spreading the infection. If the patient does touch the eyes, the hands should be washed thoroughly. Athletes in contact sports may be restricted from play. Make sure to check with the physician for guidelines.

Follow-up Treatment: Make sure the physician's orders are followed. Monitor the wound for signs of infection and remind the athlete of any medication that must be taken. If at any time the condition seems to worsen, contact the athlete's physician for further care.

Prevention: Avoid contact with inflamed eyes and their secretions. Anyone who comes in contact with a person who has symptoms of conjunctivitis should wash the hands immediately.

Sty

A sty is the result of an infection of the eyelid follicle or the subcutaneous gland, often near the eyelashes. The infection may be caused by a small piece of dirt under the eyelid. Typically, a sty is very painful; symptoms often include redness and swelling.

Immediate Treatment: Flush the eye if it is believed that the particle may still be present. Apply a moist heat pack, making sure it is not too hot for the sensitive eye area, and send the athlete to a physician for further care and diagnosis.

Follow-up Treatment: Make sure the physician's orders are followed. Monitor the wound for signs of infection and remind the athlete of any medication that must be taken. If at any time the injury seems to worsen, contact the athlete's physician for further care.

Prevention: Protective eyewear such as goggles should be worn in dusty, dirty, or windy conditions.

Hyphema

Bleeding within the anterior chamber of the eye is called hyphema. It is usually caused by a direct blow such as might occur in racquetball, tennis, squash, golf, or baseball. Symptoms include pain and redness in the anterior chamber of the eye within the first 2 hours. Vision can be partially or completely blocked.

Immediate Treatment: Cover the eye with sterile gauze and send the athlete to a physician immediately. This a serious condition; if not treated properly, permanent damage can occur.

Follow-up Treatment: Make sure the physician's orders are followed. Do not allow the athlete to return to play without written permission from the physician.

Prevention: Athletes in sports involving high-velocity objects should wear protective eyewear: goggles, glasses, or face shields as appropriate for the sport being played.

Ruptured Globe

Small objects moving at a high velocity, such as golf balls, racquetballs, or tennis balls can hit the eye and rupture the globe (the eyeball). Symptoms include severe pain, bleeding and other orbital leakage, decreased or blocked vision, and unequal pupils.

Immediate Treatment: Transport the patient to the emergency room for care by an ophthalmologist. This is a serious injury; immediate treatment by an ophthalmologist may prevent permanent damage.

Follow-up Treatment: Make sure the physician's orders are followed. Do not allow the athlete to return to play without written permission from the physician. Monitor the wound for signs of infection and remind the athlete of any medication that must be taken. If at any time the injury seems to worsen, contact the athlete's physician for further care.

Prevention: Athletes in sports involving high-velocity objects should wear protective eyewear: goggles, glasses, or face shields as appropriate for the sport being played.

Contact Lens Complications

Dirt, dust, wind, and lens displacement all can cause complications to contact lens wearers.

Immediate Treatment: Have the athlete remove the lens. Then flush the eye with saline. Once comfort to the eye is restored, the athlete may place a clean or new lens in the eye. If the discomfort returns, remove the lens and send the athlete to a physician. Glasses may need to be substituted for a while to let the eye heal.

Follow-up Treatment: Watch for signs of infection. If symptoms persist or get worse, refer the athlete to a physician for care. If a visit to the physician is necessary, make sure the physician's orders are followed.

Prevention: Advise wearers of contact lenses to keep the lenses clean and to stay out of the dust and wind. Athletes should wear protective eyewear when needed.

INJURIES TO THE NOSE

The nose is composed mostly of soft tissue, and because of its location, is susceptible to injury during sports activities (see Figure 15-14). The visible portion of the nose is a triangular-shaped composition of bone, cartilage, and skin that projects from the frontal bone of the cranium and the maxillae of the face. The sides of this projection are formed at the superior end by the two nasal bones, and at the inferior end by cartilage. The junction of the nasal bones forms the bridge of the nose, the area of the face most susceptible to fractures. At the base of the external portion of the nose are two openings (nostrils), which serve as entry to the first parts of the nasal passage. This passage is lined with mucous membranes and is separated into right and left halves by a wall of bone and cartilage called the nasal septum. The interior portion of the nasal cavity lies over the roof of the mouth (the hard palate) and contains openings to the mucous membranes of the paranasal sinuses (the air-filled spaces in the frontal, sphenoidal, ethmoidal, and maxillary bones of the cranium and the face).

Serving primarily as the air passage between the nostrils and the throat, the nose warms, moistens, and filters the air. Small hairs in the nostrils help capture foreign particles before they can enter the nasal cavity and irritate the delicate

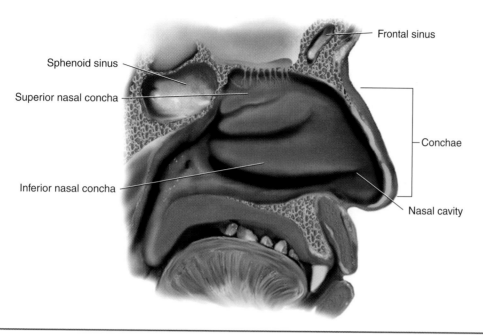

Sphenoid sinus

Superior nasal concha

Inferior nasal concha

Frontal sinus

Conchae

Nasal cavity

FIGURE 15-14 The Nose

tissues. The air then travels over the nasal conchae (bony ridges in the walls of the interior nasal cavity), which are covered with blood vessels and mucus-secreting cells that warm and moisten the air. Hairs even smaller than those found in the nostrils also cover the conchae and filter the smallest dust particles.

The nose also performs a secondary function as the organ of smell. As such, the nose receives scented vapors from the environment when air is inhaled. These vapors pass to the ends of the olfactory nerves located at the top of the nasal passage and stimulate the nerve endings to carry information about the inhaled scents to the brain for interpretation.

Nosebleeds (Epistaxis)

Nosebleeds, or **epistaxis**, caused by direct blows to the face are common in such sports as wrestling and football.

Immediate Treatment: Control the bleeding using direct pressure and a cold compress. Have the athlete sit upright, lean the head forward, and pinch the nose. Careful insertion of absorbent nose plugs in the nostrils may also help to stop the bleeding (see Figure 15-15). Small unscented tampons (when cut in half) and dental sponges make excellent nose plugs, as do

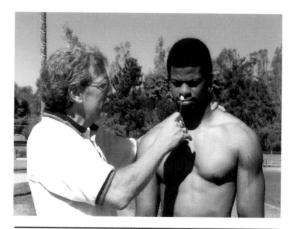

FIGURE 15-15 Forceps can be used to gently insert cotton plugs into an athlete's nose to stop epistaxis. The forceps prevent ungloved hands from coming into contact with the person's blood.

epistaxis

a nosebleed.

small rolls of sterile gauze. Be careful not to insert the plugs too far up the nose, or further injury may occur. Never force anything into the nose, and always leave some of the plug material protruding from the nose so it can be easily removed. Nose plugs should always be used with caution as they block the nasal airway. Never use a nose plug on an athlete who displays any signs of difficulty in breathing. Send the athlete to a physician if the bleeding does not stop after 5 minutes of treatment. Advise the athlete to spit out any blood that enters the throat to avoid stomach upset and caution the athlete not to blow the nose for 2 hours once the bleeding has stopped.

Follow-up Treatment: If a visit to a physician is necessary, make sure the physician's orders are followed. Furthermore, the athlete should wear protective face gear during all sports activities until told by the physician that it is okay to play without it.

Prevention: The athletes should wear protective face gear, including nose guards, during all sports activities.

Nasal Septal Deviation

Sometimes a blow to the nose can cause the septum to shift, decreasing the athlete's ability to breathe through one of the nasal passageways. Symptoms include pain, bleeding, and decreased air movement through one nostril.

Immediate Treatment: Follow the instructions for epistaxis and send the athlete to a physician for further evaluation. The deviation will be corrected by a surgeon if it is deemed necessary.

Follow-up Treatment: Make sure the physician's orders are followed. Make sure the athlete wears protective face gear during all sports activities until told by the physician that it is okay to play without it.

Prevention: Athletes should wear protective face gear, including nose guards, during all sports activities.

Nasal Septal Hematoma

The septum is the area of cartilage between the nostrils. When injured, the septum can create breathing problems. If trauma occurs to the face, and the septal area is bruised, swollen, red, painful, or infected, a septal hematoma (bleeding between the septum and the mucous membrane) may occur. The signs and symptoms of this condition are similar to those of a fracture. Sometimes the nasal passage may become blocked by swollen tissue, forcing the athlete to breathe through the mouth.

Immediate Treatment: Control any bleeding with direct pressure, being careful to avoid causing unnecessary additional pain with the pressure. Apply ice, and maintain an open airway. Do not let the athlete lie down, as this could cause blood to drain into the throat, causing choking. To help the athlete avoid an upset stomach, advise the person to spit out any blood that drains into the throat. Send the athlete to a physician for further care.

Follow-up Treatment: Make sure the physician's orders are followed. Remind the athlete of any medication that must be taken. Do not allow the athlete to return to play without written permission from the physician. If at any time the injury seems to worsen, contact the athlete's physician for further care.

Prevention: The most practical form of prevention of injuries to the nose is to wear a facemask or nose guard during any sports that may involve equipment or player contact. Further, players engaging in heavy contact sports, such as football, should have injury prevention sessions included in their training exercises. At such times, the coach instructs them in safeguard tactics to use during contact/collision activities—including those tactics that will help sports players avoid traumatic hits to the nose, as in wrestling.

Nasal Fractures

Nasal fractures occur frequently in sports. Under impact, it's possible to break or fracture bones in the nose, such as the bones at the bridge of the nose (nasal bones) and the bones at the roof of the nasal passage (conchae). Fractures of nasal bones often result from a straight-on or side-force blow against the nose. The signs and symptoms of fractured bones in the nose include deformity (anatomical distortion), crepitation, and sometimes epistaxis (a nosebleed). Other indications of injury to the nasal bones include swelling and pain. One of the best ways to determine if a fracture has occurred is to have the athlete look in the mirror and see whether the athlete thinks the nose is in normal alignment.

Immediate Treatment: Control any bleeding with direct pressure, being careful to avoid causing unnecessary additional pain with the pressure. Apply ice, and maintain an open airway. Do not let the athlete lie down, as this could cause blood to drain into the throat, causing choking. To help the athlete avoid an upset stomach, advise the athlete to spit out any blood that drains into the throat. Send the athlete to a physician for further care.

Follow-up Treatment: Make sure the physician's orders are followed. Remind the athlete of any medication that must be taken. Do not allow the athlete to return to play without written permission from the physician. If at any time the injury seems to worsen, contact the athlete's physician for further care.

Prevention: Athletes should wear face protection appropriate for the sport being played (e.g., face guards for football, lacrosse, and hockey).

INJURIES TO THE MOUTH AND JAW

The mouth of the human body is a complex structure and vulnerable to injury during contact sports. It is composed of a posterior soft palate, an anterior hard palate, mucous membranes, tongue, taste buds, and salivary glands. The lips and cheeks enclose the gums and the 32 teeth, which form the dental area of the mouth.

The major bones of the jaw are the mandible (the U-shaped lower bone) and the maxilla (the upper bone). The mandible moves forward, backward and sideways, thereby maximizing the ability of the teeth and mouth to bite and chew. The mandible and maxilla are attached to the skull by the temporomandibular joint (TMJ) and are moved by very powerful jaw muscles.

Temporomandibular Joint (TMJ) Dislocation

The jaw is prone to dislocation because of its wide range of motion. This can occur from a side blow to an open mouth. The signs and symptoms of a TMJ dislocation are a jaw locked in an open position and an overbiting of the teeth in a normal bite. Pain and deformity are also symptoms. This injury may prevent the athlete from being able to move the jaw to speak or to prevent saliva from drooling.

Immediate Treatment: Apply ice to the area and refer the athlete to a physician for further evaluation. Do not attempt to "pop" the joint back into place. The dislocation may be accompanied by a fracture, and movement may make the fracture worse.

Follow-up Treatment: Make sure the physician's orders are followed.

Prevention: Athletes and others involved in contact/collision sports should wear a facemask. They should also learn and practice tactical maneuvers that may prevent them from injury.

Jaw Fractures

Jaw fractures (fractures to the mandible or maxillae) result from direct blows to the jaw. The signs and symptoms include a possible bony displacement, abnormal movement, loss of normal bite or overbite (malocclusion), pain with movement, bleeding around the teeth, numbness of the lower lip, and point tenderness. The jaw may be "locked" in the open position and the patient may drool excessively.

Immediate Treatment: Apply ice and immobilize the athlete. Send the athlete to a physician, dentist, or orthodontist, as needed. Remember to use gloves when dealing with blood or other body fluids, including saliva.

Follow-up Treatment: Make sure the physician's orders are followed.

Prevention: Athletes and others involved in contact/collision sports should wear a facemask. They should also learn and practice tactical maneuvers that may prevent them from injury.

Dislocations and Fractures of the Teeth

One of the most common sports-related injuries to the mouth is to have teeth displaced, fractured, or knocked out. Check to see if any teeth are pushed out of place or are missing. Bleeding from an exposed tooth socket will indicate a missing tooth. Also, note any bleeding above or below the gum line of the upper and lower mouth. If tooth fragments or chips are evident along with pain and/or bleeding and loose-ness of the teeth, one or more teeth may also have fractures.

Immediate Treatment: If an athlete has a tooth knocked out, clean the tooth with water and, if possible, replace it back into the socket. Maintain pressure on the tooth to keep it in place, then send the athlete to a dentist. If unable to replace the tooth back into the socket, wrap it in moist, sterile gauze and trans-port it to the dentist along with the athlete. The tooth may also be placed and carried between the cheek and gum to keep it moist. If the tooth is kept out of water or the mouth for more than 30 minutes, the chances of saving the tooth decline rapidly. For fractures of the teeth, carefully remove any loose tooth chips or bony fragments that may impede the airway. The injured person should see a dentist immediately.

Though rare, it is possible for a dislodged tooth to be aspirated into the lung. Sometimes displaced teeth are also accompanied by a fractured jaw or concussion. Any of these medical conditions require immediate attention by a physician.

Follow-up Treatment: Make sure the physician's orders are followed.

Prevention: It is highly recommended that athletes in any type of contact sport (such as basketball, football, field hockey, or wrestling) wear properly fitted mouth guards.

Exposed Nerve

When the teeth are injured, sometimes a nerve can become exposed. It will cause intense pain that is made worse by changes in temperature. This condition requires the attention of a dentist.

Immediate Treatment: Apply some clove oil to anesthetize the area until fur-ther care can be rendered.

Follow-up Treatment: Make sure the physician's orders are followed.

Prevention: Athletes in any type of contact sport should wear properly fitted mouth guards during both practice and games.

THE SPINE

The spine (Figure 15-16) is composed of 33 cylindrical bones called **vertebrae**, which are grouped into five sections. The first seven vertebrae make up the cervical spine, which curves forward. The next 12 vertebrae curve backward, comprising the thoracic spine. The lumbar spine, like the cervical spine, curves forward and is com-posed of five vertebrae. The final two sections, the sacrum and the coccyx, create

vertebrae

the individual bone segments of the spine.

the pelvic region of the spine. The sacrum contains five vertebrae, which actually fuse together to form one bone, and the coccyx is made of four similarly fused vertebrae. The vertebrae are separated by **discs**, which are composed of concentric rings of fibro-cartilage and a central mass of pulpy tissue called the nucleus pulposus (see Figure 15-17). The discs act as shock absorbers by cushioning the vertebrae of the spinal column during movement and impact. They are relieved of pressure only when the body is recumbent (lying down).

When the cervical, thoracic, and lumbar curves of the back are in proper alignment, the body weight is evenly distributed throughout the vertebrae and the discs. Alignment refers to the proper positioning of parts in a line. When the back is properly aligned, the ears, shoulders, and hips form a straight line, resulting in correct posture. Several groups of muscles and joints help support the spine and maintain this alignment. The muscles of the thighs (hamstrings and quadriceps), buttocks, abdomen and back, as well as the joints of the hips, knees, and ankles all play important roles in the body's ability to move freely. This freedom of movement, also known as range of motion (ROM), depends on healthy, flexible muscles and joints. A healthy spine is capable of a variety of types of movement. It can move forward (flexion), and backward (extension), and from side to side (lateral flexion). The neck (cervical) and lower (lumbar) back are also capable of rotation.

> **disc**
>
> acts as a shock absorber for the spine.

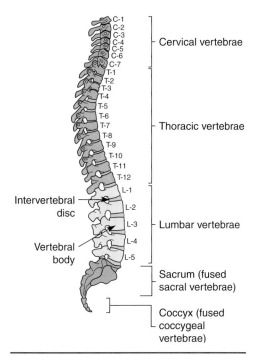

FIGURE 15-16 The Spine

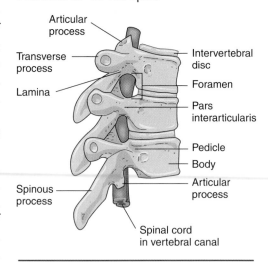

FIGURE 15-17 Intervertebral Discs, Lateral View

For those not physically fit, back injuries are among the most common injuries, because back injuries are often caused by muscular weaknesses and imbalances. For example, if the anterior muscles (the abdominals) are not strong, the strength in the posterior muscles (the muscles of the lower back) is insufficient to protect the back from injury. To prevent back injury, the musculature on the back, sides, and front of the body must have equal strength.

As an athletic trainer, extensive knowledge of the treatment and prevention of back injuries will be of great benefit. This type of expertise is very valuable, so additional training or education in back injuries beyond those found in a textbook should be pursued.

INJURIES TO THE SPINE

Contusions

Contusions to the back most frequently occur in football as a result of a direct hit. Make sure the athlete with a back contusion sees a physician to rule out the possibility of fractures and kidney or other internal injuries.

Immediate Treatment: Ice the surrounding tissues immediately for 20 minutes, followed by an hour during which the ice is off. Repeat this cycle for a 24- to 72-hour period during waking hours, or until the swelling subsides. Make sure to protect the skin by placing a cloth or towel between the ice and skin. Compression in the form of an elastic wrap may also be used. Make sure the patient's breathing is not compromised by excessive compression. Watch the athlete for signs of shock and treat accordingly. (See Chapter 17.)

Follow-up Treatment: If pain persists or does not decrease, send the athlete to a physician for further care.

Prevention: Athletes who engage in contact sports should wear rib pads and other protective pads to help prevent contusions.

Brachial Plexus Injuries

Cervical nerve stretch (also called a "burner" or a "stinger") occurs when an athlete's neck and shoulder are stretched, such as in rodeo (Figure 15-18), or when the athlete's head moves sharply to the side, such as when a football player tries to block or tackle an opponent. The cervical nerves that are stretched when a burner occurs comprise the brachial plexus (see Figure 16-9). The signs and symptoms of cervical nerve stretch include a burning sensation and pain coming down from the neck, through the arm, all the way to the base of the thumb. The athlete may complain about an electrical shock–like or burning sensation. Numbness and loss of function of the arm will generally last anywhere

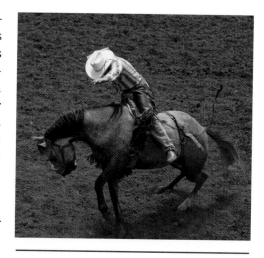

FIGURE 15-18 A cervical nerve stretch is a risk in many sports, including rodeo.

from 10 to 20 seconds; but in severe cases, these symptoms may last for days or even months. If an athlete receives repeated burners, it may result in neuritis (an inflammation of the nerves around the area), and may cause atrophy of the muscles with repeated injuries.

Immediate Treatment: Apply ice to the surrounding tissues, making sure to protect the skin from frostbite by placing a cloth or towel between the ice and skin.

The patient should also receive immediate medical attention. Send the athlete to a physician for further evaluation and suggestions for rehabilitation. Remove the ice after 20 minutes if the athlete is still waiting to see a physician. The ice can be replaced after an hour if the athlete is still waiting for a physician.

Follow-up Treatment: Make sure the physician's orders are followed.

Prevention: Athletes should be shown how to perform neck-strengthening exercises to help prevent neck injuries. Make sure the athletes are trained in preventive techniques to avoid injuries in their sport. An athlete engaged in football, hockey, rugby, or rodeo should wear a neck collar for additional protection. Warm-up stretching appropriate to the sport may also aid in the prevention of such injuries.

Abnormal Curvatures of the Spine

As a result of various conditions such as disease, poor posture, or congenital defects, the normal curves of the spinal column may become exaggerated. While these back problems are not injuries resulting from sports activity, they can affect an athlete's performance and are often detected during physical activity.

Kyphosis is an exaggerated posterior convex curvature of the thoracic spine (Figure 15-19A). A patient with kyphosis has rounded shoulders, a forward thrust of the head, and possibly a flat chest. This condition is commonly referred to as a "humpback" or "hunchback."

Lordosis is an abnormal anterior convex curvature of the lumbar spine (Figure 15-19B). This condition is sometimes known as a "swayback." The patient will have a tightness in the lower back musculature and possibly a weak abdominal area.

Scoliosis is the lateral curvature of the spine (Figure 15-19C). This condition can be aggravated by some sports such as baseball and high jumping. Scoliosis may also cause or result from unequal leg length.

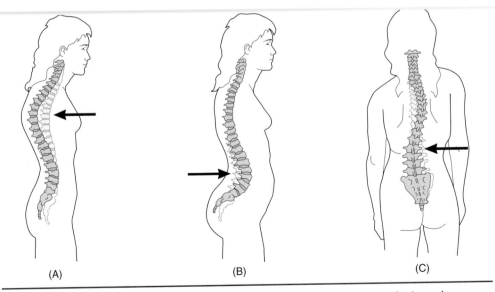

(A) (B) (C)

FIGURE 15-19 Abnormal Curvatures of the Spine: (A) Kyphosis (B) Lordosis and (C) Scoliosis

Treatment: Patients with one of these conditions should see a physician and receive appropriate physical therapy.

Prevention: These are congenital conditions, so they cannot be prevented; however, worsening of the condition may be prevented with rehabilitation.

Muscle Spasms

A muscle spasm is an uncontrolled, painful contraction of a muscle or muscle group. It can be the result of a traumatic injury, overuse, or improper lifting. Symptoms will include varying degrees of pain or discomfort, cramping, decreased range of motion, and muscle tightness.

Immediate Treatment: The best treatment for back muscle spasms is ice massage. However, if this is not possible for some reason, ice for 20 minutes using the proper skin safeguards, or massage the muscles without using ice. (See Chapter 22 for the proper massage techniques.) Before and after the massage, the patient should perform slow static stretching.

Follow-up Treatment: It is recommended that the patient sleep on a firm mattress, on the side, in a tucked position. If the patient sits for prolonged periods of time, it is suggested that a small pillow be placed behind the lower part of the back. Also, after any activities, apply ice to the back for 20 minutes. If the condition worsens or does not improve, send the athlete to a physician for further care.

Prevention: Instruct athletes to use proper body mechanics when lifting or participating in their sport. Increase strength and flexibility in all aspects of the trunk: the front, back, and sides.

Back Sprains

Most back sprains affect the ligaments of the facet joints (see Figure 15-20). Sprains are caused by improper lifting or sudden twisting motions. Overuse of the ligaments can also lead to a chronic condition in which the sprain keeps reoccurring. Signs and symptoms include localized sharp pain that is aggravated by specific movements, loss of strength, and decreased ROM. Some swelling may also be visible. **Radiating pain** will not be present with a sprain. If radiating pain is present, a disc problem is indicated.

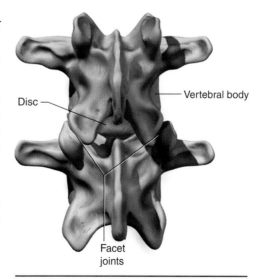

FIGURE 15-20 Posterior View of Facet Joints

Disc — Vertebral body — Facet joints

radiating pain

pain that spreads from a central point, such as the point of injury.

Immediate Treatment: Rest and ice. Put the athlete in a comfortable position and use the icing procedure (ice for

20 minutes while protecting the skin, then off for an hour) for 24 to 72 hours or until the swelling subsides. The application of ice will help decrease the pain and any spasms. If the pain is debilitating, send the athlete to a physician.

Follow-up Treatment: Advise the athlete to avoid painful motions in the activities of daily living as well as motions similar to those that caused the injury. A back brace may be applied to stabilize the back and prevent further injury. Heat may also be applied after swelling has gone down. In fact, some braces can bring heat to the injured area by trapping the body's heat with a neoprene back support. If the condition becomes worse, if pain occurs in other areas (**referred pain**), or if muscle atrophy or numbness becomes evident, send the patient to a physician for further evaluation and care. As with all sprains, maintaining strength and flexibility of the area is vital to complete healing (see Chapters 7 and 14).

Prevention: Instruct athletes to use proper body mechanics when lifting. Strengthen all aspects of the trunk muscles: the front, back, and sides.

Back Strains

Back strains can occur as the result of sudden twisting motions or an overload of a muscle or muscle group. Poor posture can increase chances of back strains because it makes the muscles work harder, to the point of fatigue. Symptoms include pain, discomfort, muscle spasms, and increased pain with motion. Radiating pain will not be present with a strain.

Immediate Treatment: Back strains are treated in the same way as back sprains: rest and ice. Follow the procedure for ice application: 20 minutes on, 1 hour off, with a towel placed between the skin and the ice, until swelling subsides. If the pain is debilitating, send the patient to a physician.

Follow-up Treatment: As with a sprain, advise the athlete to avoid motions that cause pain as well as motions similar to those that caused the injury. A back brace may also be applied to provide support and comfort. If the condition becomes worse, or if referred pain, numbness, or muscle atrophy become evident, send the patient to a physician for further evaluation and care.

Prevention: Instruct athletes to use proper body mechanics when lifting and participating in their sport. Strengthen all aspects of the trunk muscles: the front, back, and sides.

Fractures and Dislocations

Fractures and dislocations of the spine are serious injuries (see Figure 15-21). Such activities can lead to paralysis and even death. As one might imagine, they are more frequent in contact sports than in any other type of sport. They may occur from a direct blow, lifting, compression, or a fall, and may be accompanied by a sprain or strain. The symptoms of a spinal fracture or dislocation are the same: point tenderness, weakness, muscle spasms, decreased ROM, and possibly referred pain. If the injury occurs in the cervical portion of the spine, paralysis may also be a symptom and death may occur.

referred pain

pain at a location other than the injured organ or site.

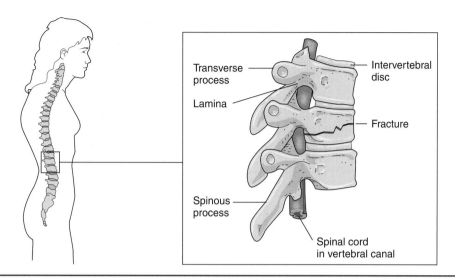

FIGURE 15-21 Fracture of the Lumbar Spine

Immediate Treatment: Follow the emergency action plan, including performing the primary survey, calling the EMS, and stabilizing the spine.

Follow-up Treatment: Make sure the physician's orders are followed. Do not allow the athlete to return to play without written authorization from the physician.

Prevention: Instruct athletes to use proper body mechanics when lifting and participating in their sport. They should also be shown how to perform strengthening exercises to help prevent spine injuries. Warm-up stretching appropriate to the sport may also aid in the prevention of such injuries. In addition, make sure the athletes are trained in preventive techniques to avoid injuries in their sport.

Intervertebral Disc Herniation

A disc that has deteriorated to the point that it pushes against a nerve is called an intervertebral disc herniation (see Figure 15-22). It most commonly refers to the spaces between the fourth and and fifth lumbar and the fifth lumbar and first sacral vertebrae. Disc herniations are caused by improper lifting, sudden twisting motions, or bending, and may accompany a sprain or strain of the back. The pressure placed on the spinal nerve causes radiating pain in the arms, legs, or back, depending on the location of the injury. Pain will increase with motion as pressure on the nerve is increased. Muscles on the involved side will become weak and may atrophy over a period of time; there will also be a decrease in reflexes on the involved side and numbness along certain dermatomes (see Figure 15-7).

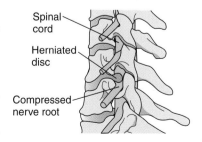

FIGURE 15-22 Herniated Cervical Disc Pressing on Nerve Root and Spinal Cord

Immediate Treatment: Put the athlete in the most comfortable position possible. To decrease the pain, apply ice using the proper procedure: 20 minutes on, with a towel placed between the skin and the ice; 1 hour off. Send the athlete to a physician for care.

Follow-up Treatment: Make sure the physician's orders are followed. Do not allow the athlete to return to play without written authorization from the physician.

Prevention: The use of proper lifting techniques, preventive tactical techniques, strengthening exercises, and warm-up stretching will all aid in the prevention of such injuries.

Spondylolysis and Spondylolisthesis

Spondylolysis is a defect in the vertebrae caused by repeated stress from hyperextension that may result in a stress fracture of the pars interarticularis (see Figure 15-23).

Athletic activities that carry a risk of this type of injury include gymnastics, football blocking, weightlifting, butterfly strokes in swimming, figure skating, volleyball spikes, and tennis serves. If the vertebrae slips forward as a result of this weakness, a condition known as spondylolisthesis results. The most common site for these injuries is in the space between the fifth lumbar and the first sacral vertebrae. Although there may be no symptoms initially, eventual symptoms of either condition include local pain and stiffness along the low back and possibly referred pain in the buttocks because of disc herniation. Pain will increase during physical activity. Numbness and weakness may also be present.

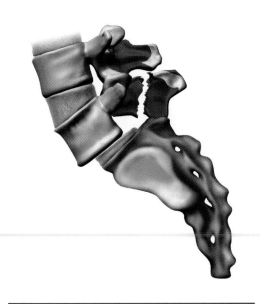

FIGURE 15-23 Spondylolysis

Immediate Treatment: Rest and ice. Put the athlete in a comfortable position and ice the area immediately for 20 minutes, followed by an hour in which the ice is off. Repeat this cycle for 24 to 72 hours during waking hours, or until the swelling subsides, or until the patient can be seen by a physician. Protect the skin by placing a cloth or towel between the ice and skin. Make sure the patient seeks a physician's care.

Follow-up Treatment: Make sure the physician's orders are followed. Advise the athlete to avoid motions that cause pain as well as motions similar to those that caused the injury. A back brace may be applied to provide support and comfort. Physical therapy will likely be a part of the prescribed treatment.

Prevention: Caution athletes to avoid extreme hyperextension of the back. Athletes should also engage in exercises that strengthen the trunk muscles, keeping in mind the importance of balance in strength among the muscle groups.

THINKING IT THROUGH

It was Friday night and the football game pit the Rubidoux Falcons against their cross-town rivals, the Columbus Titans. These games were always closely contested, so the coaches wanted to make sure that they had their best athletes on the field at all times. The winner would take home the Peach Cup, a tremendous source of pride for the school who wins it.

Twang, a sophomore defensive back, was set to start his first varsity football game and nothing was going to stop him from playing. During Wednesday's tackling drill he strained his neck a little, and it hurt to move. It was most comfortable for him when it was straight. He had put some heat on it the night of the injury because heat felt a lot better than the ice the athletic trainers would have put on. In fact, he never said anything to them because he figured they wouldn't let him play, and they didn't understand how important this game was to him.

It was coming close to the end of the third quarter and Twang's neck was hurting and getting stiff. The Titans knew Twang was a sophomore and had been running at him all night. He was holding his ground well until the final two minutes of the quarter. This is when Titan starting fullback Ralph Stein found an opening on Twang's right. Ralph put his head down, ready to run right over Twang. Twang thought this was his chance to show everyone he could go head to head with the big boys even though Ralph was a good 50 pounds heavier than he. With Ralph coming at him, Twang lowered his head and planted the top of his helmet into Ralph's numbers. They hit with a resounding "crunch." After the play was over, Ralph stumbled away as Twang lay motionless.

What are some of the concerns the athletic trainer needs to have for Twang? What would you do for Twang if you got there and he was breathing? What would you do if he wasn't breathing? What emergency steps would you take? Is there anything that could have been done to prevent this injury?

CHAPTER SUMMARY

Many times, the athletic trainer is the first person to arrive at the scene of an injury during an athletic or fitness event. Therefore, it is important to understand how an initial assessment can affect the extent of further injury and the rate of recovery. For instance, injuries to the head and spine can be serious because they can involve the brain, sensory organs such as the eyes and nose, and portions of the central and peripheral nervous systems. Injury assessment includes making primary and secondary surveys, and responding accurately and efficiently to what those evaluations reveal. Knowledge of both initial and follow-up treatment is crucial because often it is the athletic trainer or strength and conditioning specialist who will assess and treat the injury before the EMS team arrives.

Assessment, treatment, and prevention of head and spine injuries require that the first aid provider be informed about the anatomy and functions of the body. The nervous system is composed of the brain, the spinal cord, and the nerves that surround the brain and the spine. Through this system, messages are received, interpreted, and transmitted via electrical impulses throughout the body. When these impulses reach the muscles, an appropriate action occurs in response to the stimulus, such as the fight-or-flight response. Athletic trainers, athletes, and those involved in health care need to understand why any injury that affects the spine or head may also damage the body's central or peripheral nervous systems and how such damage might be observed in other body functions. Further, knowledge of the functions of organs and muscles in the body, including the parts of the eye, basic construction of the spine, and joint mechanisms of the jaw, will help the athletic trainer and other sports medicine professionals to prevent and treat injuries effectively.

STUDENT ENRICHMENT ACTIVITIES

Complete the following sentences.

1. The central nervous system consists of the _____ and _____ _____.

2. Within the autonomic nervous system, the parasympathetic system _____ the _____ of the sympathetic nervous system. The balance between these two systems is referred to as _____.

3. The _____ _____ nourishes the brain and spinal cord and assists in waste removal from these structures.

4. When a player is injured, down, and unconscious, always treat the player as though there is a _____ _____ _____ _____.

5. _____ _____ is the most common injury to the ear.

6. The three layers of the eye, from outer to inner, are the _____, the _____, and the _____.

7. The treatment for a black eye is to _____ the _____ _____ and consult a doctor for anything other than the slightest injury here.

8. Signs and symptoms of a nasal fracture include _____, _____, and _____.

9. The jaw is prone to _____ because of its wide range of motion.

10. List ten symptoms of a concussion to the head.

Write T for true, or F for false. Rewrite the false statements to make them true.

11. T F The bony portion of the head is called the skull.

12. T F The Trainer's Angel is used to remove particles from the eye.

13. T F A log roll is an injury prevention tactic used by football players when they are falling.

14. T F Noting the total time that an athlete is unconscious isn't necessary and wastes valuable time that could be applied to first aid tactics.

15. T F In football, players are not allowed to dive into other players in order to tackle them.

16. T F Following a head injury, there will be a certain amount of disorientation that is considered normal.

17. T F A cervical nerve stretch is an effective exercise for preventing injury.

18. T F Applying petroleum jelly to the outside of the ears helps to prevent cauliflower ear.

19. T F The septum is the area between the medulla and the cerebellum in the brain.

20. T F The right side of the brain controls the left side of the body and vice versa.

Complete the following exercises.

21. Explain how to treat a possible head injury as though you were explaining the procedure in the correct sequence of events to another person.

22. Get together with four other classmates and write out the steps to perform a log roll for a patient with a possible spine injury. Then demonstrate your knowledge with each group member taking a turn as the patient.

23. Write the steps for evaluating a possible concussion. Identify crucial junctures at which you would call for EMS.

CHAPTER 16

Injuries to the Upper Extremities

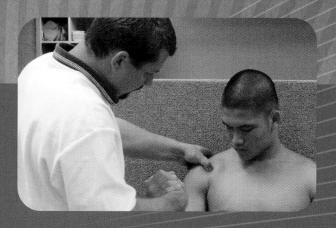

OBJECTIVES

After completing this chapter, you should be able to do the following:

1. Define and correctly spell each of the key terms.

2. Identify major bones, muscles, veins, and arteries frequently involved in upper-extremity injuries.

3. Identify commonly injured upper-extremity joints.

4. Understand and describe common upper-extremity injuries.

5. Recognize the signs and symptoms of shoulder, arm, and hand injuries.

6. Name and describe, with respect to individual sports, disorders of the upper extremities to which athletes are most susceptible.

KEY TERMS

* acromioclavicular (AC) sprain test
* apprehension test
* buttonhole deformity
* compression test
* drop arm test
* empty can test
* epicondylitis
* Finkelstein's test
* gamekeeper's thumb test

* ganglion cyst
* Hawkins-Kennedy test
* impingement
* mallet finger
* muscle rupture
* percussion test
* Phalen's test
* Speed's test
* sternoclavicular (SC) sprain test

* sulcus test
* tenosynovitis
* Tinel's sign
* valgus stress test
* varus stress test
* Volkmann's contracture
* winged scapula test

INTRODUCTION

The upper extremities are vulnerable to a variety of injuries depending on the sport being played. Participation in contact sports like rugby increases the potential for sudden onset injuries such as such as sprains, strains, dislocations, fractures, and separations to the thoracic cage, shoulder, arm, and hand. On the other hand, sports like tennis that require repetitive movements of the upper extremities increase an athlete's susceptibility to chronic stress disorders such as arthritis, bursitis, or tendonitis. As mentioned before, in treating injuries, it is important to remember to address the cause of the symptoms, not just to treat the symptoms. If symptoms do not improve after continued treatment, discuss other possible causes of such symptoms with the athlete and the coach, and explore methods of eliminating these potential causes. Athletes who participate in appropriate strength and conditioning exercises and who wear proper protective gear decrease their risk of experiencing either sudden or chronic injuries.

THE SHOULDER COMPLEX

The bones of the shoulder girdle and upper arm, along with their surrounding muscles, ligaments, tendons, and articulations, form an area commonly known as the shoulder complex (see Figure 16-1). Each shoulder girdle is composed of a clavicle (collar bone) and a scapula (shoulder blade), paired on each side of the body. These bones provide points of connection between the upper limbs and the axial skeleton, enabling a variety of movements for the arms. The clavicles articulate with the sternum (breast bone), creating the sternoclavicular (SC) joint. Articulation is another name for joint, the place where one bone joins another bone. Cartilage covers the surface of each bone at the point where the joint is formed. The scapula

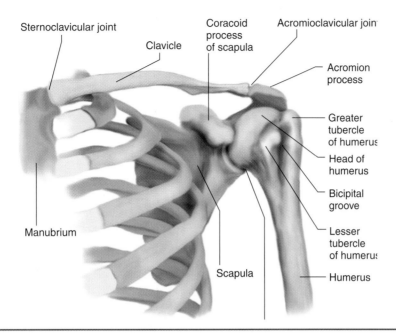

FIGURE 16-1 Bony Structures of the Shoulder Complex

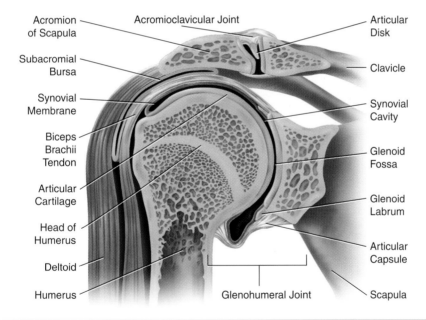

FIGURE 16-2 The Shoulder Joint

has two important surfaces called processes: the coracoid process and the acromion process. The clavicle articulates, or forms a joint, with the acromion process, forming the acromioclavicular (AC) joint. The bone of the upper arm, the humerus, is considered to be part of the shoulder complex. The point at which the scapula and the head of the humerus articulate is called the glenohumeral joint (the shoulder joint) (see Figure 16-2). The shoulder is a ball and socket joint because it consists of a bone with a ball-shaped head that articulates with the cup-shaped glenohumeral socket. The shoulder joint is capable of flexion, extension, abduction, adduction, external rotation, internal rotation, horizontal abduction, horizontal adduction, and circumduction.

The humerus is the longest and largest bone of the upper extremity (see Figure 16-3). At the proximal end, the humerus attaches to the glenoid fossa of the scapula to form the shoulder joint. At the distal end, the humerus attaches to the hinge joint known as the elbow, which connects the forearm to the upper arm. Many ligaments and tendons connect the distal end of the humerus to the proximal ends of the two bones in the forearm. Remember, ligaments attach bone to bone, and tendons attach muscle to bone. It is this group of ligaments and tendons that help to create the elbow and allow for precise movement of bones in the forearm and hand. The joints, like most joints in the body, are enclosed and protected by a common capsule and have a common synovial cavity. This cavity contains synovial fluid, which lubricates the joint and allows for flexion and extension without the discomfort of bones rubbing together.

Muscles, ligaments, and tendons surround the bones and support the joints (see Figure 16-4). The main muscles of the shoulder joint include the deltoid, supraspinatus, infraspinatus, subscapularis, teres

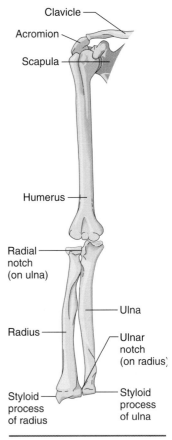

FIGURE 16-3 Bones of the Arm, Anterior View

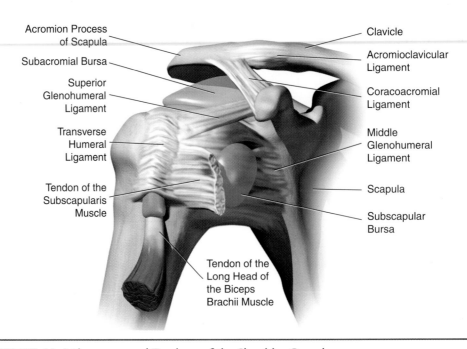

FIGURE 16-4 Ligaments and Tendons of the Shoulder Complex

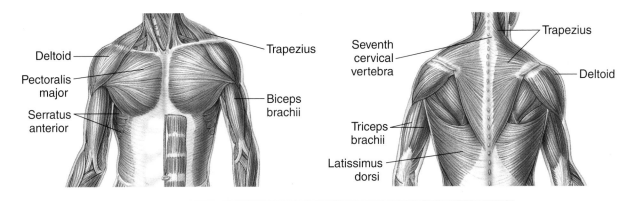

FIGURE 16-5 The Major Shoulder Muscles, Anterior (L) and Posterior (R)

major, and teres minor; the main muscles of the upper arm include the biceps brachii, the brachialis, and the triceps brachii (see Figure 16-5). These shoulder and arm muscles work together with several muscles of the back and the thoracic region of the upper body (those affecting the shoulder girdle) to make movement of the shoulder and upper arm possible. For example, although it is usually considered a thoracic muscle, the pectoralis major is significantly involved in the movement of the upper arm. Each muscle has at least one point of origin and at least one point of insertion. Some muscles, such as the pectoralis major, have more than one point of origin and/or insertion.

The main muscles affecting movement of the shoulder girdle include the trapezius, rhomboids, serratus anterior, and pectoralis major. These muscles attach the shoulder girdle to the trunk of the body. The trapezius, rhomboids, and serratus anterior affect movement of the scapula, while the pectoralis major affects movement of the humerus.

Keep in mind that muscles generally work in opposing pairs or groups according to the desired action. For example, the deltoid, a large, rounded, multifunctional muscle of the upper arm that caps the shoulder region, lifts the arm away from the body in a directly lateral movement (abduction). The deltoid is assisted in forward movement (flexion) by the pectoralis major, a large flat muscle of the thoracic region, and assisted in backward movement (extension) by the teres major and latissimus dorsi. The deltoid is paired with the latissimus dorsi of the back, and the teres minor and infraspinatus of the shoulder region. The latissimus dorsi, teres minor, and infraspinatus pull the arm down and backward in opposition to the action of the deltoid. The subscapularis also works in opposition to the deltoid by pulling the humerus down and forward. More importantly, however, the subscapularis protects the front of the shoulder joint and allows the head of the humerus to rotate inward. The primary function of the supraspinatus is to hold the head of the humerus in the glenoid cavity, although this muscle also helps the deltoid lift the arm.

The glenohumeral joint is protected on three sides by the SITS muscles: supraspinatus, infraspinatus, teres minor, and subscapularis. The subscapularis provides anterior stability to the shoulder joint; the infraspinatus and teres minor provide posterior stability; and the supraspinatus offers superior stability. These muscles, collectively known as the rotator cuff (see Figure 16-6), help to keep the head of the humerus positioned in the glenoid cavity. Injury to the rotator cuff is

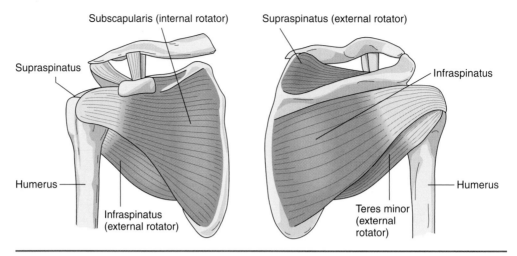

FIGURE 16-6 Rotator Cuff, Anterior View (L) and Posterior View (R)

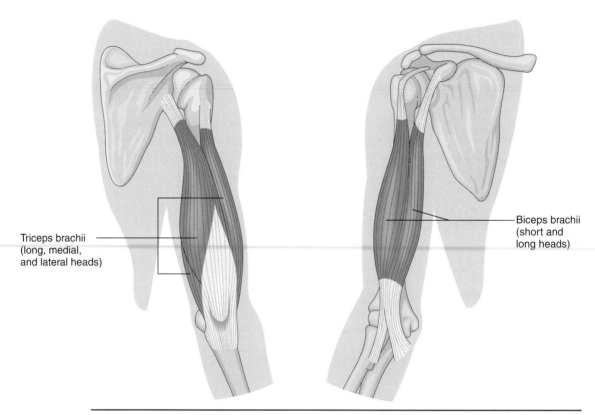

FIGURE 16-7 Muscles of the Upper Arm, Posterior View (L) and Anterior View (R)

usually confirmed with decreased range of motion and what is commonly described as a "deep ache," especially with movement, and nighttime pain (pain that wakes one up at night).

The muscles of the upper arm include the biceps brachii and the brachialis anticus on the anterior aspect, causing flexion of the arm, and the triceps brachii on the posterior aspect, causing extension of the arm (see Figure 16-7).

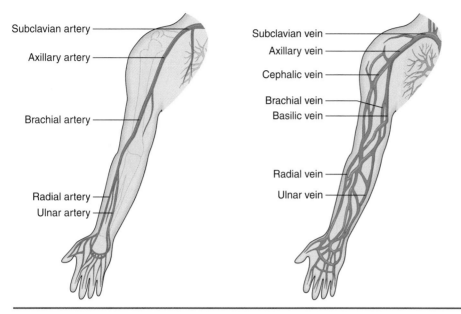

FIGURE 16-8 The Principle Blood Vessels of the Shoulder and Arm

The main arteries that supply the shoulder complex include the subclavian, vertebral, costocervical, ventral thoracic, and axillary arteries. The primary venous return includes the subclavian, vertebral, external jugular, brachiocephalic, and axillary veins. The largest vein in the body, the superior vena cava, also serves the shoulder complex. Remember, arteries carry oxygen-rich blood to the various parts of the body, and veins carry oxygen-depleted blood containing waste products back to the heart, where it is passed to the lungs to pick up more oxygen and eliminate waste products.

Many of the arteries and veins that serve the arm are continuations of those found in the shoulder complex (see Figure 16-8). For example, the subclavian arteries continue into the upper arms. On each side of the body, the subclavian artery becomes the axillary artery, which turns into the brachial artery and, at the elbow, further divides into the radial and ulnar arteries. At the wrist, the radial and ulnar arteries further divide into a network of arteries that supply the wrist, hand, and fingers. The veins follow a similar pattern. There are deep veins as well as superficial veins. The deep veins run parallel to the arteries and, as a general rule, have the same or a similar name as the arteries. The deep veins of the arm include the radial, ulnar, brachial, and axillary veins. The two main superficial veins are the basilic and cephalic veins. It should be noted, however, that some deep veins become superficial in certain areas of the arm.

The main nerves in the shoulder girdle consist of those found in the brachial plexus: the axillary, radial, musculocutaneous, median, and ulnar nerves (see Figure 16-9). These nerves then divide into additional nerves that serve the muscles of the shoulder, arm, and hand. As with the muscles and the blood vessels, these nerves are duplicated on each side of the body. The nerves can frequently become injured while playing sports. Injuries to the nerves usually create symptoms of pain, numbness, and/or tingling. Bear in mind that an athlete with cervical nerve damage may not complain of neck discomfort, but may in fact exhibit signs and symptoms of the injury distally (e.g., pain, numbness, and/or tingling in one or both upper extremities that may extend to the hands and fingers).

The major nerves of the arm include the median, radial, and ulnar nerves (see Figure 16-10). Many of the arm's nerves have anterior and posterior branches. Although numbness or tingling may be present in the fingers, the site of the injury may be in the elbow or neck.

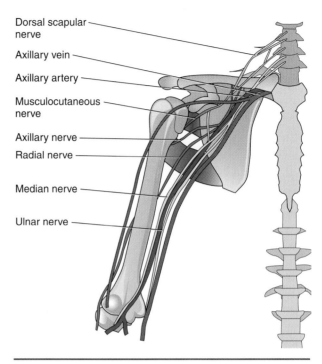

Dorsal scapular nerve
Axillary vein
Axillary artery
Musculocutaneous nerve
Axillary nerve
Radial nerve
Median nerve
Ulnar nerve

FIGURE 16-9 Brachial Plexus and Axillary Vessels, Anterior View

ASSESSING SHOULDER INJURIES

Prior to assessing any injury of the shoulder or any body part, a good history must be recorded (see the HOPS procedure in Chapter 9). This will often provide a road map to the injury. Make sure pertinent questions are asked, such as how, when, and where the injury occurred. Did the person hear anything? What care, if any, has the person had to this point? What makes it better and what makes it worse? Is this a recurring injury or the first time it has occurred? On a scale from one to ten (one least pain and ten most pain), rate the pain.

During palpation of the shoulder, ask the athlete to point with one finger to where it hurts the most and what motions make it worse now and during activity. Tap on the bone (percussion test) to see if it causes an increase in pain or point tenderness pain to check for a possible fracture. Palpate over the boney landmarks of the AC, GH, and SC joints to see if there is any point tenderness pain, crepitation, or increased laxity or spring when you compare the good side to the bad. This could be an AC or SC sprain, strain, or a contusion. Check superficial sensation of the skin. Are the color and the temperature the same? This could be a brachial plexus problem if the sensation varies. A circulation problem could be thoracic outlet syndrome; also note if the color or temperature of the skin has changed.

General Range-of-Motion (ROM) Evaluations for the Shoulder

The evaluation pictures shown in this chapter and in Chapter 18 use arrows and an isometric resistance symbol to help illustrate the motions and forces used in the evaluations. Red arrows reflect the athlete's motions, and blue arrows show the

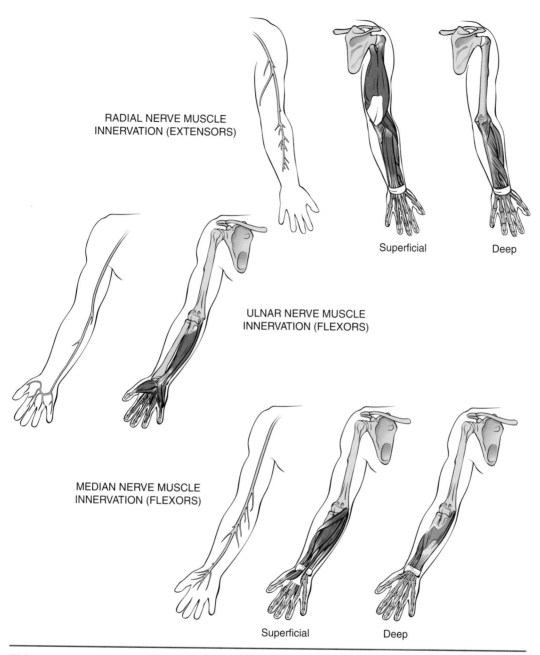

RADIAL NERVE MUSCLE
INNERVATION (EXTENSORS)

Superficial   Deep

ULNAR NERVE MUSCLE
INNERVATION (FLEXORS)

MEDIAN NERVE MUSCLE
INNERVATION (FLEXORS)

Superficial   Deep

FIGURE 16-10 Muscle Innervation in the Arm

evaluator's motions. The blue isometric resistance symbol (⊥) represents controlled isometric resistance applied by the evaluator.

ROM Test for External Rotation of the Shoulder: (See Figure 16-11.) Ask the athlete to place the hands behind the head. Instruct the athlete to externally rotate the shoulders by reaching down toward the shoulder blades as far as possible. Compare the range of motion in the uninvolved side with the involved side by noting any differences in the levels reached by the hands. Observe and compare the quality of the motion as well. You will need to step behind the athlete to evaluate results. Limited ROM on one side indicates a potential injury or deformity on that side. **Note:** A goniometer may be used to measure ROM in a joint (see Chapter 23).

ROM Test for Internal Rotation of the Shoulder: (See Figure 16-12.) Ask the athlete to grasp the hands behind the back. Instruct the athlete to internally rotate the shoulders by raising the hands as high as possible, keeping the hands behind the back. Compare the range of motion in the uninvolved side with the involved side by noting any differences in the levels reached by the hands. Observe and compare the quality of the motion as well. As with the external range of motion assessment, you will need to step behind the athlete to evaluate the results. Again, limited ROM on one side indicates a potential injury or deformity on that side.

Specific ROM Tests for the Shoulder: Specific tests may also be done to determine ROM in adduction, abduction, flexion, extension, horizontal adduction, and horizontal abduction. Ask the athlete to perform these movements through a pain-free range of motion. Compare the uninvolved side to the involved side to make your ROM assessments.

Manual Muscle Tests for the Shoulder

External Rotation Strength Test for the Shoulder: (See Figure 16-13.) With the athlete either sitting or standing in front of you, place your hands on the lateral sides of the athlete's wrists. Instruct the athlete to externally rotate the arms and push against your hands isometrically (increasing the tension of the muscle without movement of the joint). Compare the strength between the involved and uninvolved shoulders, and note any differences. Weakness on one side indicates potential injury or deformity to the infraspinatus or teres minor.

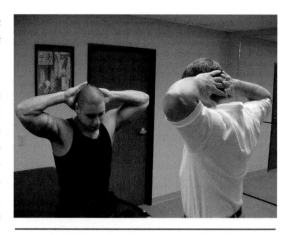

FIGURE 16-11 External ROM of the Shoulder, with Evaluator Demonstrating Hand Placement

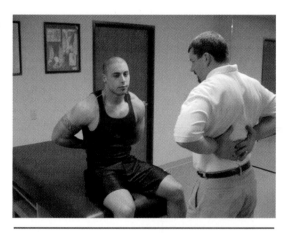

FIGURE 16-12 Internal ROM of the Shoulder, with Evaluator Demonstrating Hand Placement

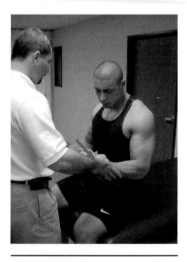

FIGURE 16-13 Shoulder Strength, External Rotation

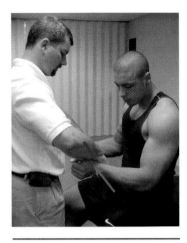 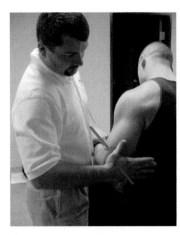

FIGURE 16-14 Shoulder Strength, Internal Rotation

FIGURE 16-15 Shoulder Strength, Extension

Internal Rotation Strength Test for the Shoulder: (See Figure 16-14.) With the athlete either sitting or standing in front of you, place your hands on the medial sides of the athlete's wrists. Instruct the athlete to internally rotate the arms and push against your hands isometrically. Compare the strength between the involved and uninvolved shoulders, and note any differences. Weakness on one side indicates potential injury or deformity to the subscapularis, pectoralis minor, or pectoralis major.

Extension Strength Test for the Shoulder: (See Figure 16-15.) With the athlete either sitting or standing, place your hand on the posterior aspect of the athlete's elbow. Instruct the athlete to push backward against your hand isometrically. Compare the strength between the involved and uninvolved shoulders, and note any differences. Weakness on one side indicates injury or deformity to the posterior deltoid.

Flexion Strength Test for the Shoulder: (See Figure 16-16.) With the athlete either sitting or standing, place your hand on the anterior aspect of the athlete's elbow and ask the athlete to push forward against your hand isometrically. Compare the strength between the involved and uninvolved shoulders, and note any differences. Weakness on one side indicates injury or deformity to the anterior deltoid.

Abduction and Adduction Strength Tests for the Shoulder: (See Figure 16-17.) With the athlete either sitting or standing, place your hand on the lateral aspect of the athlete's elbow. Apply isometric

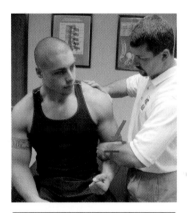

FIGURE 16-16 Shoulder Strength, Flexion

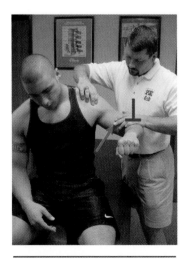

FIGURE 16-17 Shoulder Strength, Abduction

resistance to the elbow as the athlete abducts the arm. Compare the strength between the involved and uninvolved shoulders, and note any differences. Weakness on one side indicates potential injury or deformity to the lateral deltoid. To test adduction, place your hand on the medial aspect of the athlete's elbow. Apply isometric resistance to the elbow as the athlete adducts the arm. Compare the strength between the involved and uninvolved shoulders, and note any differences. Weakness on one side indicates potential injury or deformity to the latissimus dorsi and/or teres major.

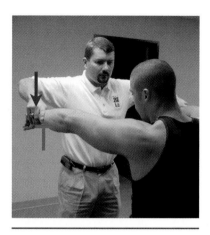

FIGURE 16-18 Shoulder Strength, Empty Can Test

empty can test

flexion of the shoulder followed by resistance to observe for weakening of the supraspinatus muscle.

Empty Can Test: (See Figure 16-18.) With the athlete sitting, instruct the athlete to extend both arms forward at a 90° angle to the body while horizontally abducting the arm to a 30° angle. The athlete must internally rotate the arms as much as possible, turning the thumbs down. Ask the athlete to hold this position as you push down on the athlete's wrists. Compare the strength between the involved and uninvolved shoulders, and note any differences. Weakness on one side indicates potential injury or deformity to the supraspinatus.

INJURIES TO THE SHOULDER

Fractures

A fracture of either the clavicle or the head (upper part) of the humerus will cause point tenderness and a decrease in the range of motion. Clavicle fractures result most commonly from a direct blow, falling onto an outstretched hand, or by landing directly on the acromion process. Such a blow can fracture the middle third of the clavicle. Contact sports, motocross, BMX, and skateboarding are sports that carry increased risk of shoulder fractures. The symptoms are pain on palpation, possibly swelling, deformity, and crepitation. The athlete will often hold the arm to one side and be unable to lift that arm. Percussion and compression tests are performed to check for signs of a fracture. These tests are performed with the understanding that if there is any possibility of a fracture, x-rays will be needed and evaluation by a physician is required.

percussion test

tapping a bone to assess the possibility of a fracture.

Percussion Test: Lightly tap the distal aspect of the athlete's involved bone with your index finger or the palm of your hand. The tapping creates a vibration that travels up the shaft of the bone. If the vibration causes pain, the test is positive (the bone may be fractured). If the test is positive, refer the athlete to a physician for diagnosis and treatment. **Note:** This test should be performed only by properly trained individuals.

compression test

compressing above and below an injury site to assess the possibility of a fracture.

Compression Test: Place one hand on either side of the injured extremity above the possible fracture site and compress the area between the hands. Repeat the procedure below the possible fracture site. Point tenderness over the possible fracture site when either superior or inferior compression is applied indicates a potential fracture. Refer the athlete to a physician for diagnosis and treatment. **Note:** Be especially careful with your hand placement on this test; *do not* place either hand directly over the suspected fracture site. This test should be performed only by properly trained individuals.

Immediate Treatment: If a fracture may exist, gently place the athlete's arm in a sling and apply a splint when possible to relieve the pain and prevent additional injury. Ice may also be applied as long as the weight of the ice does not cause more pain. Follow the steps in PRICE procedure if possible (see Chapter 14). Send the athlete to a physician for further evaluation or call the EMS. Fractures can be accompanied by great anxiety. Pain, the injury's appearance, and the realization that a season may be prematurely over can create significant stress for the athlete, leading to hyperventilation and/or mental anguish. Therefore, reassurance can be as important to the athlete's well-being as appropriate medical treatment.

Follow-up Treatment: Make sure the physician's orders are followed. If a cast is applied, instruct the athlete to keep the casting material dry.

Prevention: To prevent fractures, provide instruction in methods of falling that reduce the risk of injury. Also make sure athletes wear protective padding, such as shoulder pads, in contact sports and BMX.

Dislocations and Subluxations

Dislocations and subluxations of the shoulder are common sports injuries. Glenohumeral dislocation is so common that the finger joints are the only body parts more frequently dislocated. Once a glenohumeral joint has been dislocated, the chances of the injury recurring are as high as 80 to 90%. A dislocation of the shoulder occurs when the head of the humerus is forced or displaced from the shoulder joint. A subluxation is a partial dislocation. Symptoms of a subluxation are pain, decreased range of motion, "dead arm" (a numb and/or limp arm), a slipping sensation, and possible swelling. The athlete may experience a "popping" sensation, created by the shifting of the joint out of position and back into place. The signs and symptoms of dislocation include pain, loss of strength, loss of motion, possible swelling, and possible deformity. These symptoms can be detected by comparing the injured shoulder to the uninjured one. Watch the athlete's face for signs that pain increases with movement. X-rays will confirm the presence of a dislocation and determine whether or not a fracture exists as well. Note that because of the forces that cause a dislocation, a sprain and/or a strain of the surrounding tissues also will occur.

Immediate Treatment: *Do not* attempt to maneuver the joint back into position. Use the PRICE procedure as appropriate. Place the athlete in the most comfortable position possible. As with a fracture, pain or the injury's appearance may make the athlete anxious. Provide comfort by speaking in a reassuring tone and help the athlete control the respiratory rate by focusing on slow and steady breathing. Check for loss of sensation by asking if the patient is experiencing any numbness. Check for decreased circulation by observing for paleness, coolness, or loss of sensation. Additional circulation checks include checking the distal pulse and performing capillary refill checks by pinching the fingernails and watching to see if redness returns, indicating that the blood is returning to the fingertips. If either loss of sensation or reduced circulation is detected, a nerve, artery, or vein may be damaged and the EMS should be contacted immediately.

After checking circulation and sensation, immobilize the affected joint, and apply ice. If the weight of the ice causes the athlete more pain, reduce the amount of ice applied. Recheck circulation and sensation after splinting. Even if sensation and circulation do not seem to be impaired, the athlete will need to see a physician for treatment and possible x-rays. The possibility of a fracture along with dislocation should always be considered.

Once the dislocation is confirmed, the physician will perform a reduction, maneuvering the head of the humerus back into the joint socket. More x-rays are taken to confirm that the shoulder has been correctly repositioned, and then the shoulder is immobilized in a sling for about three weeks or as long as the physician recommends.

Follow-up Treatment: Make sure the physician's orders are followed.

Prevention: To prevent such injuries, athletes should strengthen the entire shoulder complex. Additionally, those who participate in contact sports, such as football, ice hockey, and lacrosse, should wear shoulder pads that fit properly. In all sports, coaches should teach players how to fall properly to avoid injury.

Contusions

In contact sports, the shoulders and upper arms are common sites for contusions. For example, in football, a contusion is likely to occur on the biceps where football player's shoulder pads stop on the biceps and there is still contact. Poorly fitted equipment can make this area even more vulnerable.

Contusions to the SC or AC joint can cause many of the same signs and symptoms that occur with an AC sprain: point tenderness, loss of range of motion, discoloration, and swelling (see Figure 16-19). The clavicle can also be susceptible to contusions because there is little or no protective fat padding or muscle around the area. Symptoms of a clavicle contusion include the inability to raise the arm and point tenderness. When treating a contusion, first rule out the possibility of a fracture by comparing the appearance of the uninvolved side with that of the injured side. Irregularities in appearance are possible signs of a fracture. A percussion test can also help in assessing the possibility of a fracture.

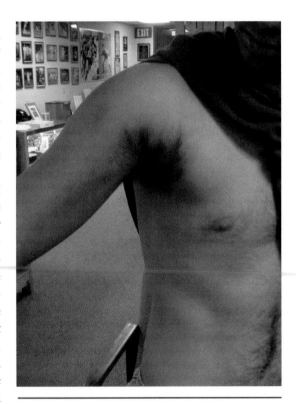

FIGURE 16-19 A Contusion

Immediate Treatment: To treat a contusion, use the PRICE procedure. Apply pressure using an elastic wrap or some other method. To rule out the possibility of fracture, refer the athlete to a physician.

If a contusion occurs to a joint, immobilize the joint. When the pain has subsided, full ROM has returned, and the strength is equal to the opposite side, the athlete may return to play with proper padding, such as a donut-shaped pad over the area of pain to disperse the pressure of any additional contact to the area. Do not re-traumatize the injury. This return-to-play criteria is based on the athlete's performance of sport-specific tests.

Follow-up Treatment: The athlete should see a physician for a possible x-ray to check for fractures. Once a fracture has been ruled out, the athlete should work on maintaining full ROM. Strength can be maintained with isometric exercises. Once the tissue has sufficiently recovered, isotonic strengthening may be done. Watch for any bruised areas that become hardened as this may indicate myositis ossificans. Pad the injured area with a donut pad as discussed above before the athlete returns to competition.

Prevention: To prevent shoulder contusions, athletes who participate in football, lacrosse, and ice hockey should wear shoulder pads with biceps extenders that fit properly. Elbow pads are also recommended for use in contact sports. Make sure the coach instructs the athletes in falling techniques to help prevent injuries.

Sprains

Contact sports commonly result in sprains of the glenohumeral joint (see Figure 16-20). For example, making a tackle in football with an outstretched arm can stretch the anterior capsule. Recall from Chapter 14 that a sprain is the overstretching and/or tearing of ligaments or other connective tissues caused by traumatic twisting of a joint. Sprains may also involve the articulating capsules or the synovial membrane.

In general, symptoms of a sprain include point tenderness, weakness, swelling, possible instability, possible deformity, and possible decreased ROM. With a glenohumeral sprain, upward movement of the arm will cause pain and a decrease in ROM. To rule out the possibility of a fracture, the athlete should be referred to a physician for possible x-rays.

Sulcus Test: Have the athlete seated with both arms relaxed. Simultaneously apply downward force to both elbows, causing inferior (downward) distraction of each humerus. Compare the involved side to the uninvolved side. A depression, or groove (also known as a *sulcus*) below the acromion is a positive sign, indicating

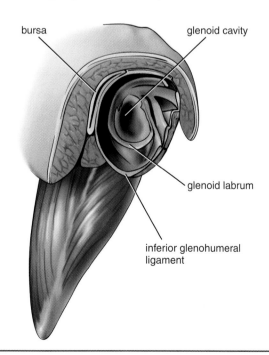

bursa

glenoid cavity

glenoid labrum

inferior glenohumeral ligament

FIGURE 16-20 Glenohumeral Ligaments, Lateral View

sulcus test

downward distraction of the humerus to assess stability, or the possibility of a sprain, of the glenohumeral joint.

multidirectional instability of the gleno-humeral joint (see Figure 16-21). **Note:** A "positive" test result means the patient probably has the condition being tested for. This test should be performed only by properly trained individuals.

Apprehension Test for Sprain of the Anterior Capsule: Stand behind the athlete, but position yourself slightly to one side so you can see the athlete's face. With the athlete's arm abducted at a 90° angle, place one hand on the athlete's wrist and use your other hand to stabilize the shoulder. Slowly and gently perform external rotation of the shoulder by pulling the athlete's wrist toward you (see Figure 16-22). Watch the face for signs of apprehension while performing this maneuver. If there is joint instability, the athlete will most likely grimace or complain that the shoulder is about to dislocate. Stop the maneuver as soon as signs of apprehension are detected; continuation of the maneuver could cause further injury. If the athlete has had a previous shoulder dislocation the test will always be positive, but the apprehension will be significant if the injury is recent. An older injury will be characterized by increased external rotation in the involved shoulder, but only minimal pain and, therefore, minimal apprehension.

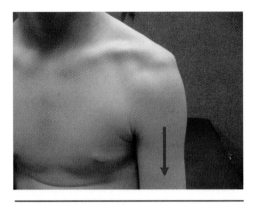

FIGURE 16-21 Positive Sulcus Test

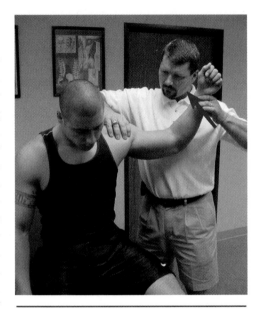

FIGURE 16-22 Apprehension Test for Sprain of the Anterior Capsule

Note: This test should be performed only by properly trained individuals.

Shoulder sprains may also occur to either the acromioclavicular (AC) or the sternoclavicular (SC) joints. The acromioclavicular sprain is commonly called an AC separation. An AC joint sprain generally occurs from a fall onto an outstretched arm, pushing the acromium upward. Such a sprain may also be caused by a direct blow to the tip of the shoulder, pushing the acromium downward. The signs and symptoms of an AC separation include superior displacement of the clavicle and point tenderness.

Acromioclavicular (AC) Sprain Test: Have the athlete remove shirt. Apply appropriate draping, allowing a clear view of the shoulder. Stand in front of the athlete and place your hands just above the elbows. Distract the humerus by pulling down on both sides simultaneously. Visible clavicular deformity in one shoulder indicates an AC sprain or, possibly, a fractured clavicle. Alternatively, you may place your thumb or finger on the clavicle and apply downward force. If the clavicle springs up when the pressure is removed, an AC sprain is indicated. If this movement of the clavicle, known as a "piano key sign," is absent, but there is pain at the distal aspect of the clavicle, a contusion (or "shoulder pointer") is indicated. **Note:** This test should be performed only by properly trained individuals.

An SC joint sprain is usually caused by a blow to the shoulder in which the shoulder is pushed backward and the sternum is forced forward. As with an AC sprain, an SC sprain may also result from an upward force, such as falling accidentally on an arm that is fully extended. Symptoms of an SC separation include pain, decreased range of motion, and increased pain with deep breathing.

Sternoclavicular (SC) Sprain Test: Stand in front of the athlete and place your thumb over the anterior proximal end of the clavicle. Apply posterior force to the clavicle. Compare the uninvolved side to the involved side, testing the uninvolved side first. Increased joint laxity on one side indicates a sprain of the SC joint. **Note:** This test should be performed only by properly trained individuals.

In assessing the degree of injury, always compare the injured side with the uninjured side, checking the uninjured side first. A first-degree, or mild, sprain will cause some point tenderness and some loss of strength. There should be no more joint laxity in the injured side than the uninjured side, and no decrease in range of motion. The lost strength will return after a short time.

A second-degree, or moderate, sprain is marked by swelling, tenderness, decreased ROM, and moderate loss of function in the injured area. When stressed for evaluation, a moderately sprained joint will exhibit some laxity when compared to the uninvolved side, indicating instability. However, the laxity will have an endpoint.

A third-degree, or severe, sprain causes a complete loss of function in the injured area, abnormal motion, and possible deformity. Local tenderness and swelling will also be present. When stressing the ligaments for evaluation, one will find an opening of the joint that appears to have no endpoint, indicating severe instability. There is no ligament resistance to the pressure you apply.

sternoclavicular (SC) sprain test

application of posterior force to the clavicle to assess stability, or the possibility of a sprain, of the SC joint.

Immediate Treatment: Use the PRICE procedure and refer the athlete to a physician for further evaluation.

Follow-up Treatment: Make sure the physician's orders are followed. The athlete may need to be fitted for a brace to add external support to the damaged ligaments. Remember when working with injuries that neoprene adds warmth; plastic and metal provide stability to the bones and ligaments; and cloth or athletic tape add stability to the soft tissues. Maintaining strength and flexibility of the area is vital to complete healing.

Prevention: Make sure that athletes wear properly fitted pads and jerseys, and make sure coaches teach athletes how to fall properly in order to minimize the risk of injury. Protect athletes by checking the event area for possible hidden dangers such as holes in the field, water on the court, etc. Also, instruct athletes in the appropriate strengthening exercises for the areas of the body that are most vulnerable to injury in the sport being played. Appropriate taping or bracing of vulnerable body parts can provide additional protection.

Strains

Muscle strains, caused by overstretching of the muscle, can affect any of the upper extremity muscles. A review of muscle strain classifications, presented more fully in Chapter 14, is provided below.

* Symptoms of a mild strain include local pain with contraction that decreases with stretching, decreased ROM, point tenderness, mild loss of function, and possible muscle spasms.

* A moderate strain is characterized by marked pain when the muscle is contracted and/or stretched, moderate swelling, point tenderness, moderate to severe loss of function, and decreased range of motion. The athlete may hear a snap or tearing sound at the time of the injury.

* A severe strain is the result of a rupture of the tendon or muscle tissue. Symptoms include a decrease or increase in ROM, severe loss of function, possible muscle spasms, and a defect in the muscle that is palpable. If pain is present with a severe strain, there will be no change in the degree of pain when the muscle is contracted or stretched.

The drop arm test may identify potential tears (strains) in the rotator cuff.

drop arm test

abduction of the arm followed by controlled lowering to assess the possibility of injury to the rotator cuff.

Drop Arm Test: Raise the athlete's arm past 90° of abduction. Instruct the athlete to slowly lower the arm. If there is a rotator cuff tear, the arm will drop down as a result of pain and weakness. A dropped arm indicates either impingement of the rotator cuff or a tear in the supraspinatus.

Immediate Treatment: Use the PRICE procedure during the first 24 to 48 hours following the injury. If pain is severe, immobilize the area to make the athlete as comfortable as possible and activate the Emergency Action Plan. A physician will need to rule out the possibility of a fracture or a complete tear.

Follow-up Treatment: After two days of rest, begin slow, static stretching of the injured area, followed by isometric and then isotonic strengthening exercises. The athlete may also appreciate the comfort of a neoprene sleeve over the area, which can add compression, support, and heat to the healing tissues.

Prevention: Proper strengthening and stretching of the upper extremity muscles will help prevent strains. See Chapter 7.

Impingement

impingement

compression of soft tissue between the ends of two or more bones because of tissue inflammation or bone displacement.

An **impingement** is the pinching of soft tissue, such as a bursa, tendon, or a nerve, between the ends of two or more bones. The joint that is probably most susceptible to impingement is the glenohumeral joint of the shoulder. Such impingement may be caused by repeated overhead activities such as throwing, tennis, swimming, and serving in volleyball. An impingement of the subacromial bursa will create symptoms of weakness in the supraspinatus muscle and point tenderness of the glenohumeral joint when the arm is elevated. The Hawkins-Kennedy Test may be used to check for the possibility of an impingement of the glenohumeral joint's subacromial bursa. A positive sign resulting from the empty can test (see page 398) may indicate weakness of the supraspinatus muscle of the rotator cuff—another common area of impingement.

Hawkins-Kennedy Test: (See Figure 16-23.) With the athlete seated in front of you, instruct the athlete to abduct the arm while bending the elbow. Place one hand beneath the athlete's elbow to stabilize it and use your other hand to apply downward force to the wrist. Pain at the shoulder joint indicates impingement of the subacromial bursa.

Nerves, such as the long thoracic nerve, may also be impinged. Such injuries may result from a muscle imbalance or trauma. The winged scapula test is used to check for possible impingement of the thoracic nerve, which serves the serratus anterior.

Winged Scapula Test: (See Figure 16-24.) Instruct the athlete to stand and have the athlete push against the wall as if doing a standing push-up. A scapula that protrudes from the ribs indicates an injury to the long thoracic nerve or a weakening of the serratus anterior on that side.

Immediate Treatment: Treat suspected shoulder or nerve impingements using the PRICE procedure to decrease inflammation. Refer the athlete to a physician for diagnosis and further treatment.

Follow-up Treatment: Once impingement is confirmed, strengthening exercises of the rotator cuff and stretching of the posterior cuff and capsule can help maintain range of motion.

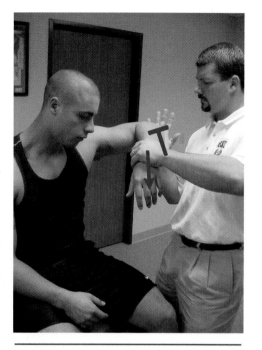

FIGURE 16-23 Hawkins-Kennedy Test

> **Hawkins-Kennedy test**
>
> compression of the supraspinatus tendon against the coracoacromial ligament to assess the possibility of impingement of the subacromial bursa.

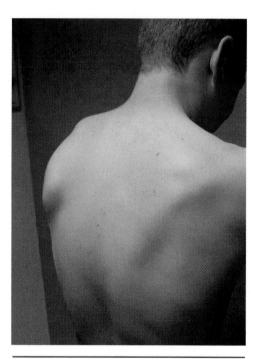

FIGURE 16-24 A Winged Scapula

> **winged scapula test**
>
> flexion of the serratus anterior to observe for weakening of that muscle as indicated by a protruding scapula.

Prevention: To prevent shoulder impingements, strengthen the rotator cuff muscles to distract the head of the humerus downward, creating more room in the glenohumeral space. (See Chapter 7.)

Tendonitis

Repeated stress to the tendons often results in tendonitis. This injury commonly affects the upper extremity tendons of those who participate in the following sports: swimming, baseball, water polo, football (some positions), discus, and other sports that involve throwing. Tendonitis may also be caused by improper body mechanics or poor conditioning. Symptoms include general soreness and point tenderness, with or without motion, and possible mild swelling. Tendonitis involving the biceps tendon is quite common among athletes who frequently move their arms in a throwing motion, baseball pitchers, tennis players, javelin throwers, and so on. This condition, called bicipital **tenosynovitis**, affects the sheath of the biceps tendon and produces anterior shoulder pain that increases with movement and palpation.

> **tenosynovitis**
>
> inflammation of the tendon sheath.

> **Speed's test**
>
> stretching or lengthening of the biceps tendon to assess the possibility of tenosynovitis.

Speed's Test: (See Figure 16-25.) Stand in front of the athlete and instruct the athlete to hold the arm at a 60° angle. Ask the athlete to attempt to flex the arm while you apply isometric resistance. If the athlete feels pain at the point of the bicipital groove the test is positive, indicating possible inflammation of the biceps tendon.

Immediate Treatment: Ice the area as soon as symptoms develop, using the proper PRICE procedure. In severe cases, resting the injured area is also recommended. For bicipital tenosynovitis, a brace that stabilizes the biceps tendon in the bicipital groove may help ease the pain and speed the healing of the injury. For tendonitis affecting the elbow or wrist, a neoprene compression sleeve may be helpful. Other types of braces may work as well.

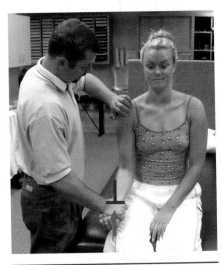

FIGURE 16-25 Speed's Test

Follow-up Treatment: Massage the area with ice for 7 to 10 minutes four times a day. If the injury does not improve within one to two weeks, the athlete should see a physician. Anti-inflammatory medicine or additional treatment, such as ultrasound therapy, may be prescribed by the physician.

Prevention: Ice applied to high-stress areas after every practice or game can help to prevent tendonitis. Proper conditioning (warm-up, pre-season and off-season) and good sport-specific body mechanics can also help prevent injury. Consult with the coaching staff regarding proper use of mechanics for the sport. Bring to their attention different ways that proper mechanics can prevent injuries.

Synovitis and Bursitis

Like all joints, the joints in the upper extremities can be affected by synovitis and bursitis. As previously noted in Chapter 14, bursitis is the inflammation of a bursa, a small sac located in the connective tissue surrounding a joint. Synovitis is the inflammation of a synovial membrane that lines a bursa. Both conditions are caused by repeated stressful motions or direct trauma. Therefore, athletes, such as baseball players, javelin throwers, tennis players, racquet-ball players, gymnasts, and swimmers are extremely susceptible to joint disorders in their shoulders (see Figure 16-26). The symptoms of synovitis and bursitis are similar to each other and include crepitation, swelling, and pain. The athlete will also experience decreased mobility of the affected area when resistance is applied.

Immediate Treatment: If no swelling is present, treatment includes the use of moist heat packs. If swelling is present, use the PRICE procedure. When applying ice to an injury, keep the ice in place for 20 minutes, then remove the ice for an hour. Repeat this cycle for 24 to 72 hours during waking hours, or until the swelling subsides. Protect the skin from frostbite by placing a cloth or towel between the ice and skin. It is also helpful to pad the affected area to prevent further injury.

Follow-up Treatment: After the swelling subsides, use moist heat treatments. To maintain mobility in the joint, advise the athlete to carefully stretch the affected joint through the pain-free range of motion. If pain increases or persists for over a week, refer the athlete to a physician.

Prevention: Make sure athletes are taught proper body and sport mechanics to avoid unnecessary stress to the joints. Instruction in sport mechanics is typically the coach's responsibility, but as the athlete's advocate, never just assume that the athlete has this information.

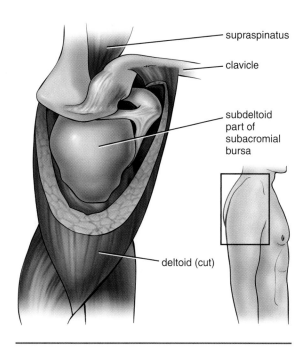

FIGURE 16-26 A Healthy Subacromial Bursa, Anterolateral View

THE ELBOW AND FOREARM

When in proper anatomical position (palms up, with arms at the sides while standing), the radius is the lateral bone of the forearm (see Figure 16-27). At the proximal end, the radius articulates medially with the radial notch of the ulna, and superiorly with the humerus. The widened, distal end of the

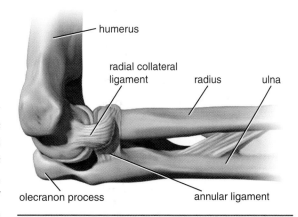

FIGURE 16-27 Elbow, Collateral Ligaments, Lateral View

radius allows for inferior articulation with the carpus, or wrist, and medial articulation with the ulna. This distal point of medial articulation is the ulnar notch of the radius. A distal projection, called the styloid process of the radius, is on the lateral side of the bone, opposite the ulnar notch.

Longer than the radius, the ulna is the medial bone of the forearm. At its proximal end, the ulna is large and forms part of the elbow joint. The most noticeable point at this proximal end is the olecranon process, which forms the tip of the elbow (see Figure 16-28). The distal portion of the ulna is small and round. A blunt projection called the styloid process of the ulna is on the medial side of the distal ulna. It is at this point that the ulna connects to the wrist.

The muscles affecting movement of the elbow include the brachioradialis, supinator, pronator teres, and the pronator quadratus. All, except for the pronator quadratus, originate on either the scapula or the humerus. As expected, they attach at some point on the radius or on the ulna in the forearm (see Figure 16-29).

The ulnar, median, and radial nerves are the primary nerves extending from the elbow region to the hand. The ulnar nerve passes through the elbow on the medial side (forming the funny bone) and the radial nerve on the lateral side. The median nerve, as the name suggests, passes through the middle of the forearm.

The elbow is supplied with blood by a number of arteries and veins that pass through the region's fossae (small hollow spaces). The primary arteries of this region are the radial and ulnar arteries. These arteries branch off from the brachial artery at the elbow and extend into the forearm and hand. The principle veins of the elbow include the cephalic, basilic, radial, and ulnar veins. The cephalic and basilic veins start in the upper arm, whereas the radial and ulnar veins begin at the elbow. All of these veins extend into the forearm and hand.

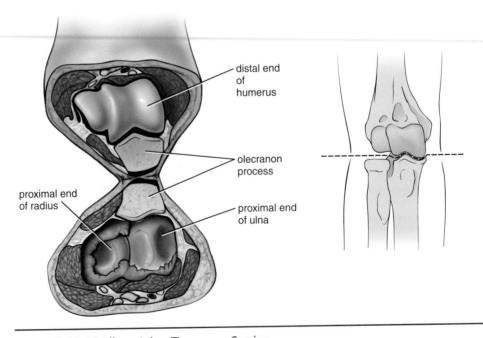

distal end of humerus

olecranon process

proximal end of radius

proximal end of ulna

FIGURE 16-28 Elbow Joint, Transverse Section

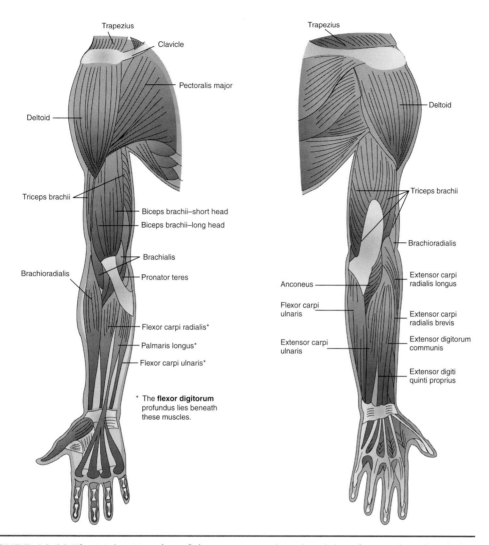

FIGURE 16-29 The Major Muscles of the Arm, Anterior View (L) and Posterior View (R)

ASSESSING ELBOW AND FOREARM INJURIES

Like all injuries, elbow and forearm injuries must be assessed using the principles of the HOPS procedure, taking care to accurately record all information and passing the information along to the appropriate members of the sports medicine team.

General Range-of-Motion Evaluations for the Elbow

ROM Test for Elbow Flexion: (See Figure 16-30.) Ask the athlete to face you with arms fully extended in anatomical position. Instruct the athlete to raise both forearms as far as possible with the hands facing palm-up. Check

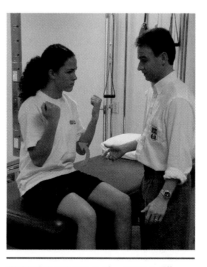

FIGURE 16-30 Active ROM, Elbow Flexion

both arms simultaneously, noting any differences. Motion should be smooth and painless. Limited ROM on one side indicates potential injury or deformity on that side.

ROM Test for Elbow Extension: (See Figure 16-31.) Ask the athlete to face you with arms fully flexed. Instruct the athlete to lower both forearms by straightening the elbows, with the hands facing palm-up. Check both arms simultaneously, noting any differences. Motion should be smooth and painless. Limited ROM on one side indicates potential injury or deformity on that side.

ROM Test for Elbow Supination: (See Figure 16-32.) Ask the athlete to face you with elbows flexed at 90° and palms facing down. Instruct the athlete to supinate the hands, keeping the elbows flexed at the 90° angle. Check both arms simultaneously, noting any differences. Motion should be smooth and painless. Limited ROM on one side indicates potential injury or deformity on that side.

ROM Test for Elbow Pronation: (See Figure 16-33.) Ask the athlete to face you with elbows flexed at 90° and palms facing up. Instruct the athlete to pronate the hands, keeping the elbows flexed at the 90° angle. Check both arms simultaneously, noting any differences. Motion should be smooth and painless. Limited ROM on one side indicates potential injury or deformity on that side.

Manual Muscle Tests for the Elbow

Flexion Strength Test for the Elbow: (See Figure 16-34.) Ask the athlete to face you with the uninvolved arm flexed at a 90° angle. Place one hand on top of the athlete's wrist and use your other hand to stabilize the athlete's elbow. Instruct the athlete to flex the arm isometrically. Compare the strength between the involved and uninvolved arms, and note any differences. Weakness on one side indicates potential injury or deformity to the biceps.

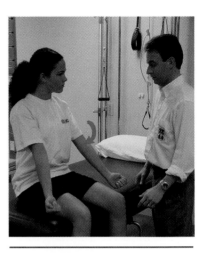

FIGURE 16-31 Active ROM, Elbow Extension

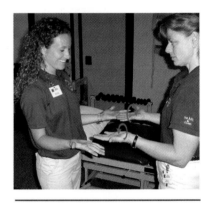

FIGURE 16-32 Active ROM, Elbow Supination

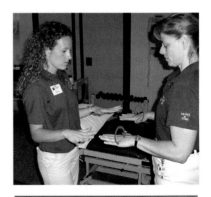

FIGURE 16-33 Active ROM, Elbow Pronation

Extension Strength Test for the Elbow: (See Figure 16-35.) With the athlete sitting or standing, ask the athlete to face you with arm flexed at an angle of 90 to 100°.

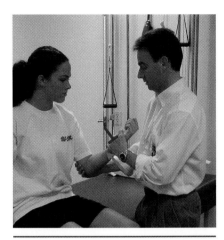

FIGURE 16-34 Biceps Strength Test

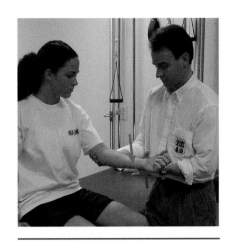

FIGURE 16-35 Triceps Strength Test

Place one hand on the back of the athlete's wrist and use your other hand to stabilize the elbow. Instruct the athlete to extend the arm isometrically. Compare the strength between the involved and uninvolved arms, and note any differences. Weakness on one side indicates potential injury or deformity to the triceps.

Supination Strength Test for the Elbow: (See Figure 16-36.) Ask the athlete to face you with arms flexed at a 90° angle and palms down. Place your hands on top of the athlete's hands, grasping the medial aspect of the hand if desired. Instruct the athlete to supinate the forearm while you provide isometric resistance. Compare the strength between the involved and uninvolved arms, and note any differences. Weakness on one side indicates potential injury or deformity to the supinator on that side.

Pronation Strength Test for the Elbow: (See Figure 16-37.) Ask the athlete to face you with arms flexed at a 90° angle and palms up. Place your hands on the bottom of the athlete's hands, grasping the medial aspect of the hand if desired. Instruct the athlete to pronate the forearm while you provide isometric resistance. Compare the strength between the involved and uninvolved arms, and note any differences. Weakness on one side indicates potential injury or deformity to the pronator quadratus on that side.

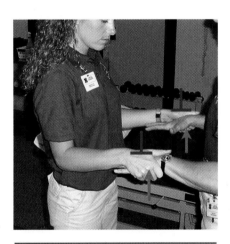

FIGURE 16-36 Supinator Strength Test

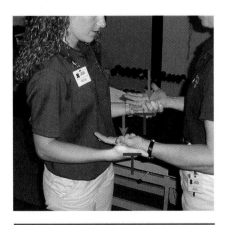

FIGURE 16-37 Pronator Strength Test

INJURIES TO THE ELBOW AND ARM

All of the injuries discussed in Chapter 14 can affect the elbows and arms. Many of these injuries are also discussed in "Injuries to the Shoulder" in this chapter. To avoid unnecessary repetition, only injuries not yet been discussed will be addressed in detail in this section.

Fractures

Fractures of the elbow often result from direct blows, or falls involving an outstretched hand, but they can also be caused by repeated stress to the bone. Elbow fractures usually affect the lower end of the humerus (see Figure 16-38).

Signs, symptoms, treatment, and prevention of fractures are discussed in detail in Chapter 14. See also "Injuries to the Shoulder" in this chapter.

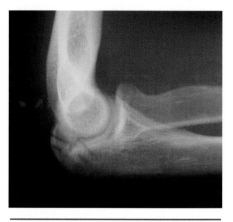

FIGURE 16-38 A Stress Fracture of the Olecranon Process

Dislocations and Subluxations

Dislocation of the elbow often occurs when an athlete falls on an outstretched arm or when a limb is twisted severely. Dislocation of the phalanges (fingers) is usually caused by a direct blow from a ball, or as the result of falling on extended fingers. Sports that carry an increased risk of these injuries include rollerblading, skateboarding, ice skating, hockey, baseball, and football.

Dislocations and subluxations are discussed in detail in Chapter 14. See also "Injuries to the Shoulder" in this chapter. To help prevent dislocations and subluxations of the elbows, athletes should strengthen the arm muscles. In addition, players of the above sports should wear elbow pads that fit properly. In all sports, coaches should teach players how to fall properly to avoid injury.

Contusions

Elbows and arms receive contusions in contact sports. Use the PRICE procedure, along with treatment guidelines for contusions outlined in Chapter 14. See also "Injuries to the Shoulder" in this chapter. To prevent elbow contusions, elbow pads are recommended for use in contact sports. Make sure the coach instructs the athletes in falling techniques to help prevent injuries.

Sprains

The most common sprains and strains of the elbow result from hyperextension. Hyperextension may occur when the athlete falls on an outstretched arm, thus overextending the elbow and tearing the capsule ligaments.

Valgus Stress Test for the Elbow: (See Figure 16-39.) Ask the athlete to face you and present the uninvolved arm, palm up. Stabilize the athlete's wrist by placing one hand on the medial aspect. Place your other hand on the lateral aspect of the elbow joint and apply medial force. Repeat the test for the involved elbow. Compare the uninvolved side to the involved side. Pain or laxity in the involved joint

---

valgus stress test

application of a medial force to the lateral aspect of a joint in an attempt to create a gap in the medial joint line, thereby testing the stability of the medial aspect of the joint.

indicates potential injury or deformity to the ulnar collateral ligament.

After this test is performed with the elbow straight, repeat with the elbow flexed at a 30° angle. The hand placement and the forces applied are the same as described above. If laxity and pain in the elbow joint also occur with this test, it confirms injury or deformity to the ulnar collateral ligament.

Varus Stress Test for the Elbow: (See Figure 16-40.) Ask the athlete to face you and present the uninvolved arm, palm up. Stabilize the athlete's wrist by placing one hand on the lateral aspect. Place your other hand on the medial aspect of the elbow joint and apply lateral force. Repeat the test for the involved elbow. Compare the uninvolved side to the involved side. Pain or laxity in the joint indicates potential injury or deformity to the radial collateral ligament.

Like the valgus test, after this test is performed with the elbow straight, repeat with the elbow flexed at a 30° angle. The hand placement and the forces applied are the same as described above. If laxity and pain in the elbow joint also occur with this test, it confirms injury or deformity to the radial collateral ligament.

In assessing the degree of injury, always compare the injured side with the uninjured side, checking the uninjured side first. See Chapter 14 for a detailed description of the degrees of sprains as well as their treatment and prevention. See also "Injuries to the Shoulder" in this chapter.

Impingement

As previously discussed, impingement is the pinching of soft tissue, such as a bursa, tendon, or a nerve, between the ends of two or more bones. The ulnar nerve may become impinged, or compressed, as a result of repeated stress to the arm. As a result, baseball players, javelin throwers, bowlers, tennis players, racquetball players, gymnasts, and swimmers are most likely to be affected by such impingements. Direct blows may also compress the ulnar nerve. Symptoms of ulnar nerve impingement include point tenderness, pain with and without motion, numbness, and possible loss of strength. Tinel's sign is used to check for possible impingement of the nerves in the elbow and wrist.

Tinel's Sign: (See Figure 16-41.) Locate the ulnar groove on the athlete's elbow and tap the ulnar nerve, located in the ulnar groove, with your forefinger. A tingling

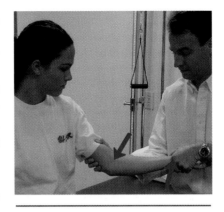

FIGURE 16-39 Valgus Test for the Elbow

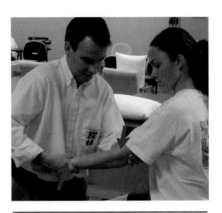

FIGURE 16-40 Varus Test for the Elbow

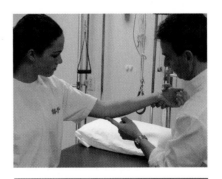

FIGURE 16-41 Tinel's Sign

varus stress test

application of a lateral force to the medial aspect of a joint in an attempt to create a gap in the lateral joint line, thereby testing the stability of the lateral aspect of the joint.

Tinel's sign

a tingling sensation produced by percussion of the ulnar nerve.

sensation that extends distally down the involved arm indicates ulnar nerve irritation, possibly caused by impingement.

To treat an ulnar nerve impingement, see "Injuries to the Shoulder" in this chapter.

Synovitis and Bursitis

The elbow is also susceptible to synovitis and bursitis. As stated previously, both conditions are caused by repeated stressful motions or direct trauma. Therefore, athletes such as baseball players, javelin throwers, bowlers, tennis players, racquetball players, gymnasts, and swimmers are extremely susceptible to disorders of the elbow.

Olecranon bursitis is the inflammation of the bursa that lies between the olecranon process and the skin (see Figure 16-42). The olecranon bursa is the most frequently injured bursa in the elbow due to its superficial location and the potential for direct contact. Like other forms of bursitis, the signs and symptoms of olecranon bursitis include pain, swelling, crepitation, decreased mobility, and point tenderness. In some cases, the swelling will be almost instantaneous.

Treatment for synovitis and bursitis involving the elbow follows the course discussed in Chapter 14. If no swelling is present, treatment takes the form of moist heat packs. If swelling is present, use the PRICE procedure with one notable exception: When applying ice to the elbow, keep the ice in place for 15 minutes, then remove the ice for an hour. Normally, ice can be applied to other areas of the body for 20 minutes, but because of the superficial location of the ulnar nerve as it passes through the elbow, the icing time should

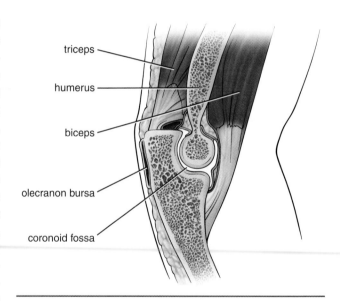

triceps

humerus

biceps

olecranon bursa

coronoid fossa

FIGURE 16-42 A Healthy Olecranon Bursa, Sagittal View

be decreased to 15 minutes for elbow injuries. Check the fingers periodically for ulnar nerve sensation while the ice is in place, and remove the ice if sensation is reduced. As with other PRICE procedures, repeat this cycle for 24 to 72 hours during waking hours, or until the swelling subsides, using the proper ice precautions. Other than the reduced icing time, the treatment should follow the course described in Chapter 14.

Biceps Brachii Rupture

The biceps brachii is the large muscle in the upper arm that assists in flexion of the elbow as well as rotation of the hands from a supine to a prone position (see Figure 16-43). This muscle can be ruptured by pulling motions. Therefore, biceps brachii ruptures occur most frequently to athletes who participate in such sports as gymnastics, rowing, and weight lifting. Although the rupture will generally occur at the point of origin, a painful bulge may appear at the fullest portion, or belly, of the muscle as a result of the tear. Symptoms include pain, a bulging biceps, and a loss or decrease of mobility. Sometimes the athlete hears a snapping sound when the **muscle rupture** occurs.

Immediate Treatment: Put the athlete in the most comfortable position possible, immobilize the upper arm, and refer the athlete to a physician for further evaluation.

Follow-up Treatment: Make sure the physician's orders are followed.

Prevention: To prevent ruptures of this muscle and others, athletes should stay within their tolerance limits when training and competing. This means they should not push themselves beyond muscle tolerance or endurance. This does not mean, however, that the overload principle should not be used in training. There is a difference between overworking a muscle to build it and pushing a muscle beyond its capability. The overload principle (discussed in Chapter 7) is the basis for all exercise training programs. For muscles to increase in strength, the workload to those muscles must increase beyond what is normally experienced without causing injury. This should be under the direction of a qualified individual.

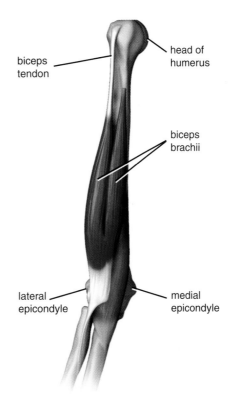

muscle rupture

a complete tear of a muscle.

FIGURE 16-43 Healthy Biceps Brachii

Epicondylitis

Epicondylitis is the inflammation of an epicondyle of the humerus and surrounding tissues. Medial epicondylitis affects the flexors and is known as "little league elbow" or "golfer's elbow." Lateral epicondylitis affects the extensors and is often called "tennis elbow." Both of these conditions are the result of chronic overuse by athletes who repeatedly twist the forearm during throwing or swinging motions. Examples of athletes who might be affected include baseball pitchers, tennis players, javelin throwers, and golfers. Athletes with epicondylitis will have pain and tenderness around the elbow. In some cases, signs of swelling may be visible. When suffering from this condition, any twisting motion will cause pain or weakness.

epicondylitis

inflammation of the medial or lateral epicondyle of the humerus and its surrounding tissues.

Immediate Treatment: Use the PRICE procedure for all forms of epicondylitis.

Follow-up Treatment: If symptoms do not improve within one to two weeks, the athlete should see a physician. When an athlete suffers from epicondylitis, you should evaluate the athlete's body mechanics. Try to find a way in which the athlete can decrease the aggravation of the elbow. For example, if the athlete is playing tennis, you might check the tennis racket for proper grip size and string tension. Wearing a brace around the forearm sometimes helps to relieve the pain of epicondylitis.

Prevention: Proper body mechanics should be emphasized to players of sports involving repeated elbow motions: javelin, tennis, racquetball, baseball, etc.

Volkmann's Contracture

Volkmann's contracture is an injury that may occur when swelling, muscle spasm, bone displacement, or a bone fracture near the elbow puts pressure on the arteries in the arm. This pressure decreases the blood supply to the hand and forearm, resulting in serious muscle damage and possibly paralysis in those parts of the body. Pain will increase when the fingers are passively extended (relaxed). The pain may be accompanied by an absence of or decrease in the brachial and radial pulses.

Immediate Treatment: This is an emergency situation. Activate the EMS.

Follow-up Treatment: Make sure the physician's orders are followed.

Prevention: As with many sports injuries, the best way to prevent Volkmann's contracture is through the use of protective padding and safe falling techniques.

THE WRIST AND HAND

The wrist is made up of eight bones, called carpals, arranged in two transverse rows. The bones are tightly bound together with synovial joints between them, allowing for little movement. Collectively, these eight bones are called the carpus.

Five metacarpals and the digits (fingers) make up the hand (see Figure 16-44). The metacarpals are the long bones of the hand and are identified as numbers one through

> **Volkmann's contracture**
>
> contracture and damage to the muscles of the forearm because of injury to their blood supply.

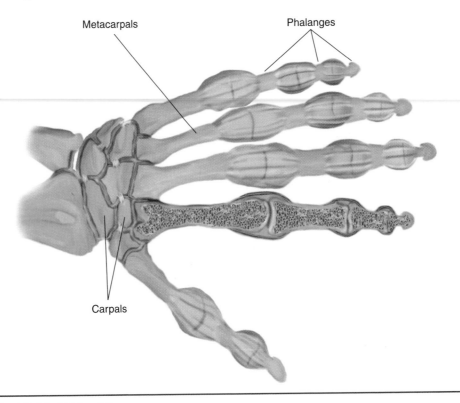

FIGURE 16-44 Hand Bones

five. The first metacarpal is the most lateral. Each digit has three phalanges, except digit number one, which only contains two phalanges. Each metacarpal articulates with one another and with the carpus. The distal end of each metacarpal, called the head of the metacarpal, articulates with the proximal end of each phalanx. Located between each phalanx are ligaments that permit a hinge type movement in the interphalangeal joints.

The wrist and hand also have muscles that allow for many different types of movement. All of the muscles originate from the distal end of the humerus and from the radius and ulna. The anterior side of the forearm contains muscles known as the flexors: flexor carpi radialis, flexor carpi ulnaris, palmaris longus, and flexor digitorum profundus. The posterior side of the forearm contains the extensors: extensor carpi radialis longus, extensor carpi radialis brevis, extensor carpi ulnaris, and extensor digitorum (see Figure 16-45).

The muscles of the wrist and hand are controlled by the median, radial, and ulnar nerves. The radial and ulnar nerves run alongside the bones for which they are named and end at the wrist; the median nerve, however, continues on through the carpal tunnel of the wrist and extends into the palm of the hand (see Figure 16-46).

Blood is supplied to the wrist and hand by the radial and ulnar arteries. The ulnar, radial, cephalic, and basilic veins transport blood from the hand, back up the forearm, to the heart and lungs for re-oxygenation. Like the nerves, the radial and ulnar blood vessels run parallel to the radius and ulna.

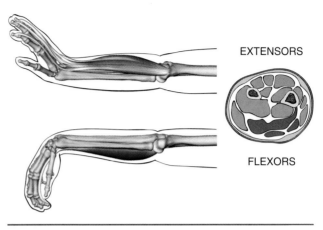

EXTENSORS

FLEXORS

FIGURE 16-45 Flexors and Extensors of the Lower Arm

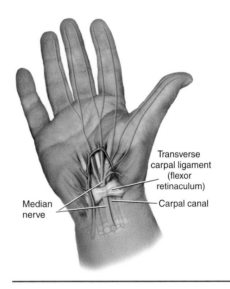

Transverse carpal ligament (flexor retinaculum)

Median nerve

Carpal canal

FIGURE 16-46 Anatomy of Carpal Tunnel

ASSESSING WRIST AND HAND INJURIES

Remember the HOPS principles when assessing wrist and hand injuries, taking care to accurately record all information and conveying it to the appropriate members of the sports medicine team.

General Range-of-Motion Evaluations for the Wrist and Hand

ROM Test for Wrist Flexion: (See Figure 16-47.) Instruct the athlete to simultaneously flex both wrists as far as possible. Compare the range of motion between the uninvolved and involved wrists. Movement should be smooth and painless. Limited ROM on one side indicates potential injury or deformity on that side.

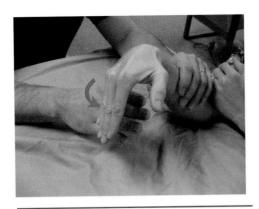

FIGURE 16-47 Active ROM, Wrist Flexion

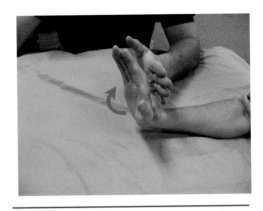

FIGURE 16-48 Active ROM, Wrist Extension

ROM Test For Wrist Extension: (See Figure 16-48.) Instruct the athlete to simultaneously extend both wrists as far as possible. Compare the range of motion between the uninvolved and involved wrists. Movement should be smooth and painless. Limited ROM on one side indicates potential injury or deformity on that side.

ROM Test for Finger Flexion: (See Figure 16-49.) Instruct the athlete to simultaneously flex the fingers of both hands as far as possible. Compare the range of motion between the uninvolved and involved hands. Movement should be smooth and painless. Limited ROM on one side indicates potential injury or deformity on that side.

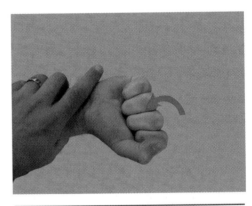

FIGURE 16-49 Active ROM, Finger Flexion

ROM Test for Finger Extension: (See Figure 16-50.) Instruct the athlete to simultaneously extend the fingers of both hands as far as possible. Compare the range of motion between the uninvolved and involved hands. Movement should be smooth and painless. Limited ROM on one side indicates potential injury or deformity on that side.

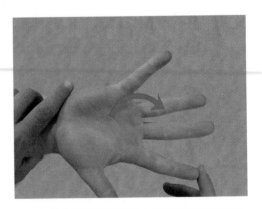

FIGURE 16-50 Active ROM, Finger Extension

Manual Muscle Tests for the Wrist and Hand

Extension Strength Test for the Wrist: (See Figure 16-51.) Place your hand on the dorsal aspect of the athlete's hand and instruct the athlete to push up against your hand as you provide isometric resistance. Compare the strength between the involved and uninvolved sides, and note any differences. Weakness

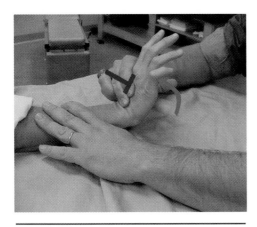

FIGURE 16-51 Wrist Strength, Extension

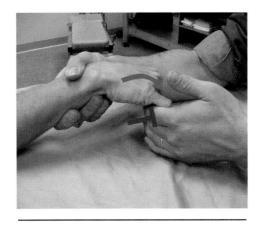

FIGURE 16-52 Wrist Strength, Flexion

on one side indicates potential injury or deformity to the extensor carpi radialis longus, extensor carpi radialis brevis, and/or extensor carpi ulnaris on that side.

Flexion Strength Test for the Wrist: (See Figure 16-52.) Place your hand on the palmar aspect of the athlete's hand and instruct the athlete to push down against your hand as you provide isometric resistance. Compare the strength between the involved and uninvolved sides, and note any differences. Weakness on one side indicates potential injury or deformity to the flexor carpi radialis and/or flexor carpi ulnaris on that side.

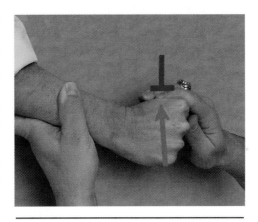

FIGURE 16-53 Wrist Strength, Radial Deviation

Radial Deviation Strength Test for the Wrist: (See Figure 16-53.) Place your hand on the radial aspect of the athlete's hand and instruct the athlete to press against your hand as you provide isometric resistance. Compare the strength between the involved and uninvolved sides, and note any differences. Weakness on one side indicates potential injury or deformity to the flexor carpi radialis and/or extensor carpi radialis on that side.

Ulnar Deviation Strength Test for the Wrist: (See Figure 16-54.) Place your hand on the ulnar aspect of the athlete's hand and instruct the athlete to press against your hand as you pro-

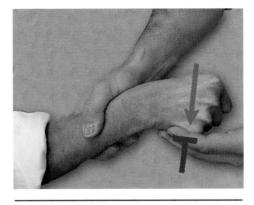

FIGURE 16-54 Wrist Strength, Ulnar Deviation

vide isometric resistance. Compare the strength between the involved and uninvolved sides, and note any differences. Weakness on one side indicates potential injury or deformity to the flexor carpi ulnaris and/or extensor carpi ulnaris on that side.

Extension Strength Test for the Fingers: (See Figure 16-55.) Place one finger on the dorsal aspect of the athlete's finger to be tested and have the athlete push the finger up into extension as you provide isometric resistance. Compare the strength between the involved and uninvolved sides, and note any differences. Weakness on one side indicates potential injury or deformity to the muscles of the finger on that side.

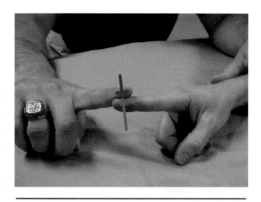

FIGURE 16-55 Finger Strength, Extension

Flexion Strength Test for the Fingers: (See Figure 16-56.) Place one finger on the palmar aspect of the athlete's finger to be tested, and have the athlete flex the finger as you provide isometric resistance. Compare the strength between the involved and uninvolved sides, and note any differences. Weakness on one side indicates potential injury or deformity to the muscles of the finger on that side.

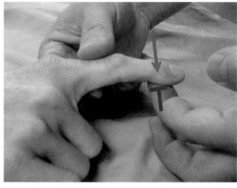

FIGURE 16-56 Finger Strength, Flexion

Abduction Strength Test for the Fingers: (See Figure 16-57.) Place one finger on the lateral aspect the athlete's finger to be tested. Place another finger on the lateral aspect of one of the athlete's adjacent fingers. Instruct the athlete to abduct the fingers as you provide isometric resistance. Compare the strength between the involved and uninvolved sides, and note any differences. Weakness on one side indicates potential injury or deformity to the muscles of the finger on that side.

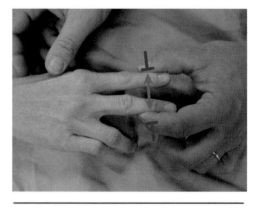

FIGURE 16-57 Finger Strength, Abduction

Adduction Strength Test for the Fingers: (See Figure 16-58.) Place one finger between the athlete's finger to be tested and the one next to it. Instruct the athlete to adduct the fingers as you provide isometric resistance. Compare the strength between the involved and uninvolved sides, and note any differences. Weakness on one side indicates potential injury or deformity to the muscles of the finger on that side.

INJURIES TO THE WRIST AND HAND

Fractures

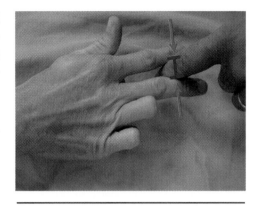

FIGURE 16-58 Finger Strength, Adduction

Fractures of the wrist and hand, such as a Colles's fracture of the distal radius, usually result from direct blows or falls involving an outstretched hand. A common injury to offensive linemen, skateboarders, rollerbladers, and ice skaters, a Colles's fracture may cause a loss or reduction of hand and wrist functions, crepitus, swelling, and in severe cases, loss of sensation.

A fracture of the navicular, also called the scaphoid, is usually caused by falling on an outstretched arm. This injury often affects offensive linemen in football. The signs and symptoms include point tenderness in the anatomical snuffbox, swelling, and pain with extension. Located at the base of the thumb, the navicular is the slowest healing bone in the body because of its limited supply of blood. Therefore, a fracture that decreases the already limited blood supply to this bone may lead to nonunion of the bone at the fracture site. "Nonunion" of the bone means the fractured portions of the bone won't heal. This condition may require surgical intervention.

A detailed discussion of the treatment and prevention of fractures may be found in Chapter 14. See also "Injuries to the Shoulder" in this chapter.

Dislocations and Subluxations

Dislocation of the wrists and phalanges (fingers) is usually caused by a direct blow from a ball, or as the result of falling on an extended hand. Sports that carry an increased risk of these injuries include rollerblading, skateboarding, ice skating, hockey, baseball, and football. Players of these sports can wear gloves and wrist guards to help prevent such injuries. In all sports, coaches should teach players how to fall properly to avoid injury.

Contusions

Like all contusions, finger contusions are usually caused by direct blows. Contusions to the fingers may cause bleeding underneath the nail bed. This can be extremely painful because of the pressure of the blood underneath the fingernail. If this occurs, the athlete should see a physician to have the blood drained from beneath the nail. Sports that carry an increased risk of contusions to the hands and fingers include basketball, volleyball, and football. Treatment should follow that described for all contusions in Chapter 14.

Sprains

Sprains to the wrist may be caused from either hyperextension or hyperflexion. Gamekeeper's thumb is a sprain of the ulnar collateral ligament, or the medial ligament of the thumb. This ligament is used in gripping, pinching, and grabbing. Gamekeeper's thumb is common among skiers, football players, and hockey players. The mechanism of this injury is usually contact that forces abduction of the thumb, resulting in stretching or tearing of the ligament.

Gamekeeper's Thumb Test: (See Figure 16-59.) Stabilize the first metacarpal of the athlete's uninvolved thumb with one hand and grasp the distal aspect of the thumb with your other hand. Bend the entire thumb down at a 45° angle and abduct the thumb. Repeat the test on the involved thumb. Increased pain or laxity of the ulnar collateral ligament of the thumb on the involved side indicates a sprain of that ligament. The absence of an endpoint indicates a complete tear (third-degree sprain) of the ulnar collateral ligament. **Note:** This test should be performed only by properly trained individuals. Other ligaments of the phalanges can be tested in a similar way by applying varus and valgus stresses to the individual ligaments of the fingers (see Figure 16-60).

In assessing the degree of injury, always compare the injured side with the uninjured side, checking the uninjured side first. See Chapter 14 for the signs, symptoms, and treatment of various degrees of sprains.

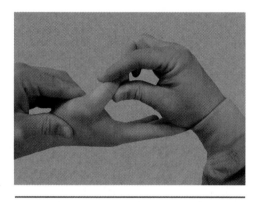

FIGURE 16-59 Gamekeeper's Thumb Test

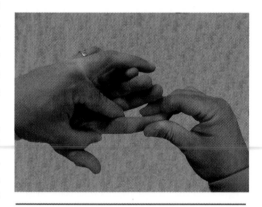

FIGURE 16-60 Ligament Stability Test—Varus/Valgus

Impingement

Like other nerve impingements, those in the wrist are most often caused by repeated stress. Signs and symptoms of such impingement include point tenderness, pain with and without motion, numbness, and possible loss of strength. Athletes such as baseball players, javelin throwers, bowlers, tennis players, racquetball players, gymnasts, and swimmers are most likely to be affected by such impingement. Treatment should follow that described in the section on shoulder impingements in this chapter.

Phalen's Test: (See Figure 16-61.) Instruct the athlete to place the backs of the hands together near the middle of the chest. The arms, elbows, and wrists will each be bent to about 90°. Grasp the athlete's palms with one hand and gently squeeze. Tingling and/or numbness in the fingers indicates nerve impingement at the wrist on that side. **Note:** This test should be performed only by properly trained individuals.

Tendonitis

Tendonitis in the wrist, fingers, and thumbs is most likely to be caused by repeated stress, or overuse. Tennis players, bowlers, discus throwers, and other athletes who make repeated motions of the wrists and fingers are susceptible to tendonitis in these areas.

Finkelstein's Test: (See Figure 16-62.) Instruct the athlete to make a fist with the thumb under the fingers and the palm facing inward. Place one of your hands around the athlete's fist and apply isometric resistance as the athlete flexes the wrist downward in an ulnar direction. Pain in the involved side indicates tenosynovitis of the thumb tendon (de Quervain's disease). **Note:** This test should be performed only by properly trained individuals.

Treatment for tendonitis of the fingers is the same as for other areas of the body. See Chapter 14, as well as "Injuries to the Shoulder" in this chapter.

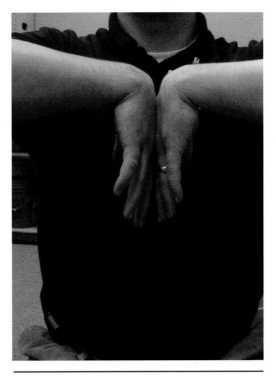

FIGURE 16-61 Phalen's Test

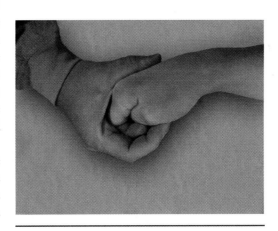

FIGURE 16-62 Finkelstein's Test

Ganglion Cyst of the Wrist

A **ganglion cyst** of the wrist is a fluid-filled sac in the synovial membrane that penetrates the tendon sheath. Also known as a herniation of the tendon sheath or joint capsule, this condition is associated with the degeneration of the tendon sheath. It often appears as a bump on the posterior aspect of the wrist. Additional symptoms include pain and decreased range of motion.

Immediate Treatment: If an athlete has a wrist ganglion cyst that does not heal spontaneously after a week, the athlete should see a physician for further evaluation. Protect the area with a donut pad while it is healing.

Follow-up Treatment: If the athlete is under the care of a physician, make sure the physician's orders are followed.

Prevention: Protective padding of the hand and wrist is helpful in preventing this injury, but spontaneous occurrences are not uncommon.

Mallet Finger

mallet finger

flexion of the distal interphalangeal joint of the finger caused by damage to the extensor tendon.

Mallet finger (Figure 16-63), or baseball finger, is a common injury in sports such as volleyball, baseball, football, and basketball. It may be caused by a direct blow to an outstretched finger, tearing the tendon along with a piece of the bone that the tendon is attached to (avulsion fracture). Mallet finger may also result when a finger is caught in an aperture such as the mesh of a jersey while the athlete is in motion. The athlete will not be able to actively extend the injured finger. Point tenderness will occur at the site of the fracture or ligament damage.

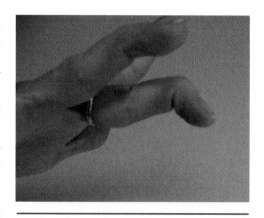

FIGURE 16-63 Mallet Finger

Immediate Treatment: The athlete should be referred to a physician for further evaluation and to check for a possible fracture.

Follow-up Treatment: Make sure the physician's orders are followed.

Prevention: There are no prevention techniques for mallet finger.

Buttonhole (Boutonniere) Deformity

buttonhole deformity

abnormal contracture of a phalange in which the proximal joint flexes and the distal joint hyperextends because of tendon rupture.

A **buttonhole deformity** is caused by a rupture of the tendon in the middle phalanx of a finger. This injury is caused by a force pushing the upper joint of the middle phalanx into excessive flexion. The athlete will experience severe pain and will be unable to fully extend the finger. There will be obvious swelling, point tenderness, and deformity.

Immediate Treatment: Use the PRICE procedure where appropriate. Refer the athlete to a physician for further evaluation and treatment.

Follow-up Treatment: Make sure the physician's orders are followed.

Prevention: Because injury occurs as a result of unique circumstances, such as the grabbing of a running back's jersey while the running back is still in motion, there is little that can be done to prevent this type of injury short of nonparticipation—which is not an option for most athletes.

THINKING IT THROUGH

The North Husky baseball team, a premiere baseball program in the southern states, had always been blessed with strong pitching. This year was no different, except for the early-season game against Melville. Mike Wilson was scheduled to start the Thursday game and was ready on Wednesday, even though his arm hurt a bit.

The arm pain resulted from a practice that followed five days of rained-out practices. After this day of throwing he had definite soreness in the back of the shoulder. Mike knew this pain meant he hadn't warmed up enough; he had felt it before, but never this bad.

Something else went wrong, too. Half the team had bad colds and were really run down. Despite warnings from the athletic trainer, the players had shared water bottles, allowing the virus to spread through the team like wildfire.

By Thursday morning Mike was sick as a dog. This was going to put Pat Cone on the mound for his first game of the season. The coach didn't really think Pat was ready, but the pickings were slim, and Melville wasn't much of a match for them. Excited and wanting the opportunity to throw, Mike convinced the coach to let him start instead of Pat, even if his arm hurt a little bit.

Mike was doing all right until the top of the sixth, when he began to struggle with his control. He wanted to finish out the game, so he figured he'd just start airing it out as hard as he could to make it through the game. This worked until he threw a fastball and failed to follow through properly. A sharp pain in the back of his shoulder told him he was in trouble; now he could hardly lift his arm.

What events led to this injury? What could an athletic trainer or coach have done to prevent this from happening? What type of injury do you think Mike suffered?

CHAPTER SUMMARY

Upper-extremity injuries affect the appendicular skeleton as well as the muscles, ligaments, tendons, blood vessels, and nerves that cover the bones. Dislocations and subluxations are as serious as fractures to an athlete because these injuries involve the soft tissues. Often, soft tissue injuries (sprains, strains, tendonitis, etc.) can result in significantly limited range of motion and require long, complex rehabilitation programs. Proper assessment of such injuries is vital to appropriate treatment. The HOPS assessment procedure provides a framework for careful and methodical injury assessment. To ensure effective continuity of care for the athlete, the information obtained from the HOPS procedure must be recorded and passed to the appropriate caregivers.

The potential for a specific type of shoulder or arm injury is directly related to the sport being played. Contact sports often result in sudden, intense, or traumatic injuries, while injuries that result from sports involving repetitive motion usually develop over time—often a surprisingly short time. In either case, appropriate strength and conditioning exercises along with proper protective gear can greatly reduce the athletes' potential for injury.

Some injuries occur frequently enough to have earned a common name, such as: Colles's fracture; golfer's elbow; tennis elbow; baseball finger; and gamekeeper's thumb. Regardless of the type of injury, applying ice to the injured area will help control pain and swelling. When possible, splinting may also reduce the athlete's discomfort. In addition, keep in mind that reassurance can be as important as pain relief to the comfort of an injured athlete.

STUDENT ENRICHMENT ACTIVITIES

Complete the following sentences.

1. The muscles affecting movement of the shoulder include the _____, _____, _____ _____, and _____ _____.

2. The major nerves of the arm include the _____, _____, and _____ nerves.

3. The glenohumeral joint is protected by the SITS muscles: the _____, _____, _____ _____, and _____, commonly called the rotator cuff.

4. The letters P-R-I-C-E in the PRICE procedure stand for _____, _____, _____, _____, and _____.

5. The _____ _____ and the _____ form the AC joint.

6. The _____ and the _____ form the SC joint.

7. The _____ nerve passes through the _____ tunnel of the wrist.

8. The biceps brachii is most often ruptured by_____ motions in sports.

9. Lateral epicondylitis is often referred to as _____ _____, while medial epicondylitis may be referred to as _____ _____ _____ or _____ _____.

10. Joint laxity is a sign of a _____ or _____ degree sprain.

Match the terms in Column A with the appropriate description in Column B.

	Column A		Column B
11.	_____ gamekeeper's thumb	A.	a sprain of the ulnar collateral ligament
12.	_____ Finkelstein's test	B.	may indicate injury to the radial collateral ligament in the elbow
13.	_____ varus stress test	C.	a wrist fracture, usually the result of falling on an outstretched hand
14.	_____ Hawkins-Kennedy test	D.	may indicate tenosynovitis in the thumb
15.	_____ head of the metacarpal	E.	the distal end of the metacarpal
16.	_____ biceps brachii rupture	F.	may indicate impingement of the subacromial bursa
17.	_____ Colles's fracture		
18.	_____ empty can test	G.	muscle damage associated with swelling near the elbow
19.	_____ buttonhole deformity	H.	caused by a rupture of the tendon in the middle phalanx
20.	_____ Volkmann's contracture		
21.	_____ valgus stress test	I.	symptoms of this condition may include a snapping sound and a bulge in the belly of the injured muscle
		J.	may indicate injury to the supraspinatus
		K.	may indicate injury to the ulnar collateral ligament in the elbow

Complete the following exercises.

22. Describe the steps and the purpose of the apprehension test of the anterior capsule.

23. Describe the difference between first-, second-, and third-degree sprains.

24. Describe the steps and the purpose of the percussion test.

25. Describe the steps and the purpose of Speed's test.

26. List *all* tests that are *not* to be performed without proper training. Research and describe where such training can be pursued.

CHAPTER 17

Injuries to the Chest and Abdomen

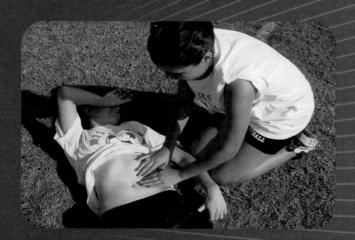

OBJECTIVES

After completing this chapter, you should be able to do the following:

1. Define and correctly spell each of the key terms.

2. Identify organs of the chest and abdomen and their respective injuries.

3. Name and define the three types of blood vessels and the three types of blood cells.

4. Identify the structure and function of the major parts of the heart.

5. Describe the path of a drop of blood as it flows through the heart.

6. Identify and describe the major parts of the respiratory system.

7. Describe the process of gas exchange.

KEY TERMS

* adipose tissue
* alveoli
* aorta
* arteries
* atria
* coronary circulation
* flail chest

* hemothorax
* hernia
* hyperventilation
* kidney
* lungs
* pancreas
* pneumothorax

* pulmonary circulation
* shock
* systemic circulation
* veins
* ventricles

THE CHEST

The thorax is another name for the chest. The bony structures of the thorax include 12 pairs of ribs, the thoracic vertebrae, the sternum, the clavicles, and the scapula. The thorax is separated from the abdominal cavity by a large muscle called the diaphragm. The heart, lungs, esophagus, trachea, major nerves, and great vessels (the **aorta**, pulmonary vessels, superior vena cava, and inferior vena cava) are protected by this structure referred to as the thoracic cage. The ribs and the diaphragm work together to bring oxygen into the body through the breathing process. Oxygen and waste products are exchanged through blood cells that are transported throughout the body via blood vessels.

> **aorta**
>
> the main artery in the body.

The Heart

Located slightly to the left of the middle of the anterior chest, the heart is a four-chambered, hollow, muscular organ (see Figure 17-1). The heart, which is about the size of a fist, is contained in the thoracic cavity of the body and is tilted slightly to the left of the sternum. It is located between the lungs and surrounded by the pericardial sac. The pericardial sac is a thin layer of tissue that surrounds the entire heart.

The natural pacemaker of the heart is located in the right atrium and is called the sino-atrial node. This node, which is influenced by the autonomic nervous system and various hormones, controls the contraction of the heart muscle through electrical impulses. The electrical activity conducted by the heart determines the pulse rate of each individual. In the average resting adult, it pumps 60 to 80 times a minute automatically. For an athlete, this range is more likely to be 40 to 60 times a minute.

The heart is composed of three layers of tissue: the smooth inner layer, called the endocardium; the muscular middle layer, called the myocardium; and the serous outer layer, called the epicardium. The heart contains four chambers: two upper and two lower chambers. The upper chambers are separated from the lower chambers by three important one-way valves. Another very important one-way valve (the

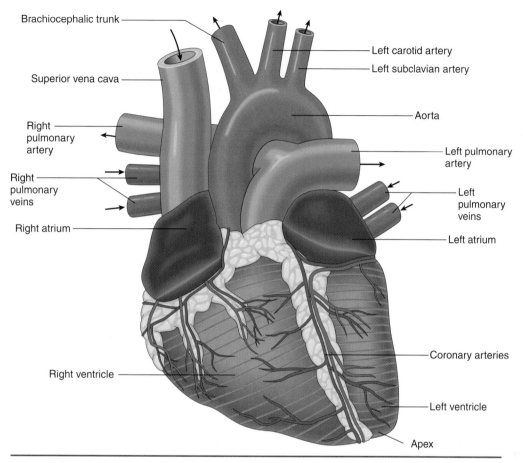

- Brachiocephalic trunk
- Left carotid artery
- Left subclavian artery
- Superior vena cava
- Aorta
- Right pulmonary artery
- Left pulmonary artery
- Right pulmonary veins
- Left pulmonary veins
- Right atrium
- Left atrium
- Coronary arteries
- Right ventricle
- Left ventricle
- Apex

FIGURE 17-1 The External Heart

atria
the upper chambers of the heart, also known as the receiving chambers.

ventricles
the pumping chambers of the heart, located inferior to the atria.

coronary circulation
the flow of blood through the muscular tissue of the heart.

pulmonary circulation
the flow of oxygen-depleted blood from the right ventricle of the heart to the lungs for reoxygenation and then on to the left atrium of the heart.

systemic circulation
the flow of oxygen-enriched blood from the left ventricle of the heart to all parts of the body (except the lungs) and the return of oxygen-depleted blood to the heart through the right atrium.

pulmonary valve) separates the heart from the lungs and prevents blood from flowing backward into the heart from the lungs. The upper chambers of the heart are receiving chambers, called **atria**. The lower chambers of the heart are pumping chambers, called **ventricles**. The right chambers are separated from the left chambers by the myocardial septum. It is important to note that the heart has its own blood supply conducted through special arteries and veins. The movement of blood through the heart is called **coronary circulation**. Good blood flow to the heart is essential because coronary circulation nourishes the heart muscle, which in turn drives the **pulmonary circulation**, which oxygenates the blood, and the **systemic circulation**, which nourishes the entire body.

THE CIRCULATORY SYSTEM

The circulatory system is often referred to as the cardiovascular system—a system composed of the heart (cardio) and the vessels (vascular). This system is divided into the pulmonary circulation, which transports blood from the heart to the lungs, and back to the heart, and the systemic circulation, which then distributes the blood to all other parts of the body. Many miles of blood vessels help accomplish this amazing process.

Blood and Blood Cells

Blood performs many important functions in sustaining life. It provides nourishment, hormones, vitamins, oxygen, and heat to the tissues, in addition to removing waste products, such as carbon dioxide, from the tissues. Blood is composed of several different types of cells, fluid, and chemical substances (see Figure 17-2). It is approximately 78% water and about 22% solids. The fluid portion of the blood, called plasma, contains many vital substances, including special proteins like fibrinogen and prothrombin. These proteins help the blood to clot, which stops active bleeding. Other substances contained in the plasma include carbohydrates, proteins, calcium, sodium, gases (such as oxygen and carbon dioxide), hormones, enzymes, and certain other substances.

Erythrocytes, or red blood cells (RBCs), make up most of the solids contained in the blood. On average, erythrocytes live only for about 120 days. Therefore, they must be constantly reproduced by the red bone marrow located in the femur, the hip, the sternum, the humerus, the vertebrae, and some of the cranial bones. The main function of erythrocytes is to carry oxygen. They are red because of a complex protein, called hemoglobin, that is contained within each red blood cell. Once oxygen attaches to an erythrocyte, the cell becomes red. The more oxygen the cells contain, the brighter red the erythrocytes become. So, when less oxygen is present, the erythrocytes become a darker red.

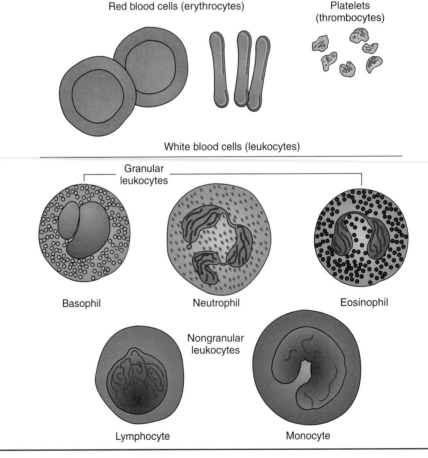

Red blood cells (erythrocytes)

Platelets (thrombocytes)

White blood cells (leukocytes)

Granular leukocytes

Basophil

Neutrophil

Eosinophil

Nongranular leukocytes

Lymphocyte

Monocyte

FIGURE 17-2 Types of Blood Cells

A platelet, or thrombocyte, is an extremely important specialized type of blood cell. This cell is produced to help coagulate, or clot, the blood. A delicate balance of platelets and erythrocytes must be maintained within the blood: Life depends on it!

Leukocytes, or white blood cells (WBCs), are another type of blood cell. There are two basic classifications of leukocytes: granulocytes, such as neutrophils, basophils, and eosinophils (leukocytes that have granules in their cytoplasm); and agranulocytes, such as lymphocytes and monocytes (leukocytes that do not have granules in their cytoplasm). Leukocytes are produced in many locations throughout the body. For example, granulocytes are produced in the bone marrow, lymphocytes are formed mostly in the lymph nodes, and monocytes are produced from the cells that line the walls of capillaries and are found in specific body organs such as the spleen. The main function of leukocytes is to fight infections. They destroy bacteria, viruses, fungi, and other pathogens. Sometimes, however, leukocytes are outnumbered by pathogens. When this happens, the leukocytes die and clump together. This collection of dead leukocytes is known as pus. If the dead white blood cells are unable to escape from the body, they form an abscess. Leukocytes are the basis of the immune system and are necessary for good health.

Blood Vessels

There are five types of blood vessels in the body: arteries, arterioles, capillaries, veins, and venules. Each type of vessel performs a specific function. **Arteries** are blood vessels that carry oxygen-enriched blood away from the heart to all the other parts of the body. Blood traveling in the arteries contains a high concentration of oxygen from the lungs. The largest artery in the body, the aorta, branches directly off the heart. The aorta then divides into arteries that nourish specific organs and tissues of the body. This is known as the systemic circulation. The pulmonary, or lung, circulation receives oxygen-depleted blood from the right side of the heart and passes it to the lungs. As the blood circulates through the lungs, it receives oxygen from the **alveoli**. The oxygen then can be transported to other body parts. Arteries contain three muscular layers: the tunica intima, or inner layer; the tunica media, or middle layer; and the tunica adventitia, or outer layer. The strength of these layers allows the arteries to receive blood that is being pumped under high pressure from the heart. Arteries further divide into smaller branches called arterioles. These arterioles join with even smaller vessels called capillaries, the smallest blood vessels in the body.

A capillary has only one thin wall that allows oxygen and nutrients to pass into and out of cells. It is at this level that the gas exchange (the process of exchanging oxygen for carbon dioxide in the blood) occurs. Tissue cells receive oxygen from the bloodstream and release carbon dioxide as a waste product. One end of each capillary is joined to an arteriole, and the other end is joined to one of many small veins, called venules.

Venules accept the blood from the capillaries and transport it directly into the veins. The **veins** are composed of three layers; however, the total thickness of the wall is thinner than an arterial wall, because of the lower pressure of the blood flow. Because veins transport oxygen-depleted blood back to the heart, they contain one-way valves that keep blood from flowing backward. Because of its low concentration of oxygen, venous blood is a deep, dark red. By contrast, arterial blood, with its high oxygen concentration, is bright red. When cuts or lacerations involve only veins

arteries

blood vessels that carry oxygen-enriched blood away from the heart to the tissues.

alveoli

microscopic air sacs within the lungs responsible for the exchange of oxygen and carbon dioxide.

veins

blood vessels that carry oxygen-depleted blood to the heart.

or venules, blood flow will be slow, either oozing or streaming. However, if an artery or arteriole is involved, the blood will flow quickly, often spurting in rhythm with the heart. The difference in blood flow, based on the type of blood vessel involved, is because of the difference in pressure. Remember that blood leaving the heart has a higher pressure due to the force of the heart's pumping action. The pressure of blood returning to the heart will be lower because it is farther away from the initial push than blood flowing from the heart. Pulses are only felt in arteries, not veins.

The Coronary Circulatory Path

An average adult has 5 to 6 quarts of blood in the body. This blood is circulated throughout the vascular system every 20 seconds. This is accomplished by the incredible pumping capacity of the heart. Figure 17-3 illustrates the path a drop of blood takes through the heart as it receives blood from the systemic circulatory system, conducts blood through the lungs for gas exchange, and returns oxygen-enriched blood to the systemic circulation, which travels to all parts of the body. Oxygen-depleted blood from the peripheral veins enters the superior vena cava (1) from the

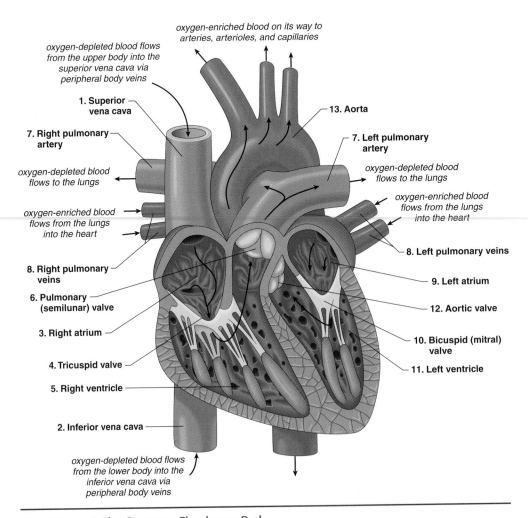

FIGURE 17-3 The Coronary Circulatory Path

head, neck, arms, and thorax. Similarly, blood from the legs and lower trunk enters the inferior vena cava (2).

The inferior vena cava and the superior vena cava both empty into the relaxed right atrium (3). Once filled, the right atrium contracts and forces blood against the tricuspid valve (4), causing the valve to open. The blood then passes through the tricuspid valve and flows into the relaxed right ventricle (5), filling the lower right chamber of the heart and causing the tricuspid valve to close.

The right ventricle contracts and the force of the blood flow opens the semilunar, or pulmonary, valve (6), marking the beginning of pulmonary circulation through the lungs. Oxygen-depleted blood enters the lungs through the pulmonary arteries (7) to exchange gases. In the gas exchange, blood receives oxygen from the alveoli (air sacs surrounded by capillaries) within the lungs, releasing carbon dioxide in the process. Oxygen-enriched blood then flows through the pulmonary veins (8) and enters the relaxed left atrium (9), which contracts and forces the blood to open the bicuspid, or mitral valve (10), and flow into the relaxed left ventricle (11).

> ## NOTE:
>
> The pulmonary circulatory path is the only place in the body where oxygen-depleted blood flows in arteries and oxygen-enriched blood is transported by veins.

Once the left ventricle is filled, the bicuspid valve closes and the left ventricle contracts. This forces the oxygen-enriched blood through the aortic valve (12) and into the aorta (13), which feeds blood into arteries, arterioles, capillaries, venules, veins, and back to the heart. This complete blood cycle occurs with every heart beat.

The Lungs

The largest organs of the chest are the **lungs**, located within the pleural cavities of the thorax. Continuous tubing that decreases in size extends from the nose and branches mid-chest into the right and left pleural cavities, creating an air passage that connects the lungs to the external atmosphere. The lungs are connected to the heart through special blood vessels. These connections provide the body with oxygen—an essential ingredient for life.

The main function of the lungs is to bring oxygen to the bloodstream and excrete carbon dioxide from the blood (see Figure 17-4). Blood is transported to the lungs through the pulmonary arteries and from the lungs to the heart by the pulmonary veins. Pulmonary circulation is the only time oxygen-depleted blood flows in arteries and oxygen-enriched blood flows in veins; for the rest of the circulatory system, arteries carry oxygen-enriched blood and veins carry oxygen-depleted blood. The exchange of carbon dioxide for oxygen occurs through the capillary walls that surround the tiny air sacs, called alveoli, which are located deep in the lungs. This process, known as the gas exchange, is initiated by signals sent from the brain to the lungs via the autonomic nervous system.

lungs
the two organs of respiration contained within the thorax.

The Ribs

Protection of the vital organs and great blood vessels is provided by 12 pairs of ribs. Anteriorly, the ribs articulate with the sternum; posteriorly they articulate with the thoracic spine (see Figure 17-5). Cartilage connects the ribs to these points of articulation, making dislocations rare; however, the ribs themselves can easily become injured. Muscle tissue, nerves, and blood vessels are between each rib. The contraction and relaxation of the thorax is the primary action of these intercostal muscles. The arrangement of the ribs is what provides the characteristic shape of the rib cage.

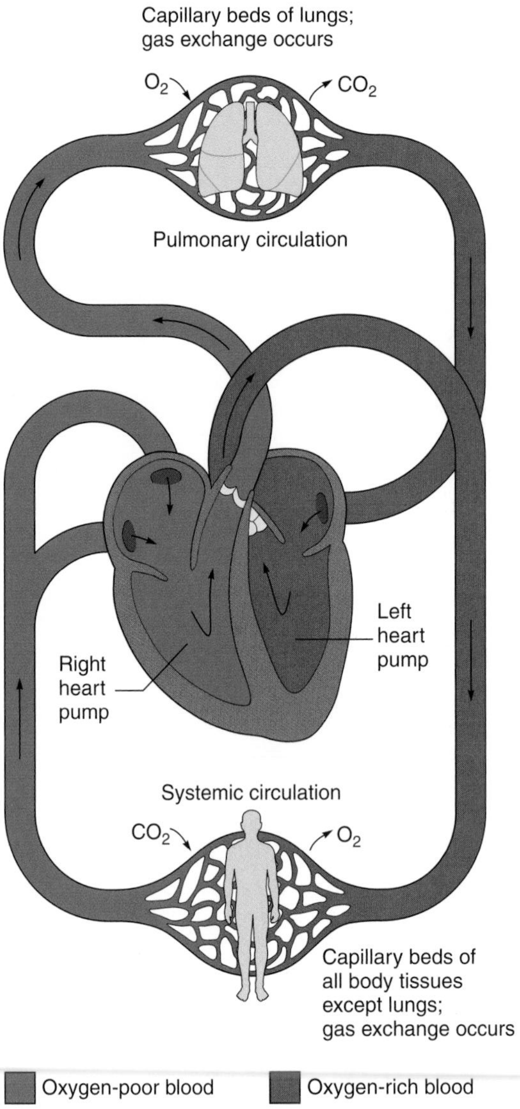

THE RESPIRATORY SYSTEM

All cells of the body need oxygen to maintain life. The human body can store enough food for weeks and enough water for five to seven days, but only holds enough oxygen to sustain life for 4 to 6 minutes. The respiratory system is responsible for carrying oxygen from the atmosphere to the bloodstream, where it can be used by the body's cells, and for expelling the waste product carbon dioxide. This intricate system consists of the nose, mouth, pharynx, larynx, trachea, bronchial tubes, alveoli, and the lungs (see Figure 17-6). During inhalation through the nose, air from the atmosphere enters the body through two openings, called nares, which are separated by cartilage called the nasal septum. The nose warms, moistens, and filters the air, reducing the amount of airborne particles and pathogens that reach the bronchial tubes and lungs.

The pharynx, or throat, is inferior to, yet connected to, the nose, allowing air to pass between the nose and mouth. It receives air from the nose as well as food and air from the mouth. The lower one-third of the pharynx is called the laryngopharynx, which provides an opening to the esophagus (the tube that leads directly into the stomach) and an opening to the trachea (the tube that leads into the bronchi within the lungs). The trachea is located anterior to the esophagus.

FIGURE 17-4 The Circulatory Path, Including Pulmonary and Systemic Circulation

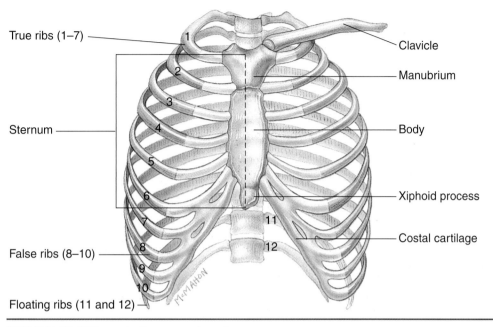

FIGURE 17-5 Thoracic Contents, Anterior

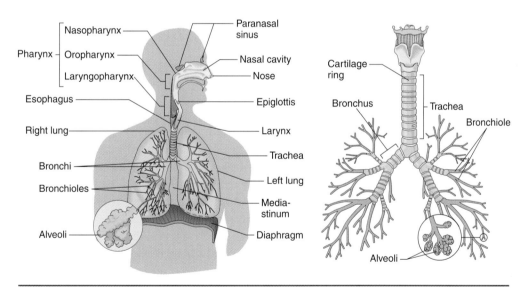

FIGURE 17-6 The Respiratory Tract

The larynx, or voice box, is located between the pharynx and the trachea. It is composed primarily of muscles and nine layers of cartilage. The largest layer of cartilage, known as the thyroid cartilage, is commonly called the Adam's apple. The larynx also houses the vocal folds, which vibrate to produce a certain pitch of sound. Located between the two vocal folds is an opening called the glottis. This opening is protected by a flap of cartilage called the epiglottis. When a person swallows, the epiglottis closes to prevent the entry of a foreign substance into the trachea and lungs.

Extending from the larynx down the center of the chest is the trachea, or windpipe. The trachea, made of C-shaped rings of cartilage, is 4 to 5 inches long in an adult. The dorsal aspect (the back) of the trachea is soft and flexible, which allows the esophagus to expand when food is present. The main function of the trachea is to allow air to pass from the atmosphere to the lungs.

The trachea divides at approximately the center of the chest into two tubes called bronchi. Each bronchus enters into a lung. The bronchi continue to decrease in diameter and form bronchioles that enter tiny air sacs called alveoli. Oxygen and carbon dioxide can easily pass through the capillary walls surrounding the alveoli, facilitating the gas exchange. Alveoli are shaped like a bunch of grapes. Because these numerous alveoli are air-filled, lung tissue is light in weight.

The lungs make up the largest part of the respiratory system. The right lung has three lobes: the superior, the middle, and the inferior lobes. Because of the position of the heart within the thoracic cavity, the left lung is slightly smaller and has only two lobes: the superior and the inferior lobes. Each lung is surrounded by a layer of thin tissue called the pleura. The pleura is a visceral lining that provides lubrication so that the lungs can inflate and deflate without friction against the ribs, which may cause irritation and inflammation. The thoracic cavity is separated from the abdominal cavity by a large muscle called the diaphragm, which is the main breathing muscle.

The Breathing Process

Breathing (respiration) consists of two phases: inspiration and expiration. These two phases form one respiratory cycle. When referring to the breathing process, another term used interchangeably with respiration is ventilation.

The process of breathing air into the lungs is called inspiration, or inhalation. During this phase of respiration, the intercostal (rib) muscles relax and the diaphragm contracts causing the chest cavity to increase in size. The lungs expand in order to accommodate the air that has been inhaled. During the gas exchange that occurs between the alveoli and the surrounding capillaries, oxygen is used by the cells, and carbon dioxide, a waste product, is produced. This exchange is also called cellular respiration. At this point the second phase of ventilation, known as expiration, occurs (see Figure 17-7).

Expiration takes place when the respiratory center in the medulla oblongata, or lower brain stem, receives a message concerning the increasing level of carbon dioxide in the alveoli from the blood. The brain then sends impulses telling the intercostal muscles to contract and the diaphragm to relax, forcing the carbon dioxide out of the lungs through the air passages. When the carbon dioxide is unable to be adequately released from the body, such as when the body is at work, the respiratory rate will increase above the normal level. This is one way in which the body attempts to adapt to, or compensate for, an abnormal condition. Although the ventilation process is mostly involuntary, a person can control the voluntary muscles and deliberately increase or decrease the respiratory rate.

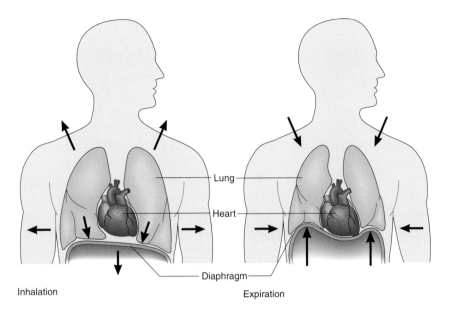

Lung

Heart

Diaphragm

Inhalation

Expiration

Nose–mouth

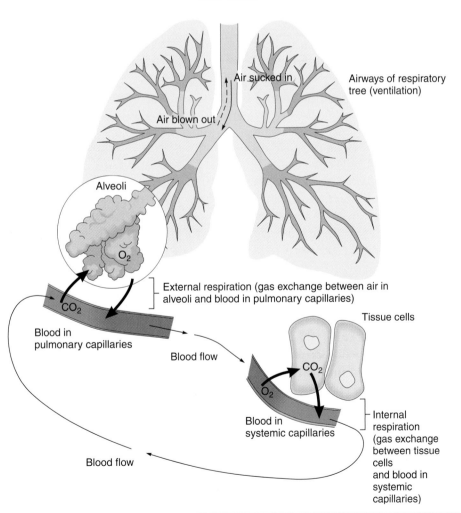

Air sucked in

Airways of respiratory tree (ventilation)

Air blown out

Alveoli

O_2

External respiration (gas exchange between air in alveoli and blood in pulmonary capillaries)

Tissue cells

CO_2

Blood in pulmonary capillaries

Blood flow

CO_2

O_2

Blood in systemic capillaries

Internal respiration (gas exchange between tissue cells and blood in systemic capillaries)

Blood flow

FIGURE 17-7 The Gas Exchange

INJURIES TO THE CHEST
Myocardial Contusions and Aortic Ruptures

A severe blow to the chest may cause a myocardial contusion, or a bruising of the heart muscle. In such a circumstance, the blow causes a disturbance in the electrical conduction system that controls the heartbeat. This injury is usually diagnosed with an electrocardiographic study and laboratory tests. If an athlete experiences a blunt trauma, it is important to check the athlete for signs of extra heartbeats or an irregular pulse rhythm. If any disturbance at all is detected in the pulse, activate the Emergency Action Plan. Those extra heartbeats may be the only early sign that a myocardial contusion has occurred. Exceptionally severe blows to the chest may also cause an aortic rupture. When this occurs, death is almost always immediate. It usually occurs from an intense forward/backward motion that fractures the aorta at the arch just before it begins it descends into the heart. In the small percentage of survival cases, immediate, fast transport to the hospital for surgery is urgent.

Immediate Treatment: Perform a primary survey to check for breathing and a pulse. Begin CPR if necessary and call the EMS. Continue to monitor the athlete's vital signs.

Follow-up Treatment: Make sure the physician's orders are followed.

Prevention: Chest padding should be worn by players of contact sports. Baseball catchers, in particular, must wear properly fitted protective chest gear.

Fractures

A fall or direct blow to the rib cage may result in one or more fractured ribs. Although usually not serious, fractured ribs (Figure 17-8) can be exceptionally painful due to the repetitive motion of the breathing process. Point tenderness that is made worse by deep breathing is the primary symptom of a rib fracture, which may be either displaced (the ends of the bone become misaligned) or nondisplaced (the ends of the bone remain aligned).

In the case of an nondisplaced rib fracture, the healing generally will occur spontaneously, without the assistance of an orthopedist. This is the nature of most rib fractures. On the other hand, if the fracture is displaced, the sharp ends of the bone may cause other complications, such as a penetrating injury to the lungs or the spleen, leading to internal bleeding.

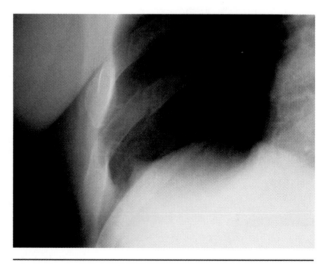

FIGURE 17-8 A Rib Fracture

Immediate Treatment: Ask the athlete to take a deep breath. If the athlete complains of a sharp pain, a fracture may have occurred. A stethoscope can be used to listen for crepitation at the site of the suspected fracture. If a fracture is suspected, send the athlete to a physician. The diagnosis will need to be confirmed by x-ray. If unable to detect a rib fracture, seek medical advice for further evaluation and diagnosis.

Wrap the athlete's ribs with a wide (preferably 6-inch) elastic wrap to support the injured area and to keep potentially broken bones from moving. Make sure to not restrict the athlete's ability to breathe. Encourage the athlete to breathe as deeply as possible. Proper taping of the ribs will reduce the amount of pain the patient experiences as a result of deep breathing.

Follow-up Treatment: Make sure the physician's orders are followed.

Prevention: To help prevent fractures, running backs, defensive backs, wide receivers, quarterbacks, lacrosse players, and hockey players should wear protective chest padding, such as rib pads.

Pneumothorax

Pneumothorax is a condition in which air has entered the space between the pleura and the chest wall, either from the lungs or the outside atmosphere. The change in pressure can cause the lung to collapse. This type of injury usually results from a penetrating object such as a fractured rib or a foreign object; however, intense impact to the chest can also cause a tear in the lung tissue inside the body. The symptoms of a pneumothorax are shortness of breath, severe chest pain, and an unequal expansion of the right and left side of the chest upon inhalation. Additionally, breath sounds will be absent or decreased on one side of the chest if a lung has collapsed.

pneumothorax
the presence of air in the thoracic cavity resulting from the perforation of the chest wall or the visceral pleura.

Immediate Treatment: Keep the athlete quiet and calm. Have the athlete sit down and think about controlling the breathing. If lung sounds are not present, call for EMS and immediate transportation to the nearest medical facility.

Follow-up Treatment: Make sure the physician's orders are followed. The athlete may be out of contact or collision sports for two to four weeks.

Prevention: Proper chest protection should be worn for all contact sports, such as football and hockey.

Hemothorax

Hemothorax is a condition in which blood collects between the lung and the chest wall in the pleural cavity. This injury is most common following an impact to the upper body, such as a violent collision to the chest area. Athletes often suffer a rib fracture during such a collision, and hemothorax can be a resulting complication.

hemothorax
blood within the pleural cavity.

A hemothorax may also result when an object, such as a fractured rib or foreign object, penetrates the pleural cavity, or when impact is severe enough to tear either the lung tissue or the pleural lining.

An athlete suffering from hemothorax will experience breathlessness, a rapid pulse, and pain in the affected side of the chest and the upper abdomen. Similar to the pressure created by air in a pneumothorax, a hemothorax can cause a lung to collapse as blood collects between the pleura and the chest wall.

Immediate Treatment: Activate the EMS. A chest x-ray will need to be taken to confirm the injury and to rule out any additional injuries.

Follow-up Treatment: Make sure the physician's orders are followed.

Prevention: Proper chest protection should be worn for all contact sports, such as football and hockey.

Hyperventilation

hyperventilation

prolonged, deep, and rapid breathing, resulting in decreased levels of CO_2 in the blood.

Breathing at a faster rate than is necessary for the proper exchange of oxygen and carbon dioxide is called **hyperventilation**. Exercise, excitement, anxiety, pain, asthma, fever, infection, and a variety of other factors, including head injuries, can lead to hyperventilation. This condition, which excessively depletes carbon dioxide from the blood, may cause chest pain, dizziness, and a numbing or tingling sensation in the lips, fingers, and toes. These symptoms can increase the patient's excitement or anxiety, which may increase the breathing rate even further. If the hyperventilation is not controlled, the athlete may have a cramping of the extremities or lose consciousness.

Immediate Treatment: Reassure the athlete, and have the athlete try to control and slow the breathing by inhaling through the nose and exhaling through the mouth. Try to calm the athlete and encourage the person to talk by asking questions. Conversation can help restore the normal breathing rate. Breathing into a paper bag in severe cases will also help to restore the oxygen-carbon dioxide balance. Stay with the athlete and allow the person to rest until symptoms subside. If at any time the situation requires someone with more experience, activate the EMS.

If the victim loses consciousness, contact the EMS and monitor vital signs. In most cases, the patient's vital signs will return to normal spontaneously after losing consciousness.

Follow-up Treatment: None required.

Prevention: This is not always a preventable condition; however, limiting anxiety and controlling breathing can help greatly.

Flail Chest

When the ribs sustain multiple fractures resulting in one or more rib segments that are not attached at either end, portions of the chest will move inward during inhalation and outward during exhalation (the actions opposite of normal breathing movement). This condition is called **flail chest**. As with any rib fracture, flail chest is a very painful condition, needing medical attention as it may be life-threatening. The ribs can puncture the heart and lungs. Symptoms include severe point tenderness, increased pain with breathing, difficulty breathing, and possible cyanosis.

Immediate Treatment: Activate the EMS. Calm the athlete as much as possible. Support the fracture site by compressing a pillow against it. This can either be held in place with a wrap or the athlete may hold it in place. Treat the patient for shock as necessary. Place the athlete in whatever position makes it easiest to breathe: right side, left side, or back.

Follow-up Treatment: Make sure the physician's orders are followed.

Prevention: Proper chest padding should be worn by players of contact sports.

Pulmonary Contusions

A pulmonary contusion is a bruise to the lung. In sports, it is usually caused by a direct blow from a ball or another player. It causes bleeding in the lung tissue, which creates swelling and makes it difficult to breathe because of the decreased lung capacity. This is an emergency. Symptoms are similar to those of a rib fracture.

Immediate Treatment: Try to reduce the pain, using compression, ice, or both. Contact EMS. Watch the athlete for signs and symptoms of shock and hyperventilation, and treat accordingly.

Follow-up Treatment: Make sure the physician's orders are followed.

Prevention: To prevent such injuries, players of contact sports should wear proper chest padding.

Blows to the Solar Plexus

Many times in sports, an athlete will receive a severe blow to the "pit" of the stomach (the solar plexus), which knocks the wind out of the athlete. A severe blow to this knot of nerves located behind the stomach can cause paralysis of the diaphragm and gasping for air. In extreme cases, respiration may temporarily stop all together.

Immediate Treatment: Encourage slow, deep breaths and reassure the athlete that relaxing will help regular respiration to resume. Let the athlete know that once normal breathing returns the athlete will feel better. If the athlete continues to have pain, the athlete should be evaluated by a physician. If the athlete has stopped breathing completely, the athlete will lose consciousness. Once consciousness is lost, the breathing should return spontaneously. However, be prepared to begin rescue breathing if the respiration does not resume naturally. Anytime an athlete loses consciousness, the EMS should be activated.

> **flail chest**
> a condition in which two or more fractures on a given rib cause the chest wall to become unstable, resulting in respiratory movements of the chest opposite to those desired.

Follow-up Treatment: If it is necessary to send the athlete to a physician, make sure the physician's orders are followed.

Prevention: Players of contact sports should wear protective chest padding, such as rib pads. Athletes should be trained in falling techniques appropriate to their sport.

Chest Contusions

As discussed in Chapter 14, a contusion is a bruise received from a sudden traumatic blow to the body, causing bleeding in the tissue. The severity of the contusion is directly related to the amount of soft tissue that has been damaged and the amount of force that has been applied to the tissue. Symptoms of a chest contusion are similar to those of a rib fracture and may include point tenderness, swelling, and pain upon movement of the rib cage. Because of the continuous movement of the intercostal muscles during respiration, contusions to the chest can also cause pain and discomfort during breathing.

Immediate Treatment: The treatment for a contusion to the rib cage consists of ice and compression. The ice should be applied for 20 minutes and then removed for one hour. The compression should be left on with and without the ice in order to decrease the swelling. Make sure the compression does not hinder normal breathing. Watch the athlete for signs and symptoms of shock and hyperventilation, and treat accordingly.

Follow-up Treatment: If signs or symptoms increase, or if they do not decrease after 24 hours, send the athlete to a physician. Make sure the physician's orders are followed.

Prevention: When the athlete is able to return to activity, protect the injured area with padding so that any future hits to the same area will be dispersed over a broader area of the chest, thereby preventing reinjury.

Side Stitches

Side stitches are spasms of the intercostal muscles brought on by a lack of oxygen during physical activity. These occur as a result of poor conditioning. Symptoms include cramp-like pains in either the left or right side.

Immediate Treatment: Stretch the affected side by having the athlete raise the arm on the involved side over the head.

Follow-up Treatment: If symptoms persist for more than an hour, send the athlete to a physician for further evaluation. If this occurs, the condition is probably the result of a more significant injury than a side stitch. In general, side stitches do not last for an hour. As with all injuries, if it becomes necessary to send the athlete to a physician, make sure the doctor's orders are followed.

Prevention: Properly conditioned athletes are less likely to experience side stitches than those who do not participate in an appropriate conditioning program. (See Chapter 7.)

THE ABDOMEN: AN OVERVIEW

The abdominal cavity (Figure 17-9) is separated from the thoracic cavity by the diaphragm and includes organs from the digestive, reproductive, lymphatic, and urinary systems. The vital organs contained within the abdominal cavity are protected from behind by the posterior ribs and the spine. However, anteriorly, only minimal protection is provided to the internal organs by the strong abdominal muscles, fascia, adipose tissue, and the peritoneum. Similar to the pleural lining of the lungs, the peritoneum lines the abdominal cavity and each organ, providing lubrication that allows the organs to move slightly without friction or irritation. The organs in the abdominal cavity are secured in place by ligaments.

The tissues of the internal organs have a rich vascular and neural supply. When injured, these muscular organs typically suffer damage to their own tissue structure, which is crisscrossed by a vast network of blood vessels and nerves. Although an injury may also involve nerves and blood vessels that branch off of an organ, the nature of the injury is not significantly different for damage to these connecting pathways than for damage to the organ itself. Either way, there is great potential for damage to organ muscle tissue resulting from impaired blood or neural circulation. Suffice it to say that the muscular tissue of the internal organs is fed by numerous blood vessels and nerves, and that injury to these delicate structures will always require evaluation and treatment by a physician.

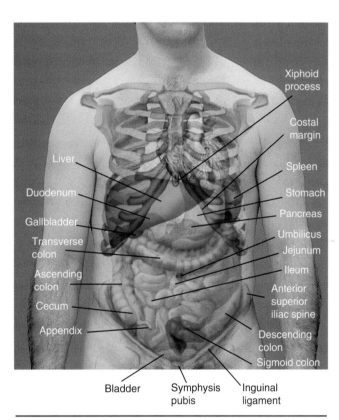

FIGURE 17-9 Abdominal Cavity, Open

The abdomen is commonly divided into four quadrants (Figure 17-10). The right upper quadrant (RUQ) contains the gallbladder and part of the liver. The left upper quadrant (LUQ) contains the spleen, pancreas, stomach, and part of the liver. The left lower quadrant (LLQ) contains some of the female reproductive organs and part of the large intestine referred to as the descending colon. The right lower quadrant (RLQ) contains the appendix, the ascending colon, and other organs of the female reproductive system. The large intestine, which is approximately 5 feet long (with a larger diameter than the small intestine), and the small intestine, which is approximately 20 feet long, are both found throughout the entire abdominal cavity. The urinary bladder is positioned midline in the lowest part of the abdomen and extends into the pelvic cavity.

The Spleen

The spleen is located in the left upper quadrant, slightly behind (posterior to) and to the left of the stomach. The spleen, which is egg-shaped, is part of the lymphatic system.

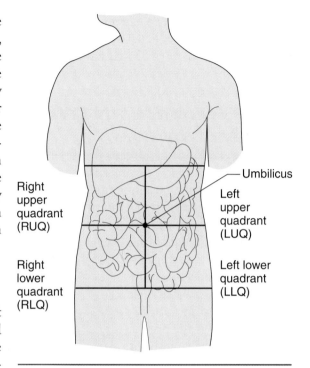

FIGURE 17-10 Abdominal Quadrants

A vascular organ, the spleen serves as a site for the production of lymphoid leukocytes, a storage site for blood, and the site for fetal blood formation. It also helps in fighting infection by digesting aged or abnormal erythrocytes. Although well protected within the abdominal cavity, the spleen can be injured as the result of either blunt or penetrating trauma.

The spleen is the most commonly injured organ in the abdominal region. The injury usually results from a blow to the left upper quadrant, the lower left rib cage, or the left side of the back. Often injury to the spleen is sustained with a fracture of the 10th, 11th, and 12th ribs on the left side. Initial pain is felt in the left upper quadrant. Referred pain may be felt in the left shoulder. The signs and symptoms of an injured spleen include shock and low blood pressure. A referred pain, called Kehr's sign, may occur approximately 30 minutes after the injury. This pain radiates to the left shoulder and one-third of the way down the left arm.

Mononucleosis (often called "mono") is an infection caused by the Epstein-Barr virus. The Epstein-Barr virus (EBV) is a virus of the herpes family and is one of the most common viruses in humans. Most people become infected with EBV, which is usually asymptomatic. Signs of mono include fever, sore throat, headaches, white patches on the back of the throat, swollen glands in the neck, feeling tired, and lack of appetite. Mono is not spread as easily as some other viruses, such as the common cold. The mono virus is found in saliva and mucus. It is usually passed from one person to another through kissing, although it may rarely be passed in other ways, such as coughing. Signs of mono usually develop four to seven weeks after initial exposure to the virus. Generally, people only get mono once.

The main concern with mono is that the spleen can become enlarged and even rupture. Although a ruptured spleen is rare in people with mono, be aware of the signs and have the athlete see a physician right away if symptoms are noticed.

Indications of a ruptured spleen include pain in the left upper part of the abdomen, feeling lightheaded, feeling like the heart is beating fast and hard, bleeding more easily than usual, and having trouble breathing.

Anyone who contracts mono should avoid sports, activities, or exercise of any kind until the physician states it is safe. Moving around too much will place the patient at risk of rupturing the spleen, especially in contact sports. It may be recommended that physical activities be avoided for about three to four weeks after the infection starts.

Mono is treated by relieving the symptoms. This can be done with rest, drinking plenty of fluids, and seeing a physician for further care.

The Liver

Affixed to the anterior abdomen and the diaphragm by several ligaments is the liver, the largest abdominal organ. Most of the liver is contained in the right upper quadrant, however, the smaller left lobe overlies into the midepigastric region and left upper quadrant of the abdomen. The liver performs many essential functions for the body. Some of those functions include producing bile (which decomposes fats) and proteins that help clot blood; storing simple sugar (in the form of glycogen) and vitamins such as A, D, and some of the Bs; and detoxifying products that are harmful to the body.

Although it is well protected by the ribs, the liver can sustain severe trauma that can be life-threatening. Because it is very large and highly vascular, injuries to the liver can result in extensive internal bleeding. A liver injury can result from a blow to the upper middle abdomen; or an impact to the right lower chest (either in the front or on the back); or a fracture of the 10th, 11th, or 12th ribs. Upper quadrant pain, followed by diffuse abdominal pain or a referred pain in the right shoulder, is a common symptom of a liver injury.

The Kidney

The two **kidneys**, located high on the posterior abdominal wall, inferior to the diaphragm, are also protected by the rib cage. The left kidney is posterior to the spleen, while the right kidney is posterior to the liver. The kidneys are part of the urinary system, which excretes waste products from the body in the form of urine.

Each kidney weighs about 6 ounces, and typically measures 4 to 5 inches long. The kidneys are suspended by ligaments and protected by **adipose tissue**. They receive their blood supply from the renal arteries that branch off from the aorta. There are about one million glomeruli, clusters of capillaries, in each kidney. Blood is filtered as it flows through the glomeruli and into tubules. The combination of the tubules and the glomeruli form nephrons, the actual functioning units of the kidney.

Injuries to the kidneys are commonly caused by a blow to the back. If an athlete has received a severe blow to the body, particularly to the back, and blood is present in the urine, a kidney injury may have occurred and the athlete should be examined by a physician.

kidney
one of a pair of organs located in the dorsal cavity of the body that are responsible for filtering blood and producing urine.

adipose tissue
fatty tissue that stores energy, insulates, and cushions.

The Bladder

Deeply inferior in the abdo-pelvic cavity lies a muscular sac called the urinary bladder. It lies inferior to the peritoneum and behind the pelvic bones. It is connected to the kidneys by two tubes called ureters. The sole purpose of the urinary bladder is to act as a reservoir for urine.

The Pancreas

The **pancreas** is a glandular organ located in the left upper abdominal quadrant, posterior to the stomach. Insulin is produced within the pancreas. This hormone regulates the level of blood sugar (glucose) through the metabolism of fats and carbohydrates.

A properly functioning pancreas is important to help the body maintain a healthy balance of blood sugar and insulin. Should the pancreas become injured or cease to produce insulin, the level of glucose in the blood may have serious negative effects on the entire body. This condition is known as diabetes mellitus. If the pancreas is unable to produce insulin, then the hormone must be introduced into the body by injections. If the amount of insulin produced by the pancreas is only slightly below normal, diet and/or oral medication may be all that is required to maintain a proper glucose level.

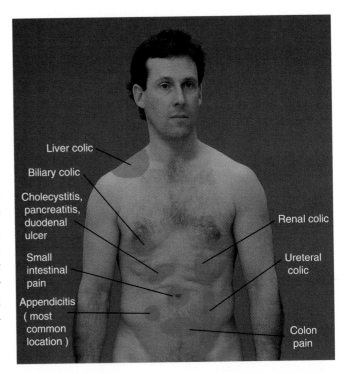

INJURIES TO THE ORGANS OF THE ABDOMEN

Overall, injuries to the internal organs of the abdomen may be divided into four major types: hernias, contusions, ruptures and lacerations, and injuries that involve internal bleeding and shock (see Figure 17-11). The following general treatments, follow-ups, and preventions for each type of injury will be equally effective no matter which of these organs has been involved.

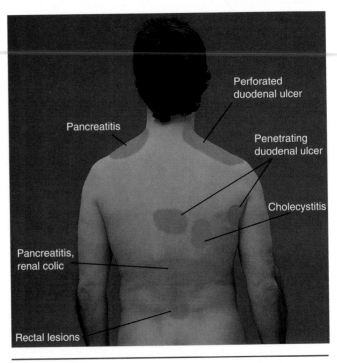

FIGURE 17-11 Common Patterns of Referred Pain

Contusions

Contusions to the internal organs occur as a result of a direct blow to the abdominal area. Because contusions produce bleeding in the organ tissue, the abdomen may feel rigid and the athlete may go into shock. Sometimes, signs and symptoms may be delayed, so if there is potential for such a contusion, based on the mechanism of the injury, make sure to communicate concerns to the athlete's family. Additional symptoms may include general pain in the area, or pain on palpation, and blood in urine or stool.

Immediate Treatment: Apply ice and compression using the proper procedures. Activate the EMS. Watch the athlete for signs and symptoms of shock and hyperventilation, and treat accordingly.

Follow-up Treatment: Make sure the physician's orders are followed.

Prevention: Protective padding should be worn by all players of contact sports.

Ruptures and Lacerations

Ruptures and lacerations of the internal organs are relatively rare in sports. When they do occur, they usually result from a severe, direct blow by a person or object. Ruptures and lacerations cause internal bleeding and, therefore, are medical emergencies. Although blood is not visible, these injuries are life-threatening. Symptoms of internal bleeding include shock, a rigid and/or distended belly, pain, nausea, and possible loss of consciousness.

Immediate Treatment: Have the athlete lie down, and make the athlete as comfortable as possible. Contact the EMS. While waiting, try to keep the athlete conscious by talking to him or her. Reassure the athlete that help is on the way.

Follow-up Treatment: Make sure the physician's orders are followed.

Prevention: Players of contact sports should wear protective padding.

Shock

A person with an abdominal injury may experience internal bleeding, which can lead to **shock**. If there is internal bleeding, the abdominal region will feel firm and will be tender to the touch. Shock can also result from other types of trauma. Signs of shock include cool, clammy, and pale skin; a weak and rapid pulse; a decreased blood pressure; dull, staring eyes; and rapid, shallow breathing. The patient may also experience nausea and vomiting, and may complain of thirst.

Immediate Treatment: If an athlete is standing and begins to show signs of shock, have the athlete lie down to prevent falling down. Do not give the athlete anything to eat or drink. If the athlete shows signs of shock, or if unsure about the severity of the injury, put the athlete in the most comfortable position possible, and cover the person with a blanket. Elevate the athlete's feet, and call the EMS. Remember, if unsure about

> **shock**
>
> a condition that occurs when an inadequate amount of blood flows through the body, causing extremely low blood pressure, a lack of urine, and other disorders; a potentially fatal condition.

the athlete's condition, it is always safest to call the EMS. It is better to have emergency personnel there and not need them, than to wish they had been called sooner.

Follow-up Treatment: Make sure the physician's orders are followed.

Prevention: When an athlete becomes injured and it looks as if shock may occur, have the athlete lie down, elevate the feet, and cover the athlete with a blanket. However, do not allow the patient to become too warm when covered with a blanket.

Hernias

An abdominal **hernia** is a lump of tissue that protrudes through the abdominal wall. It is caused by a weakness in the abdominal wall, and may occur spontaneously. Inguinal hernias occur most frequently in males, and occur in the inguinal region, commonly called the groin, while femoral hernias are more prevalent in females. Symptoms of a hernia include point tenderness and a lump that can be palpated. The size of the lump may increase during weight lifting, coughing, during defecation, or during any activity that increases abdominal pressure.

A sports hernia is an injury of the inguinal area caused by repetitive twisting and turning at high speed, causing an overuse of the groin muscles and stress on the inguinal wall. This type of hernia occurs mainly in athletes who play ice hockey, soccer, tennis, or other sports that might entail similar overuse. Although known as a hernia, in many cases an obvious hernia bulge will not be seen. Some athletes may experience groin pain for months and never find a bulge of tissue. The main symptom is groin pain that may radiate into the scrotum; this pain may linger for weeks or months. The athlete may be asked to perform sit-ups to see whether that will cause pain in the groin area. Resting the groin muscles for several weeks sometimes can resolve the problem, but in most cases surgery will be needed to reinforce the inguinal wall.

Immediate Treatment: Surgery is required, though not usually emergency surgery. If left untreated for too long, the tissue will die and a bowel obstruction may result, leading to a life-threatening condition.

Follow-up Treatment: Make sure the physician's orders are followed.

Prevention: This is not a preventable condition.

> **hernia**
>
> the protrusion of an organ or part of an organ through a wall of a cavity normally containing the organ.

THINKING IT THROUGH

The Norte Vista Braves were on their way back from a soccer game in the High Desert. The Braves had lost a tightly contested game. Everyone was a little down because this game changed the league standings.

Courtney, the starting goalkeeper for the Braves, received a hard hit to the ribs during the last minutes of the game. She never complained much, and today was no exception. Ned, the team's athletic trainer, saw what happened and checked her out before she got on the bus. He determined she might have a contusion on her rib or possibly even a fracture, so he wrapped it up and put ice on the area to control the swelling and reduce the pain. Courtney blamed herself for the loss and was pretty upset. She just wanted to be alone in the back of the bus. Ned told the girls around her to keep an eye on her during the ride home.

About 30 minutes into the trip, Megan, who was sitting next to Courtney, yelled for Ned. Something was wrong with Courtney. Ned rushed to the back of the bus to check on her. She was breathing very fast and felt cool and clammy. Then she passed out.

When traveling, what seating arrangements might be appropriate for an injured player? What do you think was wrong with Courtney? What would you do for her? Create an Emergency Action Plan for travel emergencies such as this.

CHAPTER SUMMARY

The chest and the abdomen contain the body's vital organs. Protected by the bony rib cage, the lungs bring oxygen to the blood that is pumped by the heart throughout the body via the circulatory system. In turn, this circulating blood uses specialized cells and fluid to transport life-sustaining elements such as nutrients, hormones, enzymes, proteins, and heat to all areas of the body. Red blood cells provide oxygen and specialized proteins to tissues; white blood cells deliver disease-fighting substances to infected areas. Injuries to either the lungs or heart can be instantaneously fatal.

In addition to organs of the digestive system, many other essential organs are found in the abdomen. The spleen, the main organ of the lymphatic system, serves as a site for white blood cell production and aids in the disposal of aged or abnormal red blood cells. Both the liver and the kidneys act as filtering devices to remove waste and other toxic substances from the body. However, the liver, like the pancreas, serves different body systems at the same time. That is, while the liver's primary function is to filter toxins, it also produces enzymes to help the digestive system decompose fats. Similarly, the pancreas serves the exocrine system, working with the digestive system to metabolize fats and carbohydrates, while serving the endocrine system by producing insulin, a hormone that helps regulate blood sugar levels. The internal organs of the abdomen are highly vascular and relatively unprotected. Injuries to these organs greatly increase the potential for internal bleeding, which left undetected and/or untreated can be just as life-threatening as injuries to the chest, although the effect may not be as immediate.

Complete the following sentences.

1. Plasma contains many vital substances, including special proteins like _____ and _____.

2. _____ make up most of the solids contained in the blood.

3. The thoracic cavity is separated from the abdominal cavity by a large muscle called the _____, which is the main breathing muscle.

4. The _____ is a visceral lining that provides lubrication, so that the lungs can inflate and deflate without friction against the ribs, which may cause irritation and inflammation.

Describe the following terms and list their functions.

5. arteries

6. capillaries

7. veins

8. gas exchange

9. peritoneum

Match the terms in Column A with the appropriate description in Column B.

Column A		Column B

10. _____ pneumothorax

11. _____ hemothorax

12. _____ liver

13. _____ kidney

14. _____ pancreas

15. _____ hemoglobin

16. _____ insulin

17. _____ thrombocyte

18. _____ aorta

A. produces bile, which decomposes fats; stores simple sugar, in the form of glycogen, and vitamins such as A, D, and some of the Bs

B. the largest artery in the body

C. an excretory organ responsible for the production of urine

D. a condition in which air or other gas from the lungs or outside enters the space between the pleura of the lung and the chest wall

E. a hormone that regulates blood glucose levels

F. a complex protein contained within red blood cells and essential to oxygen transportation in the circulatory system

G. a specialized type of red blood cell responsible for blood coagulation

H. a condition in which blood collects in the pleural cavity

I. a glandular organ, located in the left upper abdominal quadrant, responsible for insulin production

Complete the following exercises.

19. Photocopy and label the diagram of the coronary circulatory path.

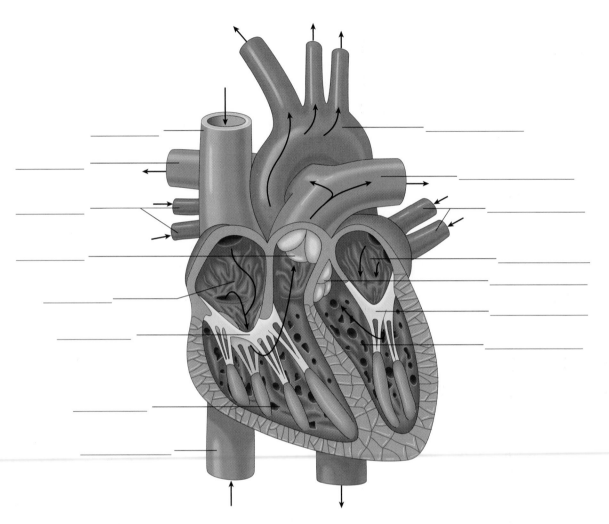

20. Draw the trunk, anterior and posterior. Shade in and identify the patterns for referred pain.

21. What is the treatment for a chest contusion?

22. What are the symptoms for a spleen injury?

CHAPTER 18

Injuries to the Pelvis and Lower Extremities

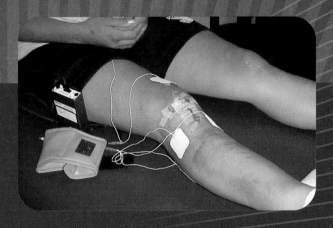

OBJECTIVES

After completing this chapter, you should be able to do the following:

1. Define and correctly spell each of the key terms.

2. Name the major bones of the pelvis and lower extremities.

3. Describe the different types of lower-extremity joints and their functions.

4. Briefly describe common injuries to the pelvis and lower extremities.

5. Discuss treatment of pelvic and lower-extremity injuries.

6. Explain potential emergencies that may result from an injury to the pelvis and lower extremities.

KEY TERMS

* anterior compartment syndrome
* anterior drawer test for the ankle
* anterior drawer test for the knee
* Apley compression test
* athlete's foot
* chondromalacia patellae (CMP)
* direct axial load
* ingrown toenail
* Lachman test
* McMurray test
* meniscal tear
* Osgood-Schlatter disease
* patella grind test
* patellar tendon rupture test
* pivot shift test
* plantar fasciitis
* posterior drawer test for the knee
* shin splints (medial tibial stress syndrome)
* talar tilt test
* tendon rupture
* Thompson test

INTRODUCTION

Many types of injuries can affect the lower half of the body. Strained, sprained, and torn ligaments, tendons, and menisci, as well as dislocations and fractures, can occur while participating in a wide range of sports. In general, the bones and muscles of the lower extremities are relatively large because they must support the whole body. Because of their size, extreme force is required to injure these bones; it is also more difficult to injure a large, strong, well-conditioned muscle than a small, poorly conditioned muscle. Therefore, to prevent injury to the soft tissues, strengthening and conditioning exercises are strongly recommended for the lower extremities. Remember: When injuries occur, treat the cause of the injury as well as the symptoms.

THE PELVIS

The pelvis (Figure 18-1) constitutes the inferior portion of the trunk. This region provides support to the vertebral column and allows articulation between the trunk and lower limbs. Formed by anterior articulations between the two pelvic bones (each composed of the ilium, ischium, and pubis) and posterior articulations between the sacrum and the pelvic bones, the bony structure of the pelvis is called the pelvic girdle. Strong ligaments create the attachments for these bones and, with the muscles and their tendons, make movement of the hip and thigh possible. Contained within the pelvic cavity is part of the urinary bladder, which descends from the abdominal cavity; the female reproductive tract, which serves as the birth canal; and numerous blood vessels and nerves, which serve the lower extremities.

The primary muscles of the pelvis (Figure 18-2) affect movement of the thigh at the hip joint and include the psoas major, iliacus, gluteus medius and minimus, adductor longus, adductor magnus, gracilis, pectineus, and the sartorius. These muscles are attached to the femur and pelvic bones through deep fascia, a fibrous protective covering, which allows a larger area of attachment and contributes to muscular movement by creating pressure, or tension, on the muscle surface.

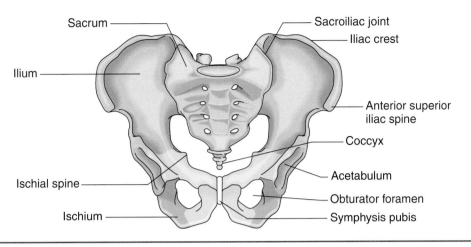

FIGURE 18-1 The Bony Structure of the Pelvis

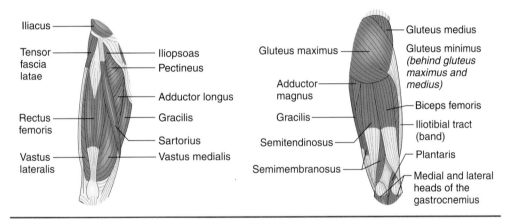

FIGURE 18-2 The Muscles of the Pelvis and Thigh; (L) Anterior, (R) Posterior

A brief description of the types of movement made possible by each muscle may enhance understanding of pelvic and lower-extremity injuries. The psoas major and the iliacus flex the thigh. The gluteus medius and the gluteus minimus abduct and medially rotate (turn inward) the thigh. The adductor longus adducts, flexes, and laterally rotates (turns outward) the thigh. The adductor magnus allows the for adduction, extension, and lateral rotation of the thigh. The gracilis adducts, flexes, and medially rotates the leg at the level of the knee. The pectineus is superior to the adductor longus and adducts the thigh. The sartorius muscle traverses the thigh from its lateral aspect to its medial aspect and flexes both the hip and the knee. The tensor fasciae latae abducts, flexes, and medially rotates the upper leg. From this description of the interrelated, or paired, action of these muscles, it is easy to understand why a sudden, severe force to the leg, resulting in overstretched muscle fibers, can result in a very painful and often debilitating injury.

Between the pelvis and the thigh lies the inguinal region, commonly called the groin. Specifically, the inguinal region is the area between the medial thigh and pubis symphysis of the pelvis. This region is a common site for hernias in males. (See Chapter 17.) Because the blood-supply needs of the large muscles and bones of the lower extremities are so great, the groin and its surrounding tissues are highly vascular

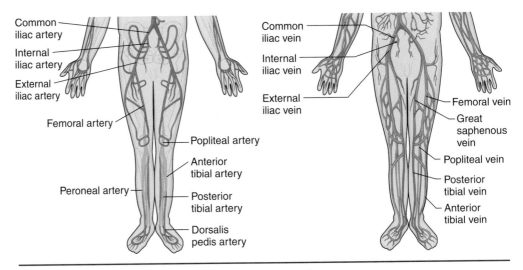

FIGURE 18-3 Arteries and Veins of the Lower Extremity

regions. Therefore, trauma to these areas may result in extensive internal and/or external bleeding.

The anterior pelvis, the groin, and the lower extremity are supplied with blood primarily by the three iliac arteries: common, internal, and external (see Figure 18-3). Near the groin, the external iliac artery branches into several arteries that supply blood to the leg, with the femoral artery serving as the primary supplier of oxygen-enriched blood to the lower leg. The common and external iliac veins are the principal pathways for the return of oxygen-depleted blood from the lower extremities to the heart.

The lateral cutaneous and femoral nerves are the principal neural pathways serving the hip and pelvic region, but numerous nerves actually serve the muscles of the pelvis and hip. On command from the brain, these nerves stimulate the muscle tissues to make movement possible (see Figure 18-27).

INJURIES TO THE PELVIC REGION

Fractures

Because the pelvic bones are so strong, injuries to the bony structures of the pelvis are rare in sports; but they do occur—particularly in contact sports. Symptoms of a pelvic fracture include possible swelling and general pelvic pain that increases when pressure is applied to the pelvis. Repeated stress or overuse of the pelvic articulations may result in a stress fracture or even an avulsion fracture. Symptoms of such fractures include localized, chronic pain and an altered gait. When a forceful collision occurs, the possibility of injury to the internal organs cannot be overlooked. Hematuria (blood in the urine) is a sign of internal injury and requires immediate evaluation and treatment by a physician.

As discussed in Chapter 16, percussion and compression tests are performed to check for signs of a possible fracture. If there is any possibility of a fracture, x-rays and evaluation by a physician are required.

Immediate Treatment: If a fracture or internal injury is suspected, treat the athlete for shock and activate the EMS. Stress or avulsion fractures may not be noticed for several days because such injuries may occur from subtle movements over a period of time. If an athlete suffers from chronic pain, the athlete should be referred to a physician for further evaluation.

Follow-up Treatment: Make sure the physician's orders are followed.

Prevention: This region is difficult to protect from traumatic injury because of the reduced range of motion that would result from protective padding, but preventive falling techniques may help prevent some impact-related fractures. Stress fractures can sometimes be prevented through proper conditioning.

Strains

Strains occur when muscle fibers are overstretched. Extreme rotation or excessive abduction of a lower limb usually causes groin strains. Symptoms of a groin injury include swelling, gradual to acute pain, and weakness.

Immediate Treatment: Apply ice using the PRICE procedure (see Chapter 14), apply compression during waking hours, and instruct the athlete to rest for 48 hours. Apply a compression wrap around the groin area to add support.

Follow-up Treatment: After two days of rest, the athlete should begin to stretch the muscles in the groin slowly, using abduction exercises such as the butterfly stretch (see Chapter 7). Applying resistance with no motion to the medial knees using the hands while adducting the knees can strengthen the groin, or pelvic, muscles. This application of resistance with no motion constitutes an isometric exercise. Once strength is gained using isometric strengthening, isotonic exercises may be added. The butterfly stretch can be changed to an isotonic exercise by applying weights to the thighs or lower legs and performing adduction with the legs. While the muscles are healing, a neoprene sleeve (Figure 18-4) can be used to add compression, support, and heat to the area.

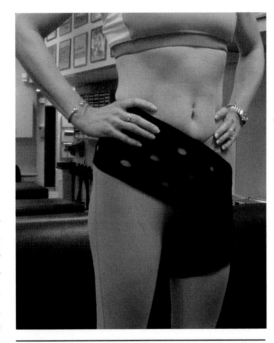

FIGURE 18-4 A neoprene sleeve can add compression, support, and heat to healing muscles.

Prevention: Strengthening and flexibility exercises such as those described above can prevent strains to the groin area.

Contusions

Trauma to the male genitalia in which the skin remains unbroken is called a scrotal contusion and can result from a hit to the groin. The athlete will feel intense pain, often accompanied by nausea, shortness of breath, inability to move, and generalized muscle spasms.

Immediate Treatment: Apply ice, using the PRICE procedure, to relieve pain and reduce swelling. To relieve the muscle spasms, the athlete should lie on his back and pull his knees to his chest.

Follow-up Treatment: If severe pain persists, send the athlete to a physician for diagnosis and treatment.

Prevention: Athletes should use athletic cups to help prevent groin injuries resulting from impact.

THE HIP AND THIGH

Each lower extremity consists of a hip, thigh, knee, lower leg, ankle, and foot. The proximal aspect of a lower extremity is commonly called the hip. The hip is a ball-and-socket joint, held together by connective tissues. The ball is formed by a large protrusion on the proximal medial femur, which articulates with the deep, bony socket (the acetabulum) in the pelvic bone (see Figure 18-5). The femur is held in the acetabulum by ligaments, tendons, and muscles. This joint allows abduction, adduction, flexion, extension, medial rotation, and lateral rotation of the femur.

The femur extends from the hip to the knee, providing the skeletal structure of the thigh (Figure 18-6). At its most proximal end, just below the head, there is an area of constriction, called the femoral neck, followed by two protrusions—the greater trochanter and the lesser trochanter. These bony projections provide areas of attachment for the muscles of the legs and buttocks. At the distal end, the medial and lateral condyles of the femur and the tibia articulate with one another, while the distal anterior surface of the femur articulates with the patella (knee cap). Although

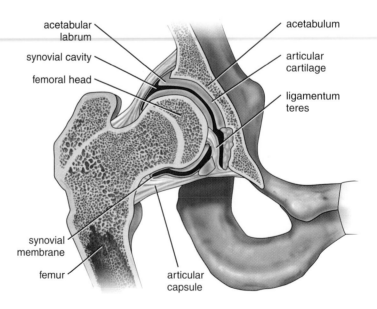

FIGURE 18-5 The Acetabulum

the femur is the largest bone in the body, requiring an extraordinary amount of force to fracture, the femoral neck is not as well protected.

Movement of the hip and thigh is achieved through muscles (Figure 18-7) that are attached to the femur and to specific areas of the pelvis. In fact, the medial and anterior muscles of the hip and thigh are the same as those of the pelvis. They make adduction and internal rotation of the thigh possible. The muscles of the posterior hip (buttocks) are the gluteals: gluteus maximus, gluteus medius, and gluteus minimus. These muscles assist in extension and lateral rotation of the thigh at the hip joint.

On the posterior thigh, the muscle group known as the

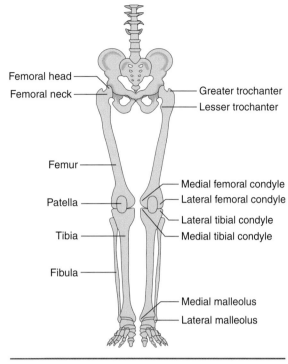

FIGURE 18-6 Bones of the Leg

hamstrings—the biceps femoris, semitendinosus, and semimembranosus—extends the hip and flexes the knee. The major anterior thigh muscles are the quadriceps: rectus femoris, vastus medialis, vastus lateralis, and vastus intermedius. All of these muscles extend the knee, with the rectus femoris also flexing the hip. The tensor fasciae latae,

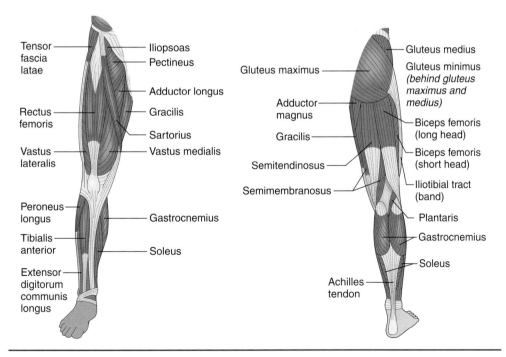

FIGURE 18-7 Muscles of the Leg

which flexes and abducts the femur, and the sartorius, which flexes both the hip and knee and laterally rotates the leg, are also important thigh muscles. Each thigh muscle connects the femur in the upper leg to the tibia or fibula in the lower leg.

ASSESSING HIP INJURIES

Like all injuries, hip injuries must be assessed using the principles of the HOPS procedure (see Chapter 9), taking care to accurately record all information and pass the information along to the appropriate medical personnel. Special tests used to assess specific conditions are presented in the injuries section of this chapter. Note that hip pain may be caused by conditions that cannot be detected through range-of-motion tests, strength tests, or even the special tests presented later in the chapter. Such conditions may include urinary tract infections, ovarian cysts, hernias, testicular torsion or ruptures, testicular cancer, and referred pain from the lymph nodes, kidneys, bladder, or bowels. Therefore, if the assessments are inconclusive, or if an injury does not heal, refer the athlete to a physician for further evaluation and diagnosis.

Range-of-Motion (ROM) Evaluations for the Hip

General Range of Motion: Instruct the athlete to perform a full squat to check general functional ROM (see Chapter 7). The motion should be smooth and painless. If the athlete complains of pain on one side, indicates pain with a grimace, or raises a heel as full flexion is achieved or attempted, decreased range of motion is indicated on that side.

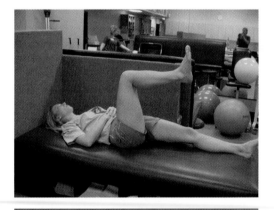

FIGURE 18-8 Active ROM, Hip Flexion, Knee Flexed

ROM Test for Hamstring Flexibility: Instruct the athlete to lie supine (on the back) and bring the knee to the chest as far as possible. Then ask the athlete to do the same thing with the leg fully extended (see Figures 18-8 and 18-9). Motion should be smooth and painless. Compare the active ROM between the uninvolved and the involved extremities, checking the uninvolved extremity first. Next, check the passive ROM by applying controlled force to create both motions (knee flexed and extended) again, first to the athlete's uninvolved leg and then to the involved leg. Compare flexibility in the hips and hamstrings by noting the endpoints. Avoid causing additional pain while

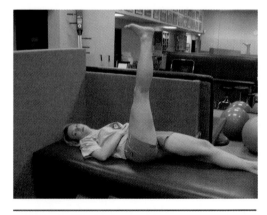

FIGURE 18-9 Active ROM, Hip Flexion, Knee Extended

performing this assessment. Limited ROM on one side indicates potential injury or deformity on that side.

ROM Test for Hip Flexor Flexibility (Thomas Test): Instruct the athlete to lie face-up on a table with the buttocks at the edge of the table and both legs hanging over the edge. Ask the athlete to flex the involved knee and bring it as close as possible to the chest (Figure 18-10). As the athlete does this, watch to see if the extended leg follows it up or stays in the same position. (The extended leg is the one being evaluated.) Repeat the test so that the involved leg is extended. Movement of the involved extended leg during the test indicates potential tightness in the hip flexor and rectus femoris on that side.

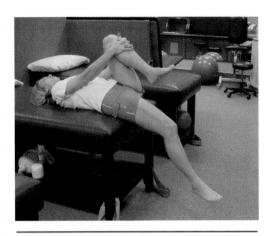

FIGURE 18-10 ROM, Hip Extension, Thomas Test

ROM Test for Internal and External Rotation of the Hip: With the athlete seated or supine (face-up), instruct the athlete to bend the uninvolved knee at a 90° angle. Check the active range of motion first, by asking the athlete to rotate the leg internally and externally (see Figures 18-11 and 18-12). Instruct the athlete to repeat the procedure on the involved hip, comparing flexibility between the two sides. Motion should be smooth and painless. Next, check the passive range of motion on both legs, checking the uninvolved leg first. Place one hand above the athlete's knee to stabilize the upper leg, and with the other hand on the distal aspect of the lower leg, apply controlled lateral force to check the pain-free ROM in internal rotation. Apply controlled medial force to the distal aspect of the lower leg to check pain-free ROM in external rotation. Limited ROM on one side indicates possible injury or deformity on that side.

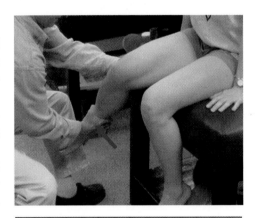

FIGURE 18-11 Passive ROM, Internal Rotation of the Hip

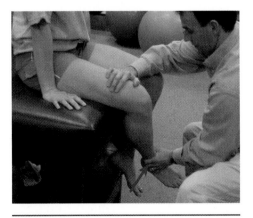

FIGURE 18-12 Passive ROM, External Rotation of the Hip

Ober's Test: Instruct the athlete lie on the involved side and ask the athlete to extend the top leg and flex the bottom leg.

Stabilize the athlete's hip with one hand and place the other hand on the medial aspect of the athlete's top leg, near the knee. Raise and slightly extend the hip while the knee is extended (Figure 18-13). Allow the leg to go back into adduction. Ask the athlete to switch sides in order to test the involved side. If the leg stays in abduction, tightness of the iliotibial (IT) band is indicated. **Note:** Avoid flexing the knee during this maneuver as it will increase stress on the femoral nerve, causing pain or tingling.

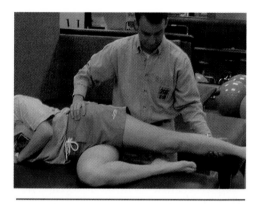

FIGURE 18-13 Passive ROM, Ober's Test

Patrick's or Faber Test: Instruct the athlete to lie supine with legs extended on the table. Place the uninvolved leg in a figure-4 position, with the heel of the leg to be tested crossed over the opposite knee (Figure 18-14). Stabilize the hip of the extended leg with one hand to prevent it from coming off the table, and place the other hand on the medial aspect of the bent knee. Slowly push down on the bent leg. Test the opposite leg in the same manner. Weakness or decreased range of motion on one side indicates potential injury or deformity to the iliopsoas on that side.

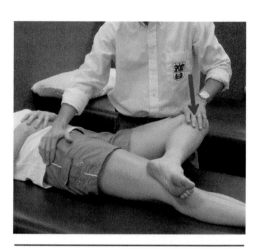

FIGURE 18-14 Passive ROM, Patrick's Test

Manual Muscle Tests for the Hip

Abduction Strength Test for the Hip: Instruct the athlete to lie on the involved side with legs extended. Stabilize the athlete's hip with one hand and place the other hand above the knee. Ask the athlete to raise the uninvolved leg to approximately a 20° angle. Apply isometric resistance to the athlete's leg by providing downward pressure as the athlete continues to elevate the leg (Figure 18-15). Make sure the athlete does not rotate the body in an attempt to use other muscles to resist the downward pressure. Note the degree of strength in the uninvolved hip. Have the athlete switch sides and test the involved hip in the same way. Weakness on one side indicates injury or deformity to the gluteus medius, gluteus minimus, tensor fasciae latae, sartorius, or piriformis on that side.

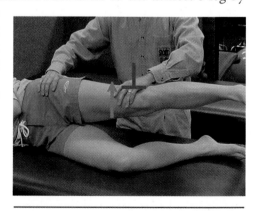

FIGURE 18-15 Hip Strength, Abduction

Adduction Strength Test for the Hip: Instruct the athlete to lie on the uninvolved side. Ask the athlete to place the upper leg in a figure-4 position (both hip and knee flexed 90°), making sure the foot is flat on the table while the knee and hip are flexed (Figure 18-16). Stabilize the upper leg by placing one hand near the distal end of the femur. Place the other hand on the lower leg at the inner aspect of the knee. Have the athlete raise the lower leg to approximately a 5° angle. Apply isometric resistance to the knee as the athlete attempts to continue to raise the leg. Make sure the athlete pushes straight up; don't allow any leaning forward or backward to use other muscles.

Note the degree of strength the athlete's uninvolved side. Ask the athlete to turn over onto the other side and then test the involved hip in the same way. Weakness on one side indicates injury or deformity to the pectineus, adductor brevis, adductor magnus, adductor longus, or gracilis on that side.

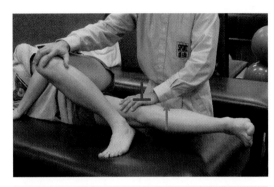

FIGURE 18-16 Hip Strength, Adduction

Extension Strength Test for the Hip (Gluteals and Hamstrings): Instruct the athlete to lie prone on the table with the legs extended. Place one hand over the gluteus maximus to stabilize the hip and feel for any deformities, and place the other hand below the knee on the posterior aspect of the lower leg (Figure 18-17). Have the athlete raise the leg so the knee is approximately 5 inches off the table. Apply isometric resistance near the knee as the athlete attempts to raise the leg further. Make sure the athlete does not rotate the hips in an attempt to use other muscles. Note the degree of strength in the uninvolved side. Test the involved side in the same manner. This test must also be performed on both legs with the knee flexed (Figure 18-18). Having the knee flexed eliminates the use of the hamstrings to compensate for possible weakness in other areas. As always, test the uninvolved side first. Again, place one hand over the gluteus maximus, but place the other hand above the knee on the posterior aspect of the thigh. Weakness on the involved side in one of these tests indicates injury or deformity to the gluteus maximus, biceps

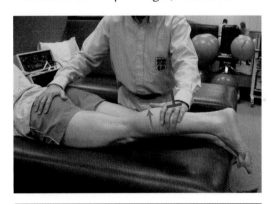

FIGURE 18-17 Hip Strength, Extension, Knee Straight

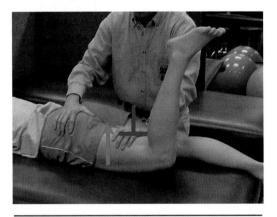

FIGURE 18-18 Hip Strength, Extension, Knee Flexed

femoris, semitendinosus, semimembranosus, or adductor magnus on that side.

Extension Strength Test for the Hip (Quadriceps): Instruct the athlete to sit at the end of the table with the knees flexed over the edge (Figure 18-19). Place one hand on the posterior side of the knee to stabilize the quadriceps and to feel for possible deformity when it contracts. Place the other hand at the distal end of the tibia. Instruct the athlete to extend the leg to approximately a 45° angle. Apply isometric resistance as the athlete attempts to fully extend the leg. Note the degree of strength in the uninvolved side. Test the involved side in the same manner. Weakness on one side indicates injury or deformity to the rectus femoris on that side.

Flexion Strength Test for the Hip: Instruct the athlete to sit at the end of the table with the knees flexed over the edge. Place one hand at the distal end of the femur above the knee and place the other hand at the distal end of the tibia to stabilize the lower leg (Figure 18-20). Have the athlete raise the upper leg slightly off the table. Apply isometric resistance to the leg with the upper hand as the athlete attempts to raise the leg further. Note the amount of strength in the uninvolved side. Test the involved side in the same manner. Weakness on the involved side indicates injury or deformity in the rectus femoris, iliopsoas, pectineus, sartorius, or tensor fascia latae on that side.

Internal Rotation Strength Test for the Hip: Have the athlete sit at the end of the table with the knees flexed over the edge. Stabilize the upper leg with one hand and place the other hand on the medial malleolus. Ask the athlete to internally rotate the leg, causing internal rotation of the hip, while applying isometric resistance (Figure 18-21). Note the amount of strength in internal rotation on the uninvolved side. Test the involved side in the same manner. Decreased strength on the involved side indicates injury or defor-

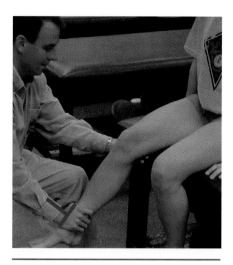

FIGURE 18-19 Hip Strength, Extension, Seated

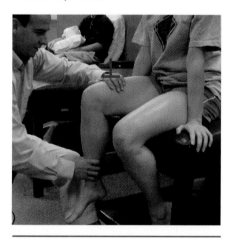

FIGURE 18-20 Hip Strength, Flexion

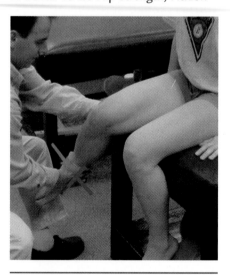

FIGURE 18-21 Hip Strength, Internal Rotation

mity in the gluteus medius, gluteus minimus, or tensor fasciae latae on that side.

External Rotation Strength Test for the Hip: Checking external rotation is similar to checking internal rotation. The athlete is in the same position, but the hand placement differs slightly: the lower hand is placed on the lateral malleolus. Ask the athlete to externally rotate the leg, causing external rotation of the hip, while applying isometric resistance (Figure 18-22). Note the amount of strength in external rotation on the uninvolved side. Test the involved side in the same manner. Decreased strength on the involved side indicates injury or deformity in the piriformis, gluteus maximus, or quadratus femoris on that side.

Trendelenburg Test: Stand behind the athlete and instruct the athlete to stand and balance on the uninvolved leg with the hands on or near the hips (Figure 18-23). Observe the athlete to see if the hips remain level. Perform the same test on the involved leg. A drop of the non-weight-bearing hip indicates weakness of the hip abductors on the weight-bearing side.

INJURIES TO THE HIP AND THIGH

All of the injuries discussed in Chapter 14 can affect the hip and thigh. Many of these injuries are also discussed in "Injuries to the Pelvic Region" in this chapter. To avoid unnecessary repetition, only injuries that have not yet been discussed will be addressed in detail in this section.

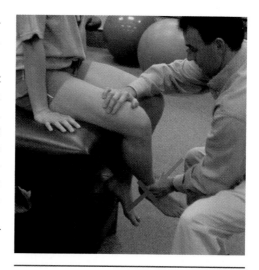

FIGURE 18-22 Hip Strength, External Rotation

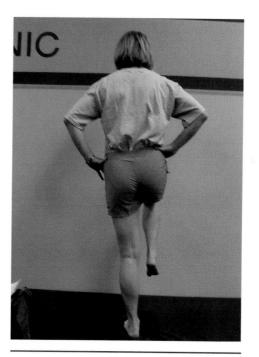

FIGURE 18-23 Trendelenburg Test

Fractures

Bones in the hip and thigh may be fractured as a result of a direct blow, twisting, or repeated stress. However, because of the size of the bones in these areas, great forces are usually required to fracture them. Participants in contact sports, motocross, BMX, and skateboarding are particularly susceptible to fractures of the hip and thigh. Fractures cause swelling, point tenderness, possible deformity, crepitation, and decreased ROM. The athlete will experience moderate to severe pain when placing weight on the injured leg.

Immediate Treatment: If the possibility of a fracture exists, treat the athlete for shock, and gently apply a splint if possible to relieve the pain and prevent additional injury. Send the athlete to a physician for further evaluation or call the EMS. Ice may also be applied as long as the weight of the ice does not cause more pain.

Follow-up Treatment: Make sure the physician's orders are followed. If a cast is applied, instruct the athlete to keep the casting material dry.

Prevention: Protective padding may help prevent fractures to the hip and thigh. Such padding is particularly important for players of contact sports and skateboarders. In addition, it is important to emphasize proper falling techniques and adherence to rules of play. Check the field of play for conditions that may increase the potential for injury.

Dislocations and Subluxations

A dislocation or subluxation of the hip, though not particularly common in sports, generally results from either a direct blow or a twisting force that displaces the head of the femur from the acetabulum. Sports that carry an increased risk of such injuries include contact sports, skateboarding, BMX, and motocross. Signs and symptoms of dislocation include complete loss of function in the injured joint, severe pain, swelling, and deformity. Symptoms of a subluxation are pain, decreased ROM, a slipping sensation, and possible swelling. The athlete may experience a "popping" sensation, created by the shifting of the joint out of position and back into place.

Compare the appearance and function of the injured side to the uninjured one, and watch the athlete's face for signs that pain increases with movement. X-rays will confirm the presence of a dislocation and determine if a fracture exists. Forces that cause a dislocation will also sprain and/or strain the surrounding tissues. In a subluxation the athlete may say that it felt as if the joint popped out and back in again, but there will probably be no deformity. Dislocations are discussed in greater detail in Chapter 14.

Immediate Treatment: Place the athlete in the most comfortable position possible, treat the athlete for shock, and call the EMS. Ice can be applied, but avoid causing additional pain from the weight of the ice. Do not attempt to splint the joint by straightening it. Only apply a splint if the joint can remain in the position it is already in. Check for loss of sensation and/ or decreased circulation in the lower extremity. If either loss of sensation or reduced circulation is detected, a nerve, artery, or vein may be damaged and this information should be given to the EMS team.

Follow-up Treatment: Make sure the physician's orders are followed.

Prevention: Advise the coaches to teach athletes how to fall properly to avoid injury. Check the field of play for conditions that may increase the potential for injury.

Contusions

Although contusions can occur anywhere, the most common area for a bruise on the lower extremities in contact sports is the quadriceps. A bruise here is often called a Charley horse. This injury, resulting from a direct blow to the quads, causes bleeding in the muscle tissue.

Immediate Treatment: Use the PRICE procedure and mild stretching through the pain-free range of motion—for example, keeping the knee fully flexed so that the heel comes in contact with the buttocks, while the ice is on (20 minutes) and while the ice is off, or performing squats to ensure flexibility. These stretching activities are vital to the prevention of further or prolonged disability. If proper stretching is not done, blood will pool in the quadriceps, leaving the area vulnerable to myositis ossificans (see Chapter 14).

Follow-up Treatment: Isometric exercises can be used to maintain strength during rehabilitation. Once the tissue has sufficiently recovered, isotonic exercises and pedaling a stationery bike will help to maintain the athlete's full range of motion. Protect the area from further injury with a thigh pad or donut pad, making sure to cover the entire area of the contusion.

Prevention: For football and hockey players, protect the area with a properly sized thigh pad so that the force of any hit on the quadriceps will be dispersed over a broader area of the thigh. Make sure that players' pants fit properly. If the pants are not tight enough, a thigh pad will shift when the leg is raised, leaving the thigh vulnerable to injury.

Sprains

Runningbacks and athletes involved in all running sports may be at increased risk of experiencing sprains of the hip. Such injuries are typically caused by sudden jerky or twisting motions of the lower extremities, causing a stretching or tearing of the ligaments. These injuries tend to be more frequent at the beginning of the season if athletes are not properly conditioned year-round. Refer to Chapter 14 for a detailed discussion of sprains.

Immediate Treatment: The treatment for any sprain is the PRICE procedure. With hip sprains, however, elevation is not an option. Give the injured athlete crutches to help with walking. If unable to determine the severity of the injury (i.e., if a fracture or severe sprain is suspected), send the athlete to a physician. Also, if the joint feels unstable (see evaluation guidelines), refer the athlete to a physician. Make sure athletes use ice techniques after practice and exercise.

Follow-up Treatment: Check the injured area again after 24 hours for any increased swelling or pain and any decrease in range of motion. If any of these signs is observed, or if symptoms do not improve within three days, send the athlete to a physician. If the injury is improving, isometric exercises can be used to maintain strength, followed by isotonic exercises to preserve full ROM. A stationary bike can be used to help increase and maintain range of motion following an injury to the hip or thigh. Cycling is also an excellent means of maintaining physical condition while under restricted play.

Prevention: Balanced strengthening and conditioning of the quadriceps and hamstrings often help to prevent sprains to the hip and thigh. Check the field of play for conditions that may increase the potential for injury.

Strains

Athletes who participate in running sports and those who play certain positions in football commonly experience muscle strains in both the hamstring and quadricep muscle groups. An overstretching of the musculature causes these strains. Most muscle strains occur at the point where the tendon meets the muscle. A more detailed discussion of strains may be found in Chapter 14.

Immediate Treatment: Use the PRICE procedure during the first 24 to 48 hours following the injury. If pain is severe, immobilize the area to make the athlete as comfortable as possible and activate the Emergency Action Plan. A physician will need to rule out the possibility of a fracture or a complete tear. When evaluating for swelling, locate a landmark on the uninvolved extremity, such as the superior aspect of the patella, and measure the girth, or circumference, of the leg about 12 to 15 inches above or below that landmark, depending on the location of the injury. Record this measurement; then compare the same point on the opposite leg.

Follow-up Treatment: After two days of rest, the athlete may begin slow, static stretching of the injured area, followed by isometric and then isotonic strengthening exercises. The athlete may also appreciate the comfort of a neoprene sleeve over the area, which can add compression, support, and heat to the healing tissues.

Prevention: Balanced strengthening and stretching of the quadriceps and hamstrings will help prevent strains. See Chapter 7.

Bursitis and Synovitis

Trochanteric bursitis (inflammation of the trochanter bursa) of the hip can be caused by a direct blow, infection, repeated stress, or other conditions such as arthritis. Bursitis will cause slight swelling and a persistent ache that is aggravated by activity. Synovitis is characterized by the same symptoms. If the affected area is not protected from another blow by the use of padding or removal from activity, the condition will gradually progress to a chronic condition. Athletes who participate in basketball, long jump, triple jump, and cross-country are particularly vulnerable to the types of stresses that can cause bursitis and synovitis of the hip. See Chapter 14 for a more detailed discussion of bursitis and synovitis.

Immediate Treatment: If no swelling is present, apply moist heat packs to the affected area. If swelling is present, use the PRICE procedure. Pad the affected joint to protect it from further injury.

Follow-up Treatment: After the swelling subsides, use moist heat treatments. To maintain mobility in the joint, advise the athlete to carefully stretch it through the pain-free range of motion. If pain increases or persists for over a week, refer the athlete to a physician.

Prevention: Make sure athletes are taught how to use the body's muscles properly to avoid unnecessary stress to the joints, and encourage the use of proper protective padding. Instruction in proper body mechanics for the sport being played is typically the coach's responsibility; however, the athletic trainer's support of these techniques is invaluable. Proper training techniques can help prevent bursitis. For instance, athletes should condition gradually and avoid training on hard or downhill surfaces that may increase the repeated stress to the joint.

THE KNEE AND LOWER LEG

The knee joint is naturally unstable and one of the most complicated—and commonly injured—joints in the body. The knee (see Figure 18-24) consists of the patella, the inferior end of the femur, the superior ends of the tibia and fibula, and several supporting ligaments and tendons. A fibrous articular capsule encloses the articulations between the femur and tibia as well as the articulation between the patella and femur. Stability is added to the knee joint by several ligaments and tendons (see Figure 18-25). Anteriorly, the patella adds support to the knee, while the collateral ligaments prevent side-to-side movements of the knee. The oblique popliteal ligament prevents overextension. The knee joint also contains menisci, which are cartilage, that add stability and act as shock absorbers.

Within the knee joint are intra-articular ligaments called the cruciate ligaments. *Cruciate* is Latin for "cross." These two ligaments cross each other, providing additional support to the knee and preventing antero-posterior motion. Another important ligament of the lower extremities, the patellar ligament or patellar tendon, helps stabilize the patella and support the knee.

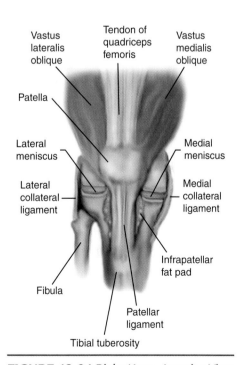

FIGURE 18-24 Right Knee, Anterior View

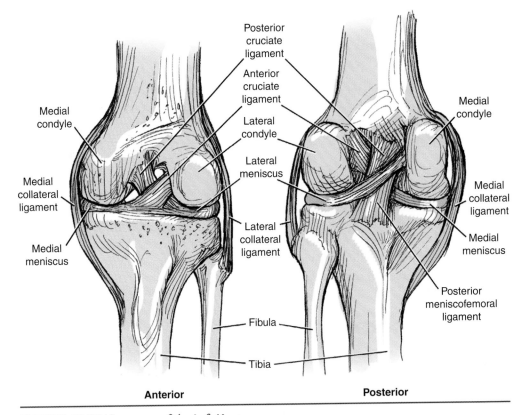

FIGURE 18-25 Ligaments of the Left Knee

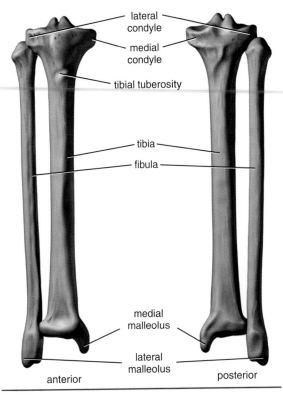

FIGURE 18-26 Bones of the Lower Leg

The anterior knee is stabilized by the quadriceps group, which enables extension of the knee. The hamstrings, plantaris, lateral and medial gastrocnemius, and popliteus are located on the posterior knee and assist with flexion. The knee is designed primarily for flexion and extension—similar to the movement of a hinge. The knee joint, however, is not a true hinge joint, in that it does allow slight rotation on the tibial axis and slight anterior and posterior glide. All of the muscles and ligaments of the knee contribute to the stability of the knee and prevent all but slight medial, lateral, anterior, and posterior movement of this joint.

The sesamoid bone that articulates with the distal end of the femur is called the patella. This bone, also known as the kneecap, is embedded within the patellar tendon, which attaches the quadriceps to the tibia at the tibial tuberosity (see Figure 18-26). The tibia, also known as the shin bone, articulates proximally with the distal end of the femur and the proximal end of the fibula. The fibula is the smaller and most lateral of the two bones in the lower leg, and it does not bear much body weight. The tibia is the larger bone and bears most of the weight. At their distal ends, the tibia and the fibula each expand to form a bony prominence. Each of these prominences is known as a malleolus. The medial, or internal, malleolus projects medially from the tibia, while the lateral, or external, malleolus projects laterally from the fibula. These malleoli articulate with the ankle.

The main muscles of the lower leg are the tibialis anterior on the front and the gastrocnemius and the soleus in the back. The soleus lies beneath the gastrocnemius and assists in plantar flexion of the foot (toes pointing downward). The gastrocnemius is a two-joint muscle, meaning that is assists in the movement of two joints: flexion of the knee and plantar flexion of the foot. The tibialis anterior assists in dorsiflexion of the foot (toes pointing upward).

The blood vessels that supply the lower leg, ankle, foot, and toes are extensions of the vessels that supply the upper leg. At the knee, the femoral artery becomes the popliteal artery. This artery then branches into four genicular arteries that serve the knee, and three main arteries that serve the lower leg: the peroneal artery, and the anterior and posterior tibial arteries. The foot is served by extensions of these arteries: the anterior tibial artery becomes the dorsalis pedis artery, and the posterior tibial artery becomes the medial plantar artery. The plantar digital arteries, extensions of the foot arteries, supply the toes with oxygenated blood.

The primary deep veins of the thigh are the external iliac and femoral veins. As with the femoral artery, the femoral vein becomes the popliteal vein at the knee. Similarly, the popliteal vein branches into the peroneal vein and the anterior and posterior tibial veins. All are considered to be deep veins. The great and small saphenous, dorsal, plantar, and dorsal digital veins are superficial veins serving the leg and/or foot. The great and small saphenous veins branch off of the femoral vein to serve both the leg and foot, and the dorsal and plantar veins (which feed the larger superior veins) serve the foot, with the dorsal digital veins serving the toes.

The lateral cutaneous and femoral nerves continue from the upper leg into the lower leg, ankle, and foot (see Figure 18-27). On the posterior aspect of the thigh, located within the gluteal muscles and descending through the hamstrings, is the sciatic nerve. These three nerves are the principal nerves of the lower extremity; however, numerous nerves supply the leg, foot, and toes. Each of these principal nerves divides into numerous smaller branches to innervate the entire lower extremity.

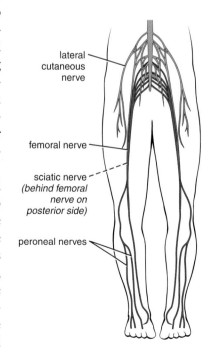

FIGURE 18-27 Primary Nerves of the Lower Extremity

ASSESSING KNEE INJURIES

When assessing knee injuries, remember to apply the principles of the HOPS procedure, taking care to accurately record all information and pass the information along to the appropriate medical personnel. Special tests used to assess specific knee conditions are presented in the injuries section of this chapter.

Range-of-Motion Evaluations for the Knee

ROM Test for Knee Extension: Instruct the athlete to lie in the supine position with legs fully extended. Place one hand on the medial side of the athlete's uninvolved ankle and use the other hand to stabilize the knee (Figure 18-28). Carefully extend the knee through the pain-free passive range of motion. Motion should be smooth and painless. Note and document any laxity in the uninvolved side. Test the involved side in the same manner. Limited range of motion on the involved side indicates possible injury or deformity on that side.

ROM Test for Knee Flexion: Instruct the athlete to lie in the supine position. Place one hand on the heel of the uninvolved foot and use the other hand to stabilize the knee. Flex the knee through the pain-free passive range of motion (Figure 18-29). (**Note:** The hip will also need to be flexed to achieve full flexion of the knee.) Motion should be smooth and painless. Note and document any laxity in the uninvolved side. Test the involved side in the same manner. Limited range of motion on the involved side indicates possible injury or deformity on that side.

Manual Muscle Tests for the Knee

Extension Strength Test for the Knee: Instruct the athlete to lie in the supine position with both knees bent to about 90° (Figure 18-30). Stabilize the uninvolved leg by placing the forearm behind the athlete's uninvolved knee, and

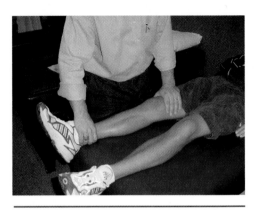
FIGURE 18-28 Passive ROM, Knee Extension

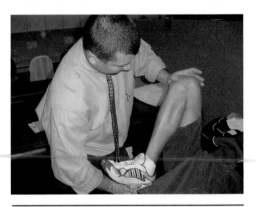
FIGURE 18-29 Passive ROM, Knee Flexion

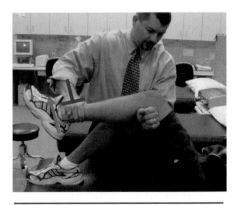
FIGURE 18-30 Knee Strength, Extension, Athlete Supine

resting that forearm on top of the athlete's involved leg. Place the other hand on the anterior portion of the ankle. With the knee at full flexion, ask the athlete to raise the lower leg while applying isometric resistance. Feel for any strength changes and look for deformities as the athlete extends the leg through the ROM. Test the involved knee in the same way. Compare the strength of the quadriceps in both legs and note any differences. Weakness in the involved knee indicates injury or deformity of the quadriceps. This test may also be performed with the athlete seated. However, this will limit the range of motion because the table will interfere with flexion.

Flexion Strength Test for the Knee: Instruct the athlete to lie in the prone position with both legs extended. Place one hand at the distal end of the athlete's tibia; with the other hand, palpate the hamstring area and feel for deformities (Figure 18-31). With the uninvolved leg at full extension, apply isometric resistance at the ankle as the athlete brings the leg into full flexion. Feel for any differences in strength and look for deformities as the leg goes through full ROM. Test the involved side in the same way. Compare the strength of the hamstrings in both legs and note any differences. Weakness in the involved knee indicates injury or deformity of the hamstrings. This test may also be performed with the athlete seated. However, this will limit the range of motion because the table will interfere with the available ROM.

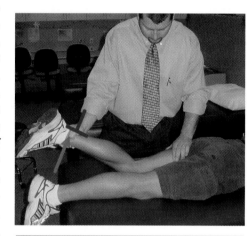

FIGURE 18-31 Knee Strength, Flexion, Athlete Supine

INJURIES TO THE KNEE AND LOWER LEG

All of the injuries discussed in Chapter 14 can affect the knee and lower leg. Many of these injuries are also discussed in previous sections of this chapter. To avoid unnecessary repetition, only injuries that have not yet been discussed will be addressed in detail in this section.

Fractures

Patellar fractures are very rare, but the possibility of their existence should never be overlooked. These usually occur from a direct blow, but may also be caused by repeated stress. Fractures of the tibia and fibula are more common. Like patellar fractures, these fractures may be caused by direct blows or repeated stress. Avulsion fractures may occur to the knee and ankle where the ligaments attach to the bones. Sports that carry an increased risk of fractures to the knee and lower leg include contact sports, cross-country, skateboarding, BMX, and motocross. If there is reason to suspect a fracture or if unsure about an evaluation, refer the athlete to a physician for diagnosis and treatment. See Chapter 14 for a detailed discussion of the symptoms and treatment of fractures. See also "Injuries to the Hip and Thigh" in this chapter.

Protective padding for players of contact sports and sports involving high-velocity objects, such as baseball and hockey, can help prevent fractures of the bones of the knee and lower leg. Skateboarders will also benefit from such padding. Proper falling techniques should be emphasized and the field of play checked for conditions that may increase the potential for injury. Make sure appropriate rules of play are followed.

Dislocations and Subluxations

Dislocation or subluxation of the patella may result from sudden internal rotation of the trunk while the foot is planted, causing lateral dislocation of the patella. Patellar dislocation or subluxation may also be caused by a direct blow (see Figure 18-32). Such injuries are most likely to affect offensive guards, as well as basketball, soccer, and volleyball players. The signs, symptoms, and treatment of subluxations and dislocations are discussed in Chapter 14. Also see "Injuries to the Hip and Thigh" in this chapter. In addition to taking the preventive techniques already mentioned, advise athletes to strengthen the quadriceps to avoid such injuries.

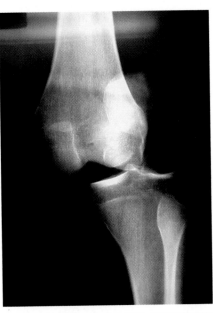

FIGURE 18-32 A Dislocated Knee

Apprehension Test for the Patella: Instruct the athlete to sit and extend the legs on the table. Place the thumbs on one side of the athlete's uninvolved patella and the index fingers on the other side. Make sure the leg muscle is relaxed, and then push medially and laterally on the patella (Figure 18-33). Repeat the test on the involved patella. Note any differences in the athlete's response to the two tests. If the athlete complains of increased pain or winces when the pressure is applied to the involved patella, a possible subluxation of the patella is indicated.

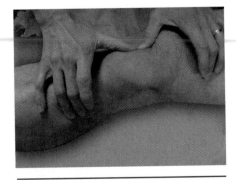

FIGURE 18-33 Apprehension Test for the Patella

Contusions

Contusions to the knees and lower legs can occur in many sports, especially soccer. Such contusions may also be a problem for runningbacks. Contusions to the knee can be prevented in football, volleyball, softball, and wrestling through the use of knee pads. For proper protection, the pads should be worn correctly; football players who wear their knee pads too high won't be properly protected from knee contusions. Refer to Chapter 14 for a detailed discussion of contusions.

Sprains

Sprains of the knee ligaments can be of first, second, or third degree. The most commonly sprained ligament in the knee is the medial collateral ligament (MCL). This is usually caused by a lateral force, which results in a valgus (knock-kneed) stress on the knee. Next most common are sprains to the anterior cruciate ligament (ACL). Torsion or an anterior blow usually causes these sprains. There are other ligaments in the knee that may be sprained as well, such as the lateral collateral ligament (LCL) and the posterior cruciate ligaments (PCL), but the MCL and the ACL typically are the most vulnerable.

A ligament sprain in the knee will cause swelling, point tenderness, decreased strength, loss of function, possible decreased ROM, and possible joint instability. The athlete may actually hear a "pop" when a severe sprain occurs. The degree of symptoms will depend upon the severity of the injury. It is important to look at the mechanism of injury when evaluating the severity of the injury. For example, if the MCL is involved and the mechanism was a lateral blow, the ligament is likely sprained, whereas if the blow is medial, it is more likely a contusion. Likewise, if the LCL is injured from a medial blow, it is likely to be sprained, but if the blow is lateral, the LCL is probably only contused.

Sports that carry an increased risk of sprains to the knee include basketball, soccer, football, and wrestling. Refer to Chapter 14 for a more detailed discussion of the symptoms, classifications, treatment, and prevention of sprains. See also "Injuries to the Hip and Thigh" in this chapter.

Prevention of knee sprains is similar to prevention of other knee injuries: advise athletes to strengthen the quadriceps, check the playing field for hidden dangers, and make sure the athletes are instructed in proper falling techniques appropriate to their sport. Sometimes, knee braces are also used in injury prevention for athletes who play sports or positions that make the knee vulnerable to injury, such as for offensive linemen; however, schools of thought vary on the effectiveness of preventive knee braces. If a sprain does occur, the sprained knee can be protected from further injury with a hinged knee brace. Different braces provide different levels of support, so selection of a brace should be based on the amount of support needed.

Valgus Stress Test for the Knee:
Instruct the athlete to either sit or lie down with the legs extended and relaxed (Figure 18-34). Place one hand on the medial aspect of the athlete's ankle and the other hand on the lateral side of the knee. Extend the athlete's leg so it is straight. Simultaneously apply medial force to the knee and lateral force to the ankle to create tension on the medial collateral ligament (MCL). Note the degree of laxity in the MCL. Test the involved side in the same way. Compare the laxity of the MCL in both legs and note any differences. Excessive laxity in the involved knee with or without pain indicates a potential sprain or tear of the MCL.

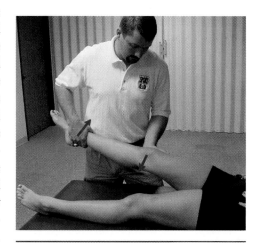

FIGURE 18-34 Valgus Stress Test, Full Extension, Athlete Prone

After this test is performed with the leg straight, it also needs to be performed with the knee flexed at a 20 to 30° angle (Figure 18-35). The hand placement and the forces applied are the same as described above. If laxity and pain in the medial knee joint also occur with this test, it confirms injury or deformity of the MCL.

The placement of the hands may be altered if there are injuries to the ankle as well. If the ankle is injured, placing a hand on the ankle or foot will cause additional pain. Observe the athlete and talk over the situation to find a suitable location for hand placement that limits the amount of pain, but still allows the test to be performed.

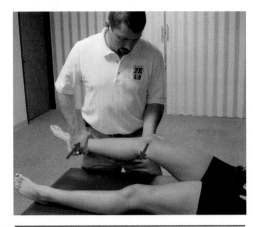

FIGURE 18-35 Valgus Stress Test, 20° Flexion, Athlete Prone

Varus Stress Test for the Knee:
Instruct the athlete to either sit or lie down with the legs extended and relaxed. Place one hand on the lateral aspect of the athlete's ankle and the other hand on the medial side of the knee (Figure 18-36). Extend the athlete's leg so it is straight. Simultaneously apply lateral force to the knee and medial force to the ankle to create tension on the lateral collateral ligament (LCL). Note the degree of laxity in the LCL. Test the involved side in the same way. Compare the laxity of the LCL in both legs and note any differences. Excessive laxity in the involved knee joint with or without pain indicates a potential sprain or tear of the LCL.

After this test is performed with the leg straight, it also needs to be performed with the knee flexed at a 20 to 30° angle (Figure 18-37). The hand placement and the forces applied are the same as described above. If laxity and pain in the lateral knee joint also occur with this test, it confirms injury or deformity of the LCL.

As with the valgus stress test, the placement of the hands may be altered if there are injuries to the ankle as well. If the ankle is injured, placing a hand on the ankle or foot will cause additional pain. Observe the athlete and talk over

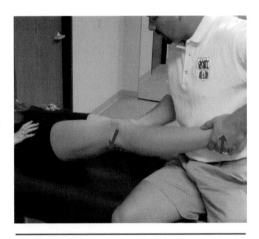

FIGURE 18-36 Varus Stress Test, Full Extension, Athlete Prone

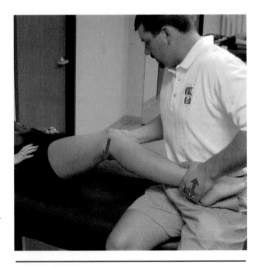

FIGURE 18-37 Varus Stress Test, 30° Flexion, Athlete Prone

the situation to find a suitable location for hand placement that limits the amount of pain, but still enables the test to be conducted.

Anterior Drawer Test for the Knee:
Instruct the athlete to lie in the supine position with legs extended. The hamstrings and surrounding muscles must be relaxed. Flex the uninvolved knee to approximately a 90° angle, keeping the foot flat and straight on the table (Figure 18-38). Stabilize the foot by gently sitting on it while performing the assessment. Place both hands behind the proximal end of the athlete's tibia and pull anteriorly. Watch to see if the tibial plateau pulls anterior to the patellar plane. As with all the tests, compare the uninvolved side with the involved side. This test needs to be performed with the foot in three different positions: straight, internally rotated, and externally rotated. The foot is rotated internally and externally to determine if there is any rota-

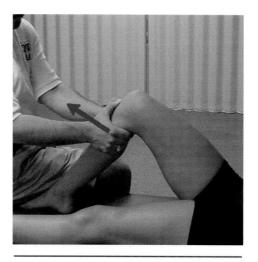

FIGURE 18-38 Anterior Drawer Test, Foot Straight, Athlete Prone

tional instability. Excessive laxity in the involved joint with or without the athlete experiencing pain indicates a sprain or tear of the anterior cruciate ligament (ACL).

    This test can also be performed with the athlete seated. Hand placement and the forces applied are the same as described above. The evaluator will need to stabilize the athlete's foot by placing it between the evaluator's legs or feet during the test.

Posterior Drawer Test for the Knee: Instruct the athlete to lie in the supine position with legs extended and relaxed. Bend the uninvolved knee to approximately a 90° angle, keeping the foot flat and straight on the table (Figure 18-39). Look at the proximal tibia for a dropping off of the tibial plateau where it meets the femur. This condition is known as posterior sag, and if present in the involved knee, but not the uninvolved knee, indicates a sprain or tear to the posterior cruciate ligament (PCL). Stabilize the foot by gently sitting on it. Place both hands at the proximal end of the tibia and push posteriorly. Watch to see if the tibial plateau pushes posterior to the patellar plane. Note and compare the uninvolved side to the involved side. Laxity in the joint with or without the athlete experiencing pain indicates a sprain or tear to the PCL.

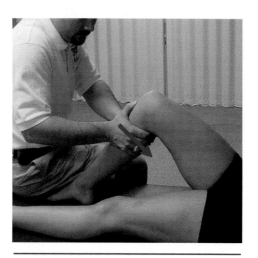

FIGURE 18-39 Posterior Drawer Test, Foot Straight, Athlete Supine

Lachman Test: This test is an alternate method of determining the integrity of the

---

anterior drawer test for the knee

application of anterior force to the proximal posterior aspect of the tibia to assess the stability of the ACL.

posterior drawer test for the knee

application of posterior force to the proximal anterior aspect of the tibia to assess the stability of the PCL.

Lachman test

application of anterior and posterior force to the proximal posterior tibia to determine the stability of the ACL and PCL.

ACL and/or the PCL. Instruct the athlete to lie in a supine position with the uninvolved knee flexed 20 to 30°, making sure the hamstrings are relaxed (Figure 18-40). Place one hand on the upper leg to stabilize the femur and place the other hand around the middle of the lower leg. Apply anterior force to the lower leg to check for damage to the ACL. Also apply posterior force to check for damage to the PCL. Repeat the test on the involved side. The difference in the amount of laxity between the uninvolved and involved knee joints determines the degree of sprain or tear of the ACL or PCL.

For larger athletes, or if the evaluator has small hands, the evaluator can place his or her knee (see Figure 18-40) or a 4-inch bolster under the athlete's thigh to create 20 to 30° of flexion. This will make it easier for one hand to stabilize the athlete's upper leg while using the other hand to move the lower leg anteriorly and posteriorly.

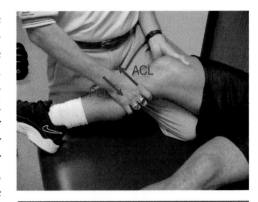

FIGURE 18-40 Lachman Test, with Athletic Trainer's Knee Under the Athlete's Thigh to Create 20 to 30° of Flexion

Pivot Shift Test: Instruct the athlete to lie in the supine position with legs extended and relaxed. Place one hand on the bottom of the foot and lift the leg so the hip is at approximately a 45° angle. Place the other hand on the lateral side of the knee to supply minimal medial pressure (Figure 18-41). Perform the pivot by internally rotating the

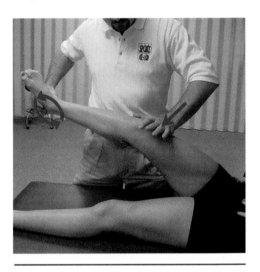

FIGURE 18-41 Pivot Shift Test

> **pivot shift test**
>
> internal rotation of the ankle combined with medial force to assess the stability of the ACL.

ankle, keeping the knee fully extended. Perform the shift by flexing the knee 20 to 40° while using one hand on the foot to apply a simultaneous rotational medial force and **direct axial load**. If the ACL is damaged, the tibia will sublux in the fully extended position. As the knee is flexed between 20 and 40° the ACL will reduce and produce a palpable shift or "clunking" noise, indicating a possible tear of the ACL.

> **direct axial load**
>
> direct pressure applied to the long axis of a body or limb.

Strains

Muscle strains affecting the knee and lower leg commonly occur in the gastrocnemius, soleus, and quadriceps muscles. The most common mechanism of injury is dynamic overload (quick motion with considerable force), such as that experienced by jumpers, basketball players, and runners who make sudden stops and pivots. An overstretching of the musculature can also cause these strains. As previously stated, most muscle strains occur at the point where the tendon meets the muscle. The best way to avoid such strains is to strengthen and properly stretch the muscles of the leg, paying particular attention to the muscles listed above and maintaining balance of strength.

Tendon Ruptures

A **tendon rupture** is a complete or near complete tearing of a tendon. Symptoms of a tendon rupture include immediate pain, swelling, and deformity. A complete rupture will result in loss of motion in that extremity. If the rupture is incomplete, the athlete will be able to extend the extremity, but it will be extremely painful. Palpation will increase the pain. A patellar tendon rupture will most likely occur from an eccentric contraction of the quadriceps or a violent motion.

Patellar Tendon Rupture Test: Instruct the athlete to attempt to extend the lower leg. Inability to extend the lower leg indicates a complete rupture of the patellar tendon; the quadriceps and the tibia are no longer connected to each other. If the athlete can extend the lower leg, but pain, swelling, and deformity are present, an incomplete rupture is indicated.

Immediate Treatment: Use the PRICE procedure. Stabilize the foot and calf with a splint, if possible, or assist the athlete into the most comfortable position possible, and help the athlete maintain that position. Refer the athlete to a physician for further evaluation and treatment.

Follow-up Treatment: Make sure the physician's orders are followed.

Prevention: To avoid patellar tendon ruptures, makes sure athletes gradually increase flexibility and strength in the quadriceps and apply the concept of balanced strength to all conditioning efforts.

Tears of the Meniscus

A **meniscal tear** can result from a rotation or twisting of the knee, which causes damage to the cartilage. There may or may not be severe pain or loss of motion when the meniscus is torn. Upon injury to the meniscus, the athlete may feel a locking of the knee and the inability to fully flex or extend the leg. In each case there is the possibility of point tenderness at the site of the tear.

McMurray Test: Instruct the athlete to lie face-up with the legs extended and relaxed. Place one hand on the bottom of the athlete's foot and the other hand on the anterior portion of the leg, slightly beneath the patella. Position the hand on the patella so that one finger can be used to feel the medial joint line and another finger can be used to feel the lateral joint line (Figure 18-42). The hand on the foot is used to rotate the ankle internally and externally and to flex and extend the leg.

Begin the test by fully flexing the knee and internally rotating the foot

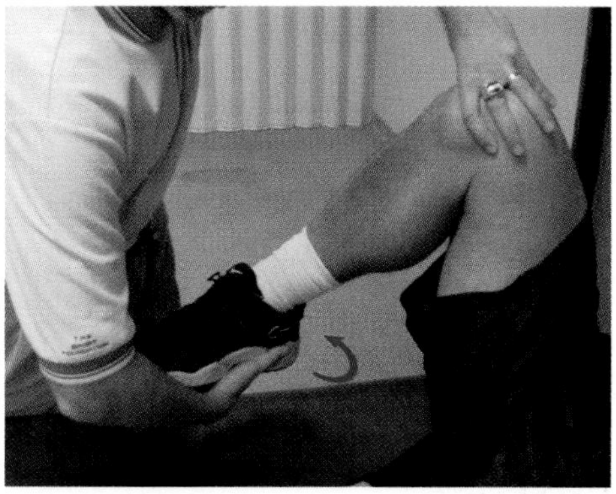

FIGURE 18-42 McMurray Test, Knee Fully Flexed, Foot Internally Rotated with Slight Varus Stress

tendon rupture

a complete tear of a tendon.

patellar tendon rupture test

extension of the lower leg to assess the integrity of the patellar tendon.

meniscal tear

a partial or complete tear of a meniscus.

McMurray test

compression of the meniscus of the knee combined with internal and external rotation while the patient is face-up to assess the integrity of the meniscus.

(Figure 18-43). The following motions are done in a fluid manner, almost as one continuous motion. Extend the knee, keeping the foot internally rotated. Flex the knee again, externally rotating the foot at full flexion. Extend the knee once more with the foot externally rotated, and flex the knee again, internally rotating the foot at full flexion (Figure 18-44). A "pop" felt on the lateral or medial joint line during internal or external rotation of the foot indicates a tear of a meniscus.

The evaluator must be able to distinguish between a joint line pop and a patellar pop. In many cases there will only be one good chance for this evaluation without the athlete becoming apprehensive about what is happening. If there are injuries to the foot or ankle, hand placement must be moved to a location above the injury site. **Note:** Often the physician will rely on the athletic trainer's evaluation of this test in forming a diagnosis, rather than repeat the test, because by the time the athlete reaches the physician, edema (swelling) may inhibit the ability to perform the test.

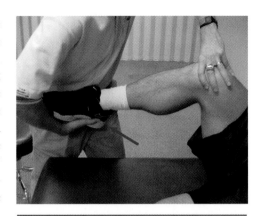

FIGURE 18-43 McMurray Test, Knee Flexed 90°, Foot Internally Rotated

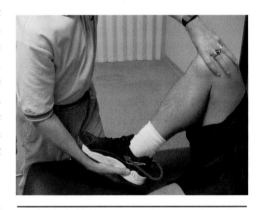

FIGURE 18-44 McMurray Test, Knee Fully Flexed, Foot Externally Rotated with Slight Valgus Stress

Apley compression test

compression of the meniscus of the knee combined with internal and external rotation on a patient who is face-down to assess the integrity of the meniscus.

Apley Compression Test: This test is also used to determine damage to the meniscus. Instruct the athlete to lie face-down, flexing the knee at a 90° angle. Place one hand on the bottom of the athlete's foot, near the heel, and the other hand on the upper leg, near the distal end of the femur. Push down on the foot while rotating it internally and externally (Figure 18-45). As with most of the tests, compare the uninvolved side with the involved side. If there is a torn meniscus the athlete will feel pain or hear an audible "clunk." Damage to the medial meniscus is indicated if the these signs are present when the knee is internally rotated, and damage to the lateral meniscus is indicated if the signs appear during external rotation.

Immediate Treatment: The treatment for this type of injury is the PRICE

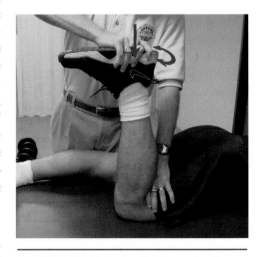

FIGURE 18-45 Apley Compression Test

procedure. Any athlete with a possibly torn meniscus should be referred to a physician.

Follow-up Treatment: Make sure the physician's orders are followed.

Prevention: Inspect all playing surfaces for holes, water, and other hazards that could create an environment where torsion to the knee is likely to occur.

Tendonitis

Patellar tendonitis is a condition in which the tendon that attaches the patella to the quadriceps becomes inflamed. This is caused by repeated forceful extension of the knee, causing inflammation, which in turn causes pain. Sports presenting increased risk of this injury include those that involve jumping, such as basketball, high jump, volleyball, and long jump. Bicyclists may also suffer from patellar tendonitis if the bicycle seat is too low, causing undue stress on the patellar tendon. Patellar tendonitis may also be caused by running downhill or down stairs. Symptoms include pain or soreness over the patellar tendon, possible mild swelling, and crepitation of the patellar region. The pain will increase during activities such as going down stairs, jumping, and sudden slowing from a run. Patellar tendonitis may be indicated when knee extensions against resistance with and without motion produce pain in the involved side. These symptoms may also be indicative of patellofemoral stress syndrome.

Immediate Treatment: Use the PRICE procedure immediately. For patellar tendonitis, the athlete should perform gradual, slow stretching of the quadriceps, followed by strengthening exercises. Leg extensions, when held for a moment at the top of the extension, will help to strengthen the quadriceps. Remember to advise the athlete to remain within the pain-free range of motion whenever strengthening is being used as a treatment.

Follow-up Treatment: For patellar tendonitis, apply compression to the knee by having the athlete wear a neoprene sleeve with a patellar cutout. Also, ice the knee after any practice, and ice massage the knee three to four times a day for 10 minutes (see Chapter 22). If the condition does not improve within 7 to 10 days, refer the athlete to a physician. It is important to identify the source of the injury (stairs, running, etc.) and to avoid activities that will further aggravate the injury during the healing process. Once the pain is gone, heat may be applied to the injured area prior to exercise, followed by ice after the activity.

Prevention: Proper conditioning, meaning a slow progression in intensity and duration of exercises, is vital to preventing patellar tendonitis. Strengthening should focus on the quadriceps; strong quads will protect the tendons and ligaments of the patellar region. In addition, maintaining flexibility in the hamstrings and quads will reduce stress on the patellar region. Once an athlete develops patellar tendonitis, a more severe case can be prevented by applying ice at the first sign of pain and immediately following exercise. Do not allow the athlete to wait until arriving home.

Bursitis

The prepatellar bursa, located anterior to the patella, is extremely susceptible to bursitis. As with all forms of bursitis, the inflammation may be caused by a direct blow, infection, repeated stress, or other conditions. Sports that carry an increased risk of prepatellar bursitis include basketball, wrestling, volleyball, and running sports. To help athletes avoid this condition, make sure they are taught how to use the body's muscles properly to avoid unnecessary stress to the joints and encourage the use of knee pads.

Osgood-Schlatter Disease

Osgood-Schlatter disease

inflammation or irritation of the tibia at its point of attachment with the patellar tendon.

Osgood-Schlatter disease is a condition of the tibial tubercle, which is where the patellar tendon attaches to the front of the tibia. This disorder usually involves a genetic predisposition and occurs during adolescence as a result of repeated stress to the patellar tendon, which causes it to pull away from the tibia at the point of attachment. Repeated irritation causes swelling and point tenderness (Figure 18-46). The athlete with Osgood-Schlatter disease may complain of pain when kneeling, jumping, or running, as well as pain upon contact. When the knee is flexed at 90° there will be pain and possibly a bump at the point where the patellar tendon inserts into the tibial tubercule at the tibial tuberosity (see Figure 18-25). Although the bump created by this condition remains permanent, the pain usually subsides when the athlete stops growing and the bone hardens—usually when the athlete reaches age 18 or 19.

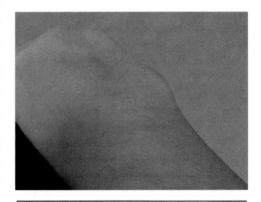

FIGURE 18-46 Osgood-Schlatter Disease

Immediate Treatment: The treatment for this injury includes the application of ice after activity, using the PRICE procedure. In addition, some type of 1/2-inch thick, C-shaped, closed-cell foam or felt pad should be placed around the area of injury to disperse the pressure of any contact. A donut pad will also work, but a C-shaped pad fits the knee area better. Protect the area with such a pad as soon as symptoms develop to prevent the condition from getting worse. Caution the athlete to try to avoid unnecessary kneeling, running, and direct contact as much as seems practical. Refer the athlete to a physician for further diagnosis and treatment. This condition may require extensive periods of rest.

Follow-up Treatment: Once this condition develops, treatment will be ongoing until the bone hardens. Symptoms will likely be sporadic and should be treated as described above when they arise.

Prevention: Athletes with this disorder may want to reconsider participation in certain sports, as some sports will obviously tend to cause more pain than others. A meeting with the athletic trainer, the coach, the family, the team physician, and the athlete is also recommended to discuss alternative sports and activities. Ultimately, whether to participate or not should be the adult athlete's decision.

Chondromalacia Patellae

Chondromalacia patellae (CMP) is a gradual degenerative change that occurs to the cartilage beneath the patella and on the surface of the femur. A type of patellofemoral stress syndrome, this degeneration is caused by acute trauma, repeated micro-trauma, or an improper alignment of the patella within the femoral groove, or path of articulation. The patella is manipulated by four different muscles (the quadriceps); if muscle strength is not balanced in each direction, then the patella can be pulled toward the edge of the groove instead of being centered, causing the irritation known as CMP. Any type of compression force will aggravate this condition. The athlete with CMP will complain of a dull ache around the patella that becomes worse during squats, going down stairs, or sitting for long periods of time. Deep squats may also cause pain. An athlete with this injury may have recurrent swelling in the patellar region. Stiffness around the knee after sitting for a prolonged period of time is another symptom. This stiffness is sometimes called a "theater sign" because of the stiffness experienced after sitting in a theater. Crepitation or popping can be heard during range-of-motion testing.

> **chondromalacia patellae (CMP)**
>
> abnormal softening of the cartilage beneath the patella.

Patella Grind Test: Instruct the athlete to sit with the legs fully extended on the table. With the muscles of the athlete's thigh relaxed, place the web (the area between the thumb and index finger) of one hand at the superior pole of the patella. Ask the athlete to flex the muscles of the thigh. As the athlete does this, push the web of the hand down and forward (Figure 18-47). If the athlete reports pain on one side, injury or deformity to the underside of the patella is indicated. As with all such assessments, make sure to compare the uninvolved side to the involved side.

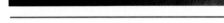

FIGURE 18-47 Patella Grind Test

> **patella grind test**
>
> application of inferior force to the superior aspect of the patella as the quadriceps are flexed to assess the condition of the cartilage beneath the patella.

Immediate Treatment: At first signs or symptoms, use the PRICE procedure immediately following activity. Do not allow the athlete to wait until arriving home.

Follow-up Treatment: Continue the PRICE procedure as needed for pain. Use a neoprene sleeve on the medial side of the patella, with a C-shaped pad placed between the sleeve and the skin to help to add support, comfort, and warmth to the area. The pad will help support the patella in the proper position and reduce the source of irritation. Work at gently strengthening the quadriceps to balance the muscle pull. Also work on increasing quad and hamstring flexibility. Refer the athlete to a physician for treatment if symptoms don't improve within 7 to 10 days.

Prevention: In many cases, a weak vastus medialis oblique (VMO) muscle causes the improper alignment. Strengthen the quadriceps muscles and minimize movements (squats, running downhill, bicycling with a seat that is too low, etc.) that aggravate the condition.

Shin Splints (Medial Tibial Stress Syndrome)

The term "**shin splints**," or **medial tibial stress syndrome**, describes a variety of conditions characterized by pain and irritation or inflammation in the lower leg, usually on the anterior aspect, or shin. The pain may develop or worsen during periods of exercise. The pain is caused by activity, such as running, that tightens the posterior leg muscles and causes undue stress on the tibia or fibula at the points of muscle attachment. The injury can result from improper conditioning of the gastrocnemius/soleus complex (posterior muscles of the lower leg).

Immediate Treatment: Use the PRICE procedure immediately after exercise. As with other soft tissue injuries, waiting until the athlete gets home to apply ice will only lengthen the healing process and increase the pain.

Follow-up Treatment: Ice massage the shin three to four times a day, for 7 to 10 minutes each time. This should be followed by gradual stretching of the anterior and posterior muscle groups of the lower leg. Stretching must be static (without a bounce), slow, and controlled. The athlete may also strengthen the muscles on the anterior side of the leg (the tibialis anterior) by doing toe taps. Toe taps are performed in a seated position with the feet flat on the floor. The toes are then raised and lowered in a tapping motion. Posterior strengthening of the gastrocnemius and soleus muscles can be done with heel raises. Heel raises are performed in a standing position with the feet flat on the floor. The heels are then raised and lowered by rising up on the toes. If the symptoms do not decrease in 7 to 10 days, send the athlete to a physician for further evaluation and to rule out the possibility of a stress fracture or anterior compartment syndrome. To prevent reinjury upon return to play, make sure the athlete progresses slowly in returning to normal activities.

Prevention: Proper conditioning of the anterior and posterior muscle groups will help prevent shin splints. Posterior strengthening can be done with heel raises, and posterior flexibility can be maintained or increased with the gastrocnemius-soleus stretch (see Chapter 7). Anterior strengthening can be done with toe taps, while anterior flexibility can be improved by kneeling on the floor and sitting on the heels of the feet. Then, grasp the distal portion of the foot from behind and gently stretch the tibialis anterior by pulling up on the foot. Shoes that fit properly are also important for preventing injuries. For example, shoes need to have supportive arches. Shoes break down over time; the cushions and the arch deteriorate, increasing the potential for injury. Therefore, shoes need to be replaced before the deterioration causes problems to the wearer.

Anterior Compartment Syndrome

Anterior compartment syndrome is the swelling of the compartment, or muscular area, between the tibia and the fibula. Primarily an injury of overuse, anterior compartment syndrome can also result from a direct blow. Runners, soccer players, and swimmers are particularly prone to this type of injury because of the repetitive foot motions required for these sports. Although the symptoms of anterior compartment syndrome can mirror the symptoms of severe shin splints, this syndrome is a medical emergency because the increased pressure can lead to permanent neural, muscular, or vascular damage.

The symptoms of anterior compartment syndrome include swollen, hot, red skin on the front of the leg, along with numbness and reduced range of motion in the ankle. Additional symptoms include limited dorsal flexion of the foot, limited extension of the great toe, and numbness or tingling in the web between the first and second toe. Symptoms are usually relieved with rest after about 20 minutes, but will resume if exercise is started again. The athlete may also experience mild foot drop and an increase in the girth of the foot.

Immediate Treatment: Apply ice using the PRICE procedure, and rest the leg. Do not elevate the leg or apply compression as either of these could aggravate the condition. If any of the above signs or symptoms are present, refer the athlete to the physician immediately. Be aware that the symptoms of this injury can be confused with those of a stress fracture or shin splints. When in doubt, always refer the athlete to a physician.

Follow-up Treatment: Make sure the physician's orders are followed.

Prevention: Proper gradual conditioning of the anterior compartment muscles using dorsiflexion exercises, such as toe taps, will help prevent anterior compartment syndrome. Improperly fitting shoes and/or the surface on which the athlete is participating may also affect this condition. Check to make sure that athletes wear properly fitting shoes with correct arch support and train on conducive surfaces.

THE ANKLE AND FOOT

The ankle, or tarsus, is composed of seven tarsal bones and joins the lower leg to the foot (see Figure 18-48). One of the tarsal bones, the talus, moves freely with the tibia and fibula. The remaining six tarsal bones are firmly connected to each other and

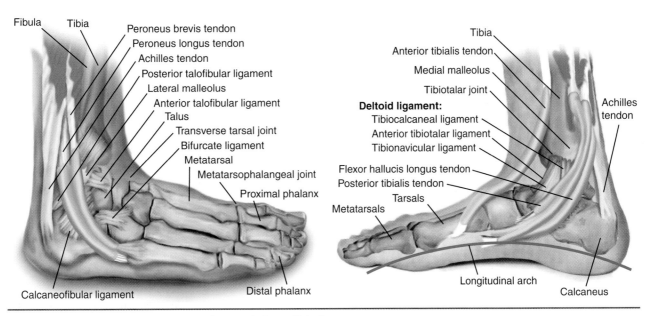

FIGURE 18-48 The Ankle; (L) Lateral View, (R) Medial View

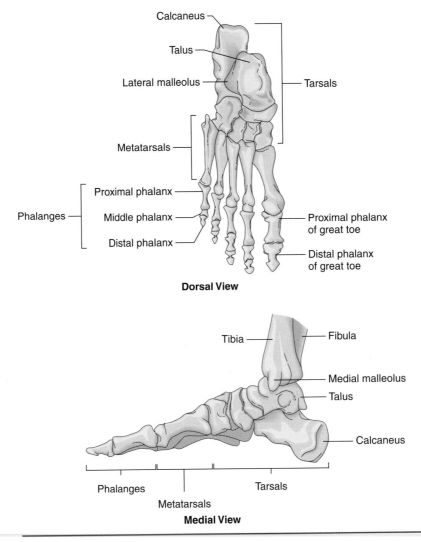

FIGURE 18-49 Bones of the Foot

form a platform on which the talus rests. The foot consists of the tarsus, metatarsus (instep), and phalanges (toes) (see Figure 18-49). The calcaneus, or heel bone, is part of the tarsus and helps to support the weight of the body. Muscles that move the foot connect to the calcaneus via the Achilles tendon.

The five metatarsal bones form the instep of the foot. This is similar to the anatomy of the hand. Each of the five metatarsals articulates with the tarsus. They are numbered one to five, beginning on the medial side. The heads of the metatarsals form what is known as the ball of the foot. Ligaments bind the tarsals and metatarsals together, forming the arches of the foot. There are actually two arches in the foot: a longitudinal and a transverse arch.

Similar to the phalanges that comprise the fingers of the hand, the phalanges of the toes are the most distal bones in the foot. There are three phalanges in each toe except the great toe, which has two. The proximal phalange of each toe articulates with a metatarsal.

Muscles that move the ankle, foot, and toes are extensions of the muscles of the lower leg. These muscles allow for moving the foot upward (dorsiflexion) or downward (plantar flexion). They also permit the sole of the foot to be turned inward (inversion) or outward (eversion). The primary invertor muscle is the tibialis posterior, and the primary evertor muscle is the peroneus longus. The dorsal flexors are the tibialis anterior, peroneus tertius, and the extensor digitorum longus. The plantar flexors are the gastrocnemius (large calf muscle), soleus, and the flexor digitorum longus.

ASSESSING ANKLE AND FOOT INJURES

As with all assessments, remember the principles of the HOPS procedure. Special tests used to assess specific ankle and foot conditions are presented in the injuries section of this chapter. Please note that though there are times when the initial assessments can be performed with the shoes on, the best and most complete assessments are made when the athlete's shoes are removed.

Range-of-Motion Evaluations for the Ankle/Foot

ROM Test for Ankle Inversion: Instruct the athlete to lie supine or sit on a table with the feet hanging off the edge (Figure 18-50). Unlike most of the tests, in this case testing both sides at the same time allows for a direct comparison to be made of the

range of motion. Ask the athlete to turn both ankles in, so the soles of the feet begin to face each other. Observe and compare the quality of the motion as well as the range of motion. This tests the active range of motion. Next, check the passive ROM by applying controlled force to the feet as the ankle goes through the ROM described above. Limited ROM on one side indicates potential injury or deformity on that side.

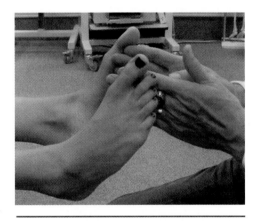

FIGURE 18-50 Active ROM, Ankle Inversion with Evaluator Indicating Endpoint

ROM Test for Ankle Eversion: Instruct the athlete to lie supine or sit on a table with the feet hanging off the edge (Figure 18-51). As with the inversion test, testing the uninvolved and involved sides at the same time allows for a direct comparison to be made of the range of motion. Ask the athlete to turn both ankles out, so the soles of the feet face away from each other. Observe and compare the quality of the motion as well as the range of motion. This tests the active range of motion. Next, check the passive ROM by applying controlled force to the feet as the ankle goes through the ROM described above. Limited ROM on one side indicates potential injury or deformity on that side.

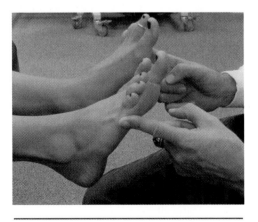

FIGURE 18-51 Active ROM, Ankle Eversion with Evaluator Indicating Endpoint

ROM Test for Plantar Flexion of the Ankle: Instruct the athlete to lie supine or sit on a table with the feet hanging off the edge. Test the active ROM on both sides at the same time by asking the athlete to extend both ankles so the toes extend as far away from the body as possible (Figure 18-52). Next, check the passive ROM in both sides by applying controlled force to the feet as the ankles go through the ROM described above. Limited ROM on one side indicates potential injury or deformity on that side.

ROM Test for Dorsiflexion of the Ankle: Instruct the athlete to lie supine or sit on a table with the feet hanging off the edge. Test the active ROM on both sides at the same time by asking the athlete to flex both ankles so the toes move closer to the body (Figure 18-53). Next, check the passive ROM by applying controlled force to the feet as the ankle goes through the ROM described above. Limited ROM on one side indicates potential injury or deformity on that side.

Manual Muscle Tests for the Ankle/Foot

Inversion Strength Test for the Ankle: Instruct the athlete to lie supine or sit on a table with the feet hanging off the edge. Test both sides at the same time by making the hands into fists and placing them together between the athlete's feet, near the toes (Figure 18-54). Apply isometric resistance as the athlete pushes medially against the hands at the same time. Weakness on one side indicates potential injury or deformity to the tibialis anterior.

Eversion Strength Test for the Ankle: Instruct the athlete to lie supine or sit on a table with the feet hanging off the edge. Place the hands on the outer aspect of both the athlete's feet, near the toes, in order to test both sides at the same time. Apply isometric resistance as the athlete presses laterally, or into eversion, against the hands (Figure 18-55). Weakness on one side indicates potential injury or

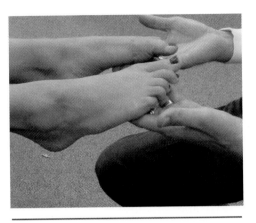

FIGURE 18-52 Active ROM, Plantar Flexion of the Ankle

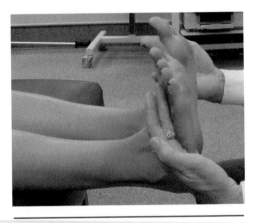

FIGURE 18-53 Active ROM, Dorsiflexion of the Ankle

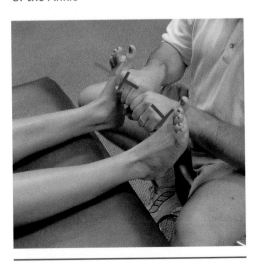

FIGURE 18-54 Ankle Strength, Inversion

deformity to the peroneus tertius, peroneus longus, and peroneus brevis.

Plantar Flexion Strength Test for the Ankle: Instruct the athlete to lie supine or sit on a table with the feet hanging off the edge. Place the hands on the underside (plantar aspect) of both the athlete's feet in order to test both sides at the same time (Figure 18-56). Apply isometric resistance to the feet as the athlete pushes downward, away from the body. Weakness on one side indicates potential injury or deformity to the gastrocnemius, soleus, and plantaris.

Dorsiflexion Strength Test for the Ankle: Instruct the athlete to lie supine or sit on a table with the feet hanging off the edge. Place the hands around the distal portion of the athlete's feet (backs of the hands facing the athlete) in order to test both sides at the same time (Figure 18-57). Apply isometric resistance as the athlete pulls the feet back toward the body. Weakness on one side indicates potential injury or deformity to the tibialis anterior.

INJURIES TO THE ANKLE AND FOOT

Fractures

Fractures of the ankle and foot usually result from a combination of plantar flexion and inversion. For example, if an athlete jumps up and then lands on an uneven or slippery surface, such as a gopher hole, someone else's shoe, or water, the ankle is likely to fracture and/or sprain. Basketball, soccer, volleyball, and football are sports that carry increased risk for such fractures. Symptoms of a fracture include swelling, point tenderness, and decreased ROM. The athlete will experience moderate to

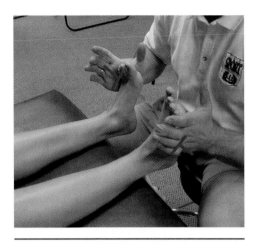

FIGURE 18-55 Ankle Strength, Eversion

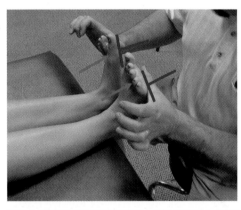

FIGURE 18-56 Ankle Strength, Plantar Flexion

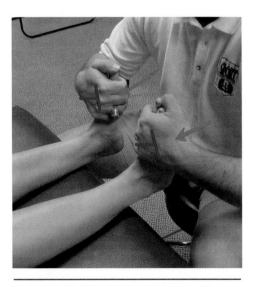

FIGURE 18-57 Ankle Strength, Dorsiflexion

severe pain when placing weight on the injured leg. A detailed discussion of the treatment and prevention of fractures may be found in Chapter 14.

Dislocations and Subluxations

Dislocation or subluxation of the ankle is usually the result of a twisting motion. The risk of such injuries is increased in basketball, soccer, volleyball, football, and baseball. Signs and symptoms of a dislocation include complete loss of function in the injured joint, severe pain, swelling, and deformity. See Chapter 14 for a discussion of the treatment and prevention of dislocations and subluxations. See also "Injuries to the Hip and Thigh" in this chapter.

Contusions

Heel contusions that result from direct blows and improperly fitted shoes are also common. Athletes such as basketball players and long jumpers are prone to heel contusions as a result of the jumping activities involved in their sports. The primary symptom of a heel contusion is point tenderness around the heel. During follow-up care, using a donut or heel pad over the area of tenderness can relieve the pain. The donut should be used to disperse the pressure on the foot away from the point tenderness. If the pain seems severe or does not go away in three or four days, the athlete should consult a physician for further evaluation. A complete discussion of contusions may be found in Chapter 14.

Sprains

The ankle sprain is one of the most common injuries to the body. It has been found that 85% of ankle sprains involve inversion of the ankle. Stepping on a rock or someone else's foot, stepping in a hole, landing off balance, or anything that causes the ankle to turn inward may cause sprains. Signs and symptoms of an ankle sprain include possible decreased ROM, possible deformity, crepitation, point tenderness, loss of function, possible instability, possible abnormal motion, and immediate swelling. (See Chapter 14 for a detailed discussion of the signs, symptoms, and treatment of sprains.)

talar tilt test

inversion of the foot to determine the stability of the ankle joint.

Talar Tilt Test: Instruct the athlete to sit or lie on a table with the feet hanging over the edge. Place the uninvolved ankle joint at a 90° angle, and stabilize the foot by holding the heel or the medial aspect of the foot with one hand. Invert the foot to determine the degree of laxity in the ankle joint (Figure 18-58). Test the involved ankle in the same way. Compare the degree of laxity between the two ankle joints. Increased laxity on the involved side indicates potential injury or deformity to the calcaneofibular ligament, and possibly the anterior and posterior talofibular

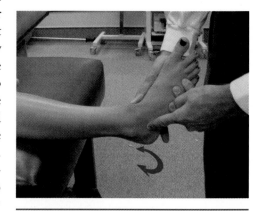

FIGURE 18-58 Talar Tilt Test

ligaments. The degree of injury to the deltoid ligament can be determined in much the same way, by everting the foot instead of inverting it.

Anterior Drawer Test for the Ankle: Instruct the athlete to sit or lie on the table in the supine position with the feet hanging over the edge. The athlete's foot should be relaxed and in slight plantar flexion. Stabilize the uninvolved ankle by placing one hand over the tibia and fibula near the distal end of the athlete's leg and use the other hand to grasp the heel. Apply anterior force to the heel and note the degree of laxity in the ankle joint (Figure 18-59). Test the other ankle in the same way. Compare the degree of laxity in both ankles.

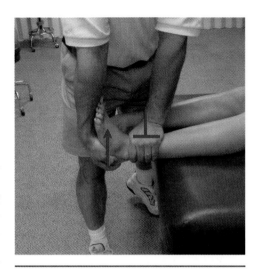

FIGURE 18-59 Anterior Drawer Test for the Ankle

anterior drawer test for the ankle

application of anterior force to the heel to assess the stability of the ankle joint.

Increased laxity on the involved side indicates a sprain or tear of the anterior talofibular and calcaneofibular ligaments.

A sprained ankle may be braced to prevent further injury. Remember—different braces provide different levels of support, so selection of a brace should be based on the amount of support needed. Proper strengthening and conditioning of the muscles of the lower extremities may help to prevent ankle sprains. Check the field of play for conditions that may increase the potential for injury. Supportive ankle braces may be used to prevent ankle sprains in sports that involve jumping, such as volleyball and basketball.

A sprain of the big toe is more commonly referred to as "turf toe." This sprain is caused from a continuous kicking or pushing-off motion. Sprains of this type commonly occur in sports where athletes wear light, flexible shoes and participate on inorganic surfaces, such as artificial grass. Signs and symptoms of turf toe include pain with motion and possible swelling. Running, jumping, pushing-off, and other resistive forces will also be painful. The risk of turf toe can be reduced by taping the big toe to add proper support and by adding sole supports to make the shoe firmer. See Chapter 14 for a detailed discussion of the treatment of sprains.

Tendon Ruptures

The Achilles tendon can be ruptured by activities that require abrupt stops and starts, such as quick push-offs or sudden back-peddling. Achilles tendon ruptures commonly occur in athletes over the age of 30 with a past history of tendonitis in this area. At the time of the injury, the athlete may feel a sudden snap that feels like a hit to the calf muscle. Symptoms of a tendon rupture include immediate pain, swelling, and deformity. A complete rupture will result in loss of motion in that extremity. If the rupture is incomplete, the athlete will be able to extend the extremity, but it will be extremely painful. Palpation will increase the pain.

Thompson test

compression of the calf muscle while observing for plantar flexion to assess the stability of the Achilles tendon.

Thompson Test: Instruct the athlete to lie in the prone position, with the feet hanging over the edge of the table. Place one hand on either side of the involved leg with the thumbs in the middle of the calf muscle. Carefully squeeze the calf muscle with the palms of the hands. The foot should move into plantar flexion. Little to no movement of the foot indicates a ruptured Achilles tendon or possibly a strain of the gastrocnemius.

Immediate Treatment: Use the PRICE procedure. Stabilize the foot and calf with a splint, if possible, or assist the athlete into the most comfortable position possible, and help the athlete maintain that position. Refer the athlete to a physician for further evaluation and treatment.

Follow-up Treatment: Make sure the physician's orders are followed.

Prevention: Proper warm-up and stretching of the calf musculature is the best way to prevent problems with the Achilles tendon. The gastrocnemius and the soleus can be stretched using the respective stretches presented in Chapter 7 or by doing heel raises.

Tendonitis

The overstretching or overuse of the Achilles tendon causes Achilles tendonitis. The signs and symptoms of this injury include chronic soreness, pain with dorsiflexion, pain with plantar flexion against resistance, possible mild swelling, and crepitation. Sports that involve any kind of jumping activity such as basketball, running, high jump, and long jump present an increased potential for Achilles tendonitis. Without properly conditioning, this type of injury occurs at the beginning of participation in running sports. This is why freshmen frequently suffer these types of injuries.

Immediate Treatment: Use the PRICE procedure immediately. For Achilles tendonitis, the athlete should begin gradual, slow stretching of the gastrocnemius and soleus muscles. Heel lifts will help relieve the stress to the Achilles tendon. Remember to advise the athlete to remain within the pain-free range of motion whenever strengthening is being used as a treatment.

Follow-up Treatment: For Achilles tendonitis, continue the PRICE procedure until symptoms subside. Ice massage the area three to four times a day for 10 minutes. Apply a neoprene sleeve during activity to increase compression, support, and heat to the injured area. Apply ice after activity. Refer the athlete to a physician if symptoms do not improve within 7 to 10 days.

Prevention: Proper conditioning and warm-up exercises (heel raises or the gastrocnemius and soleus stretches) will help prevent Achilles tendonitis.

Bursitis and Synovitis

Achilles bursitis may be caused by repeated stress to the bursa behind the Achilles tendon. Basketball players, soccer players, and jumpers are particularly susceptible to this condition because of the repeated stress their ankles receive during training and competition. The ankle may also be affected by synovitis. Refer to "Injuries to the Hip and Thigh" in this chapter and Chapter 14 for a review of the signs, symptoms, treatment, and prevention of bursitis and synovitis.

Ingrown Toenail

An **ingrown toenail** is a condition in which the skin extends over the edge of the nail while the nail grows into the nail bed, causing pain and possible infection. Two common causes of ingrown toenails are shoes that fit too tightly and toenails that are trimmed incorrectly. Participants of all sports are susceptible to this condition.

Immediate Treatment: The treatment for an ingrown toenail is to soak the toe in a warm saltwater solution a few times a day, and to cut a "V," centered, in the top edge of the nail. Cutting the nail in a "V" shape will encourage the nail to grow inward, away from the tender skin on the edges of the toe. If the problem does not improve in 3 to 5 days, the athlete should be referred to a physician. Diabetics with ingrown toenails or any foot condition should never be treated by anyone other than a physician or podiatrist.

Follow-up Treatment: Monitor the toe for signs of infection and blood poisoning (see Chapter 14). If symptoms of either condition are present, refer the athlete to a physician. If a physician becomes involved in the athlete's care, make sure the athlete follows the doctor's orders.

Prevention: To prevent this condition, athletes should wear well-fitted shoes and properly trim their toenails. Always trim a toenail by cutting straight across the nail, or use the slight V-shape described in the treatment above. Do not cut down the sides of the nail as this will allow sharp edges of the nail to cut into the tender skin along the sides of the toe.

> **ingrown toenail**
> a toenail that has grown into the skin of the toe.

Athlete's Foot

Athlete's foot is an extremely contagious fungal condition of the foot caused by a buildup of moisture and heat in darkness. The symptoms of athlete's foot include extreme itching, with a possible rash, pimples, or blisters (Figure 18-60). When the pimples or blisters are opened, a yellowish serum will come out.

Immediate Treatment: There are a number of treatments available for athlete's foot. After showering, make sure feet are dry and powdered before putting on shoes and socks. There are also a variety of over-the-counter antifungal creams available.

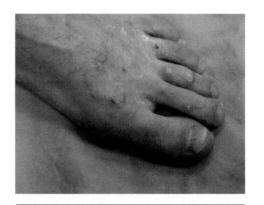

FIGURE 18-60 Athlete's Foot with Calluses from Ingrown Toenails

> **athlete's foot**
> a fungal infection of the foot.

Follow-up Treatment: If symptoms do not improve after two weeks, advise the athlete to consult a physician for further treatment.

Prevention: Prevention is the best cure. Make sure socks are always clean and dry. Using a medicated, antifungal powder on the feet may also help prevent the occurrence or recurrence of athlete's foot. In addition, instruct athletes to always wear shower shoes when using public showers and when walking around the locker room, as many people contract the fungus walking barefoot in these areas.

Plantar Fasciitis

plantar fasciitis

inflammation of the fibrous membranes, or connective tissue, in the sole of the foot.

Plantar fasciitis is an inflammation of the fibrous membranes supporting, covering, and separating the muscles of the sole of the foot. It is caused by repeatedly standing on the toes, resulting in stress to the supporting tissues and tightness in the gastrocnemius-soleus complex. Signs and symptoms include point tenderness, which increases with pressure, on the bottom of the foot, in front of the heel, and along the longitudinal arch. Pain may also increase when raising up on the toes (heel raises). Runners and aerobic exercisers are particularly susceptible to plantar fasciitis. The athlete may have pain in the morning that is particularly severe when getting out of bed, but that subsides as the day goes on. The pain subsides because the tissue warms with activity, reducing the pain.

Immediate Treatment: Use the PRICE procedure.

Follow-up Treatment: The treatment for this injury includes ice massage, stretching, taping, or orthotics to give support to the arch.

Prevention: Proper warm-up and conditioning that involves stretching the arch of the foot can help prevent this condition. One conditioning technique involves stretching the arch and the gastrocnemius-soleus complex by bracing the ball of the foot on a raised area (approximately 3 inches high) and leaning forward to apply weight to the ball of the foot. Wearing shoes (both athletic and street shoes) that have proper arch supports will also help prevent plantar fasciitis.

THINKING IT THROUGH

Alameda was playing an away game at Clearcreek. Near the end of the first half, the basketball game was starting to get a little sloppy and physical. This is when Julia stole the ball and took off like a flash toward the other end of the court for what looked like an easy layup. Maggie was at the other end of the court waiting to defend her. Julia was going full tilt, but Maggie was prepared to take the charge. Just as Julia went up, Maggie turned to protect herself. Wham! Her elbow hit the middle of Julia's thigh, and Julia went down in pain. She tried to get back up, but was a little wobbly. Coach Winn came out to make sure she was okay. Since neither school had an athletic trainer, he was responsible for providing any necessary first aid. Once the coach got there, Julia was able to get up and limp off to the locker room for halftime.

During halftime she sat with her leg extended and listened to the coach's words of inspiration. Fifteen minutes later, halftime was over and Julia tried to jog out, but limped noticeably instead. Coach Winn had her try to run forward, backward, and side to side, but she couldn't do it. It was just too painful. On top of that, the leg was starting to get tight and was losing range of motion.

What should Julia have done at halftime? Can you think of anything that could have made her more comfortable? What can be done to protect her thigh from getting hit again? If she loses her ROM, how can she get it back? How can she maintain her ROM?

CHAPTER SUMMARY

The pelvis and lower extremities provide support and mobility to the body as a whole. Because of the size of the bones and muscles in the pelvis and hip, sports-related fractures to the pelvic and hip areas are not as common as they are in other parts of the body. Such injuries do occur, however, and when they do, excessive internal and external bleeding is a life-threatening possibility.

While fractures are painful and often frightening, soft tissue injuries in the pelvis and lower extremities can be just as painful and debilitating as a fracture. Proper padding, detailed instruction in falling techniques, and extensive stretching and conditioning exercises are essential to preventing such injuries.

The hip, knee, and ankle are susceptible to the same types of injuries that affect the upper-extremity joints. Conditioning, support, and strength training for the surrounding muscles, tendons, and ligaments are the best strategies for preventing and/or recovering from injuries to these joints. Understanding the complicated anatomy and physiology of the pelvis and lower extremities can help in understanding the nature of certain significant injuries and will assist in preventing many injuries, as well as indicating appropriate first aid for the injuries that do occur.

STUDENT ENRICHMENT ACTIVITIES

Complete the following sentences.

1. The six major components of the lower extremity are the _____ , _____ , _____ _____ , _____ , _____ , and _____ .

2. An injury that causes bleeding in the muscle tissue is called a(n) _____ .

3. In determining the extent of swelling due to a quadricep strain, the _____ leg should be examined first, because _____ .

4. The _____ moves freely with the tibia and fibula.

5. The _____ _____ is used to determine whether or not the Achilles tendon has ruptured.

6. Unlike the hip, which is a _____ and _____ joint, the knee is usually considered to be a _____ joint, even though it allows for slight movements other than flexion and extension.

7. Symptoms of an ankle sprain include decreased range of motion, _____ , _____ , point tenderness, and _____ _____ .

8. _____ _____ is a sprain of the _____ _____ caused by continuous kicking or pushing motions.

Write the letter of the correct answer.

9. The _____ is not one of the bones that make up the knee.

   A. femur
   B. tibia
   C. fibula
   D. patella
   E. acetabulum

10. The fibula

    A. allows rotation of the hip.
    B. is the inner, larger bone of the lower leg.
    C. articulates with the femur proximally and with the talus distally.
    D. provides little weight-bearing support.
    E. articulates with the ulna.

11. Toe taps may be used in the treatment of

    A. turf toe.
    B. disco fever.
    C. shin splints.
    D. Achilles tendon ruptures.
    E. scrotal contusions.

12. A Charley horse affects the

    A. quadriceps.

    B. biceps.

    C. Achilles tendon.

    D. aorta.

    E. soleus.

Describe the symptoms and causes of the following conditions.

13. MCL sprain

14. ACL sprain

15. CMP

16. patellar tendonitis

17. plantar fasciitis

Write T for true, or F for false. Rewrite the false statements to make them true.

18. T   F   Donut pads are used to protect the buttocks from contusions.

19. T   F   A groin injury may cause shortness of breath in males.

20. T   F   The knee is a naturally stable joint.

21. T   F   Osgood-Schlatter disease usually occurs during adolescence.

22. T   F   The external iliac vein carries oxygenated blood to the toes.

23. T   F   Anterior compartment syndrome is an injury of overuse.

Rewrite this paragraph, filling in the blanks with the appropriate part of the lower extremity.

24. The anatomy of the lower extremity is similar to that of the upper extremity; the heaviest bone (the _____) is the most proximal, connected distally by a hinge joint (the_____) to a pair of lighter bones (the _____ and _____), that are connected to a compressed arrangement of small flat bones (the _____), that create an interface between the phalanges (_____) and the rest of the extremity.

CHAPTER 19

Environmental Conditions

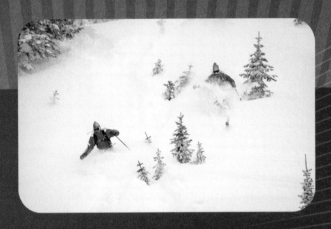

OBJECTIVES

After completing this chapter, you should be able to do the following:

1. Define and correctly spell each of the key terms.

2. Identify the signs and symptoms of conditions caused by exposure to extreme environments.

3. Describe methods to prevent or minimize the effects of environmental conditions.

4. Describe methods of handling emergencies associated with extreme environmental conditions.

5. Describe what to do during a thunderstorm.

KEY TERMS

* convection
* evaporation
* flash-to-bang method
* heat cramps

* heat exhaustion
* heatstroke
* humidity
* hypothermia

* psychrometer
* radiation
* relative humidity
* 30/30 rule

INTRODUCTION

The treatment and prevention of injuries that have been caused by motion and impact are significant aspects of sports medicine; however, many other factors are equally important to this profession. The preceding chapters on athletic injuries have focused largely on injuries caused by mechanical force such as a blow or torsion, but mechanical injuries like fractures, sprains, and contusions are not the only problems that may affect an athlete's health and participation. Environmental conditions may also produce circumstances that can become dangerous to an athlete or any individual. Environmental conditions such as heat, humidity, moisture, and cold can impair the body's ability to function properly. Under extreme conditions, these factors can be life-threatening.

ENVIRONMENTAL CONDITIONS AFFECTING ATHLETES

The human body is capable of adapting to a variety of changes in both internal and external conditions. The process that allows the body to adapt in this way is called homeostasis. One example of homeostasis is the body's ability to maintain a core temperature that protects the functions of vital body systems despite external and internal influences. However, conditions occasionally arise that may prevent the body from maintaining this optimum internal environment; such conditions may lead to health complications. External environmental extremes, such as heat and cold—particularly in damp or windy conditions—are among those conditions that may create health problems for athletes in the course of routine practice or competitive play.

Heat is an important product of chemical activities constantly taking place inside the body, such as the metabolic process that converts food into energy. Muscle contractions also produce heat through the burning of calories—another chemical activity. Thus, when the body is exercising and the muscles are working, heat is constantly generated within the cells. Even when the body is at rest, the slight involuntary contraction of skeletal muscles generates heat. When the brain detects that the body's temperature has fallen below normal, it sends signals to the skeletal muscles to contract, or shiver. In normal circumstances this shivering produces enough heat to warm the body back to normal temperature. The heat is then dispersed throughout the body via the circulatory system.

The heat-regulating center of the body, known as the hypothalamus, lies within the brain. By monitoring nerve impulses from temperature receptors in the skin and the flow of blood to the brain, the hypothalamus tracks and controls the amount of body heat lost. In many ways, the hypothalamus does the same thing for the body that a thermostat does when it controls the temperature in a room.

The body cools itself in a variety of ways. Approximately 80% of total heat loss occurs through the skin (see Figure 19-1). When the blood temperature rises, the hypothalamus sends signals via nerve impulses to dilate (expand) the blood vessels in the skin. This increases the amount of heat lost through **convection** and **radiation**. The hypothalamus also sends nerve impulses to the sweat glands to stimulate perspiration, which leads to heat loss through **evaporation**. Evaporation cools the body by eliminating body heat whenever the air temperature equals or exceeds the body's temperature.

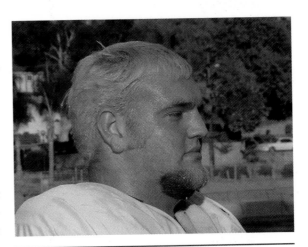

FIGURE 19-1 Perspiration is one way the body cools itself.

In order for its various temperature-regulating mechanisms to function properly, the body must be well fed, hydrated, rested, and kept in good physical condition through regular exercise. Should the body temperature fall outside of the optimum range, a variety of complications may result, some of which can be fatal.

ENVIRONMENTAL HEAT STRESS

The likelihood for a person to suffer from heat disorders increases with temperature and humidity. In high humidity the body cannot cool itself as well as it can in less-humid conditions because perspiration does not easily evaporate—one of the primary ways in which cooling takes place. When the external air is hot and humidity is high, the athletes' bodies are not able to cool by evaporation, so the athletes may experience heat disorders, such as cramps, heat exhaustion, and heat stroke.

Exertion leads to perspiration. This perspiration (sweat) depletes the body of water, as does urination. Adequate hydration is necessary to maintain optimal body temperature. If eliminated fluid is not replaced, dehydration will result. Fluids can be replaced by drinking water or sports drinks. The loss of 2% or more of the body's weight because of water loss impairs athletic performance and increases the risk of heat-related illnesses. However, fluid absorption is limited by

convection

a method of heat loss in which the layer of heated air next to the body is constantly being removed and replaced by cooler air, such as by a fan.

radiation

the release of rays in different directions from a common point; the transfer or loss of heat by or from its source to the surrounding environment in the form of heat waves or rays.

evaporation

a method of heat loss in which a liquid changes from a liquid to vapor, as with perspiration.

how quickly the fluid can leave the stomach and enter the intestines. It has been found that cold drinks leave the stomach quicker and do not cause stomach cramping.

The rate at which perspiration evaporates is strongly influenced by **humidity**. Humidity is the amount of moisture that is in the air. Both heat and humidity should be monitored during athletic activity because both affect the body's ability to cool itself. Sweat becomes an insulating factor when it cannot evaporate, such as when humidity is high. In these conditions sweat doesn't cool—but instead makes the body even hotter. A cotton t-shirt soaked with sweat can also be an insulator and keep the heat in. On days with high humidity and heat, t-shirts might be changed halfway through practice. This will cool athletes by removing the insulation and letting their bodies cool down. When the humidity exceeds 70%, players should be more closely monitored for heat-related problems. Refer to Figure 19-2 for precautions that should be taken when certain temperature/humidity thresholds are reached. **Relative humidity** is a figure that is based on the difference between the amount of water vapor in the air and the maximum amount the air could contain at the same temperature and is used to calculate the Heat Index. Devised by the National Weather Service, the Heat Index (also referred to as "apparent temperature") is an accurate measure of how hot it really feels when the relative humidity is combined with the actual air

humidity

moisture in the air.

relative humidity

a measurement of moisture in the air based on the difference between the amount of water vapor in the air and the maximum amount the air could contain at the same temperature.

Temperature and Humidity Training Guidelines

Temperature	Humidity	Procedures
80–90°F	<70%	Carefully observe athletes with special weight considerations.
80–90°F	≥70%	Athletes should rest and drink water frequently (10 min. every hour).
90–100°F	<70%	Athletes should rest and drink fluid frequently (10 min. every hour). Clothing should be changed when it becomes wet because dampness becomes an insulator under these conditions. All athletes should be carefully observed for signs of heat-related illness.
90–100°F over 100°F	≥70%	Discontinue or shorten practice, or move the practice to a climate-controlled location (i.e., a gym). Have the athletes change into cooler clothing if possible. Athletes should rest and drink water frequently (10 min. every hour). Clothing should be changed when it becomes wet to avoid insulating effects. All athletes should be carefully observed for signs of heat-related illness.

FIGURE 19-2 Training Guidelines for Hot and Humid Weather

Heat Index

Temperature (°F)

Relative Humidity (%)	80	82	84	86	88	90	92	94	96	98	100	102	104	106	108	110
40	80	81	83	85	88	91	94	97	101	105	109	114	119	124	130	136
45	80	82	84	87	89	93	96	100	104	109	114	119	124	130	137	
50	81	83	85	88	91	95	99	103	108	113	118	124	131	137		
55	81	84	86	89	93	97	101	106	112	117	124	130	137			
60	82	84	88	91	95	100	105	110	116	123	129	137				
65	82	85	89	93	98	103	108	114	121	128	136					
70	83	86	90	95	100	105	112	119	126	134						
75	84	88	92	97	103	109	116	124	132							
80	84	89	94	100	106	113	121	129								
85	85	90	96	102	110	117	126	135								
90	86	91	98	105	113	122	131									
95	86	93	100	108	117	127										
100	87	95	103	112	121	132										

Likelihood of Heat Disorders with Prolonged Exposure or Strenuous Activity

☐ Caution ▢ Extreme Caution ▢ Danger ▢ Extreme Danger

Source: National Weather Service. http://www.nws.noaa.gov/on/heat/index.shtml.December 2006.

FIGURE 19-3 The Heat Index

temperature (see Figure 19-3). The Heat Index combines air temperature and humidity to determine how hot it actually feels. A high Heat Index reduces the body's ability to cool itself. In other words, 70% relative humidity is easier to tolerate at 80° than it is at 90°. A **psychrometer** can be used to determine the relative humidity (see Figure 19-4).

psychrometer

an instrument used to measure relative humidity.

Sunburn

Sunburn is a potential hazard for anyone who participates in outdoor activities without proper protection. Sunburns are caused by ultraviolet (UV) rays from the sun and can cause skin cancer and premature aging of the skin. Symptoms of sunburn include red and painful skin and may appear 2 to 8 hours after exposure. Severe sunburns often

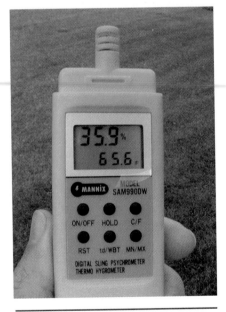

FIGURE 19-4 Relative humidity can be measured with a psychrometer, such as this digital sling psychrometer.

cause swollen skin, blisters, fever, chills, and headaches. In most cases the symptoms will decrease within the first 72 to 96 hours.

Some circumstances increase the likelihood of getting a sunburn. For example, skin damaged by a previous burn is more susceptible to sunburns than undamaged skin. Likewise, lightly pigmented skin is more susceptible to sun damage than skin with dark pigmentation. Certain medications can increase sensitivity to the sun, so individuals who take medication should check the labels for potential side effects. Snow and water can also increase the risk of sunburn because of reflection of the UV rays.

Immediate Treatment: Treat a sunburn like any burn, based on the severity of the injury. Applied topically, cold compresses and 1% hydrocortisone or aloe vera products can provide relief to mild burns. Moderate to severe burns should be evaluated and treated by a physician.

Follow-up Treatment: If symptoms do not improve in four days or if signs of infection or blood poisoning are present, refer the athlete to a physician.

Prevention: Individuals who participate in outdoor activities should wear adequate sunscreen. Sunscreen should be applied to all exposed skin at least 20 to 30 minutes before exposure. An SPF (sun protection factor) of 15 or higher is recommended. Swimmers and athletes prone to excessive sweating should use a waterproof sunscreen. Hats and proper clothing are also good methods of sun protection, as is gradual exposure to the sun. Overcast skies do *not* provide protection from sunburn as one might expect. Although sunlight is blocked by cloudy skies, the damaging UV rays are not.

HEAT-RELATED ILLNESS

Heat-related illness is a preventable sports problem. It is an accumulation of body heat that results when the body's ability to cool itself is overwhelmed. Heat problems can be caused by inadequate heat acclimatization, inadequate fitness level, higher body fat, dehydration, illness or fever, presence of gastrointestinal distress, salt deficiency, inadequate meals or insufficient energy intake, skin conditions (e.g., sunburn, skin rash, abrasions, infections, etc.), ingestion of medications or dietary supplements, overly motivated athletes, and athletes reluctant to report problems.

Heat Cramps

Heat cramps (muscle cramps) are painful spasms of skeletal muscle, most commonly occurring in the gastrocnemius, or calf muscle, but possibly in the abdominals as well. When one or more athletes complain of cramping and the weather is warm or humid, suspect heat (dehydration) rather than activity as the source of the problem. Heat cramps are caused by a lack of fluid volume and in most cases can be

heat cramps
muscle spasms resulting from dehydration.

prevented by drinking the proper amount of fluid. When the athletes themselves control fluid intake, overhydration is rare. Therefore, it is better to let athletes drink as much water or sports drinks as they would like during practice and not schedule hydration breaks. This way, athletes will learn how much fluid they need. However, always be aware of those not drinking. Make sure there is an unlimited supply of cool water or sports drinks available to the athletes. Each athlete should have a separate water/sports drink bottle to prevent the spread of illness. The bottles should be cleaned daily.

Immediate Treatment: Stretch the area and massage it. Keep the athlete hydrated. If cramps are severe, treat the injury as if it were a muscle strain.

Follow-up Treatment: If the athlete is in the sun, move the athlete to a shaded area and have the person drink water or a sports drink until the cramping stops.

Prevention: The best ways to prevent heat cramps and other heat-related disorders are described in the guidelines on the following pages.

Heat Exhaustion

heat exhaustion

a physical reaction to heat exposure resulting from dehydration and characterized by profuse sweating and extreme weakness or fatigue; can lead to heatstroke.

Heat exhaustion is a condition in which the body becomes dehydrated from water and/or electrolyte loss. Symptoms of this condition include extreme weakness, exhaustion, and sometimes unconsciousness. Additional symptoms may include headache, dizziness, hyperventilation, dilated pupils, nausea, vomiting, clammy skin, and profuse sweating. The internal body temperature of a person suffering from heat exhaustion is usually near normal, but may be as high as 102°F. Improperly treated, heat exhaustion can lead to heatstroke.

Immediate Treatment: Individuals affected by heat exhaustion should replenish lost fluid by drinking water or a sports drink. The athlete should lie down in a cool, shaded place with feet elevated and should be withdrawn from further activity for the remainder of the day. If the athlete does not recover fully within 30 minutes, send the athlete to a physician. If symptoms worsen at any time, call the EMS. It is important to replace the same amount of fluid that is lost. The amount of fluid lost can be determined by weighing athletes before and after practice. Most of the weight lost during practice or play is fluid weight.

Follow-up Treatment: Make sure the physician's orders are followed.

Prevention: Heat exhaustion can be prevented in the same way as heat cramps. See the guidelines for preventing heat-related disorders on the following pages.

Heatstroke

Heatstroke is a medical emergency that can lead to permanent brain damage or death. It may occur suddenly without any other symptoms, or it may arise from heat exhaustion. An athlete suffering from heatstroke may become disoriented, collapse, and lose consciousness. Heatstroke is characterized by hot, dry, flushed skin and a high internal body temperature, usually above 105°F. Athletes with dark skin may turn ashen, rather than appearing flushed. The symptoms of heat exhaustion, with the exception of sweating, will also likely be present. The most important symptom differentiating heat exhaustion from heat stroke is that an individual experiencing heatstroke stops sweating. The absence of perspiration is a sign of serious dehydration, which is a major medical emergency.

heatstroke

elevated body temperature such that the body's internal organs begin to shut down because of excessive heat.

Immediate Treatment: If an athlete is suffering from heatstroke, get the EMS on the scene as fast as possible. While waiting for the EMS to arrive, cool the athlete by removing unnecessary clothing and elevate the athlete's legs to prevent shock. Fan the athlete and apply cold packs or cloths to areas with a rich blood supply, such as the groin, armpits, and head. Wrapping the athlete in cool, wet sheets or towels is also recommended. The objective is to lower the body temperature as quickly and safely as possible to prevent death or serious brain damage, which can occur in minutes. Continue to monitor the athlete's temperature, making sure that it does not fall below 102°F. If the temperature falls too rapidly, hypothermia may result.

Follow-up Treatment: Make sure the physician's orders are followed.

Prevention: All heat-related illnesses can be prevented using the guidelines on the following pages.

A summary of heat-related illnesses and their treatment is shown in Figure 19-5.

GUIDELINES FOR PREVENTING HEAT-RELATED DISORDERS

1. Keep a record of each athlete's weight before and after practice. Athletes should wear similar clothes each time they weigh in or weigh out. Weight loss in excess of 3% of body weight from sweating should be noted.

2. Athletes who lose more than 3% of their body weight during practices should be observed for signs of heat exhaustion because of excessive water loss. If an athlete loses more than 7% body weight during one practice or game, the athlete should be sent to a physician.

3. Check the percentage of body fat for each athlete. Athletes who have a low percentage of body fat will be more likely to experience heat cramps because of the lower level of fluids in their body. (Information for obtaining body fat measurements is presented in Chapter 5.)

HEAT-RELATED ILLNESSES

HEAT CRAMPS	HEAT EXHAUSTION	HEATSTROKE
Signs and Symptoms ＊ Muscle cramps ＊ Heavy and/or salty sweat ＊ Not adequately acclimatized to the heat ＊ Insufficient sodium ＊ Fatigued and dehydrated ＊ Eating irregularly, inadequate meals ＊ Previous history of cramping	*Signs and Symptoms* ＊ Physical fatigue ＊ Dizziness ＊ Dehydration ＊ Profuse sweating ＊ Headache ＊ Nausea ＊ Vomiting ＊ Diarrhea ＊ Stomach or intestinal cramps ＊ Persistent muscle cramps	*Signs and Symptoms* ＊ Dizziness ＊ No or less sweating ＊ Light-headedness ＊ Lack of coordination ＊ Irritability ＊ Confusion ＊ Seizures ＊ Decreased blood pressure ＊ Coma ＊ Rising body temperature ＊ Death
Treatment ＊ Reestablish normal hydration status ＊ Replace sodium losses ＊ Light stretching ＊ Massage of the involved muscles	*Treatment* ＊ Rest in a cool, shaded area ＊ Elevate legs ＊ Rehydrate, drink small amounts of fluid often ＊ Remove excessive clothing and equipment	*Treatment* ＊ Call 911 ＊ Remove unnecessary clothing ＊ Immerse in ice water ＊ Spray the body with water ＊ Wrap in cool wet towels or cool body with ice packs ＊ Monitor ABCs
Return to Play Once all signs and symptoms are gone and the athlete is able to move at a preinjury pace, the athlete may return to competition. Continue observation for any other signs or symptoms that may arise.	*Return to Play* The athlete should not resume exercise until rested at least two hours or more. Athletes should be symptom-free, fully hydrated, and cleared by a physician before returning to play. Gradual return to full-intensity training and competition is recommended.	*Return to Play* The athlete must be completely asymptomatic and cleared by a physician.

FIGURE 19-5 Summary of Heat-Related Illnesses

4. Check the weather forecast for the area before practice and competition. Two good Internet sources of weather information are The Weather Channel at http://www.weather.org and Intellicast at http://www.intellicast.com.

5. Be aware of the duration and intensity of practice in hot or humid weather (see Figure 19-6). Use the Temperature/ Humidity Training Guidelines and the Heat Index to make decisions about athletic participation in hot or humid weather. If practice is held in hot or humid weather, look out for symptoms of overheating, which are not always easy to identify. At-risk athletes may

consider a "heat pill," which once swallowed transmits body temperature to an electronic sensor, taking the guesswork out of monitoring core temperature. Moving practice indoors during hot days can be a possible solution if conditions are better inside. However, moving inside to an area that is hotter and more humid, like a non-air-conditioned weight room, will cause more harm to the athletes.

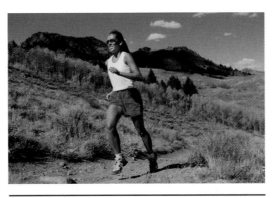

FIGURE 19-6 Exposure to environmental heat increases the potential for dehydration.

6. Use acclimatization strategies to help the athletes become accustomed to temperature and environmental conditions that may change between in- and off-season. For example, if the athletes practice during the off-season in a cool, climate-controlled environment, and practice during the season in an outside environment with heat and humidity, the athletes will not be properly acclimatized to the type of environment in which they will be expected to compete. It can take up to two weeks to become properly acclimatized; make sure all athletes are aware of this. Some areas of the country provide challenges with acclimatization because of environmental differences within a region. For example, a competition may be in a desert region, whereas school and practice sessions for the athletes may be in the mountains where it is cooler.

7. Select practice clothing and summer or winter uniforms in accordance with the temperature and the humidity of that particular day. Black or dark-colored, thick fabrics absorb heat; so light-colored, lightweight, or vented fabrics are preferred for hot or humid weather. Plastic and rubber retain heat. Therefore, never let an athlete practice or perform while wearing plastic or rubber clothes. These clothes do not allow the body's cooling systems to work properly because they interfere with the process of evaporation.

8. Make sure athletes change shirts that become soaked with sweat, because these sweat-soaked shirts become insulators in hot weather and do not allow sweat to evaporate and cool the body. In this situation, it is best to have the athletes change shirts and put on dry ones. This way, the sweat will evaporate from the body and the athletes can stay cool.

9. Have athletes avoid caffeine, alcohol, and carbonated beverages.

10. Be sure the athletes replenish every lost pound with 20 ounces of fluid.

11. Thirst is not an adequate indicator for water needs during exercise. By the time a person is thirsty, that person is already 2% dehydrated.

12. Be sure athletes drink fluids before exercising: 17 to 20 ounces 2 to 3 hours before, and 7 to 10 ounces 10 to 20 minutes before.

13. During exercise, have athletes drink 7 to 10 ounces of fluid every 10 to 15 minutes; always keep water available.

14. Remind athletes that water from cold fluids empties from the stomach faster than water from warm fluids.

15. Athletes should monitor the color and volume of their urine. Passing light-colored urine is normal. If the urine is dark yellow and has a strong odor, the athlete needs to drink more fluids. Note that taking a large number of vitamins can change both the color and odor of the urine.

16. An athlete with a fever is more susceptible to heat problems because the body's core already has an increased temperature.

17. Make sure athletes drink plenty of water or sports drinks before, during, and after exercise to replace lost fluid (see Figure 19-7). During light to medium exercise, the average fluid loss is 1.5 to 2.5 liters (51 to 85 ounces) per hour. During intense exercise or activities, such as football, the rate of fluid loss can be even greater. **Note:** The fluids athletes are given to drink during practice should also be provided at competitions. If athletes are not given sports drinks during practice, sports drinks should not be provided during sporting events. Use water instead.

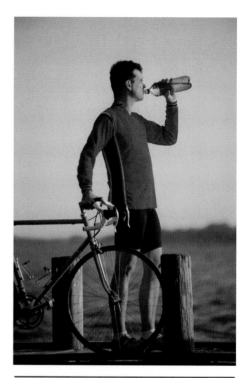

FIGURE 19-7 To avoid dehydration it is important to replace the same amount of water that is lost.

18. Some sports drinks provide an advantage over water because they contain important electrolytes as well as water. Both water and electrolytes, such as sodium, potassium, and chloride, are lost from the body when an athlete perspires. In solution, these electrolytes conduct electrical charges important to nerve conduction, muscle contraction, and fluid level regulation. Since electrolytes are so important to proper body function, many athletes choose to rehydrate with a sports drink containing these vital substances. However, some sports drinks may contain inappropriate amounts of certain substances or even undesired substances; therefore, it is important to read labels carefully or consult a dietitian when choosing a sports drink. Electrolytes can also be replaced by eating certain foods. For example, athletes can boost potassium intake by eating potatoes, oranges, or bananas, or drinking orange juice.

19. Salt can be added to water or sports drinks at $1/2$ teaspoon per quart. However, salt, or sodium chloride, is so plentiful in the American diet that there is generally no need to supplement the diet with this electrolyte.

20. Remind athletes that a well-balanced diet with limited fat consumption is important in preventing heat problems because it provides the body with the nutrients needed to help compensate for changing temperatures.

WINDCHILL

Temperature (°F)

Calm / Wind (mph)	40	35	30	25	20	15	10	5	0	−5	−10	−15	−20	−25	−30	−35	−40	−45
5	36	31	25	19	13	7	1	−5	−11	−16	−22	−28	−34	−40	−46	−52	−57	−63
10	34	27	21	15	9	3	−4	−10	−16	−22	−28	−35	−41	−47	−53	−59	−66	−72
15	32	25	19	13	6	0	−7	−13	−19	−26	−32	−39	−45	−51	−58	−64	−71	−77
20	30	24	17	11	4	−2	−9	−15	−22	−29	−35	−42	−48	−55	−61	−68	−74	−81
25	29	23	16	9	3	−4	−11	−17	−24	−31	−37	−44	−51	−58	−64	−71	−78	−84
30	28	22	15	8	1	−5	−12	−19	−26	−33	−39	−46	−53	−60	−67	−73	−80	−87
35	28	21	14	7	0	−7	−14	−21	−27	−34	−41	−48	−55	−62	−69	−76	−82	−89
40	27	20	13	6	−1	−8	−15	−22	−29	−36	−43	−50	−57	−64	−71	−78	−84	−91
45	26	19	12	5	−2	−9	−16	−23	−30	−37	−44	−51	−58	−65	−72	−79	−86	−93
50	26	19	12	4	−3	−10	−17	−24	−31	−38	−45	−52	−60	−67	−74	−81	−88	−95
55	25	18	11	4	−3	−11	−18	−25	−32	−39	−46	−54	−61	−68	−75	−82	−89	−97
60	25	17	10	3	−4	−11	−19	−26	−33	−40	−48	−55	−62	−69	−76	−84	−91	−98

Frostbite Times   ☐ 30 minutes   ☐ 10 minutes   ☐ 5 minutes

Source: National Weather Service. http://www.nws.noaa.gov/on/windchill/index.shtml. December 2006.

FIGURE 19-8 Windchill Exposure Risks Associated with Wind and Cold Temperatures

ENVIRONMENTAL COLD STRESS

Just as humidity can increase the problems caused by heat, wind and moisture can complicate performance in cold weather. The effect of wind in cold temperatures is known as the windchill factor (see Figure 19-8). The velocity of wind cools the air, making temperatures even cooler than the thermometer reads. Moisture can also increase the effects of cold because it limits the body's ability to conserve heat. When participating in any cold-weather sport—such as skiing, skating, and snowboarding—or conditioning program held in a cold climate, precautions must be taken against cold, wind, and moisture. If precautions are not taken, the athletes, as well as coaches and athletic trainers, can suffer from hypothermia or frostbite. Even when precautions are taken, it is important for everyone to keep moving as long as they are exposed to the cold. The effects of moisture, whether from rain or perspiration caused by exertion, can usually be overcome as long as the body is active and not just standing around. However, once an athlete stops moving and remains exposed to the cold while damp with perspiration, the body may lose significant heat. Athletes who perspire profusely in cold conditions, whether because of overexertion or too many clothes, may also suffer dramatic heat loss.

Hypothermia

Hypothermia occurs when the body's core temperature drops below 95°F. Symptoms of hypothermia include shivering, slurred speech, confusion, loss of motor control, and loss of memory. In severe cases, shivering will stop, muscles will turn rigid, skin will become blue, respiration and pulse rates will decrease, and consciousness will decrease or may be lost. Death can occur if hypothermia is not properly treated.

hypothermia
an unusually low body temperature capable of causing cardiac arrest and problems with the central nervous system.

Immediate Treatment: Remove any of the athlete's wet clothing and replace it with dry clothing if possible. Attempt to move the athlete to a warmer environment. Apply heat to the axillary regions (armpits), neck, and groin. Place blankets both over and beneath the athlete. If the athlete cannot get warm, or if symptoms do not improve within 10 minutes, or if uncomfortable about the situation, contact the EMS. If body temperature drops below 90°F at any time, contact the EMS immediately. Monitor vital signs and prepare to perform CPR if necessary. Even in cases where symptoms improve quickly and contacting the EMS is not necessary, if symptoms beyond shivering are present the athlete should see a physician. Symptoms such as slurred speech, confusion, and loss of memory or motor control, even if temporary, suggest neural impairment and should be assessed by a physician.

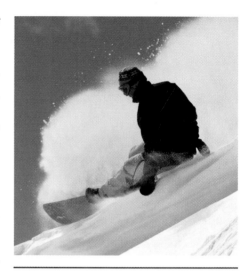

FIGURE 19-9 Wearing protective clothing and monitoring weather reports are essential to the comfort and safety of cold-weather athletes.

Follow-up Treatment: Make sure the physician's orders are followed. Even if the athlete recovers within the 10-minute period and seems stable, continue to observe the athlete for signs of confusion or any other symptoms of hypothermia. Send the athlete to a physician if anything seems out of the ordinary or if signs of neurological impairment are present.

Prevention: Keep the athletes warm and dry. Advise them to wear hats, gloves, and extra socks in cold weather (see Figure 19-9). Instruct athletes to keep a change of clothes handy and to work out with a buddy in case conditions arise in which a lone athlete would have trouble recovering. Monitor windchill factors and watch weather reports for approaching storms and freezing conditions. Since blood circulation plays an important role in warming the body, make sure the athletes are aware that shoes fitting too tightly impair circulation.

Frostbite

Frostbite is the freezing of skin and other tissues that results in reduced blood flow and potentially permanent damage to affected areas. Symptoms include aching, tingling, or numbness of the affected area, and white or grayish skin that is hard and crusty. Mild cases of frostbite are often called frostnip, which is less damaging than frostbite. In cases of frostnip the skin is pale, cold, waxy, and firm. If severe, frostbite may result in the loss of a limb.

Immediate Treatment: Contact the EMS. For mild to moderate cases of frostbite, remove any jewelry or restrictive clothing from the affected area and attempt to slowly warm the affected areas using blankets or body heat, taking care *not* to rub the injured tissue. For severe cases, rapid rewarming is necessary; place the affected area in hot water (100 to 108°F), or use a hot water bottle or moist hot cloths (again, 100 to 108°F). Transport the athlete to a hospital as soon as possible.

Follow-up Treatment: Make sure the physician's orders are followed.

Prevention: Cover vulnerable areas, such as the nose, ears, fingers, toes, and extremities. Keep the athlete warm and dry.

LIGHTNING

Lightning is one of the top-three causes of weather-related deaths. Always check weather conditions before going outside. Obtain a weather report each day before practice or an event. Be aware of National Weather Service thunderstorm watches and warnings, and watch the sky for potential thunderstorms.

Have a lightning safety plan ready, and designate people to monitor the weather and make decisions about removing athletes from the site. Know where the nearest shelter is and how long it takes to get there.

Use the **flash-to-bang method** to estimate how far away lightning is occurring. Count the seconds between a flash of lightning and the bang of thunder. Divide this number by five to learn how many miles away the lightning is occurring. If the time between the lightning flash and the bang of thunder is 30 seconds or less (6 miles), immediately seek shelter. Activities should not resume until 30 minutes after the last audible thunder. This is known as the **30/30 rule**.

Immediate Treatment: If someone is struck by lightning, call for help and get medical attention as quickly as possible. If the victim has stopped breathing, begin rescue breathing. If the heart has stopped beating, give CPR. If the person has a pulse and is breathing, address any other injuries.

When a person has been hit, check for burns in two places. There will be burns at both the point of entry and the point of exit. Lightning can also cause nervous system damage, broken bones, and loss of hearing or eyesight. An athlete struck by lightning will not carry an electrical charge and will not shock anyone providing first aid.

Follow-up Treatment: Be sure any physician's orders are followed.

Prevention: Check the forecast and watch the sky before practice or events. While outside, look for darkening skies, flashes of lightning, or increasing wind. These may be signs of an approaching thunderstorm.

Use the flash-to-bang method and the 30/30 rule. Find a safe shelter. A sturdy building is the safest place to be. Avoid sheds, picnic shelters, baseball dugouts, and bleachers. If no sturdy building is nearby, a hardtop vehicle with windows closed will offer some protection. Don't wait for rain to seek shelter. Many people take shelter from the rain, but one can be struck by lightning even before the rain.

Once inside a suitable shelter, get everyone in the lightning-safe position. Have people crouch on the ground with their weight on the balls of the feet, feet together, and head lowered and ears covered.

If you are unable to find a safe shelter, avoid isolated trees or other tall objects. Never take shelter under a tree. Avoid bodies of water, sheds, fences, convertibles,

flash-to-bang method

a manner of estimating the proximity (miles away) of dangerous lightning by counting the seconds between a flash of lightning and the bang of thunder. Dividing the number of seconds by five gives the miles away.

30/30 rule

a rule that states if the flash-to-bang calculation is 30 seconds or less, people should seek shelter and not resume outdoor activity until 30 minutes after the last audible thunder.

tractors, bikes, and motorcycles. Avoid leaning against vehicles, and get off and away from bicycles and motorcycles. Get out of the water, which is a great conductor of electricity. Do not stand in puddles of water, even if wearing rubber boots. Do not hold on to metal items such golf clubs, fishing rods, tennis rackets, or tools. Do *not* stay in a group. Stay several yards away from other people.

THINKING IT THROUGH

Zack Valadez is a great golfer. He is also extremely superstitious. No matter how hot or humid it is, he won't drink water while he plays. Although he might drink a soda from time to time while golfing to quench his thirst, he never drinks water during practice or a round. Several years ago he found that when he drank water before playing, he felt bloated and he didn't shoot as well.

Zack was enjoying the annual winter golf outing in Fort Myers, Florida, an event he always attended with a group of college golfers from Ohio. It was their opportunity to get out and have some fun before the season began. This year, the weather in Ohio had been so cold they had practiced in a climate-controlled indoor range all winter; they hadn't played a round outdoors since late October. The trip to Florida brought a welcome change—warm weather. The weather has always been great on these trips, but this winter was just a little warmer than usual and more humid, too. It rained almost every day at about 11 a.m. for about 15 minutes. Then the humidity would rise, making the afternoons less comfortable than usual.

On Friday, they started playing at about noon, following the usual rainstorm. Zack had worked out on the stair-stepper that morning and worked up a good sweat. The workout left him no time to grab anything but a nondiet cola to drink before he met up with his buddy, Blair, on the green. They got off to a great start, but by 2:30 in the afternoon the weather was starting to wear on Zack: his cotton shirt was soaked with sweat. The temperature was in the high 80s and the humidity was close to 90%! About halfway through the second 18, Blair noticed that Zack was acting differently.

What are some of the signs of heat-related illnesses? What can be done to prevent heat-related emergencies? What first aid procedures are appropriate for someone with heatstroke? Heat exhaustion? How would you establish an Emergency Action Plan for a golf course in a different town?

CHAPTER SUMMARY

The body has a variety of methods for increasing or decreasing heat loss or gain in order to stabilize its internal temperature. The body's core temperature remains constant because the brain "tells" the body to continuously make small adjustments in metabolic rate, muscular activity, perspiration, and superficial circulation. When the body becomes chilled, heat production is augmented by a slight increase in the metabolic rate, shivering, and other semiconscious activities. At the same time, the body prevents additional heat loss by limiting perspiration and causing the superficial blood vessels to constrict, shunting the blood and heat away from the surface of the skin and the extremities.

Still, the body can only do so much to protect itself against environmental factors such as extreme heat and cold. The use of good judgement, along with the guidelines offered in this chapter, will help athletes be able to work out and compete in the most comfortable and sensible ways possible.

There is very little that can be done about the weather; we just do our best to respond to and work with it. However, when thunderstorms are present, athletic trainers and coaches must have a lightning safety plan that determines where people will go for safety and how much time it will take to get there.

STUDENT ENRICHMENT ACTIVITIES

Complete the following sentences.

1. The elements that contribute to heat-related illnesses are changes in _____ and _____.

2. Body temperature is reduced primarily through the _____.

3. A(n)_____ can be used to determine relative humidity.

4. Sunscreen with a minimum SPF rating of _____ is recommended to prevent sunburn.

5. The loss of body water impairs _____ _____ and increases the risk of _____- _____ _____.

6. The average water loss is _____ to _____ liters per hour of light to medium exercise.

7. The process in which athletes become accustomed to temperature and environmental conditions expected for the season is called _____.

Match the environmental condition in Column A with the appropriate procedure or precaution in Column B. (Hint: More than one may apply.)

Column A	Column B
8. _____ 80–90°F; ≥70% humidity	A. Carefully observe athletes with special weight considerations.
9. _____ 80–90°F; <70% humidity	
10. _____ >100°F	B. Athletes should rest and drink water frequently (10 min. every hour).
11. _____ 90–100°F; <70% humidity	C. Clothing should be changed when it becomes wet.
12. _____ 90–100°F; ≥70% humidity	D. Discontinue or shorten practice, or move the practice to a climate-controlled location (i.e., a gym). Have the athletes change into cooler clothing if possible.

Write circle T for true, or F for false. Rewrite the false statements to make them true.

13. T   F   There is no relationship between the type of uniform worn and the temperature and humidity of the day.

14. T   F   Sweat-soaked shirts do not help athletes stay cool on hot, humid days.

15. T   F   Cold drinks leave the stomach quicker but also cause stomach cramping.

16. T F It is only necessary to drink water before and during periods of exercise.

17. T F Athletes with a low percentage of body fat are more likely to experience heat cramps.

18. T F Some athletes can take up to two weeks to become properly acclimatized.

19. T F A body temperature above 105°F is a symptom of heatstroke.

20. T F An athlete experiencing heatstroke will stop perspiring.

21. T F When the relative humidity is 75% and the air temperature is 92°F, the heat index is 116°F.

Complete the following exercises.

22. List five symptoms associated with heat exhaustion.

23. It is a hot, dry day in August. Football practices are going twice a day. What are all the steps the athletic trainer should take to prevent heat illnesses in practice?

CHAPTER 20

Medical Conditions

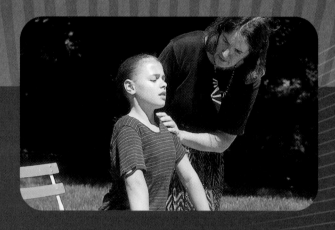

OBJECTIVES

After completing this chapter, you should be able to do the following:

1. Define and correctly spell each of the key terms.

2. Describe methods to prevent medical conditions from becoming emergencies.

3. Identify the signs and symptoms of medical conditions that require immediate treatment.

4. Describe methods of handling emergencies associated with preexisting medical conditions.

KEY TERMS

* appendicitis
* asthma
* diabetes mellitus
* diabetic coma
* epilepsy
* insulin shock

INTRODUCTION

The treatment, recognition, and prevention of medical conditions are things that the sports medicine team should be aware of and know how to handle. This chapter will establish an understanding of the medical conditions that are part of the daily life of athletes. These preexisting medical conditions in most cases will not stop an athlete from participating, but the athlete will need to be monitored and proper emergency procedures will need to established.

MEDICAL CONDITIONS AFFECTING ATHLETES

Athletes are not always in perfect health, even when injury-free. Like everyone, athletes experience headaches, colds, flus, and other common ailments. It is also possible for an athlete to have a medical condition that can create health disturbances during the course of practice or play. Often such medical conditions can be managed so well through medication and other treatments that it is impossible to detect the condition with simple observation. This is why thorough and accurate documentation of health histories is so important to the athletic trainer. Accurate and up-to-date health records allow athletic trainers to prepare in advance for emergencies that may affect their athletes.

Diabetes Mellitus

Diabetes is a general term used to describe conditions characterized by the excretion of too much urine. Although diabetes may result from insufficient levels of ADH (antidiuretic hormone, the hormone that limits urine production), it is often caused by high blood glucose (sugar) levels (see Figure 20-1). When high blood sugar is the cause of excess urine production, the condition is known as **diabetes mellitus**. This disease is

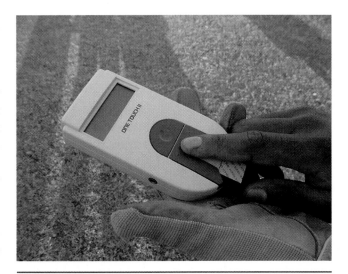

FIGURE 20-1 Diabetic athletes should monitor their blood sugar levels frequently.

> **diabetes mellitus**
>
> excess urine production caused by high blood glucose (sugar) levels.

characterized by the inability to make enough insulin, or the inability to use it properly. As noted in Chapter 17, insulin is a hormone produced in the pancreas. This hormone regulates the level of blood sugar (glucose) in the body and is vital for proper metabolism of blood sugar.

In general, individuals with diabetes mellitus have symptoms of extreme thirst, frequent urination, and possible blured vision and weight loss or gain. They will lose sugar and protein in their urine and the sugar levels in the blood will be high. Untreated or improperly managed, diabetes mellitus can progress to a condition known as diabetic ketoacidosis. Symptoms of diabetic ketoacidosis, which generally develop gradually, include abdominal pain, nausea, headache, blurred vision, irritability, flushed dry skin, rapid weak pulse, decreased blood pressure, frequent urination, and fruity-smelling breath. With the onset of these symptoms loss of consciousness may occur rapidly, followed by a coma. A **diabetic coma** is a life-threatening condition, so early detection is essential. If the athlete has any of the signs or symptoms of diabetic ketoacidosis, activate the EMS system. Although diabetes mellitus can create some very serious health problems for athletes who have been diagnosed with this condition, diabetics can usually lead very normal lives with proper treatment.

diabetic coma

coma induced by a lack of insulin in the body, resulting from diabetic ketoacidosis.

Immediate Treatment: Treatment for diabetes requires a doctor's care. In most cases, the athlete will have been advised by a physician as to what to do if symptoms resulting from diabetes start to occur. Often the symptoms can be controlled through diet, but sometimes oral medication or insulin is needed to control diabetes. If an athlete goes into a diabetic coma, treat the athlete for shock, contact EMS, and monitor vital signs. If the athlete is under the care of a physician for diabetes, follow the physician's instructions in the event any of the above symptoms occur. These instructions should be recorded as part of the athlete's health history in the files. Be aware of how to proceed with treatment *before* the situation arises.

If an athlete has not been diagnosed with diabetes but begins to display any of the above symptoms (either of diabetes in general, or diabetic ketoacidosis), instruct the athlete to consume a small amount of sugar and to consult a physician for diagnosis and treatment. If symptoms do not resolve within 10 minutes of consuming sugar, or if the symptoms become worse, contact EMS. **Note:** Although diabetic ketoacidosis is characterized by high blood sugar, it is still often recommended to provide a small amount of sugar to the athlete in the event diabetic symptoms occur. This is because only a physician can diagnose high blood sugar versus low blood sugar. It is unlikely that a small amount of sugar will cause increased harm to an athlete with high blood sugar, and it will certainly help a person with low blood sugar—it may even save the athlete's life.

Follow-up Treatment: Make sure the physician's orders are followed.

Prevention: Diabetics must adhere to daily diet and medicinal regimes and regular blood glucose testing. Diabetics are often advised to eat a carbohydrate snack about 30 minutes prior to activity to help control blood sugar levels.

Hypoglycemia and Insulin Shock

If an athlete has diabetes mellitus, participation in intense exercise will burn energy and deplete the blood sugar level. If this is not anticipated correctly, the athlete could easily experience hypoglycemia (low blood sugar). Likewise, if too much insulin is produced or taken into the body, the excess insulin will cause the level of blood sugar to fall below normal. Symptoms of hypoglycemia, which generally have a sudden onset, include headache, nausea, weakness, loss of motor coordination, profuse perspiration, and anxiety.

Left untreated, hypoglycemia can lead to **insulin shock**, convulsions, coma, and death. The signs and symptoms of insulin shock include weakness, moist and pale skin, drooping eyelids, a rapid bounding pulse, normal to shallow breathing, and unconsciousness. Because insulin shock is a life-threatening condition, hypoglycemia requires immediate treatment.

insulin shock

shock caused by an overdose of insulin.

Immediate Treatment: Hypoglycemic athletes should consume sugar at the onset of symptoms. Make sure the food being consumed contains true sugar, not a substitute like those found in diet sodas. Most insulin-dependent diabetics carry some type of sugar with them at all times as a precaution. Candy or orange juice should be readily available in the event a reaction occurs. If symptoms do not resolve within 10 minutes of consuming sugar or if the symptoms become worse, contact the EMS.

If the athlete experiences insulin shock, immediately give the athlete a small amount of sugar and contact the EMS.

Follow-up Treatment: If the athlete is sent to a physician, make sure the physician's orders are followed.

Prevention: The diabetic athlete should eat a carefully planned diet that includes snacks before exercise. Suggest that such athletes eat a carbohydrate snack, such as cheese and crackers, about 30 minutes prior to activity to help maintain proper blood sugar levels.

Asthma

Asthma is a disease marked by recurring temporary constriction of the bronchi and bronchioles in the lungs. People who suffer from this disease have lungs that are unusually sensitive to airborne irritants and allergens. Irritation of the delicate tissues causes the interior lining of the lungs to swell and secrete a thick mucus. The swelling and mucus secretion combine to reduce the size of the air passages and restrict the flow of oxygen to the bloodstream. Symptoms of an asthma attack include wheezing, shortness of breath, and coughing. Often these symptoms are caused by an increase in activity, but such attacks may also result from an allergic reaction to a plant, an animal, a food, or smoggy conditions. Depending on their severity, asthma attacks are potentially life-threatening. Although the disease can often be managed with the use of an inhaler

asthma

a lung disorder that causes breathing difficulty, wheezing, and coughing, and that can lead to airway obstruction.

(Figure 20-2) that has been prescribed by a physician, inhalers do not always work. The devices may be depleted of medication, the medication may have expired, or the attack may be so severe that the medication is not strong enough to treat the problem.

Immediate Treatment: The athlete should sit down with arms elevated and supported by a pillow on a table. This position will make it easier for the athlete to breathe. Contact the EMS. Encourage the athlete to use the inhaler. The athlete should also attempt to drink water, perform controlled breathing, and relax.

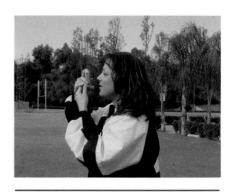

FIGURE 20-2 Athletes with asthma must keep their inhalers available at all times.

Follow-up Treatment: Make sure the physician's orders are followed.

Prevention: To prevent asthma attacks, athletes and others who have been diagnosed as asthmatics are encouraged to use an inhaler prescribed by their physician. These inhalers should be kept readily available at all times. However, athletes must also be aware of any legal restrictions on the use of inhalers during competition. Decisions about the best way to manage the athlete's condition during competition should be made by the athlete, the physician, and the athlete's parents or guardian in the case of minors.

Seizure Disorders (Epilepsy)

epilepsy

a group of nervous system disorders that involve disturbed rhythms of the electrical impulses that fire throughout the cerebrum, resulting in seizure activity or abnormal behavior.

Epilepsy is a term that describes a group of nervous system disorders that involve disturbed rhythms of the electrical impulses that fire throughout the cerebrum, resulting in seizure activity or abnormal behavior. An epileptic seizure can range from a minor attack, called a petit mal or absence seizure, to a major episode, which is called a grand mal or generalized tonic-clonic seizure. During a grand mal seizure, the individual will usually shake uncontrollably, fall to the ground, and lose consciousness. The person may defecate and/or urinate, bite the tongue, or experience some other type of injury as a result of the uncontrolled muscle spasms or shaking. Grand mal seizures often last from 2 to 5 minutes. In petit mal seizures, the affected person rarely falls, and the muscular contractions may be less severe. These seizures are characterized by the sudden stopping of activity for several seconds to a few minutes due to loss of awareness of the immediate surroundings or even a loss of consciousness. Whether or not consciousness is lost, the patient may have no memory of the seizure after it is over. Partial, or focal, seizures are also possible. In these seizures, only a portion of the body is affected and loss of consciousness may or may not occur.

Seizures often can be controlled with medication, allowing those with seizure disorders to participate in a wide range of sports with little, if any, increased risk to their health. However, people who are prone to seizures generally are advised to avoid scuba diving, swimming alone, and participating in sports at great heights. This caution is because of the increased risk of injury if a seizure takes place during the activity.

Immediate Treatment: The main concern is to make sure that the victim of a seizure does not incur harm. Clear the area around the person who is having the seizure so the person cannot get hurt or hurt anyone else. Make sure the victim's airway remains open. Contact the EMS.

Follow-up Treatment: Make sure the physician's orders are followed.

Prevention: Athletes who take medication for a seizure disorder should follow the prescription in accordance with the physician's orders. In a school setting, medications must be kept and administered according to school policy. The athletic trainer should always be aware of athletes who are susceptible to seizures by making sure that health histories are thoroughly conducted and documented.

Appendicitis

The vermiform appendix is a narrow worm-shaped tube that attaches to the cecum, a portion of the large intestine. If the appendix becomes inflamed, symptoms similar to those of an intestinal flu virus may result. This condition, known as **appendicitis**, causes symptoms such as pain in the lower right quadrant of the abdomen, nausea, vomiting, fever, and either diarrhea or constipation. The symptoms of appendicitis usually appear suddenly—over a period of 2 to 3 hours. Additionally, when the symptoms are caused by appendicitis, the athlete will usually find some relief by bringing the knees to the chest. The sudden onset of abdominal pain should always be treated with great caution because if the appendix bursts, the infection will spread into the abdominal cavity. This can be life-threatening.

> **appendicitis**
> inflammation of the appendix, producing sudden onset of abdominal pain and other flu-like symptoms.

Immediate Treatment: Contact the EMS. Surgery is often required.

Follow-up Treatment: Make sure the physician's orders are followed.

Prevention: This is not a preventable condition.

Genetic Heart Conditions

On rare occasions, an athlete may have a genetic heart defect and not be aware of it. The presence of such a defect may cause the athlete to suffer cardiac arrest with or without a precipitating injury. Under such conditions, the physical exertion that is put forth in practice or play may stress the heart muscle to the point that it is unable to meet the demands of the body, causing a myocardial infarction (a heart attack). On the other hand, a direct blow to the chest may cause damage to a heart that is already weakened or compromised in some way, such as a heart with a valve defect. These instances are quite rare, but it is important to remember that they can occur and to be prepared for them.

Immediate Treatment: Regardless of the cause or underlying condition of the heart, cardiac arrest is always treated the same way: contact the EMS and begin CPR. This is a life-threatening emergency.

Follow-up Treatment: Make sure the physician's orders are followed.

Prevention: This is not a preventable condition.

Common Viruses

Common illnesses, such as a cold or influenza, are generally not considered to be emergencies. However, they can still pose a threat to the athlete's health and performance. In fact, because of their contagious nature, these illnesses can threaten the health and performance of an entire team! There is no cure for the common cold, or for influenza. Treatment for either type of virus generally focuses on palliative measures, aimed at making the patient more comfortable. Both viruses can cause respiratory symptoms such a runny or stuffy nose, sore throat, headache, cough, and fatigue. If fever or body aches are present, the illness is more likely to be a flu virus than a cold, but there are exceptions to this rule of thumb. Some flu viruses affect the gastrointestinal tract, causing nausea, diarrhea, vomiting, dizziness, fever, and chills. People suffering from such viruses will experience great discomfort and should be monitored carefully. Dehydration is always a possibility when vomiting, diarrhea, or high fever is present.

Immediate Treatment: Because antibiotics are not effective against viruses, the primary means of relief are rest, over-the-counter (OTC) cold and flu remedies, and time—most of these viruses last no more than a few days. If symptoms do not improve after five days or if the athlete has a fever or severe diarrhea, the athlete should be referred to a physician. In all cases, make sure the athlete stays hydrated, especially when vomiting or diarrhea occur. Further, the athlete should be advised of the regulations that apply to the use of OTC medications and participation in specific events. Some medications have been banned at certain levels of competition, and an athlete's use of these medications could lead to disqualification. In a school setting, OTC medications may not be allowed on school grounds, or may only be dispensed by the school nurse.

Follow-up Treatment: Make sure the physician's orders are followed, if applicable. Observe the athlete closely during practice and competition for signs of relapse.

Prevention: One of the primary ways to prevent the transmission of a virus is to practice good hygiene. Athletes should wash their hands frequently and avoid sharing towels or water bottles. An entire team can be taken down if contaminated water bottles are shared. Flu shots can also aid in the prevention of influenza.

THINKING IT THROUGH

Is was a hot, dry, and smoggy day in Riverside, California, where the Poly Bears were competing against the M.L. King Sharks. Richard, the star runner for the Bears, was ahead of the pack at the $2^1/2$-mile mark when his breathing became labored. Richard is an asthmatic and had left his inhaler at home, in a rush to make it to school that day. Even though his breathing became labored, he was determined to keep the pace up and win the event.

The Poly Bears had set up emergency stations at each $^1/_2$-mile mark to look for any type of medical condition. The medical station at mile $2^1/_2$ could see Richard was having trouble.

What should the person at that medical station do? If Poly was the home team, how could they have prepared for this situation? If Richard does have an asthma attach, what are the first aid procedures?

CHAPTER SUMMARY

The sports medicine team will encounter medical conditions almost daily among the athletes they work with. Some of these conditions can be controlled, such as asthma and diabetes. The team must also be prepared for other conditions, such as acute appendicitis or a seizure that may occur unexpectedly and require immediate action and treatment by the sports medicine team. Proper emergency procedures must be set up ahead of time for all the different conditions and events, from the golf course to the swimming pool. If the team is not properly prepared, the conditions can turn into an uncontrolled medical emergency.

Not enough can be stated about the importance of gathering a proper, accurate, up-to-date, and complete medical history for each athlete. Having this history will help prepare the sports medicine team for most medical emergencies. It is essential that the athletic trainer, coaches, and other members of the sports medicine team are informed about the athlete's medical conditions. Additionally, being aware of emergency procedures is the best way of preparing for the sudden onset of medical conditions that can lead to emergency situations.

STUDENT ENRICHMENT ACTIVITIES

Complete the following sentences.

1. Moist and pale skin, drooping eyelids, and shallow breathing are all symptoms of _____ _____.

2. The _____ and the _____ temporarily constrict during an asthma attack.

3. The vermiform appendix is a _____ _____-_____ tube that attaches to the cecum.

4. A direct blow to the chest can cause _____ to a heart that is already weakened.

Describe the medical treatment for the following medical conditions.

5. diabetes

6. hypoglycemia

7. asthma

8. common viruses

9. seizure

10. appendicitis

Write out a proper emergency plan for the following sports.

11. football

12. golf

CHAPTER 21

Taping and Wrapping

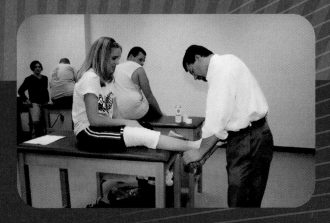

OBJECTIVES

After completing this chapter, you should be able to do the following:

1. Define and correctly spell each of the key terms.

2. Understand the proper use and storage of athletic tape.

3. Discuss the importance of taping techniques in the prevention and treatment of athletic injuries.

4. Describe potential pitfalls of taping techniques.

5. Discuss the purpose of several different taping techniques.

KEY TERMS

* athletic adhesive tape
* backcloth
* bony prominences
* fasciitis

* ischemia
* optimal support
* prophylactic strapping
* tension

* tensile strength
* stirrup

ADHESIVE TAPE IN THE PREVENTION AND TREATMENT OF ATHLETIC INJURIES

athletic adhesive tape

cloth tape backed with adherent, used in preventing and supporting athletic injuries.

There is no doubt that there are a number of broad and varied uses for **athletic adhesive tape**, and not all are related to injury prevention or treatment. Athletic adhesive tape has been put to many imaginative uses: as nametags on lockers, shirts, and football helmets; to improve the grip on a baseball bat; to prevent socks from sliding down; as a temporary splint on a cracked crutch or cane; and as a patch over the tear on the fabric of a tackling dummy. However, athletic adhesive tape is best used for its intended purpose: the prevention and treatment of athletic injuries. Examples of such use are listed below.

* Temporarily or permanently closing lacerations

* Preventing blisters on areas of skin exposed to repeated friction

* Holding bandages, protective pads, dressings, and splinting devices in place

* Securing splints for small fractures

* Supporting bony anatomy and relieving stress on adjacent or supportive soft tissue

* Restricting motion to support and eliminate stress on ligaments

* Restriction of motion and compression to support muscle, tendon, or stress injuries

The basic principle of taping is that all taping is based on common sense combined with a sound understanding of the anatomy and kinesiology of the parts involved and an accurate assessment of the problem and/or injury. It is then easy to understand what must be protected, restricted, or supported. With this information, basic taping procedures can be applied with adjustments and refinements being made through trial and error and feedback from the athlete.

Before beginning any taping procedure, put the athlete in a comfortable position that can be maintained until the procedure is finished. Do not allow the athlete to move the extremity during the taping procedure. In addition, the athletic trainer should minimize the amount of personal strain and fatigue that can be encountered while taping an athlete, especially to the back. Position the table at a comfortable height and maintain good postural alignment.

Athletic taping does not prevent injuries, although in some cases the taping procedure can decrease the severity of the injury. Injuries are prevented through proper conditioning and athletic techniques. If an athlete is throwing curve balls improperly, taping the elbow is not going to help. The atheltic trainer should look at other avenues for prevention. Instead of taping the ankles of an entire basketball team to prevent sprains, the athletic trainer may institute an ankle strengthening program, or have players change to high-top shoes or a type of preventive ankle brace. Athletic taping and wrapping are just part of the arsenal the athletic trainer has to offer to the athlete.

With all taping and wrapping procedures:

* If pain or soreness doesn't decrease or go away, a further evaluation and diagnosis will be needed.

* Adequate circulation is crucial. If the extremity changes color or starts to get cold, the taping or wrapping is probably too tight and must be redone to the athlete's recommendations.

TAPING GUIDELINES

The best taping procedure is done directly on shaved skin. Taping every day may cause the skin to become irritated. Underwrap and skin adherent prior to taping are often used to prevent this. If the procedure is done using underwrap, it is still best to start the taping procedure with the tape directly on the skin to add security.

Ask athletes if they are allergic to either the tape or skin adherent. If an athlete comes to you after practice and complains of itching or a rash where the tape was, this is a sign of an allergy to the tape or tape adherent.

A properly prepared area to be taped should clean and dry, and all oils should be removed for better adhesion. Cover all cuts and blisters with an adhesive bandage containing some type of skin lubricant. Then apply skin lubricant and foam padding on any friction or pressure areas before applying the underwrap.

The Need for Quality in Athletic Adhesive Tapes

Athletic users of adhesive tape consume large quantities in a unique manner: athletic trainers, coaches, athletic training students, etc., constantly use adhesive tape directly off the spool rather than cutting predetermined lengths and then applying them piece by piece.

Probably the greatest single use of adhesive tape by the athletic trainer is in **prophylactic strapping** of the ankle. This preventative taping is done daily, usually in a short time before practice or games. Applications of adhesive tape to other parts of the body such as the hand, wrist, shoulder, and knee are, of course, done during this same short time period. So it becomes crucial that adhesive tape be applied with ease, speed, and consistency. It is not enough that it be easy to work with; it must also afford protection and stability to the part being strapped.

prophylactic strapping

taping that helps to prevent or decrease the severity of injuries.

Use and Storage of Athletic Tape

Tearing adhesive tape is a simple procedure to learn, but is often complicated by the tape twisting, lotion on the hands, or a fingernail used to start the tear. For proper tearing, the adhesive tape is held firmly on each side of the point of the proposed tear line, and the free end is pulled away at an angle so the force crosses the lines of the fabric of the **backcloth** at a sharp angle (Figure 21-1). The tear then occurs sequentially through the backcloth. The more quickly and deftly this maneuver is done, the more even the edges will be.

Increased **tensile strength** of tape may be achieved by one of three techniques. The first is to fold over the leading edge of the tape (Figure 21-2). This increases the tear resistance on that edge. A second method is to twist the tape into a cord (Figure 21-3). The third method is *layering*, using successive pieces of tape in exact overlap to increase the tensile strength in an area of stress (Figure 21-4). This layered strip of tape can then be used as a basic support strip.

Supportive and specialty tapes should be stored in a cool, relatively dry place. High temperatures, above 70 to 75°F, will alter the character and consistency of the latex adhesive masses, increasing the unwind **tension** on the roll and making the tape difficult to work with. Therefore, tape should be kept in a cool place and in its container for as long as possible; avoid exposing the tape to direct or constant airflow and high temperature.

THE PURPOSE OF TAPING

The purpose of athletic taping is to support the bony anatomy as well as control the stresses in the adjacent connective and supportive soft tissue. Stresses can be associated with overuse, which can result in injuries such as tendonitis, **fasciitis**, sprains, strains, and in some cases, synovitis. For example, taping the plantar fascia can reduce the discomfort associated with plantar fasciitis. This same taping can also reduce the stresses on the posterior tibialis tendon while controlling the discomfort associated with tendonitis of this muscle tendon unit. This is sometimes referred to as "shin splint," the

backcloth

the cloth layer of athletic tape.

tensile strength

the ability of fabric or tape to resist tearing, based on thread count.

tension

the degree to which tape is stretched.

fasciitis

inflammation of a sheet of connective tissue covering or binding together body structures (fascia).

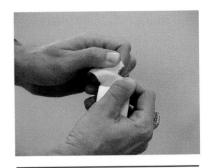

FIGURE 21-1

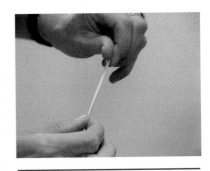

FIGURE 21-2

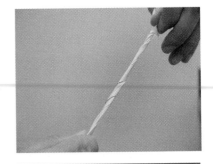

FIGURE 21-3

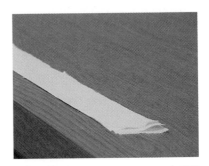

FIGURE 21-4

catch-all term used for all pain in the lower leg. The goals of the taping procedures are to decrease any harmful movement and add support and strength to the injured or potentially injured area, while allowing pain-free motion.

Supportive strapping for sprains is a universal supplement to the treatment and rehabilitation programs of joint injury. The support allows a maximization of functional activity in a graduated program so that adequate healing and a return of functional capability are achieved at the same time. During the rehabilitation program, there should be limited, if any, activity that produces pain, either immediate or delayed.

Some muscle and tendon strains might be made more comfortable or functional through routine taping. A snug taping around the forearm may reduce the discomfort of lateral epicondylitis (tennis elbow). A snug taping or wrapping around the upper thigh may reduce the symptoms of a hamstring strain and allow participation. A snug wrapping and taping around the groin and back (hip spica) will reduce the discomfort of a groin strain (a strain of the rectus femoris, sartorius, iliopsoas, or hip adductors).

The theory is that a tight wrap will reduce the pull at that point of the muscle belly or at its attachment and will reduce the level of discomfort. A trial taping will dictate which procedure should be used and how helpful it becomes. Make sure the wrap is comfortable and does not hinder circulation.

TAPING PITFALLS TO AVOID

There are several potential difficulties that inexperience may cause. For example, if the tape folds over, it is difficult to tear at the fold. It is better to either use scissors or tear the tape at a fresh edge. Another potential difficulty is turning corners over irregular anatomy: keeping the tape smooth and wrinkle-free can be difficult. When using nonelastic tape, turns with the tape must be anticipated to make the tape smooth and wrinkle-free and not affect the angle of pull. Sometimes too much focus is placed on the pattern of the procedure, causing the tape to be too loose or too tight.

Excessive pressure over **bony prominences** may not be felt immediately, but will create an aching discomfort when the tape is on for an extended period of time. Similarly, excessive tightness around soft tissue parts may also produce discomfort and interfere with circulation.

Blisters may be caused by excessive traction on a portion of the skin for a prolonged time. This is most common at the Achilles area in a taping procedure involving the ankle. Excessive tension is applied to the tape, beginning with the edge of attachment, causing **ischemia** at that point. When taping over pre-wrap, remember that the best adhesion is between skin and tape. When the taping procedure extends beyond the pre-wrap, the traction will be greatest where there is no pre-wrap, and the risk of blister formation is increased.

Easy removal of adhesive tape is accomplished by using bandage scissors or a specially constructed tape cutter (Figure 21-5). A bit of lubricant on the

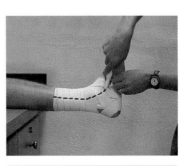

FIGURE 21-5

> **bony prominences**
>
> protrusions of bone, such as the lateral malleoli.

> **ischemia**
>
> reduced or obstructed blood circulation.

blunt edge of the scissors or cutter will allow sliding under the edge of the tape with ease. Move the scissors or cutter along the natural channels or in areas of greatest soft-tissue cushion, taking care to avoid bony prominences. Peel the tape off directly back against itself at an angle as close to 180° as possible. Careful observation while removing the tape will allow the athletic trainer to stop if evidence of blistering or skin being pulled off with tape is seen. Cut around these areas and remove the tape carefully.

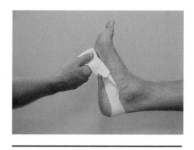

FIGURE 21-6

The sole of the foot requires special caution in the removal of tape because the adhesion of the tape can be quite strong and the callous tissue may be stripped away with the tape (Figure 21-6). If this begins to occur, stop and pull the tape from the opposite direction. Alcohol will remove the residue of tape adherent, and tape remover will remove any of the adhesive mass that remains on the skin. An ordinary skin cream may be used to keep the skin in good condition. If irritation from repeated tapings does occur, various topical ointments and preparations may be prescribed, and pre-wrap may be used until the skin is healed.

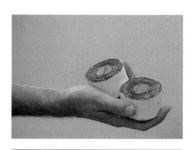

FIGURE 21-7

Note: Specially prepared tape has been used throughout this chapter to help illustrate the taping techniques. The tape edges have been colored with black for illustrative purposes (Figure 21-7).

BASIC ANKLE STRAPPING

1. The athlete's skin is prepared in the usual manner and a layer of underwrap is applied. Tape of 1¹/₂" width will be used, although 2" tape may be used on individuals with larger ankles. The athlete is positioned comfortably on the table, the leg extended, the foot in neutral (neither turned in nor out) and dorsiflexed (toes to nose) slightly to approximately a 90° angle (Figure 21-8).

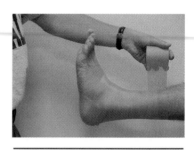

FIGURE 21-8

2. The first strip of tape is applied around the leg above the ankle. This is the first of two anchor strips for **optimal support**. The leg at this point is not cylindrically shaped; therefore, the tape must be angled slightly. This slight angling allows the tape to conform smoothly to the shape of the leg (Figure 21-9).

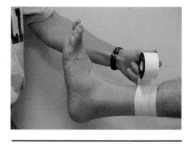

FIGURE 21-9

> **optimal support**
>
> when half of the first anchor is taped to the underwrap and half directly to the skin.

3. Two more anchors are applied at the instep; the first is applied over the hook of the fifth metatarsal. The tape is applied quite snugly, but not so tightly as to compromise circulation, or to exert undue pressure on the hook of the fifth metatarsal (Figure 21-10).

4. Care must be exercised here to ensure that the tension is not so great as to cause discomfort to the athlete when walking, during running, in practice, or a game situation. The overlap in adhesive taping is usually one-half to two-thirds of the previous strip. The two upper anchors and two lower anchors have been applied. This delineates the area of the preventive ankle taping (Figure 21-11).

5. The first **stirrup** strip is applied. It begins on the medial (inside) aspect of the ankle and continues down, over, and behind the medial malleolus, under the foot and arch, up the lateral (outside) aspect of the foot, over and behind the lateral malleolus, and torn off at the upper anchor (Figure 21-12).

6. The first horizontal strip is started on the medial (inside) aspect of the lower anchor, carried over and below the medial malleolus, behind the Achilles tendon (Figure 21-13).

7. The strip is then brought around the ankle, over and below the lateral malleolus, and across the dorsum (upper part) of the foot. The tape is torn off where the strip was started. Figure 21-14 shows one stirrup and one horizontal strip.

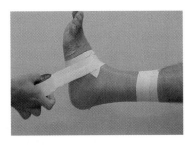

FIGURE 21-10

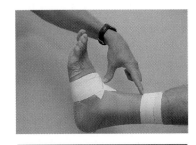

FIGURE 21-11

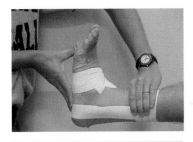

FIGURE 21-12

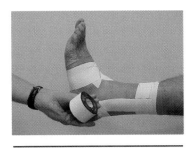

FIGURE 21-13

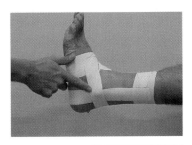

FIGURE 21-14

stirrup

a general term describing strips of tape applied from one side of the ankle to the other, passing beneath the heel.

8. Successive sets of interlocking stirrups and horizontal strips are applied, again overlapping the tape one-half to two-thirds of its width. The tape should be smooth and snug, with all pieces overlapped and joined. Figure 21-15 shows the completed portion of the closed basket weave with four sets of interlocking stirrups and horizontal strips.

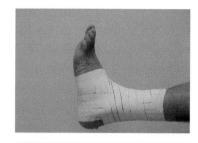

FIGURE 21-15

9. The heel lock strip is begun by attaching the tape to the lateral (outside) aspect of the heel, coming across the dorsum (top) of the foot and angling underneath the arch (Figure 21-16).

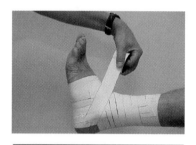

FIGURE 21-16

10. This heel lock strip should then cross on the outside of the heel, and progress behind the heel to come up over and above the medial malleolus (Figure 21-17).

11. The strip is continued around the ankle and brought down the inside of the heel. It should then wrap under the arch and pass just anterior to the lateral malleolus (Figure 21-18).

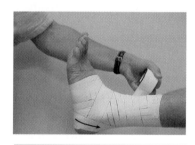

FIGURE 21-17

12. By continuing around the ankle, the strip is brought back to the starting point (Figure 21-19).

13. The spiral is completed and the tape is torn off. This strip of tape provides a lateral heel lock to the closed basket weave. The tape is continued upward in spiral fashion until the cylindrical portion of the lower leg is passed (Figure 21-20).

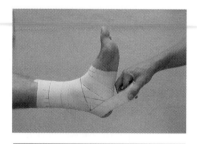

FIGURE 21-18

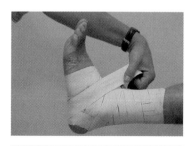

FIGURE 21-19

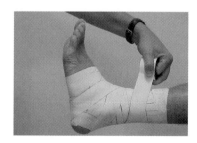

FIGURE 21-20

14. A new strip is applied in the angle fashion described at the beginning of this taping procedure. This is a finish strip that ties in all of the ends. For additional support, more heel locks may be applied. In fact, a medial heel lock may be utilized, beginning on the medial aspect of the heel and using the same pattern as the lateral heel lock, but in a reverse manner (Figure 21-21).

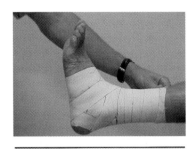

FIGURE 21-21

COMBINATION ELASTIC AND NONELASTIC TAPE ANKLE STRAPPING

Elastic tape and nonelastic tape can be combined in ankle taping when a great deal of control is not necessary. Combination taping is used for an overnight compression period or for the normal activities of daily living.

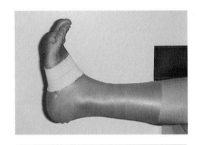

FIGURE 21-22

1. The skin is prepared as usual, the tape adherent applied, and a layer of underwrap material wrapped over the extremity for the entire course of the taping procedure. An elastic tape anchor is applied at the upper portion of the foot (Figure 21-22).

2. Beginning on the medial aspect, nonelastic tape is applied in a series of three or four stirrups. Care is taken to ensure that the stirrup strips do not extend over the hook of the fifth metatarsal, and that the last two stirrup strips are angled slightly forward to fit the contours of the leg, allowing the tape to be applied smoothly (Figure 21-23).

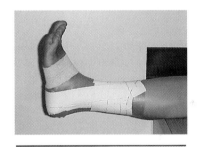

FIGURE 21-23

3. An elastic tape anchor is applied at the arch. It is begun over the hook of the fifth metatarsal (Figure 21-24).

4. The strip is wrapped around the ankle to the lateral (outside) aspect of the heel and across the dorsum (top) of the foot, completing a heel lock. Additional heel lock patterns may be performed if additional protection is desired (Figure 21-25).

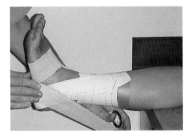

FIGURE 21-24

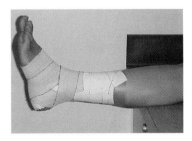

FIGURE 21-25

5. The elastic tape is then spiralled up the leg to the top of the underwrap, where it is torn off (Figure 21-26).

   Note: While 1½"- and 2"-width tapes are illustrated and recommended, 1"-width tape will be easier to handle and will conform better on smaller-bodied athletes.

   In addition, an underwrap has been used in many procedures, but taping directly to the skin in conjunction with the use of tape adherent will provide optimum stabilization and increase the life of the taping procedure.

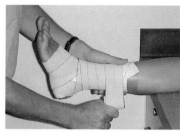

FIGURE 21-26

LOWER TIBIA TAPING

Pain in areas of the lower leg (shin splints/medial tibial stress syndrome) can be any of various painful conditions of the shins caused by inflammation of the surrounding muscles. These conditions frequently occur among runners.

   Adding a compression wrap around the shin area may provide some relief. It is important to first determine if the soreness is on the medial or lateral aspect of the tibia. If the soreness is on the medial side of the tibia, the taping should pull the tape medially; the opposite should be done if the soreness is on the lateral side.

   As with all taping procedures, if pain or soreness doesn't decrease or go away, a further evaluation and diagnosis will be needed.

   The taping procedure can be done using elastic tape with continuous circumferential wrapping from the top of the malleolus to the base of the calf. As with all procedures, ensuring adequate circulation is important. If the extremity changes color or starts to get cold, the taping is probably too tight and must be redone with the help of the athlete's specifications (Figure 21-27).

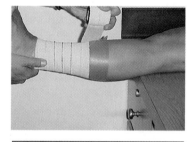

FIGURE 21-27

   An alternative technique, used when additional strength is desired, is applying single and overlapping nonelastic strips, starting from the top of the malleolus to the base of the calf (Figure 21-28).

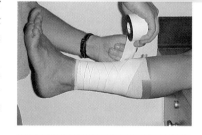

FIGURE 21-28

TURF TOE TAPING

Turf toe is a sprain of the first metatarsophalangeal (MTP) joint. The objective of this taping procedure is to limit dorsiflexion and/or abduction of the first MTP joint.

1. The skin is prepared in the usual fashion and anchor strips are applied using 1" nonelastic tape around the proximal phalanx of the toe and 2" elastic tape around the arch (Figure 21-29).

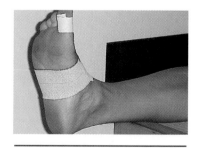

FIGURE 21-29

2. A series of nonelastic tape strips are applied in a fan-shaped pattern, starting at the distal anchor and ending at the proximal anchor (Figure 21-30).

3. A circumferential wrap using elastic tape is applied from toe to arch. A tie-down anchor is then applied over the toe area to complete the procedure (Figure 21-31).

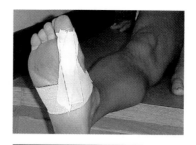

FIGURE 21-30

ARCH TAPING

Taping of the arch is useful for supporting the ligaments, small muscles, and plantar (sole) aspects of the foot. It is also useful to a great percentage of people suffering from shin splints on the medial (inside) aspect of the leg. This condition is usually a result of overuse, through excessive running and pounding. The skin is prepared in the usual manner: it is cleansed and tape adherent is applied from the heads of the metatarsals to well up over the heel.

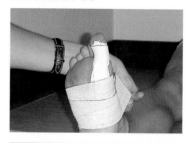

FIGURE 21-31

1. Apply a section of taping pad to a 6" strip of elastic tape (Figure 21-32).

2. The cushioned tape is secured to the heel to help prevent blistering (Figure 21-33).

3. The first strip of 1" nonelastic tape is applied from beyond the heads of the metatarsals, and extended over the heel approximately 1 to 1¹/₂" beyond the rounded contour of the heel. There is a bit of tension applied to this strip of tape and the foot is held in a semi-relaxed position. Subsequent strips of tape are applied in a similar manner; however, they are fanned to the medial and lateral borders of the foot, respectively (Figure 21-34).

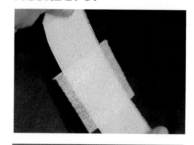

FIGURE 21-32

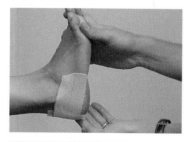

FIGURE 21-33

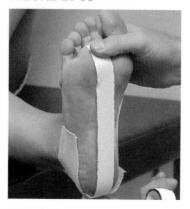

FIGURE 21-34

4. The fan pattern extends from the head of the first metatarsal to the head of the fifth, and all strips converge at the heel, where they go over the rounded contour into a single unit. Usually, six strips of tape are used: five in the fanning procedure and one additional supporting strip over the center of the fan pattern. This reinforcement lends strength and the ability to withstand the forces that are applied to it while running.

The foot is then relaxed and the adhesive tape is pressed upward and contoured to the skin. By tightening the tape, the height of the arch is increased (Figure 21-35).

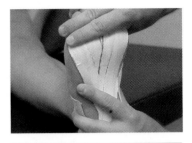

FIGURE 21-35

5. The next strip of tape begins just beyond the head of the first metatarsal and runs diagonally across the plantar aspect of the foot to the lateral portion of the heel, where it traverses around the heel to lock in the end of the fan strips. Then the strip is brought forward over the medial aspect of the foot to the origin of the tape (Figure 21-36).

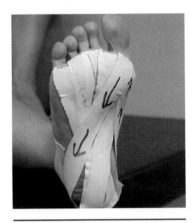

FIGURE 21-36

Additional overlapping strips of tape are used in a similar manner from the head of the first metatarsal. Additional support strips may be applied in the same manner from the head of the fifth metatarsal and returned to the head of the fifth metatarsal. These strips of tape lend reinforcement to the arch support and secure the ends so that the tape does not slip.

6. Because of the unusual contour of the forefoot over the heads of the metatarsals, it is easier to anchor these ends down by using short strips of 1" tape; usually two strips will suffice. Covering the distal end of the taping will anchor them in place and provide a very neat appearance. The ends are carried singly to the dorsum of the foot and tacked down (Figure 21-37).

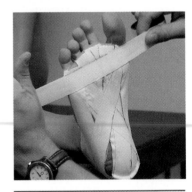

FIGURE 21-37

7. A second strip is applied in an overlapping and like manner (Figure 21-38).

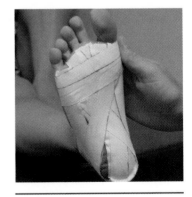

FIGURE 21-38

8. Once these two strips have been applied, the forefoot and mid-foot then resume more regular contours where 1¹/2" nonelastic tape can be used as an arch support or an arch lifting. This tape is started on the dorsum of the foot, extended over the lateral border under the plantar surface, and then wrapped over the medial border of the foot to its origin, where the strip is torn off.

Three or four of these overlapping strips complete the arch support taping procedure (Figure 21-39).

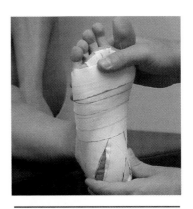

FIGURE 21-39

9. The procedure is completed with circumferential wrapping with elastic tape beginning at the forefoot and ending at the arch (Figure 21-40).

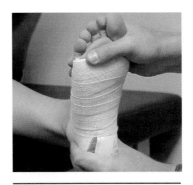

Care must be exercised when removing the arch support taping. An easy method of removal is to cut the support strips just distal to the medial aspect of the heel, and then run the cutter or scissors down the medial aspect of the foot. *Remember the previous caution about removing tape from the sole of the foot:* remove the tape slowly, close to a 180° angle to the skin, and if there is any evidence of callous tissue being pulled away from the plantar aspect of the foot, stop and reverse the direction of the pull.

FIGURE 21-40

BASIC KNEE STRAPPING

The next series of photos demonstrates a basic strapping for support of the knee joint for medial and/or lateral sprains of the knee. The athlete is positioned standing on a table so that the knee is at a comfortable height for the athletic trainer. The skin is prepared in the usual manner, being shaved and prepared with tape adherent. A lift is put under the heel so that the knee joint is at an angle of approximately 20° of flexion.

1. Two distal anchor strips have been applied just above mid-calf using 3" elastic tape. The second pair of anchor strips is applied at mid-thigh. The athlete may assist by cutting the tape as shown in Figure 21-41.

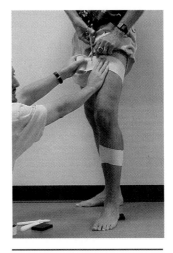

FIGURE 21-41

2. The first support strip is applied by beginning at the lateral aspect of the leg, passing under the patella (kneecap), and crossing over the medial aspect of the knee to the proximal anchor on the medial aspect of the thigh. The tape is tacked down first, and a few inches run off before the firm tension is applied. The tape is tacked down at the proximal anchor in a similar manner, allowing the end to retract before it is tacked down. Allowing the end to retract reduces the risk of traction blisters at these points in the taping procedure (Figure 21-42).

3. The second support strip begins on the medial aspect of the calf, passes under the patella, and wraps over the lateral aspect of the knee to the proximal anchor strip on the lateral aspect of the thigh (Figure 21-43).

4. The third support strip begins on the medial aspect of the calf, crosses the knee joint at the joint line, goes above the patella, crosses the thigh, and attaches to the proximal anchors on the lateral aspect of the thigh (Figure 21-44).

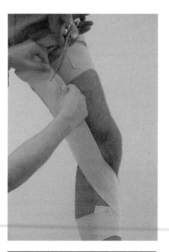 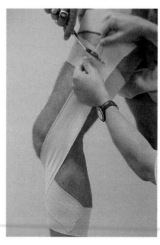 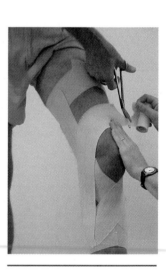

FIGURE 21-42   **FIGURE 21-43**   **FIGURE 21-44**

5. A similar strip is applied in like manner from the lateral aspect of the leg and is completed at the medial aspect of the thigh on the proximal anchor (Figure 21-45).

6. This completes one set of medial and lateral support strips. It is easy to see why the taping procedure can be called an X method of taping, because an X is created across the medial and lateral joint lines. Subsequent and overlapping strips of elastic tape are applied over the medial and lateral aspects of the leg. Two to three sets of these overlapping elastic strips usually suffice (Figure 21-46).

7. Next, a series of support strips is applied using nonelastic tape. The first strip is applied on the medial knee. The leading edge of the tape is folded over so that it crosses the knee. By placing the folded edge at a point of stress, the tensile strength at this point is increased to resist tearing as the knee is flexed and extended (Figure 21-47).

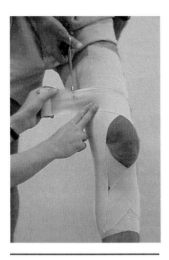

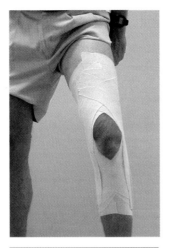

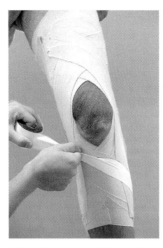

FIGURE 21-45   **FIGURE 21-46**   **FIGURE 21-47**

8. A number of sets of the nonelastic tape are applied in the same manner as that described with the elastic tape, folding the leading edge of the elastic tape as it crosses the joint line (Figure 21-48).

9. Additional medial support can be given by a series of overlapping vertical strips, traversing from the calf to the thigh, with the leading edge of the tape folded. Three such overlapping strips are applied to the medial aspect of the knee. To maintain good tension and stability at the joint line where it is most critical, these support strips must be spaced evenly (Figure 21-49).

10. Next, a strip of elastic tape that is long enough to go around the knee joint is cut. A small slit is cut into each end of the tape (Figure 21-50).

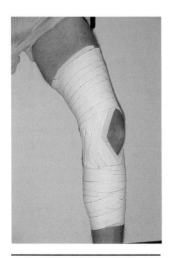

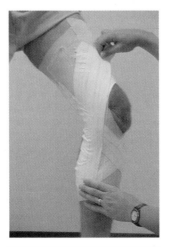

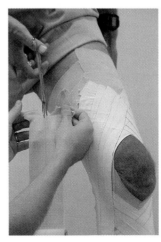

FIGURE 21-48   **FIGURE 21-49**   **FIGURE 21-50**

11. Cotton, felt, or foam padding is applied to the center of this elastic tape. This will act as a cushion as the tape is applied and pulled behind the knee in the popliteal space. Several foam pads are shown (Figure 21-51).

12. The padded portion of the tape is put behind the knee. The medial tails are tacked temporarily while the lateral tails are split and stretched.

    The split ends are then brought above and below the patella (kneecap), with a fair degree of tension. Care must be exercised that tension is not so great as to compromise blood flow by pressing too hard in the popliteal space behind the knee where, in fact, the major vessels and nerves lie (Figure 21-52).

13. The lateral tails are in place, and now the medial portion of the popliteal band is picked up, split, and its tails are brought forward to above and below the patella (Figure 21-53).

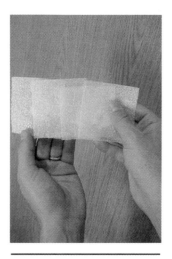 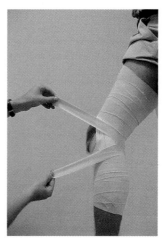 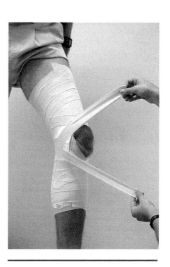

FIGURE 21-51 **FIGURE 21-52** **FIGURE 21-53**

14. The popliteal band is now completed and the support strips are well anchored at the points of most stress at the joint line (Figure 21-54).

15. A cover is then applied with elastic tape, beginning proximally and working downward. This is not necessary for all athletes, but is required for those who must put on a tight pant, as in football. If this cover tape is applied from distal to proximal points, the elastic tape will roll and then slide the pant up the leg. However, if the tape is applied from proximal to distal points, this effect is minimized.

    Tape is applied on the proximal portion and is then cut as it crosses just above the patella. It is begun again just below the patella and extended to the most distal portion of the taping procedure (Figure 21-55).

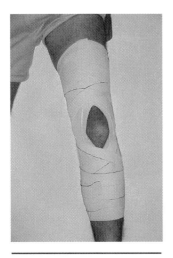

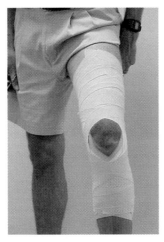

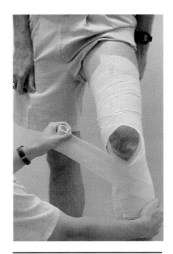

FIGURE 21-54   **FIGURE 21-55**   **FIGURE 21-56**

16. To enhance anterior-posterior support, a series of medial and lateral spiral strips are applied to cover tapes as illustrated in Figure 21–55. The first strip is started on the lateral aspect of the leg and extended behind the knee over the popliteal pattern (Figure 21-56).

17. The first strip continues its spiral, ending on the medial aspect of the thigh (Figure 21-57).

18. A corresponding strip is applied in the opposite direction. Two to three sets of the spiral strips should be adequate (Figure 21-58).

19. To secure the nonelastic tape, 1¹/₂" tape can be used (Figure 21-59).

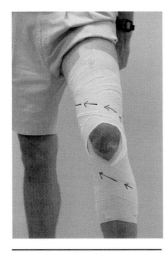

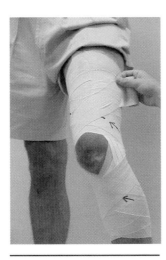

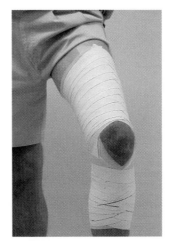

FIGURE 21-57   **FIGURE 21-58**   **FIGURE 21-59**

ACHILLES TENDON TAPING

This taping procedure restricts the degree of dorsiflexion at the ankle joint. To determine the appropriate degree of restriction and tension, the position of the knee and ankle will be determined through progressive degrees of increased extension. In effect, the tape will tend to act as a second Achilles tendon and take some of the stresses of walking and/or running to allow participation by individuals affected by tendonitis. This, of course, would only be used with an individual who can demonstrate being functional with the taping procedure applied. It certainly would be of no value on anyone incapacitated by both the injury and the taping procedure.

1. The underwrap is applied from the knee to the ankle. A slight bend in the knee is necessary for this tape application, as is a degree of plantar flexion at the ankle.

   The proximal anchors are applied using elastic tape. This is done smoothly and snugly, avoiding excessive tension to compromise any venous or lymphatic flow. Similarly, elastic anchors are applied over the heads of the metatarsals and the mid-foot (Figure 21-60).

2. The first support strip of nonelastic tape is applied from the proximal to the distal anchor. Slight knee flexion and plantar flexion is maintained so that there is a small degree of tension across this first support strip, which is not yet adhered to the skin and underwrap (Figure 21-61).

3. Additional pieces of tape are applied in fan shapes, fanning on the heads of the metatarsals as well as over the calf, coming to a common point over the heel and increasing in strength as the tape is layered. The tape is contoured to the plantar aspect of the foot (Figure 21-62).

4. The support strips are then crimped at the Achilles. This crimping wrinkles the tape, increasing the tensile strength and constructing a secondary support for the Achilles tendon (Figure 21-63).

5. Elastic tape is then applied at the heads of the metatarsals and wrapped upward in a spiral fashion with a figure-8 around the ankle, securing the nonelastic portions of the taping procedure.

   The elastic tape is extended up the leg to the proximal anchors where it is cut with scissors (Figure 21-64).

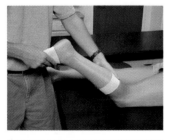

FIGURE 21-60

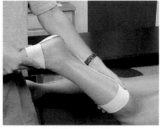

FIGURE 21-61

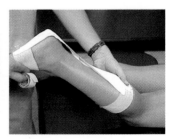

FIGURE 21-62

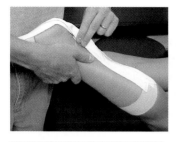

FIGURE 21-63

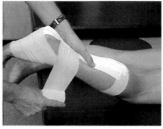

FIGURE 21-64

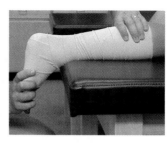

FIGURE 21-65

6. The ankle is now supported in a position of plantar flexion. The degree of dorsiflexion, the position and motion that will cause stretch and strain on the Achilles tendon, is restricted. Pressing firmly on the plantar aspect of the foot should demonstrate that the angle is effectively limited to 90° dorsiflexion (Figure 21-65).

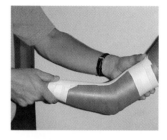

FIGURE 21-66

ELBOW TAPING

This taping procedure is for a sprain of the elbow joint occurring when the elbow has been forcibly extended beyond its limits. The skin is prepared in the usual manner, tape adherent is applied, and a layer of underwrap is applied over the limits of the taping procedure. Elastic tape is used as proximal and distal anchors.

1. The angle at which the elbow is held must be determined by trial and error. There is always a bit of slippage in the taping procedure, so the angle selected should be slightly more acute than that angle where discomfort begins so as to allow for slight slippage. A series of nonelastic support strips is then applied between the two anchors (Figure 21-66).

2. The support strips are fanned and overlapped, forming an X or a butterfly pattern with the strips overlapping in the anticubital space (Figure 21-67).

3. Seven to nine support strips are usually sufficient. The "butterfly" may also be prefabricated and applied as a unit (Figure 21-68).

4. Elastic tape is spiraled circumferentially over the support tape, completing the procedure (Figure 21-69).

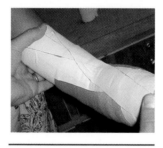

FIGURE 21-67

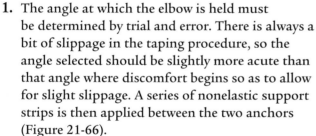
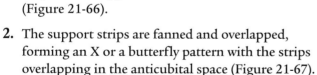
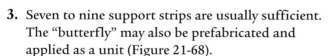

FIGURE 21-68

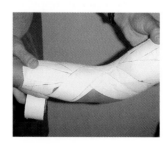
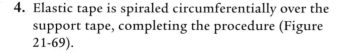

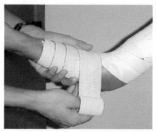

FIGURE 21-69

WRIST STRAPPING

The principle of strip taping may be used to protect a sprained wrist by applying strips across the dorsum (the back of the hand) and the volar (palmar) aspect of the hand. The most secure taping is done by taping directly to the skin. However, the skin may be prepared in the usual manner: tape adherent is applied and underwrap is applied from the knuckles to well above the wrist joint, approximately 5″ up the forearm.

1. Anchor strips of nonelastic tape are used at the base of the knuckles and at the upper portion of the taping procedure (Figure 21-70).

2. A series of four or five overlapping strips of 1½″ nonelastic tape are placed on the dorsum of the hand, between the two anchor strips (Figure 21-71).

3. Two additional strips are placed in an X fashion to reinforce these longitudinal strips (Figure 21-72).

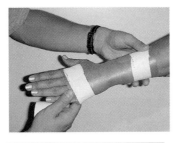
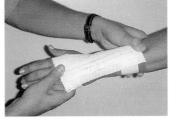
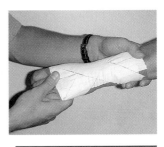

FIGURE 21-70   **FIGURE 21-71**   **FIGURE 21-72**

4. Similarly, a series of longitudinal strips and reinforcing X patterns are applied to the volar, or palmar, aspect of the wrist (Figure 21-73).

5. Additional support for the wrist taping may be achieved through the use of longitudinal strips of ½″ nonelastic tape, placed between the fingers and pulled up on the dorsal and the volar aspect of the tape procedure. First, small pieces of foam material are placed between the fingers and the web space to provide cushioning and reduce chafing or abrasion between the web space and the fingers. Mild tension is applied, but not so tightly as to compromise the blood flow or irritate the web space between the fingers (Figure 21-74).

6. Figure 21-75 shows three of the longitudinal reinforcement strips in position. These strips will hold the taping procedure in place at the knuckle line.

7. *All* of these strips are held in position by a circumferential wrapping of 2″ elastic tape, beginning proximally and working down toward the base of the knuckles. Again, care is taken not to pull the tape too tightly in the web space between the thumb and the first finger as the blood flow in this area could be compromised (Figure 21-76).

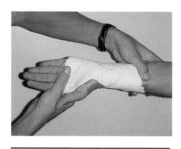

FIGURE 21-73

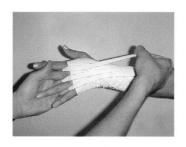

FIGURE 21-74

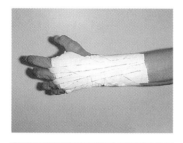

FIGURE 21-75

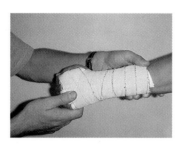

FIGURE 21-76

THUMB TAPING

1. The simplest protection for the sprained thumb is merely to tape it to the adjacent index finger. A strip of 1" tape is circumferentially wrapped around the thumb and index finger (Figure 21-77).

2. After one or two turns have been taken around the thumb and index finger, a strip of ½" tape is wrapped around the space between the thumb and index finger. The shape created by this taping procedure gives rise to its name: butterfly taping for the thumb (Figure 21-78).

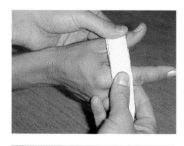

FIGURE 21-77

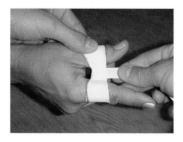

FIGURE 21-78

FINGER TAPING

A sprained joint of one finger may be protected by taping that finger to its neighbor. The little finger, however, is only taped to its neighbor when it is the injured finger, because tying the little finger to the ring finger reduces full hand span.

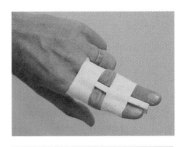

FIGURE 21-79

1. A piece of foam is placed between the two fingers, and 1" tape is circumferentially wrapped between the index finger and the middle finger (Figure 21-79).

2. If it is necessary to maintain the useful function of each of the fingers, a single joint may be taped. In this procedure, two anchor strips of $1/2$" tape are then placed across the sides of the joint in an X pattern, very much like the taping procedure for the knee joint (Figure 21-80).

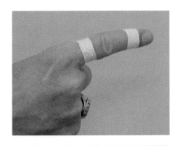

FIGURE 21-80

3. The strips of tape are overlapped and fanned (Figure 21-81).

4. Anchor strips are then applied around the ends of the X-taping to secure them in position. This taping procedure reinforces the collateral ligaments of the interphalangeal joint of the finger (Figure 21-82).

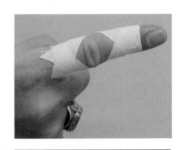

FIGURE 21-81

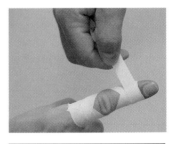

FIGURE 21-82

RESTRICTION OF THUMB FLEXION, EXTENSION, AND ABDUCTION

If an athletic activity makes it necessary to protect an injured thumb while maintaining its usefulness, a strip taping procedure may be used. The skin is prepared in the usual manner: tape adherent is applied, and the hand and wrist are wrapped with underwrap.

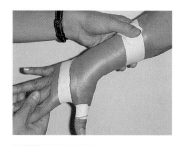

FIGURE 21-83

1. Assuming that the thumb has been injured in such a way that causes flexion and abduction to be painful, an anchor strip of 1" tape is placed just above the first joint of the thumb, just above the knuckles of the hand and approximately 4" above the wrist bones (Figure 21-83).

2. The first strips of tape traverse across the back of the thumb, the hand, and the wrist. Successive overlaps of strips in this direction will reduce the amount of flexion to the thumb (Figure 21-84).

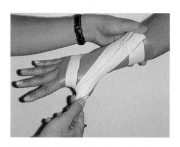

FIGURE 21-84

3. Similarly, strips applied from the back of the thumb across the dorsum of the hand will reduce the amount of abduction that the thumb may go through (Figure 21-85).

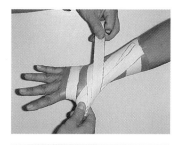

FIGURE 21-85

4. An anchor strip of 1" tape is placed around the ends of tape on the thumb. Elastic tape is then used as a cover, beginning proximally above the wrist joint and working down across the hand in a figure-8 pattern around the thumb and the back of the hand (Figure 21-86).

5. Care is taken not to pull the tape too tightly in the web space between the thumb and the first finger. Tape applied too tightly in this area will compromise the blood flow to the thumb (Figure 21-87).

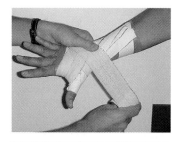

FIGURE 21-86

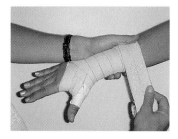

FIGURE 21-87

BASIC ANKLE WRAPPING

There are times when an athletic trainer will need to apply an elastic wrap to an injured area for compression and support or to keep an ice bag in place. Elastic wraps come in widths from 2″ to 6″ and lengths from regular to extra-long. Which of these different sizes and lengths to use will be determined by the area wrapped. Elastic wraps can be washed and reused.

An elastic wrap must be snug but not cut off circulation. The muscles being wrapped should be at their maximum contraction during the wrapping procedure to decrease problems with circulation. When using the elastic wrap, overlap each turn with about 50% of the wrap. Always check with the athlete for any concerns over circulation, and teach athletes what to look out for when circulation is decreased, such as an abnormally cold feeling, and have them squeeze the fingertips to check for adequate circulation with an elbow or hand wrap.

The wraps can be anchored and supported by 1½″ athletic tape and/or elastic tape over the top of the taping procedure. To make sure the wraps stay up, spray the skin with a tape adherent prior to applying the wrap.

This next series of pictures demonstrates a fundamental method for wrapping the ankle. For the most effective and efficient procedure, the patient should be seated with the leg fully extended and the foot flexed at a 90° angle.

1. Using a 3″ or 6″ wrap, depending on the size of the ankle, start wrapping around the bottom of the foot and move toward the heart (Figure 21-88).

2. Keep circling up, making sure that the edges of the wrap do not roll up. Always verify that the patient does not feel any numbness or discomfort during the procedure (Figure 21-89).

3. Once the top is reached, secure the wrap with tape or the clips that came with the wrap. Then pinch the patient's toenail to check for circulation. On all wrap procedures, check for adequate circulation (Figure 21-90).

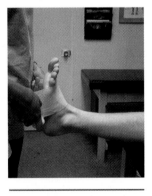

FIGURE 21-88

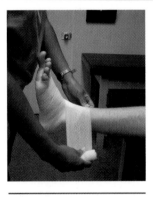

FIGURE 21-89

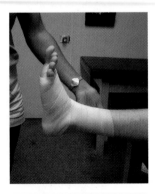

FIGURE 21-90

4. Horseshoes can also be used around the medial and lateral malleolus to prevent edema in those areas (Figure 21-91). Once again, start from the bottom and go up, following the procedure described above (Figure 21-92).

5. Plastic wrap can be used to ice-wrap an ankle (Figure 21-93). This will help reduce any swelling, but should be removed after 20 minutes. When using plastic wrap, remember to always start at the bottom of the ankle and move toward the base of the calf.

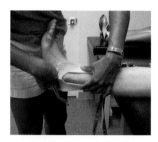

FIGURE 21-91

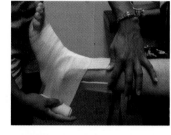

FIGURE 21-92

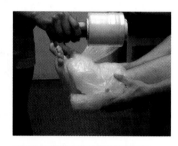

FIGURE 21-93

CALF AND KNEE WRAPPING

Injuries to the calf and knee are common in both contract and noncontact sports, many of which involve much running, jumping, and twisting. Minor sprains and strains can be aided through wrapping techniques. For the most successful wrapping jobs, the athlete should be standing, with the knee slightly bent.

Gastrocnemius (Calf) Wrap

1. Start at the bottom of the calf and move upward. Depending on the size of the leg, a 3" or 4" wrap can be used (Figure 21-94).

2. Secure the wrap at the top using either tape or clips.

3. To add cold to the area, an ice bag can be placed next to the skin and covered with the elastic wrap. Never put any analgesic under the wrap, as this could cause burns (Figure 21-95).

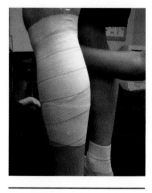

FIGURE 21-94

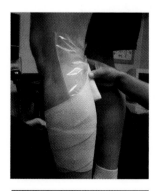

FIGURE 21-95

Knee Wrap

1. Start from the middle of the calf and move upward to the middle of the thigh (Figure 21-96). Depending on the size of the leg, either a 4" or 6" wrap can be used.

2. Make sure that the wrap allows for the desired amount of movement, but supplies enough security to stabilize and protect the knee.

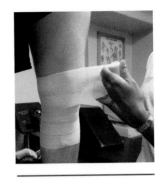

FIGURE 21-96

THIGH, GROIN, AND BACK WRAPPING

The following wrapping procedures are useful for adding support to an injured area. By adding pressure but not immobilizing the region, wrapping can aid an injured joint or muscle, allowing the athlete to participate in sports and everyday activities. For the optimal results, the athlete should be standing during the process.

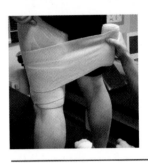

FIGURE 21-97

Hamstring/Quadriceps Wrap

1. Start at the base of the knee and move upward (Figure 21-97). Depending on the size of the leg, use either a 4" or 6" extra-long wrap.

2. Keep wrapping up the leg, and secure at the top. Added security can be gained by continuing the wrap around the waist. As with all wrapping procedures, spray tape adherent can also be used to prevent the wrap from sliding (Figure 21-98).

3. A layer of plastic can be placed underneath the wrap to insulate heat, but never put any analgesic on the skin under the wrap.

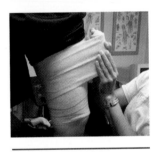

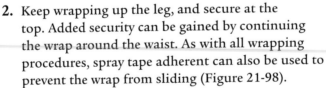

FIGURE 21-98

Groin Wrap

1. Turn the athlete's foot inward while pulling the wrap up. Depending on the size of the leg, use either a 4" or 6" extra-long wrap (Figure 21-99).

2. Continue wrapping around the waist (Figure 21-100). Wrap in the opposite direction for a hip flexor, also called a "hip spica."

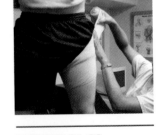

FIGURE 21-99

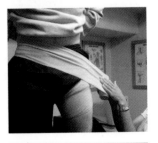

FIGURE 21-100

Back Wrap

Using a 6″ wrap, circle around the trunk of the body. This procedure will add support to the lower back (Figure 21-101).

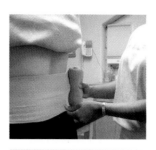

FIGURE 21-101

ELBOW, HAND, AND THUMB WRAPPING

The upper extremities are commonly injured from their frequency and variety of use. Basic wrapping procedures can help reduce pain by limiting the ROM of the specific region and/or providing protection and support to the injury.

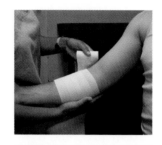

FIGURE 21-102

Elbow Wrap

Using a 4″ wrap, start at the middle of the forearm and then work up to the middle of the bicep (Figure 21-102).

Hand Wrap

Start at the knuckles and work toward the wrist (Figure 21-103). A 2″ wrap should be used for this procedure.

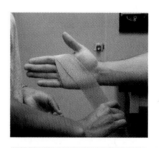

FIGURE 21-103

Thumb Wrap

1. Using a 2″ wrap, start at the knuckles and move toward the thumb.

2. Lasso the wrap around the thumb, pulling inward, making sure not to cut off circulation. Continue wrapping to the wrist and secure the end (Figure 21-104).

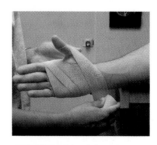

FIGURE 21-104

MOLESKIN

Moleskin is a soft, self-adhesive padding that is used to relieve pain caused by friction between the skin and the athlete's shoes. This friction can cause a variety of conditions such as turf toe, bunions, and plantar fasciitis. Moleskin is typically made of cotton flannel and is available in precut strips (Figure 21-105) or in rolls. Following are specific uses for moleskin.

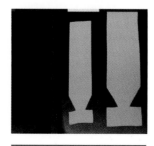

FIGURE 21-105

* Turf toe: Attach the moleskin to the toe and pull back to correct tension (Figure 21-106).

* Bunion: Attach the moleskin to the toe and pull out to correct tension (Figure 21-107).

* Plantar fasciitis: Attach the moleskin to the heel and pull forward (Figure 21-108).

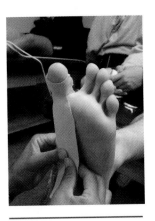

FIGURE 21-106

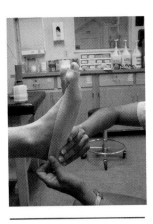

FIGURE 21-107

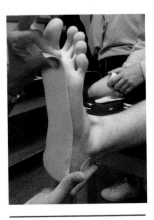

FIGURE 21-108

TAPING SUPPLIES

When outfitting an athletic training room, first establish a budget and understand the supplies needed. This can be accomplished using the athletic training pyramid. A tape pyramid (Figure 21-109) can be used to determine quantities needed when establishing the yearly inventory and proposed budget. For example, the tape pyramid shows that for every case of heel and lace pads, buy:

* 1 skin lubricant

* 1 case of 3" tear stretch

* 3 cases of 1" tear stretch

* 2 cases of 1" non-tear stretch

* 2 cases of 2" non-tear stretch

* 2 cases of 3" non-tear stretch

* 3 cans of taping adherent spray

* 3 zip cutters

* 4 cases of pre-wrap

* 16 cases of 1$\frac{1}{2}$" athletic tape

* 4 cases of 2" tear stretch

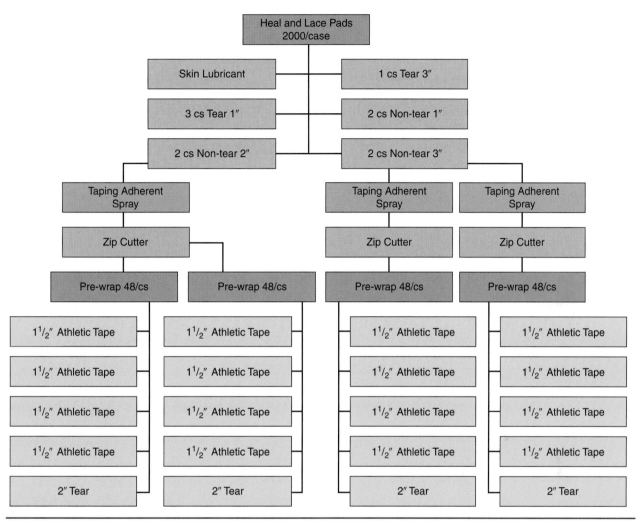

FIGURE 21-109 Tape Pyramid

THINKING IT THROUGH

Emilee is an outside hitter for the Carroll High School volleyball team. Last year she sprained her ankle and went through an extensive rehabilitation program with the athletic trainer, Craig Wall. For the competitive season, Emilee and Craig decided to add extra support. She had tried some of the ankle braces but decided she preferred the tape procedure that Craig applied.

What kind of taping methods will Craig use for Emilee's ankle? How much tape will it take to make it through the season? The season lasts three months, with three practices and two games each week. What supplies will Craig need other than the tape for this procedure? What would be the cost difference if Emilee had used a brace instead of taping for practices and for games?

CHAPTER SUMMARY

A wide variety of taping products are useful to the athletic trainer. It is important to keep in mind the purpose of a particular taping technique. Is the tape being applied to prevent blisters, to restrict motion, or to compress an injury? Often joints and extremities are taped to provide support. Avoid excessive pressure in all tape applications. It is easy to interrupt circulation, especially around any bony prominence. Typically a combination of elastic and nonelastic tape is used when a great deal of control is not necessary, as in overnight compression and support of everyday activity. Remember that tape should be reapplied if it becomes loose or wet, and whenever changes in activity or injury occur. Finally, the use of scissors, lubricants, and underwrap may make tape removal easier.

STUDENT ENRICHMENT ACTIVITIES

Write T for true, or F for false. Rewrite the false statements to make them true.

1. T F Prophylactic strapping means preventative taping.

2. T F Tape should be removed by pulling quickly at a 90° angle to the skin.

3. T F The best stabilization is achieved when tape is applied directly to the skin.

4. T F Scissors are not usually used in tape removal.

5. T F Tape should be stored in a cool, dry place with temperature below 70°.

6. T F It is not possible to apply tape too tightly.

7. T F Underwrap requires the use of adherent.

8. T F Tape should be of a high enough quality that it will provide protection and stability.

Complete the following exercises.

9. Name three purposes of athletic tape application.

10. Name three common pitfalls encountered by inexperienced tapers.

11. List the three ways in which the tensile strength of tape may be increased.

12. List at least two types of specialty tape.

Have your instructor observe your demonstration of the following taping techniques and provide comments and a score for each one.

13. basic ankle strapping

14. basic knee strapping

15. taping of fingers

16. shoulder strapping

17. combination elastic and nonelastic ankle strapping

18. shin splint taping

19. thumb restriction

20. wrist strapping

Complete the following exercise.

21. Photocopy the following page and use the chart to put together a possible budget for your school for taping supplies. Choose one sport and the number of athletes that will be participating. Use a catalog or the Internet to find prices for your budget line items. Decide where the money will come from for your budget.

Possible Budget

Item	Size/Amount	Unit Cost	Total Cost
1¹/₂" tape (24 rolls per box)			
pre-wrap (48 rolls per box)			
3" tear elastic tape			
2" tear elastic tape			
1" tear elastic tape			
3" non-tear elastic tape			
2" non-tear elastic tape			
1" non-tear elastic tape			
tape adherent			
heal and lace pads			
blister pads			
zip cutters			
scissors			
4" × 4" gauze sponges			
2" non-adhesive tape			
assorted adhesive bandages			
peroxide			
skin lubricant			
2" elastic wrap			
4" elastic wrap			
6" elastic wrap			
6" double length elastic wrap			
sling			
tongue depressors			
cotton swabs			
nail clipper			
ice bags			

CHAPTER 22

Return to Play

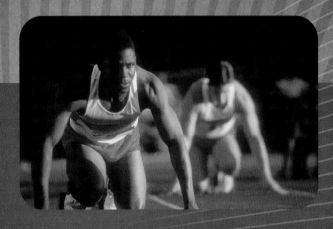

OBJECTIVES

After completing this chapter, you should be able to do the following:

1. Define and correctly spell each of the key terms.

2. Explain when is appropriate to restrict participation and when to refer an athlete to a physician.

3. Recognize the five psychological stages of recovery.

4. Identify methods for assessing return-to-play potential for athletes with upper-extremity injuries.

5. Identify methods for assessing return-to-play potential for athletes with lower-extremity injuries.

6. Identify methods for assessing return-to-play potential for athletes with back and trunk injuries.

7. Describe the athletic trainer's responsibility in responding to abnormal behaviors on or off the field of play.

KEY TERMS

* acceptance
* anger
* apathy
* bargaining
* coping mechanisms
* denial

* depression
* diagnosis
* grimace
* pain threshold
* plateau
* proactive

* prognosis
* psychological fitness
* restricted participation
* self-esteem

WHO MAKES THE DECISION?

Deciding whether an athlete may return to play following an injury can be difficult. After recovering from any major injury, an athlete must provide written proof of a physician's permission to return to play before resuming athletic activities. After a minor or first-degree injury, the athletic trainer must decide whether or not the athlete may return to play. The person with the highest level of medical training is responsible for this decision.

In most cases, removal from play results from a musculoskeletal injury. Such injuries cause pain and reduce range of motion, impairing athletic performance and normal activities. Often minor (first-degree) to moderate (second-degree) soft tissue injuries do not require a physician's care, but major (third-degree) injuries to either the bones or soft tissues must be evaluated by a physician and, therefore, will require written authorization from a physician before the athlete can resume sports activities. Any questions at all about returning to play after a mild or moderate injury must be resolved by a physician.

Additional circumstances that require a physician's written permission before the athlete can return to play include:

* Head injuries (with or without loss of consciousness)

* Spinal injuries

* Trauma to the internal organs

* Any injury or illness in which the athlete was referred to a physician for further evaluation and treatment

* Any injury or illness that the person making the evaluation is unsure of

restricted participation

engaging in athletic activity while injured, but in a restricted manner that prevents an injury from becoming worse.

When a soft tissue injury is minor to moderate or after a severe injury has healed, an athlete can be allowed to engage in **restricted participation**. Restrictions may include limitations on types of activity, prevention of certain motions with protective taping, or other cautionary measures, depending on the sport. For example, if a baseball player injures a shoulder, the athlete may be allowed to run but not hit; a football player with an injured thumb may be able to play with the thumb immobilized with tape. The determination to restrict participation or allow an individual to return to

Guidelines for Authorizing and Restricting Participation

Type of Injury	Return to Play	Restrict Practice	Remove from Play
head or spine	physician	physician	athletic trainer, contact EMS
internal organs	physician	physician	athletic trainer, contact EMS
soft tissue			
mild (1st degree)	athletic trainer[*†]	athletic trainer[*†]	athletic trainer[*]
moderate (2nd degree)	athletic trainer[*] or physician	athletic trainer[*] or physician	athletic trainer[*] or physician
severe (3rd degree)	physician	physician	athletic trainer[*] or physician

[*]If uncomfortable with making the decision, refer the athlete to a physician.

[†]Unless the athlete was referred to a physician for evaluation or treatment, in which case written permission from the physician is required.

Note: Certified athletic trainer may also act under the orders of a physician.

FIGURE 22-1 Guidelines for Determining Who Should Authorize and Restrict Participation

play following an injury is based on the athlete's ability to perform certain physical activities related to the specific sport. These activities are described later in this chapter. The duration of restricted play, which may range from one play to an entire season, is defined by the severity of the injury and the athlete's ability to regain the degree of strength, skill, and conditioning required for a particular activity. Generally, a physician will make the decision as to whether restricted practice is appropriate for a given athlete; however, if an injury is mild and a physician's care is not required, an athletic trainer may permit the athlete to continue practice under certain restrictions if it is in the athlete's best interest (see Figure 22-1). In deciding if restricted practice will be of benefit to the athlete, the athletic trainer and the physician must consider the long-term effects of repeated injuries and give the athlete's best interests the highest priority.

> **NOTE:**
>
> If the athlete loses consciousness for any period of time, the athlete must be checked by a physician before being cleared for practice or play.

PHYSICAL CONSIDERATIONS

An athlete's physical fitness should be carefully considered when determining ability to return to play after recovering from an injury that has required restricted participation or removal from play. The athletic trainer is the athlete's advocate; the athletic trainer is responsible for protecting the athlete from situations that might cause additional harm. Therefore, assessment of both physical and **psychological fitness**, as well as any decision regarding activity restrictions, should always be based on the athlete's immediate safety and long-term well-being. Refer the athlete to a physician immediately if any of the following situations occur:

* You feel uncomfortable about your ability to recognize the symptoms of an injury. (Remember, only physicians can diagnose. Athletic trainers must be able to recognize the situations that require a doctor's expertise.)

psychological fitness

the mental and emotional ability to perform in competition without undue strain on other aspects of one's life.

* You believe the athlete's condition is not improving at the expected rate.

* You notice that activities are causing the athlete unexpected pain. (Do not rely on the athlete to tell you about experiencing pain; the athlete may be attempting to avoid further restrictions.)

* You believe the athlete is not coping well psychologically with the disability produced by the injury.

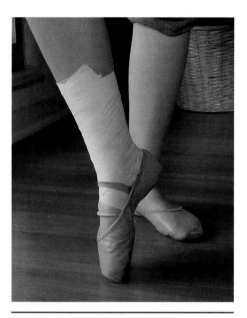

FIGURE 22-2 Taping may enhance an athlete's ability to participate while injured.

If taping or bracing may help the athlete to pass the return-to-play tests, taping the injury can be done (see Figure 22-2). (See Chapter 21.) The goal of the athletic trainer is not to keep the athlete out of play, but to make sure no additional injuries occur as a result of the athlete's continued participation. With that in mind, the athlete's failure to perform any simple functional test should result in removal from participation. When in doubt, remove the athlete from participation.

General Assessment Procedures

Since the decision to return an athlete to play is based on that athlete's ability to perform certain physical activities, the procedures for assessing an athlete's suitability for participation must be straightforward and nondiscriminatory. Athletes (or their parents or guardian) must not feel that the athletic trainer or physician is making a random decision to exclude the athlete from participation. Therefore, share return-to-play information with the athletes and coaches (and in the case of minors, the parents or guardian) so they will understand the criteria used to make this decision before an injury occurs. These predetermined drills, or procedures, allow the athletic trainer to make an impartial decision as to what is in the athlete's best interest. An athletic training student will never make a return-to-play decision. As a student, the best way to learn is by watching the athletic trainer's decision-making process.

The assessment procedure varies, depending on the the part of the body that is injured; however, certain elements are common. When using any of the assessment drills in this chapter, make sure to take these steps:

1. Write down a complete history of the incident: find out how (the mechanism of injury), when, and where the injury occurred. This history *must* be included in the injury log.

2. Look at the injury and compare the injured side to the uninjured side.

3. Explain to the athlete what is being looked at or felt for and take into consideration any abnormalities the athlete claims to have had before the injury happened.

4. Palpate the injury to feel for deformities (see Figures 22-3 and 22-4).

5. Ask if the injured player can feel the area being palpated and if there is any numbness, unusual sensations, or feelings of weakness, and if both sides of the body feel the same.

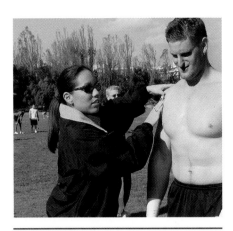

FIGURE 22-3 Palpate the uninvolved side first.

Assessing Return-to-Play Potential for Athletes with Upper-Extremity Injuries

To determine if an athlete with an upper-extremity injury can return to play, assess the athlete's ability to perform the following procedure, taking care to check for full, pain-free range of motion (ROM) and full, pain-free strength:

1. Ask the athlete to perform arm and wrist circles, to flex and extend both elbows, and to raise the arms over the head (see Figure 22-5). This will demonstrate the athlete's full, pain-free range of motion (ROM).

2. Ask the athlete to perform 10 push-ups (see Chapter 5). This will demonstrate the level of strength in the athlete's upper extremities.

3. Ask the athlete to catch an object tossed to the right, left, and midline. This will demonstrate the athlete's reflex abilities. Again, the injured area may be taped or braced to try to help the athlete perform the above tasks.

4. Ask if the athlete feels capable of returning to play or if there is anything that you, as the athletic trainer,

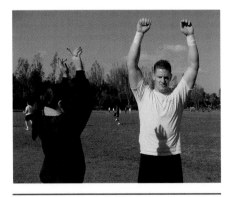

FIGURE 22-4 Then palpate the involved side.

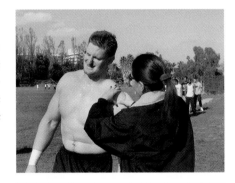

FIGURE 22-5 The athlete raises his hands over his head as part of a ROM assessment.

should know before the athlete returns to competition. The athlete may not feel psychologically capable of participating. Something other than physical factors, such as family, romantic, or job-related problems, may be a part of the reason that the athlete does not feel up to participating.

If the athlete can perform these tests without any pain (or unspoken indications of pain such as a **grimace**, clenched teeth, or intensified breathing) and feels able, the athlete may return to play.

Assessing Return-to-Play Potential for Athletes with Lower-Extremity Injuries

To determine if an athlete with a lower-extremity injury can return to play, assess the athlete's ability to perform the following activities, taking care to check for full, pain-free range of motion (ROM) and full, pain-free strength:

1. Ask the athlete to walk forward and backward. This will demonstrate the ability to walk without a limp.

2. Ask the athlete to perform 10 squats. This will demonstrate the level of strength in the athlete's lower extremities (see Chapter 7).

3. Ask the athlete to run forward and backward at half speed without limping. This will demonstrate the ability to avoid limping when the stress of running is applied to the limb.

4. Ask the athlete to run in a figure-8 pattern without limping. This will demonstrate the ability to avoid limping when still more stress is applied to the limb and tests the limb's ability to withstand stress from a different angle.

5. Ask the athlete to hop for approximately 5 yards on the uninvolved (uninjured) extremity and then approximately 5 yards on the involved one (see Figure 22-6). Differences in the athlete's ability to hop on one side will indicate reduced function in the injured extremity that would prohibit the athlete's return to play. Again, if necessary, tape or brace the injured area to try to help the athlete perform the above tasks.

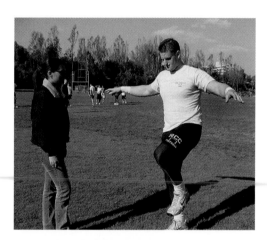

FIGURE 22-6 The athlete hops on one foot to demonstrate the degree of function in that extremity.

6. Have the athlete run through some sport-specific drills.

7. Ask if the athlete feels capable of returning to play or if there is anything that you, as the athletic trainer, should know before the athlete returns to competition.

If the athlete can perform the activities without any pain (or unspoken indications of pain) and feels able, the athlete may return to play.

Assessing Return-to-Play Potential
for Athletes with Injuries to the Back or Trunk

To determine if an athlete with an injury to the back or trunk can return to play, assess the athlete's ability to perform the following activities, taking care to check for full, pain-free range of motion (ROM) and full, pain-free strength:

1. Ask the athlete to stand and slowly bend from the waist to touch the toes. Instruct the athlete to bend backward from the waist as far as possible, and then to twist the body at the waist as far to the right as possible, and then as far to the left as possible. This will demonstrate the athlete's full, pain-free range of motion.

2. Ask the athlete to bend from the waist to touch the toes and straighten up again while you apply a slight resistance with your hand against the back as the athlete rises (see Figure 22-7). Then, ask the athlete to bend forward again from the waist while you apply the same amount of resistance with your hand against the chest. This will demonstrate the level of full, pain-free range of motion in the athlete's upper body.

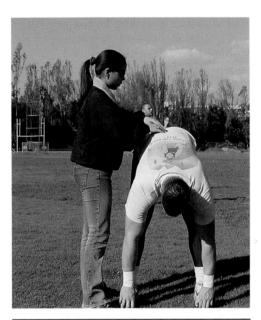

FIGURE 22-7 The athlete bends over to touch his toes to demonstrate the ROM in the upper body.

3. Ask the athlete to perform 10 push-ups to demonstrate capability for full, pain-free, upper-body strength.

4. Ask the athlete to perform 10 squats. This will demonstrate the level of strength in the athlete's lower extremities.

5. Ask the athlete to walk forward and backward. This will demonstrate the ability to walk without a limp.

6. Ask the athlete to run forward and backward at half speed without limping. This will demonstrate the ability to avoid limping when the stress of running is applied to the limb.

7. Ask the athlete to run in a figure-8 pattern without limping. This will demonstrate the ability to avoid limping when still more stress is applied to the limb and tests the limb's ability to withstand stress from a different angle than running in a straight line.

8. Ask the athlete to hop for approximately 5 yards on the uninvolved (uninjured) extremity and then approximately 5 yards on the involved extremity. Differences in the athlete's ability to hop on one side will indicate reduced

function in the injured extremity that should prohibit the athlete's return to play. Again, one can tape or brace the injured area to try to help the athlete perform the above tasks.

9. Have the athlete run through some sport-specific drills.

10. Ask if the athlete feels capable of returning to play or if there is anything that you, as the athletic trainer, should know before the athlete returns to competition.

If the athlete can perform the activities without any pain (or unspoken indications of pain) and feels able, the athlete may return to play.

Follow-up Procedures

Once an athlete has returned to play, watch the athlete both on and off the field or court. Look for any changes in the athlete's movements. Does the athlete limp or avoid using the injured area? Valuable information can be gained through particularly close observation of the athlete during active participation, as opposed to the time in-between a play or activity (see Figure 22-8). Although it is important to watch the athletes at all times, activity during the actual sport is most likely to produce pain and determine whether or not to participate. Remember that every athlete has a different **pain threshold** or tolerance for pain. It is important to know

pain threshold

the point at which pain affects performance.

the athletes and how they react to pain and injury. If unsure of an athlete's pain threshold, talk with the coaches; the coaching staff should be able to give a background of the athlete. Discourage athletes from playing while they are in pain because they are at greater risk of further injuring themselves. Of course, some pain is derived from almost any sport. Pain is acceptable as long as it does not jeopardize the athlete or teammates during practice or in an event. If signs of pain see noticed in an athlete who has just returned to play, or if something just doesn't seem right, inform the coach of the

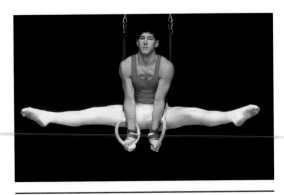

FIGURE 22-8 Careful observation of athletes during active participation will provide valuable information regarding the level of pain that is being endured.

decision to pull the athlete back out of play for reassessment.

Not all injuries will be obvious at first. An athlete may get injured, "shake off" the pain between plays, and continue as if nothing happened (see Figure 22-9). In many cases this is completely acceptable; however, sometimes an athlete's determination to finish out a game or a practice may cloud judgement regarding the severity of an injury. For example, if an athlete has suffered a concussion, the injury may cause light-headedness and leave the athlete feeling somewhat dazed. The athlete may not realize the potential severity of the injury and continue to play, thinking that the dazed feeling will wear off. However, the concussion may be made worse by continued play. This is why it is so important to watch the athletes carefully during all phases of athletic activity; although symptoms of an injury are usually immediate, sometimes their onset and/or resulting complications can be delayed.

At times, after an athlete is removed from play, the athlete may try to influence the athletic trainer into returning him or her to activity. *Do not return an athlete to play against better judgement!* Never let an athlete impose a feeling of guilt about taking him or her out of a game—or even a practice. Remember, it is the injury that takes the athlete out, not the athletic trainer or coach. The most important responsibility of the athletic trainer is to protect the athletes; let them return to participation as soon as they can perform the required drills, indicating that they can function safely—no sooner.

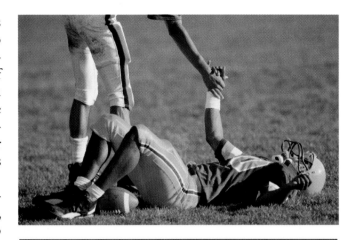

FIGURE 22-9 A downed athlete may not realize the severity of certain symptoms and try to "shake off" the discomfort of an injury to stay in the game.

PSYCHOLOGICAL CONSIDERATIONS

An athletic trainer must always be aware of the mental status of the injured athlete. Watch the athlete for signs of trying to "tough it out" and play through the injury out of pride or in the spirit of competition. Conversely, an athlete may also try to use an injury as an excuse to be removed from play. For example, a severe blow might make an athlete reluctant to risk getting hit that hard again. Or, the athlete may perceive not receiving enough attention and may fake an injury to get the desired attention. The athlete, the athletic trainer, the coach, and any other interested parties such as the parents must deal with this situation together. The athlete must be made to understand that this behavior is unacceptable: it draws the athletic trainer's attention away from the other athletes who may really need it, and makes it difficult for the athletic trainer to take that athlete seriously when an injury does occur. Regardless of whether an athlete is playing up (exaggerating) an injury or playing it down (minimizing), the athletic trainer is not there to cast judgement, but to facilitate the athlete's needs.

When an athlete has been restricted or removed from play, or has been advised of a permanent disability, the athlete may have a mental battle to overcome as well as a physical one (see Figure 22-10). If competitive activity is restricted for only a short time (the duration of a play or a single event), the athlete's confidence or motivation to resume activity is not likely to change significantly. These athletes are generally ready and excited to get back to the game as soon as they can perform the necessary physical and mental maneuvers. But when an athlete is out of competition for an extended time, psychological **coping mechanisms** often emerge in response to the stress of the change in lifestyle. The athlete may experience

coping mechanisms

defense mechanisms; the psychological or physical methods by which an individual adjusts or adapts to a challenge or stressful situation.

something similar to the five psychological stages defined by Dr. Elisabeth Kubler-Ross in her timeless book, *On Death and Dying*. In this book, Dr. Kubler-Ross describes the stages of adjustment typically experienced by those faced with the stress of death or great loss. For many athletes their sport is central to their lives. Restriction or loss of ability to participate in that sport represents a significant loss to them. An athletic trainer can more effectively address the psychological needs of an athlete's rehabilitation by becoming familiar with these stages. Plan for and work toward the athlete's psychological recovery as well as the physical rehabilitation. If an athlete is physically fit but not mentally ready, a return to full potential is unlikely. The following stages of psychological recovery from athletic injuries have been adapted from the stages of adjustment, or coping mechanisms, described in Dr. Kubler-Ross' book.

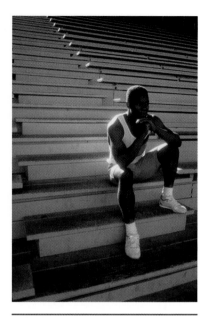

FIGURE 22-10 Injured athletes often must overcome mental or emotional challenges to their recovery as well as physical ones.

Denial

denial

refusal to believe that which is true or real.

The **denial** stage usually occurs first. More than likely the athlete will experience denial when told of the severity of the injury. While the physician will provide the athlete with a **diagnosis** and **prognosis**, other vital information may be left for the athletic trainer to explain to the athlete. Such information may include a description of the anatomy involved in the injury and the importance of the athlete's role in the rehabilitation process. At this time the athlete may start to face the reality of the injury. This may begin with the athlete realizing the possibility of not being up and moving tomorrow—maybe not for the rest of the season. Help direct the athlete's focus away from the injury by pointing out opportunities for increasing attention to other significant areas of life, such as more study time or more family time. One of the most powerful motivations to rehabilitation is the hope of returning to play. An athletic trainer can enhance this motivation by reassuring injured athletes that they are still a part of the team and finding or creating opportunities for involvement that are suited to the injury. Helping other players understand game plans, assisting with equipment inventory or maintenance, and providing moral support to their teammates are all excellent ways of keeping injured athletes active and involved while they work through their rehabilitation.

diagnosis

identification of the nature of a disease or condition based on scientific assessment.

prognosis

an estimate of a chance for recovery; a prediction of the likely outcome of a disease or injury.

The most important response to the denial stage is reassurance. It is the athletic trainer's responsibility to reassure that the athlete will survive the pain and sense of loss, and that the athletic trainer will be there to help.

Anger

anger

frustration, bitterness, or hostility.

During the **anger** stage the athlete is mad at the world. The athlete is also mad at the athletic trainer, the bearer (or co-bearer with the physician) of news that is least welcome and the person who is making the athlete grind through exercises not directly competitive and often very painful. In some cases the athlete may now want to play more than ever. Be aware of anyone else with whom the athlete may be angry and help minimize this response by explaining to the athlete that the injury is not anyone's fault. Help the athlete work through this anger in positive ways such as increasing repetitions of exercises or simply allowing the athlete to "shout it out, then put it away." An injured athlete needs to understand that teammates, coaches, athletic trainers, physicians, family, and friends are there to help because they care and are concerned. The athlete may need to be reminded not to jeopardize these relationships with misdirected or inappropriate anger. Reassure these athletes that support will be there even when they blow up, but remind them that support and recovery are a lot easier when hostility is kept under control.

Be constant yet realistic with encouragement. Try to avoid cliches like, "this hurts me as much as it hurts you" unless willing to truly experience some of the athlete's pain firsthand. Also, even if the same type of injury has been experienced, saying, "I know how you feel" may only increase an athlete's anger. Although the physical pain may have been similar, keep in mind that the personal and/or psychological situations may be polar opposites. Instead, be objective in support by offering observations geared to the athlete. Try supportive statements like, "I can see this is difficult for you," or "I've seen you play. I know you can do this."

Bargaining

Injured athletes sometimes feel they will be able to negotiate with someone who will allow them to return to play earlier than they should. They will play one person against the other using half-truths and **bargaining** to accomplish their goals. At this stage athletes may go from doctor to doctor until they find one who will say what the athlete wants to hear. In some cases an athlete may find someone who will say exactly that but who will not then bear the responsibility for complications or further (sometimes permanent) injury that often results from returning to play too soon.

Only physicians can offer a prognosis. Tell an athlete how long an average injury might take to heal, but avoid giving the athlete specific recovery estimates. When a physician is involved with the case, the physician will tell the athlete how long rehabilitation is expected to last. However, for minor to moderate soft tissue injuries in which a physician's care was not required, the athletic trainer may have to provide this information. When providing general estimates to an athlete, always give the most conservative estimate possible for rehabilitation time. Do not allow the athlete to try to persuade you to grant permission to return to play too soon. In most cases the athlete will hear the short side of the estimate. In other words, when the athlete is told "three to six weeks," "three weeks" is all the athlete will hear.

Other indications of the bargaining stage include the athlete's realization that some of the attention gotten as an active part of the team may decline. This realization often intensifies the bargaining process, yet remember to stay consistent and not give the athlete information that might backfire later. Better to not say the athlete will be ready to return to play after three weeks, because this statement cannot be guaranteed.

Frequently, when bargaining fails, the athlete will experience or return to the anger stage. It is the athletic trainer's job to recognize these stages of psychological recovery and help the athlete work toward the final stage, acceptance. Never allow an athlete to return to play against better judgement.

> **bargaining**
>
> attempting to make a deal with an authority figure in an attempt to change the outcome of a situation.

Depression

depression

extreme feelings of sadness or hopelessness.

Depression can result from a variety of life situations—not just injuries. Mild cases, known as "the blues," may resolve themselves on their own, but such cases may also lead to more-serious emotional distress. Prolonged depression may lead to emotional instability and destructive behaviors. Be alert to intense changes in the athlete's moods, such as increased sadness or unrealistic cheerfulness. Never hesitate to discuss concerns with more-experienced professionals—an athlete's life may depend on gut instincts.

plateau

a period in the process of rehabilitation in which no significant improvement or progress is shown.

Some rehabilitation programs are long and tedious, often reaching **plateaus** that can last for weeks. These plateaus may consist of extended periods during which no increase in strength or range of motion is noted. All kinds of setbacks can occur during these periods, including weight gain, loss of **self-esteem**, **apathy**, or trouble at home or school because the athlete feels that no one understands.

self-esteem

pride in oneself; self-respect.

As compassionately as possible, without dismissing or generalizing the sense of loss or despair, let the athlete know that many people have gone through similar tragedies and that others will experience tragedy in the future. As a professional, keep in mind that, in many cases, injured athletes have too much time to think and feel sorry for themselves. This is one of the main reasons to change the workout routine frequently and add excitement to long rehabilitation programs. There are many ways to work the same muscle, so add variety. Stay ahead of the athletes; if self-pity or boredom is sensed make an extra effort to work together with those around the athlete to keep his or her attitude focused in a positive direction. Keep in mind the influence of your positive attitude, as the injured athlete's time with you will be dramatically increased throughout the recovery period. Try to minimize the athlete's negative ideas and influences.

apathy

lack of interest or concern.

Acceptance

acceptance

coming to terms with the outcome of one's prognosis.

Acceptance is the stage in which athletes are able to fully understand and appropriately deal with the extent of their injuries, as well as their responsibilities in the recovery process. This understanding includes coming to grips with the time frame of restricted participation, or even the possibility they may never return to their particular sport and need to find other activities through which they can channel their energies. This stage often signals the beginning of the athlete's recovery from a psychological standpoint. Remember, in order to be ready for competition, and everyday life, one must be physically and psychologically fit.

If the athlete is going to return to the sport, confidence and determination must be addressed and emphasized during the acceptance stage. The athletic trainer must provide and encourage as many activities as possible to bring the injured athlete closer to a competitive setting. An unexpected play, crowd noise, teammates asking the injured athlete's opinion on strategies, and post-game celebrations can all contribute to rebuilding an injured athlete's confidence and desire to return to play.

Some athletes whose injuries require an extended recovery period do not experience any of the stages described above; others may experience only some of the stages; still others may experience each stage but not necessarily in the order listed. There is no set order for these stages of adjustment and no definite period of duration for any stage. Sometimes even athletes with short-term restrictions experience some of these stages. Furthermore, in a long rehabilitation program, the athlete may go from one stage to another and back again. In any case, the athletic trainer must be **proactive**, anticipating and preventing as many obstacles to recovery as possible. Stay alert to possible relapses throughout the recovery process, and make the rehabilitation program as exciting as possible, constantly moving toward positive goals. Listening and being aware of athletes' psychological, as well as physical, needs during the rehabilitation process can help determine the best ways to help them return to play. Recognize personal limitations when assessing physical injuries; if unsure or unable to properly address the psychological aspects of an injury, refer the athlete to someone with a higher level of training.

proactive

acting in advance to avoid or manage an anticipated difficulty.

UNDERSTANDING AND RESPONDING TO ABNORMAL BEHAVIORS

Sometimes, outside influences may affect an athlete's mental status in a negative way, whether or not the athlete has been injured. Effects on an athlete's mental status are often revealed through subtle to overt changes in behavior (see Figure 22-11).

These problems must be addressed. Although athletic trainers should note such problems, they are not expected to solve them. Overall, the athletic trainer is expected to notify the appropriate members of the sports medicine team and any other individuals as necessary of any potentially serious problems or issues an athlete is experiencing. Recall from Chapter 2 on athletic training that the team members who should be notified include the team physician, the coach, the athlete, the athlete's family, and the school or team administration. In the best interest of the athlete, as well as the athletic trainer, it is important to record such notification, and follow up with the appropriate people until one is confident the situation is being properly handled.

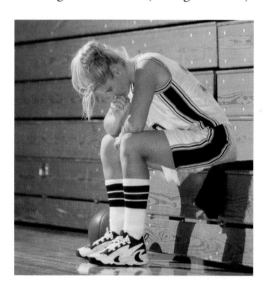

FIGURE 22-11 Influences outside the sports setting may cause depression, agitation, mood swings, and other unexpected behaviors. Athletic trainers should alert the appropriate sports medicine team members of such changes in personality and follow up to make sure the athlete's needs are being addressed.

Athlete's don't live in the locker room. In our high-tech society, they may be tempted to experiment with artificial enhancement of their natural abilities or to speed the recovery process following an injury. A wide variety of stimulants, ranging from herbal extracts to illegal drugs, are readily available to athletes who are unaware of potential danger. Diuretics and laxatives are frequently abused by people looking for quick solutions to weight control. Perhaps the most dangerous of all artificial enhancements is the use of steroids. These drugs are illegal without a prescription and are banned in almost all competitions. Further, steroids can lead to sexual disfunction, organ damage, depression, mood swings, stunted growth, and other serious physical and psychological consequences. Use of steroids and other illegal substances can also damage one's career—leading to humiliation, depression, and loss of potential income.

It is the duty of a sports medicine professional to make sure that the athletes are aware of the complications and side effects of artificial enhancement. Reinforce the athletes' self-image and good sense by talking about their natural strengths and developing more challenging workout routines that will help athletes achieve goals naturally.

Aside from performance enhancements, outside influences create an immeasurable impact on an athlete's mental status and subsequent behavior. Jobs, grades, scholarships, families, friends, and lovers all have a dramatic affect on an athlete's self-image, concentration, athletic performance, and everyday actions. The athletic trainer may be the member of the sports medicine team in closest contact with the athletes. Again, while it is not the athletic trainer's responsibility to solve personal problems, awareness of the impact of such concerns will help to better guide and motivate the athletes. Also be aware that it is the responsibility of the athletic trainer and coach to report any suspected abuse of an athlete, either physical or behavioral, to the appropriate authorities. Becoming familiar with various resource agencies, such as tutoring facilities, financial aid contacts, and legal, medical, and mental health clinics is an excellent way to help athletes resolve personal issues and get on with their lives.

THINKING IT THROUGH

In August of last year, Tracy, a cheerleader, was at the top of a pyramid when she lost her balance and fell. On landing, she twisted her knee and felt a pop in the joint. The doctor told her it was too swollen to take an x-ray, so he sent her home, telling her to stay off of it for a couple of weeks, apply ice to help decrease the swelling, and then come back and see him again. After two weeks the swelling had gone down, but she had lost some of her range of motion and strength in her knee.

Tracy was a senior, and the year was very important to her in getting a cheerleading scholarship. When her mother called the doctor's office she was told they would have to wait a week because the doctor was all booked up. So, three weeks after the injury, Tracy was finally able to get her knee evaluated by her doctor.

After examining the knee and the x-rays he ordered, the doctor felt there might be a tear in the ACL. He told Tracy he wanted her to see an orthopedist as soon as possible. Tracy was completely frustrated; she could see her season and scholarship fading away. On top of that, the doctor said her insurance did not cover physical therapy. She would have to do basic rehabilitative exercises at home.

After another week Tracy still hadn't heard anything from the medical group, so her mother called to check on the appointment with the orthopedist. They said the orthopedist couldn't see Tracy until the following week. That meant it would be a full five weeks after the injury before Tracy could finally get in to see the orthopedist, obtain a diagnosis, and begin treatment so she could plan her future.

What are some of the emotional stages Tracy could be going through? How might you help her through them? When she completes her rehabilitation, what will determine if she can participate in cheerleading again?

CHAPTER SUMMARY

The decision to allow an athlete to return to play or to restrict participation is never easy and should not be taken lightly. Serious injuries require written permission from a physician before an athlete may return to play. Remember that it is the athletic trainer's duty to protect the athlete's immediate safety and long-range health considerations. Never let an athlete, a coach, or a parent influence a judgement regarding restricted participation. Understanding Dr. Kubler-Ross's theory of grief and responding compassionately to the needs of each stage is one of the best ways to help an injured athlete prepare psychologically to return to play. Don't hesitate to refer the athlete to someone with more experience if unprepared to deal with any element—physical or psychological—of the athlete's injury or recovery.

Assessment tests can help determine an athlete's ability to return to play. In addition to general assessment procedures, specific tests for strength and ROM of upper and lower extremities provide objective information about an athlete's physical condition. Information provided by the athlete is subjective; often the athlete's perception of physical condition is strongly influenced by psychological factors, such as the desire to play, fear of injury, or personal issues, which can distort the real situation. Communicating the goals and results of assessment tests can help athletes and their families understand the reasoning behind the decisions about restricting participation.

Athletes may discuss things with an athletic trainer that they won't discuss with their families, friends, or coaches. An athletic trainer may hear or observe things that no one else could. For example, evidence of abuse or injury is never confidential. While it is important not to violate an athlete's trust in the ability to talk to you (gossip is never pretty), it is your personal and professional responsibility to alert appropriate members of the sports medicine team of behavior that you feel might be harmful to the athlete or to others.

STUDENT ENRICHMENT ACTIVITIES

Complete the following sentences.

1. Major injuries to the _____, _____ or _____ _____ require a physician's written permission before the athlete can return to play.

2. Assessment of strength in lower extremities includes an athlete's ability to perform _____ squats.

3. Athletes may make you feel _____ about taking them out of a game or even a practice.

4. As an athletic trainer, you are the athlete's _____.

5. Athletes who are experiencing intense anger in response to an injury may need to be reminded that they should not _____ important relationships with misdirected or inappropriate anger.

Match the terms in Column A with the appropriate description in Column B.

Column A	**Column B**
6. acceptance	A. An athlete may go from doctor to doctor or try to make a deal in an attempt to change the outcome of the situation.
7. denial	
8. depression	B. The athlete may demonstrate inappropriate or misdirected behavior.
9. anger	C. In this stage confidence and determination must be emphasized if the athlete is to return to play.
10. bargaining	D. An athlete is unable to accept the reality of the situation or injury at hand.
	E. The athlete feels emotional distress or "the blues."

Write T for true, or F for false. Rewrite the false statements to make them true.

11. T F Mental status can significantly impact general behavior and athletic performance.

12. T F Athletes who have experienced trauma to internal organs must have a physician's written permission to return to play.

13. T F If the athletic trainer is not sure how to properly assess a physical injury or psychological issue, the athletic trainer should take a guess.

14. T F Discounting is one of the five stages of adjustment.

15. T F Athletic trainers should offer athletes a prognosis.

Complete the following exercises.

16. List five general assessment procedures.

17. List three situations in which you should immediately refer an athlete to a physician.

18. Describe three types of artificial enhancements that athletes may be tempted to try.

19. Interview one of your local coaches. Ask how this coach determines if an athlete can return to play.

20. Interview a local athletic trainer and ask the same question.

CHAPTER 23

Therapeutic Modalities

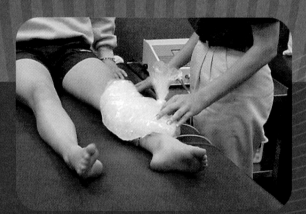

OBJECTIVES

After completing this chapter, you should be able to do the following:

1. Define and correctly spell each of the key terms.

2. Discuss the purpose of therapeutic modalities.

3. Explain the legal implications associated with the use of therapeutic modalities.

4. List the different types of modalities discussed in this chapter, and explain how they are used.

5. Discuss several safety considerations involved with the use of therapeutic modalities.

KEY TERMS

- cryotherapy
- diathermy
- electrical modality
- electrical muscle stimulation (EMS)
- fluidotherapy
- galvanic stimulation
- hydrocollator pack
- ice massage

- ice pack
- ice water immersion
- interferential stimulation (IFS)
- intermittent compression
- iontophoresis
- massage
- mechanical modality
- muscle spasm/pain cycle

- paraffin bath
- thermotherapy
- traction
- transcutaneous electrical nerve stimulation (TENS)
- ultrasound therapy
- vapo-coolant spray
- whirlpool bath

THERAPEUTIC MODALITIES AND THEIR USE IN REHABILITATION

Rehabilitation is the application of physical exercise following an illness or injury to restore optimal health and function to an individual. When rehabilitation is successful, debilitated individuals are often able to return to their activities of daily living with little to no adjustments in routine. In cases where function cannot be restored completely, rehabilitation will also include education in methods of compensating for the loss of function. Much of this healing and restorative process is made possible by the use of therapeutic modalities.

The term *therapeutic modalities* describes various methods and agents used to manipulate circulation (bloodflow) in the treatment of muscles and joints. The purpose of therapeutic modalities is to improve or restore an individual's range of motion, regain strength, cope with pain, and engage in daily activities and athletic endeavors at an optimal performance level. Although the methods in this chapter are used most frequently in the treatment of injuries and medical conditions, some forms of therapy may also be used to condition and stimulate muscles and joints. It is important to understand how such therapy can benefit individuals, and how to use the modalities safely. Therapeutic modalities can be divided into five general categories—cryotherapy, thermotherapy, electrical modalities, mechanical modalities, and pharmacologic agents—depending on the mode of stimulation. This chapter provides an introduction to various therapeutic modalities used in physical rehabilitation.

LEGAL IMPLICATIONS ASSOCIATED WITH THE USE OF THERAPEUTIC MODALITIES

Therapeutic modalities can provide great benefits in the rehabilitative process, but they must be properly used. For some modalities, proper use involves extensive training. For the protection of the client as well as the healthcare provider, it is vital to understand some of the limitations that apply when working with therapeutic modalities. Because regulations concerning the use of therapeutic modalities vary from state to state, athletic trainers, physical therapists, and physical therapist assistants should check the specific laws of the state in which they will practice. Going beyond the scope of practice constitutes negligence.

Awareness of the laws concerning use of therapeutic modalities is key in the process of rehabilitation. It is essential to document all therapeutic treatments to ensure continuity of care and to track treatment or outcomes. Such documentation may also be used as part of a defense in a lawsuit to provide evidence regarding the nature of treatments (Figure 23-1).

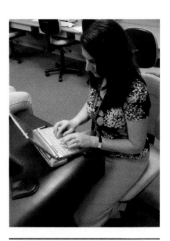

FIGURE 23-1 The use of all therapeutic modalities must be documented.

THE USE OF MODALITIES

Injuries such as sprains and strains increase bloodflow to the involved tissues, resulting in inflammation and edema. Symptoms of inflamed tissues include pain, heat, and redness. Because of this local trauma, vessels in the injured area are unable to meet the needs of the tissue's oxygen demands. Additional tissue breakdown, or damage, results from the lack of oxygen to the tissues and may cause muscle spasms and increased edema. The muscle spasm then causes additional pain, which can increase the spasms, and so on. This syndrome, called the **muscle spasm/pain cycle**, leads to decreased mobility.

Therapeutic modalities are used to stop, slow down, or otherwise interrupt the muscle spasm/pain cycle. For example, to interrupt the cycle for a strain or sprain, ice—a method of cryotherapy—can be applied to the inflamed area. The cold will cause vasoconstriction in blood vessels serving the muscle tissue, decreasing local inflammation and edema, as well as stopping or slowing the muscle spasm/pain cycle. As useful as modalities can be, however, it is important to know that the misuse or overuse of modalities can create an effect opposite to that which is intended: misapplication of a modality may aggravate a condition rather than provide relief.

> **muscle spasm/ pain cycle**
>
> a debilitating syndrome in which pain caused by injury produces muscle spasms that increase pain and spasms in a cyclical manner.

Choosing a Modality

There is a wide range of therapeutic modalities to choose from to achieve the best results. That is, after assessing an individual's needs, the athletic trainer must determine whether including exercise or various applications of heat, cold, and electrical or mechanical stimulation will be most effective in regulating bloodflow to specific areas of the body. Three important factors to consider when selecting a modality to treat an injury or disease process are:

1. Is this modality safe for use on this type of injury?

2. Will use of this modality contribute significantly to the rehabilitation process and the total recovery of the person?

3. Is the person applying the modality trained and authorized to use it safely and efficiently?

Patients may not be familiar with the instruments and techniques used in athletic training, physical therapy, and rehabilitation. This can be a source of stress for the patient. Therefore, always put the patient at ease by explaining all procedures.

METHODS OF HEAT OR COLD TRANSFER

Modalities using temperature variation to manipulate circulation in the muscle tissues include those that use heat (thermotherapy) and those that use cold (cryotherapy). **Thermotherapy** uses heat to increase the temperature of a body region in order to cause blood vessels to dilate (vasodilation), increasing bloodflow to those tissues. Heat is also used to decrease pain and muscle spasms, as well as to increase flexibility of the tissues. **Cryotherapy** uses cold to reduce the temperature of body tissue in order to cause blood vessels to constrict (vasoconstriction), decreasing bloodflow to the area and reducing pain, edema, and muscle spasms.

The body can be heated or cooled through the following means:

* **Conduction:** a method of heat transfer by direct contact with another medium (examples: heat packs or ice packs)

* **Convection:** a method of heat transfer that takes place indirectly through a secondary conductive medium, such as air or liquid (examples: fluidotherapy, whirlpool baths, paraffin soaks)

* **Radiation:** a method of heat transfer by or from its source to the surrounding environment in the form of waves or rays (examples: infrared ultraviolet light, laser, or electrical stimulating modalities)

* **Conversion:** a method of heat transfer that takes place through other forms of energy, such as sound, electricity, or chemicals (examples: ultrasound, diathermy, or heating/cooling ointments)

* **Evaporation:** a method of heat transfer that takes place when a liquid is converted to a gas (examples: perspiration or vapo-coolant sprays)

thermotherapy

treatments involving the use of heat to increase circulation in order to improve flexibility and decrease pain and muscle spasms.

cryotherapy

rehabilitative treatments involving the use of cold to decrease circulation in order to decrease pain, muscle spasms, inflammation, and edema.

CRYOTHERAPY

Methods of cryotherapy include ice massage, cold water immersion, ice packs, and vapo-coolant sprays. Because of the cold that is involved in cryotherapy, the patient may experience slight discomfort when it is first applied. As with all procedures, make sure to clearly explain the procedure in advance so the patient knows what to expect.

In most applications of cryotherapy, the length of the treatment corresponds to the depth of the tissue that the cold sensation must reach in order to be of benefit. Cooling the tissue can decrease bloodflow, reducing muscle spasms, pain, and edema. These therapeutic effects are achieved when cold is applied to the skin for 20 to 30 minutes, causing vessels of the involved tissue to constrict. Cooling an area for less than 20 minutes does not reach a therapeutic level, and applications lasting more than 30 minutes can actually increase bloodflow. After 30 minutes of cryotherapy, the body defends itself in much the same way as it responds to cold stress, causing the vessels to dilate. When cryotherapy is used at a therapeutic depth, the person will experience three phases of sensation:

1. A cold sensation lasting 0 to 3 minutes

2. Mild burning and aching lasting 2 to 7 minutes

3. Relative numbness lasting 5 to 12 minutes

Guidelines for Cryotherapy

To ensure the safety of the client or patient, cryotherapy must be applied according to certain guidelines. Be aware of these safety considerations:

1. Never apply any form of cold on an open wound without a protective covering.

2. Never apply any form of cold to anesthetized skin.

3. Except for vapo-coolant sprays, do not apply cryotherapy to patients with decreased circulation, diabetes, or cardiac conditions.

4. Monitor the patient for signs of cold allergy, or Raynaud's phenomenon, a condition in which the arteries and arterioles of an extremity constrict excessively. This constriction, which may be caused by the application of cryotherapy, causes reduced arterial bloodflow. Symptoms include blue, gray, or purple-colored skin in the fingers or toes, accompanied by numbness or burning and tingling sensations. If any of these symptoms are present, discontinue cryotherapy and refer the patient to a physician.

5. To avoid further injury to the tissues, always monitor the time for which cryotherapy is applied; applications should not exceed 30 minutes.

Ice Packs

ice pack

ice, placed in a plastic bag, applied to an injury to decrease circulation, pain, edema, muscle spasms, and inflammation.

The most common form of cryotherapy, **ice packs** are portable and easy to apply (see Figure 23-2). They are frequently used in the treatment of acute injuries and first-degree burns. Crushed ice placed inside a wet towel is another way to cool the tissues using ice but it can be uncomfortable and wet for the patient.

Ice, by itself, is only capable of cooling by conduction. A wet towel adds to the cooling action of the ice by cooling through convection as well. Reusable ice bags wrapped in towels may also be used. Again, if the towels are dry, the cooling benefits of the treatment are reduced, whereas the wet towels increase the cooling action.

For acute injuries, wrapping a wet elastic wrap around the injury

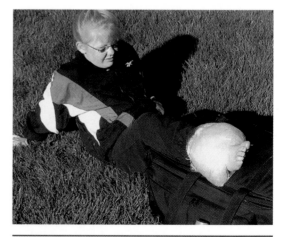

FIGURE 23-2 An ice pack is the easiest method of applying cryotherapy.

site before applying the ice can enhance the effect of the ice in reducing edema by compressing the area. The ice bag is then placed over the wrapped injury for a treatment time of 20 to 30 minutes, leaving an hour between treatments. The wet elastic wrap is used only when the injured person is conscious and awake. Compression should not be used when the injured person is sleeping.

With or without compression, ice packs should not be left on for more than 30 minutes at a time. All of the other cryotherapy guidelines apply to ice packs as well. Be aware of any signs of abnormal pain, even after the treatment is finished. Rash-like symptoms may result from undesirable effects of an ice pack or ice water immersion. If this occurs, discontinue treatment and refer the client to a physician for further evaluation.

To apply an ice pack:

1. Fill a plastic bag with enough crushed ice to mold around the injured area. Squeeze as much air out of the bag as possible. This will allow the ice to conform better around the injury. Or, obtain a reusable ice pack from the freezer.

2. Explain the procedure to the patient.

3. Expose the area to be treated, draping the patient for modesty as appropriate.

4. When possible, use a wet elastic wrap or towel and place it between the ice bag and the patient's skin for best results. This is especially important if using a reusable or chemical ice pack, as burns may result if the packs are placed in direct contact with the skin. If neither a wet towel nor elastic wrap are available, placing the ice pack directly on the skin is acceptable.

5. Leave the ice in place for 20 to 30 minutes, checking with the patient periodically for signs of undue discomfort or cold allergy.

6. Leave the treatment area clean and dry when finished. Wipe up any water drops from the floor to prevent others from slipping. Discard towels in the place designated by the facility.

Ice Massage

Ice massage is commonly used for chronic tendonitis, chronic bursitis, and muscle strains. It may also be used prior to a workout to increase range of motion. Performed by massaging the affected area with ice, this is the only form of cryotherapy in which ice is applied directly to the skin (Figure 23-3). The usual treatment time is 7 to 10 minutes for a 5-inch-square area. This treatment can be done two to four times per day and should be performed in accordance with the cryotherapy guidelines.

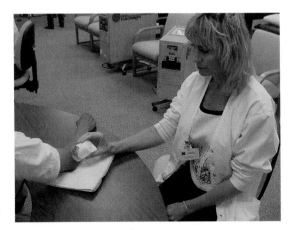

FIGURE 23-3 Ice massage is the only form of cryotherapy in which ice is applied directly to the skin.

> **ice massage**
>
> direct application of ice to the body to obtain a therapeutic numbing effect; used to decrease circulation, inflammation, muscle spasms, and pain in a local area.

To perform ice massage:

1. Prepare the ice by freezing a disposable cup three-quarters full of water, forming a cylinder of ice. Peel the cup from around the upper portion of the ice, exposing just enough of the ice to massage onto the area to be treated. The cup will shield the fingers from the cold as the procedure is performed. (**Note:** Styrofoam cups work best because of their insulating capabilities.)

2. Explain the procedure to the patient.

3. Expose the area to be treated, draping the patient for modesty as appropriate. Place towels around the patient to catch water drops.

4. The edges of the ice cups can be smoothed prior to the treatment by rubbing the exposed top on the hands before placing it on the injured area.

5. Slowly massage the ice over the injury in overlapping stokes, taking care not to cause the patient undue discomfort by the pressure of the strokes. Remove more of the styrofoam or paper from the cup as the ice melts.

6. After 7 to 10 minutes of treatment, dry the patient's skin and assist the patient from the treatment table. If draping was necessary and the patient's movements are hampered, assist the patient in getting dressed.

7. Leave the treatment area clean and dry when finished. Wipe up any water drops from the floor to prevent others from slipping. Discard used towels in the place designated by the facility.

Vapo-Coolant Sprays

vapo-coolant spray

an aerosol coolant used to quickly lower the temperature of superficial body tissues and decrease pain.

Vapo-coolant sprays have the ability to reduce muscle spasms and increase range of motion, but the effects of such sprays are momentary and superficial. These products distribute a fine cooling spray when the can is inverted and the nozzle is pressed (Figure 23-4). Vapo-coolant sprays are usually used in combination with stretching techniques to help break the muscle spasm/ pain cycle of soft tissue injuries. The most common use of vapo-coolants is in the treatment of lumbar strains, cervical strains, and hamstring injuries. These sprays are not applied to broken skin or to patients who are allergic to the spray. Treatments are applied as often as recommended by the physician or therapist.

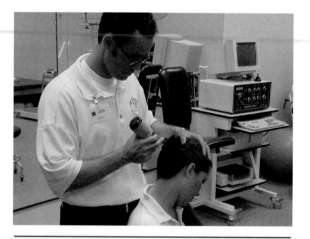

FIGURE 23-4 Vapo-coolant sprays can provide rapid pain relief to the superficial tissues.

To apply a vapo-coolant spray:

1. Make sure the room is well-ventilated and that no sparks or flames are present. Some of these products are flammable.

2. Explain the procedure to the patient.

3. Expose the area to be treated, draping the patient for modesty as appropriate.

4. Hold the nozzle of the bottle at a 30 to 45° angle, 12 inches from the patient's skin.

5. Spraying in one direction only, cover the entire muscle in a slow, sweeping manner. Avoid frosting the area by keeping the spray moving; never hold the spray in place over one area.

6. After a series of sprays, the therapist should passively stretch the area. Repeat four times, allowing the area to re-warm between each series of sweeps.

Ice Water Immersion

Ice water immersion of an injury requires the use of a small bucket or whirlpool bath filled with ice and cold water. The injured body part is immersed into the water (see Figure 23-5). Typical treatments last for 10 to 20 minutes. Longer treatments or colder water could lead to over-cooling of the tissues and may result in frostbite. Best suited for injuries to the hands, elbows, and feet, ice water immersion may be repeated throughout the day during waking hours, leaving an hour

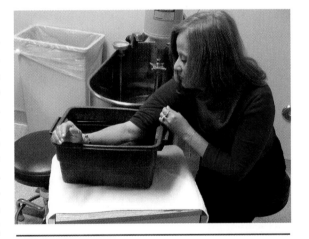

ice water immersion

the cooling of tissues through submersion in ice cold water; used to decrease circulation, inflammation, muscle spasms, edema, and pain in the treated area.

FIGURE 23-5 Water for cold water immersion therapy is kept at 50 to 60°F.

between treatments, as recommended by the physician or therapist. Ice water massage should be applied in accordance with the guidelines for cryotherapy.

To perform ice water immersion:

1. Fill a clean bucket or whirlpool with a mixture of ice and water to achieve a water temperature of 50 to 60°F.

2. Explain the procedure to the patient.

3. Expose the affected extremity.

4. Cleanse the area to be treated with soap and water, drying it thoroughly.

5. Explain the procedure to the patient.

6. To make the treatment more tolerable for the patient, neoprene caps may be placed on the toes or fingers of the extremity prior to immersion. Without the caps, the cold is felt most intensely in these areas.

7. Immerse the affected extremity into the cold water for 10 to 20 minutes.

8. Withdraw the extremity from the bath, gently drying it with clean towels.

9. To prevent infection, the container should always be cleaned with disinfectant and thoroughly dried with clean towels, or according to facility guidelines, after each use.

10. Leave the treatment area clean and dry when finished. Wipe up any water drops from the floor to prevent others from slipping. Discard used towels in the place designated by the facility.

Whirlpool Baths

whirlpool bath

a therapeutic bath of heated or cooled water in which all or part of the body is exposed to forceful, massaging currents in the water.

The **whirlpool bath** combines heated or cooled water with a massaging action to increase the treatment's effectiveness (see Figure 23-6). Whirlpools use both conduction and convection to achieve their therapeutic benefits. Conduction is achieved through the direct contact between the skin and the water. Convection occurs when the water swirls around the surface of the skin, facilitating heat exchange. Hot whirlpool baths can increase the elasticity of muscles and decrease pain and muscle spasms; cold whirlpool baths reduce edema, muscle spasms, and pain. Range-of-motion exercises may also be done in a whirlpool. Whirlpool baths should last 15 to 30 minutes.

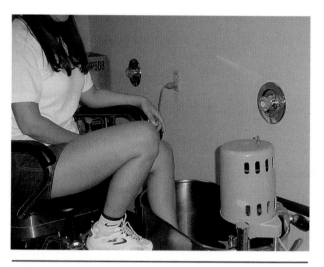

FIGURE 23-6 Therapeutic effects can be achieved in whirlpool baths using either heated or cooled water.

Remember that cold decreases circulation to reduce edema, pain, muscle spasms, and inflammation. Heat increases circulation to improve flexibility, reduce pain, and relieve muscle spasms. See the temperature table in Figure 23-7.

Temperatures for Whirlpool Baths

Description	Temperature	Effects
Cold whirlpool	55–65°F	Decreased bloodflow
Hot whirlpool (for extremities)	100–110°F	Increased bloodflow
Hot whirlpool (for full body)	94–100°F	Increased bloodflow

FIGURE 23-7 Temperatures for Whirlpool Baths

General guidelines for administering a whirlpool bath treatment follow:

1. Check to make sure that all electrical outlets have a ground fault circuit interrupter.

2. Check to see that the whirlpool is at an appropriate temperature, according to the chart in Figure 23-7.

3. Explain the procedure to the patient.

4. Expose the area to be treated. For full-body whirlpools, the patient will wear a swimsuit.

5. For the sake of hygiene, all immersed skin should be cleansed with soap and water prior to immersion.

6. Immerse the affected extremity or the entire body into the water for 15 to 30 minutes.

7. Instruct the patient not to operate the whirlpool's "on" or "off" switches, particularly when in the bath. Operation of any electrical appliances while in water may result in electrocution.

8. Ask the patient if the temperature is within a tolerable range.

9. Check back after 5 minutes to see how the patient is tolerating the temperature. Some people become light-headed in a heated full-body whirlpool.

10. Withdraw the extremity from the bath and provide the patient with a clean, dry towel. In the case of full-body immersion, assist the patient in exiting the bath and provide a clean, dry towel. Provide any additional assistance necessary.

11. Leave the treatment area clean and dry when finished. Wipe up any water drops from the floor to prevent others from slipping. Discard used towels in the place designated by the facility.

12. Cleanse and maintain the whirlpool according to manufacturer and facility guidelines. Such maintenance is vital in keeping the whirlpool, and the patients, free from infection. Expect the following instructions:

    * Empty the tank after each use.

    * Thoroughly scrub inside of the tank with a commercial disinfectant.

    * Rinse the tank with clear water and dry it with towels following the use of disinfectant.

THERMOTHERAPY

Heat therapies provide comfort by increasing circulation and decreasing localized pain, edema, muscle spasms, and joint stiffness. Heat also increases collagen elasticity to the area where the heat is applied. When recommended by a physician, thermotherapy may also be used to treat infections. The heat increases bloodflow to the area, promoting healing. To reduce the risk of cross-infection, Universal Precautions must be used when treating patients with open wounds or infections.

Methods of thermotherapy include moist heat packs, warm whirlpool baths, fluidotherapy, and paraffin baths. Moist heat packs are the most common form of heat therapy. Dry heat packs may also be used, but moist heat tends to penetrate the tissues better. When applying heat, keep in mind that superficial heating methods, such as heat packs and whirlpools, provide heat penetration to a depth of approximately 2 centimeters into the tissue. Deep-heating treatments, like ultrasound, can penetrate to a depth of approximately 5 centimeters, depending on the setting used.

Because heat is comforting to most people, there is less need to prepare the patient for initial discomfort as with cryotherapy, but professionalism still requires that the procedure be explained so the patient knows what to expect.

Guidelines for Thermotherapy

1. Never apply heat to an area where any loss of sensation exists; burns could occur without the client being aware of it.

2. Never apply heat immediately after an injury. Heat will increase swelling in the acute phase.

3. Never apply heat directly to the eyes or the genitalia, as burns may occur.

4. Never apply heat to the abdomen if there is a possibility that the patient is pregnant. The heat could injure the fetus.

5. Never apply any form of heat on an open wound, a burn, or over an area of malignancy. Infected areas should also be avoided unless the treatment is approved by a physician. Heat may aggravate these conditions.

6. To reduce the risk of complications, do not use thermotherapy on patients with a history of reduced thermal regulation or diabetes.

7. To avoid further injury to the tissues, always monitor the time for which thermotherapy is applied, and use appropriate padding or towels.

Moist Heat Packs

hydrocollator pack

a moist heat pack used to increase circulation and flexibility as well as to decrease pain and muscle spasms in the treated area.

Moist heat packs, or **hydrocollator packs**, are a method of heating through conduction. The major benefits of using moist heat packs is relaxation of the muscle area and reduction in the muscle spasm/pain cycle. They are used for subacute to chronic pain (Figure 23-8).

One of the primary limitations of moist heat packs is that the deeper tissues, insulated by the layer of fat just beneath the skin, do not receive the effects of the heat therapy. However, a great deal of heat may be transmitted to the

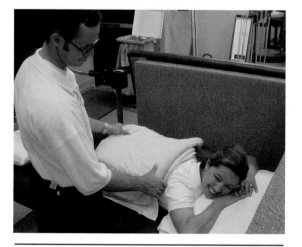

FIGURE 23-8 Moist heat packs are an easy way to reduce pain and muscle spasms.

superficial tissues during this treatment, so make sure to place several layers of dry towels between the patient's skin and the heat pack. Many commercial heat packs come with protective coverings that help protect the skin, but additional protection is considered wise. To prevent bacteria from growing in the heat packs, they should be cleaned and the water in them replaced once a week or according to manufacturer's guidelines. The treatment time for a heat pack is usually 15 to 20 minutes.

To apply a heat pack, use the thermotherapy guidelines and follow these steps:

1. Prepare the moist heat pack according to manufacturer's directions.

2. Explain the procedure to the patient.

3. Expose the area to be treated, draping the patient for modesty as appropriate.

4. To avoid burning the patient, place two or more layers of towels between the heat pack and the patient's skin.

5. Ask the patient if the temperature of the heat pack is within a tolerable range, and make adjustments as necessary.

6. Leave the pack in place for 15 to 20 minutes, checking with the patient periodically for signs of undue discomfort. As the heat pack starts to cool, layers of the towels may be removed, allowing more of the heat to reach the skin. Always check back after doing so to make sure the patient is comfortable at all times and to ensure that the pack is not too hot or too cold.

7. Leave the treatment area clean when finished, discarding used towels in the place designated by the facility.

Fluidotherapy

Using cellulose particles and the circulation of air, **fluidotherapy** utilizes much higher temperatures than those used in water modalities. In spite of its name, no water is used in this method of thermotherapy; therefore, fluidotherapy is often referred to as a "dry" whirlpool. The fluidotherapy unit disperses the cellulose particles in a whirlwind of hot air. Because of the size of the fluidotherapy units, treatment is usually limited to extremities (see Figure 23-9). Like other heat

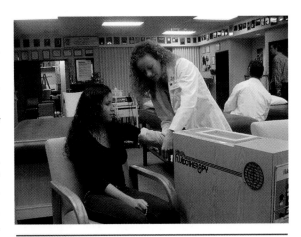

FIGURE 23-9 Fluidotherapy is often called a "dry" whirlpool.

> **fluidotherapy**
>
> a "dry" whirlpool, in which cellulose particles are dispersed in a whirlwind of heated air to decrease pain and muscle spasms as well as to increase flexibility and circulation in the treated area.

modalities, fluidotherapy helps to decrease pain, muscle spasms, and edema, and increase flexibility and bloodflow. The temperature of the treatment usually ranges from 102 to 120°F. The treatment time is 15 to 20 minutes. The patient is allowed to exercise and perform ROM activities during the treatment. Treatment should follow thermotherapy guidelines. Fluidotherapy should not be used on uncovered wounds or areas with extremely poor circulation.

General instructions for performing fluidotherapy follow:

1. Explain the procedure to the patient.

2. Expose the area to be treated.

3. Cleanse the affected extremity with soap and water. Dry it thoroughly.

4. Make sure the fluidotherapy unit is plugged in and set to the temperature recommended by the manufacturer or facility.

5. Insert the affected extremity in the fluidotherapy unit and turn the power switch to the "on" position. Instruct the patient to perform ROM exercises, as recommended by the physician or therapist.

6. After 15 to 20 minutes of treatment, or the length of time recommended by the manufacturer, withdraw the affected extremity from the unit.

7. Leave the treatment area clean and dry when finished.

8. To prevent infection and ensure safe use, follow the manufacturer's instructions for cleaning and maintaining the fluidotherapy unit.

Paraffin Bath

paraffin bath

the immersion of a body part in melted paraffin to increase circulation and flexibility as well as to decrease pain and muscle spasms.

The **paraffin bath** consists of a mixture of seven parts wax to one part mineral oil and is maintained at a temperature of 118 to 127°F. Plastic bags, paper towels, and cloth towels are also needed to provide this treatment. The paraffin remains on the skin, retaining the heat and allowing it to reach a deep-tissue level. The paraffin bath is often used for treating chronic inflammation injuries, such as arthritis, bursitis, tendonitis, and epicondylitis, of the hands, wrists, elbows, ankles, and/or feet. It may also be used for subacute sprains and strains and/or loss of ROM in the distal extremities. It should not be used on open wounds or areas with extremely poor circulation. Special caution should be made to make sure that any part of the body that comes in contact with the paraffin bath is cleansed prior to treatment; this will avoid contaminating the paraffin mixture. Also, the patient should be closely observed for signs of discomfort or potential burns during the treatment. All thermotherapy guidelines should be followed.

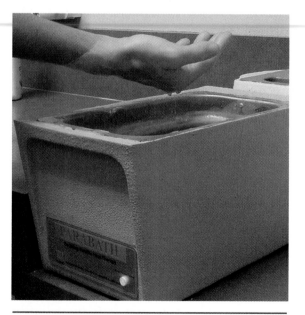

Application of the paraffin bath treatment can be accomplished in several ways. The most common methods of applying the paraffin mixture are dipping and soaking (see Figure 23-10). Always use caution when administering a

FIGURE 23-10 A paraffin bath can be applied as either a "dip" or a "soak."

paraffin bath—burns may result if the paraffin is too hot. If applying the paraffin to the hands, it is important to warn the patient that the paraffin treatment will temporarily make the hands slippery, creating the potential for items to be dropped accidentally.

General guidelines for administering a paraffin dip follow:

1. Heat the paraffin mixture (seven parts paraffin to one part mineral oil) to 118 to 127°F, according to the manufacturer's instructions.

2. Explain the procedure to the patient.

3. Cleanse and dry the affected extremity before immersing it in the paraffin mixture.

4. If the dipping method is used, the cleansed extremity is then dipped into the paraffin bath and quickly pulled out. Repeat six times until the coating is approximately ¼ to ½ inch thick. If applying paraffin to the hands, make sure to keep the fingers apart and in the same position during each dip. This technique allows the wax to dry and form a solid cover. To achieve the full effect of the treatment, all areas of the extremity must be equally covered with paraffin.

5. When the dipping is complete, cover the coated extremity with a plastic bag and wrap it in a towel. The paraffin treatment is left on for 15 to 20 minutes or until heat is no longer generated.

6. Peel off the wax with the aid of a tongue depressor, and put the wax back into the container for re-use.

7. Proper hygiene requires that the paraffin in the container be changed periodically. Follow the manufacturer's guidelines.

8. Leave the treatment area clean when finished.

The paraffin soak is similar to the paraffin dip. The difference is that after the extremity is dipped six times and the wax coating has dried, the extremity is placed in the hot wax container for 15 to 20 minutes. The process of convection, obtained from the heat of the surrounding paraffin, makes the heating benefits of this technique last longer than the dip.

ELECTRICAL MODALITIES

Electrical modalities use electricity to influence healing by stimulating the body tissues. Like the other therapeutic modalities, electrical modalities are used to speed the healing of tissues. Because electrical modalities penetrate deeper into the tissues than other modalities, they are among the most effective in terms of decreasing healing time. In general, low-voltage stimulation is used to help control pain and high-voltage stimulation is used to increase bloodflow. General instructions for the electrical modalities follow, but should *not* be interpreted as sufficient instruction for therapeutic use in any environment.

electrical modality

rehabilitative treatment that uses electrical current to achieve therapeutic effects.

Guidelines for Electrical Modalities

Administration of electrical modalities requires special training beyond the scope of this book. Furthermore, procedures will vary according to the modality and equipment used. Some general guidelines follow:

1. Follow the physician or therapist's orders for all electrical modalities.

2. Make sure the equipment is in proper working order, is plugged in, and is powered through a circuit served by a ground fault interrupter.

3. Explain the procedure to the patient.

4. Expose the area to be treated.

5. Cleanse the treatment area with soap and water or alcohol. Then, dry it thoroughly. (Cleansing the patient's skin of dirt and oils will ensure proper adhesion of the electrode pads.)

6. Place electrode pads according to the manufacturer's instructions.

7. Avoid prolonged point contact when using ultrasound.

8. Follow the manufacturer's instructions for use of all equipment. Improper use may cause burns.

9. Turn the treatment channel(s) off before carefully removing the adhesive electrodes from the patient's skin.

10. Leave the treatment area clean when finished.

11. To prevent infection and ensure safe use, follow the manufacturer's instructions for cleaning and maintaining the unit.

12. Never use an electrical modality on an open wound.

13. Do not use electrical modalities on a patient with a pacemaker without approval from a physician. The electrical current may interfere with the pace of the heart set by the pacemaker.

14. Avoid high-fluid areas of the body (the eyes, ears, genitals, brain, spinal cord, heart) when using electrical modalities. The electrical current may be intensified by high concentrations of fluid, causing burns.

15. Avoid using electrical modalities over the carotid arteries as this could change blood pressure and cause the patient to faint.

16. Electrical modalities should never be used on the trunk of a pregnant patient. Their use on the extremities is permitted upon approval by the physician.

17. Stop the treatment if the procedure increases the patient's pain.

Ultrasound Therapy

Ultrasound is a high-frequency sound wave converted to heat (see Figure 23-11). Because it is one of the deepest penetrating heat sources available and can reach depths of 3 to 5 centimeters, ultrasound is one of the more commonly used modalities. Frequently used for subacute pain, inflammation, and muscle spasms, **ultrasound therapy** is applied with a sound head. A coupling medium is also used to help the sound waves penetrate the skin and stimulate the bloodflow in the treated area.

There is a wide variety of coupling mediums available, including water-soluble creams and conductive gels. The coupling medium ensures an airtight contact between the skin and the ultrasonic waves generated by the mechanical head; it also reduces

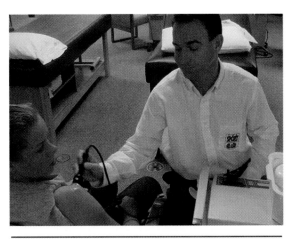

FIGURE 23-11 Ultrasound is an effective and frequently used method of thermotherapy.

ultrasound therapy

the application of sound waves to a body area to increase circulation and flexibility as well as to decrease pain and muscle spasms in that area.

friction against the skin, which allows the sound head to glide smoothly over the body surface and provide an even distribution of heat. When using the water-soluble medium, the skin should be thoroughly washed and dried before applying the medium to prevent air bubbles that hamper the flow of the sound waves to the skin.

When using ultrasound, the sound head is moved in a slow, circular pattern or a stroking method. The sound head must be kept in constant motion; if left in one spot for a prolonged time, the patient could be burned, or the ultrasound head can be damaged.

The intensity of the ultrasound varies according to the depth and density of the tissue and the type of the injury. Controls on the ultrasound machine allow the user to change settings to adjust to various depths and intensities. For example, 0.1 to 0.8 watts/cm² is regarded as low intensity, while 0.8 to 1.5 watts/cm² is medium intensity, and 1.5 to 3.0 watts/cm² is high intensity. The duration of an ultrasound treatment is 3 to 8 minutes. These treatments can range from daily use to three times per week.

Ultrasound cannot be applied to high-fluid areas of the body, such as the eyes, ears, genitals, brain, spinal cord, or heart. Reproductive organs in women who are pregnant must also be avoided. Acute injuries and areas with extremely poor circulation should not be treated with ultrasound. The epiphyseal plate areas in children, stress fractures, open wounds, hemhorrages, and infected, inflamed, or malignant areas also should not be treated with ultrasound. Ultrasound therapy should not be applied to an area that exceeds 3 to 4 inches in diameter in one treatment. If the area treated is larger than 3 to 4 inches, then the tissue does not receive the concentration of ultrasound needed for adequate treatment; in such cases, the ultrasound application will require more than one treatment.

Because airtight contact between the skin and the sound waves is so important, ultrasound therapy is applied underwater to irregularly shaped body areas such as wrist, hand, elbow, ankle, and foot. The water provides an airtight coupling that allows the sound waves to travel at a constant velocity to the extremity, so no additional coupling medium is necessary. To accomplish this, the extremity is fully immersed in the water and the ultrasound head is positioned approximately 1 inch from the body part that will be treated. As with other ultrasound treatments, the sound head should be moved slowly in a circular or stroking pattern to cover the treatment area. Air bubbles that attach to the skin must be wiped away continually.

Phonophoresis uses ultrasound waves to drive therapeutic agents, such as a 10% hydrocortisone or dexamethasone, into body tissues. In this method, the therapeutic agent is used along with the coupling medium. The machine setting for this type of ultrasound treatment is usually 50%, pulsed (not continuous), with an intensity of 2.0 watts/cm². Another common setting is 100%, continuous, with an intensity of 1.5 watts/cm².

Ultrasound can also be combined with electrical muscle stimulation. This treatment combines the deep heating effect of ultrasound stimulation and the benefits of muscle contractions provided by electrical muscle stimulation. The duration of this treatment is generally 5 to 15 minutes.

Electrical Muscle Stimulation (EMS)

electrical muscle stimulation (EMS)

also known as neuromuscular stimulation (NMS); the use of electrical stimulation to re-educate injured muscles, strengthen healthy muscles, and slow the effects of atrophy in a given area.

The primary uses of **electrical muscle stimulation (EMS)**, or neuromuscular stimulation, are to re-educate injured or impaired muscles, slow the effects of atrophy, and increase the strength of healthy muscles through electrical stimulation. The EMS machine consists of pads, wires, and the control unit. The pads are placed on the patient's skin at both ends of the muscle (see Figure 23-12). Wires attached to these pads connect to the control unit, which is used to set the intensity and duration of the treatment. EMS should not be used over carotid arteries, cardiac pacemakers, high fluid areas, or a pregnant uterus. Duration of treatment is generally 10 to 20 minutes.

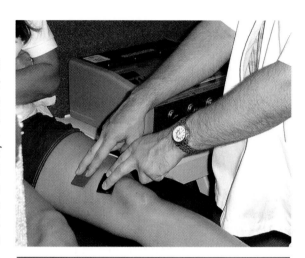

FIGURE 23-12 The therapeutic effects of EMS depend largely on the polarity of the current.

Galvanic Stimulation

galvanic stimulation

the use of a direct electrical current to regulate circulation as well as to decrease pain, edema, and muscle spasms in a given area of the body.

This modality uses a high- or low-voltage galvanic, or direct, current for therapeutic purposes. **Galvanic stimulation** is used in the treatment of contusions, sprains, strains, and acute edema. In this treatment, the patient is connected to the galvanic stimulator through the attachment of two positive pads and one negative pad connected to the machine by wires (see Figure 23-13). The patient will

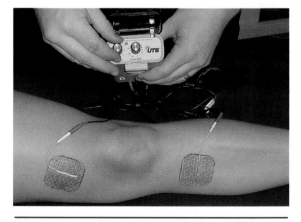

FIGURE 23-13 Medical galvanism uses direct current to regulate bloodflow.

experience a change in circulation to the body part between the electrodes. Galvanic stimulation may also speed the elimination of cellular waste products. It should not be used over a cardiac pacemaker, the carotid arteries, high fluid areas, or a pregnant uterus. Follow the physician's, therapist's, or manufacturer's guidelines in the use of galvanic stimulation. This modality may also be used with heat packs or ice packs. Duration of treatment is generally 10 to 20 minutes.

The physiologic responses in the body, such as vasodilation, that result from galvanic stimulation depend on the polarity of the current, as shown in Figure 23-14.

Polarity and Galvanic Stimulation Effects	
Negative Polarity	**Positive Polarity**
Vasoconstriction	Vasodilatation
Hardens tissues	Softens tissues
Local analgesic	Increases nerve excitability
Decreases nerve excitability	Increases venous and lymphatic return

FIGURE 23-14 Polarity and Its Effects on Galvanic Stimulation

Interferential Stimulation (IFS)

Interferential stimulation (IFS) uses interfering electrical currents to regulate bloodflow, reduce pain, decrease edema, relieve muscle spasms, and strengthen muscle tissue. Used in the treatment of contusions, sprains, strains, and a variety of other injuries, IFS uses two generators and four electrodes to produce two currents that act on the tissues simultaneously. The patient is connected to the generators through the attachment of pads, or electrodes, connected to the units by wires. The four pads are placed in a square pattern in which two pairs of opposing pads will each produce a current that will intersect with each other at a midpoint, causing interference. This interference then causes the currents to spread from the point of intersection to the surrounding tissues. The patient should feel only a slight vibrating sensation beneath and between the pads. IFS may also be used in conjunction with heat packs or ice packs (see Figure 23-15).

Settings used for IFS should follow the physician's, therapist's, or manufacturer's guidelines. IFS therapy

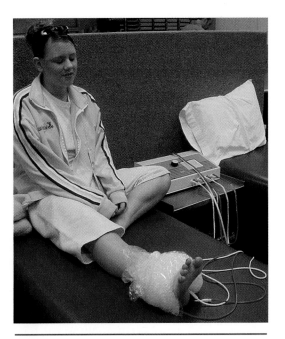

FIGURE 23-15 Interferential stimulation uses two "interfering" electrical currents to achieve therapeutic effects.

interferential stimulation (IFS)

the use of interfering electrical currents to increase circulation and flexibility as well as to decrease pain and muscle spasms in a given area of the body.

may be done once a week or several times a day, depending on the physician's or therapist's recommendations and should last an average of 15 minutes per treatment. IFS should not be used over carotid arteries or high fluid areas, for undiagnosed pain, or for prolonged periods. Individuals with a pacemaker and women who are pregnant should not use an interferential device without consulting a physician.

Iontophoresis

iontophoresis
the administration of ionized medications to the tissues through the use of an electrical current.

Similar to the way in which phonophoresis uses ultrasound to drive therapeutic agents into the skin, **iontophoresis** uses electricity to drive medications, such as dexamethasone and hydrocortisone, through the skin and into superficial tissues. A painless treatment, iontophoresis uses an electrical current that passes from the positive electrode to the negative electrode to administer the ionized medications to the tissues. Pads and wires are used to connect the patient to the machine (see Figure 23-16). One pad

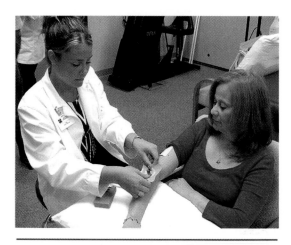

FIGURE 23-16 Iontophoresis drives ionized medications into superficial tissues.

delivers the medication, and the other pad serves as a ground. This modality can be used for superficial tendonitis and bursitis to decrease edema, inflammation, and pain. Iontophoresis should not be used on pregnant women without a physician's approval, or over the eyes, carotid arteries, unhealed wounds, pacemakers, or new scar tissue. Treatment time ranges from 5 to 10 minutes, once per day, or as recommended by the manufacturer, physician, or therapist.

Transcutaneous Electrical Nerve Stimulation (TENS)

This modality is used primarily for pain control. Electrodes are placed on the skin over the painful area to block the sensation of chronic or acute pain (see Figure 23-17). The

transcutaneous electrical nerve stimulation (TENS)
the use of electrical current to block the sensation of pain to a given area of the body.

use of **transcutaneous electrical nerve stimulation (TENS)** can cause a muscle contraction, so this modality must be used with caution. TENS does not have to be administered continually to be effective. Often, a 30-minute to 1-hour application will relieve pain for hours after the treatment. However, stimulation of the muscle must be controlled or it will cause undesired tension. The use of TENS therapy may allow a patient to perform therapeutic exercise without pain. The TENS electrodes must not be placed over the

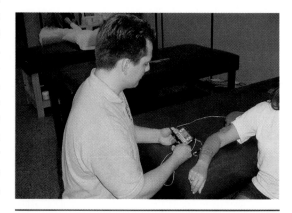

FIGURE 23-17 TENS is often effective in reducing pain in a treated area.

carotid arteries, metal implants, high fluid areas, the abdomen of a pregnant woman, or where there is a pacemaker. Additional contraindications include undiagnosed pain, hypertension, diabetes, or an allergic reaction to the tape, gel, or electrodes.

Diathermy

Therapeutic **diathermy** uses a high-frequency electrical current to heat the body's tissue. Diathermy will increase the bloodflow and tissue metabolism; it also decreases deep muscle spasms. This treatment can be used for chronic sprains and strains, limited ROM, and subacute inflammations, such as bursitis, epicondylitis, tendonitis, and arthritis—but it is not used for acute inflammation, hemorrhages, or nondraining infections, or in body areas where moisture, casts, metal implants, or screws are present. Metal and moisture will concentrate the current and may cause burns. Additional areas to avoid include epiphyseal plates, open wounds, and areas with extremely limited circulation, or malignancy. Diathermy should not be used on pregnant women, hemophilia patients, or patients with pacemakers without physician approval.

Properly used, diathermy will heat the tissues to 104 to 112°F at a depth of about 2 inches from the skin's surface. The treatment time is 20 minutes. The patient should feel only the sensation of mild warmth when undergoing diathermy. Any moisture resulting from the treatment should be removed with a clean towel as the treatment is being performed.

> **diathermy**
>
> the therapeutic use of a high-frequency electrical current to increase circulation and flexibility as well as to decrease pain and muscle spasms in a given area of the body.

MECHANICAL MODALITIES

Mechanical modalities, such as intermittent compression, traction, and massage therapy, assist in healing by exerting pressure to the soft tissues, increasing circulation and/or distracting (pulling) bony structures. This pressure can be applied manually or with a device. Joint mobilization and myofascial release, performed by osteopaths, chiropractors, physical therapists, and certified athletic trainers are also mechanical modalities, but are beyond the scope of this text because of the amount of training required to use them. General instructions for the mechanical modalities follow, but should *not* be interpreted as sufficient instruction for therapeutic use in a professional environment.

> **mechanical modality**
>
> rehabilitative treatment that uses external force to increase or decrease circulation and reduce pain.

Guidelines for Mechanical Modalities

Like the electrical modalities, administration of mechanical modalities requires special training beyond the scope of this book. However, some general guidelines follow:

1. Follow the manufacturer's instructions for use of all equipment.

2. Frequent circulation checks of extremities are important when applying traction.

3. Stop the treatment if the procedure increases the patient's pain.

Intermittent Compression

Intermittent compression is used to control or reduce edema following an acute injury to an extremity. In this treatment, the injured extremity is placed inside a

> **intermittent compression**
>
> the periodic application of compression to a part of the body to reduce edema in that area.

compression sleeve and, if possible, elevated above the patient's heart. This sleeve is then inflated periodically to a specific pressure that forces excessive fluid from the area of injury (see Figure 23-18).

There are four parameters that may be adjusted on intermittent compression devices: compression time, inflation pressure, temperature, and treatment time. Manufacturers will make recommendations for compression times, which will vary from machine to machine. Frequently, inflation of 30 to 40 seconds is followed by 30 to 40 seconds of deflation.

Manufacturers' recommendations for pressure settings vary from machine to machine. They commonly recommend pressure settings of 50 to 90 mm/Hg, but

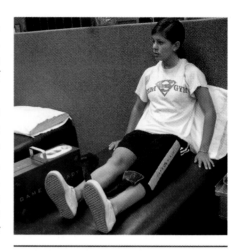

FIGURE 23-18 Intermittent compression with cold can be used to help reduce edema.

because arteriole capillary pressure is approximately 30 mm/Hg, any pressure that exceeds this figure should help reduce the swelling. Furthermore, the machine's pressure must not exceed the patient's diastolic blood pressure. Too much pressure may cause the patient additional discomfort, so always ask how the treatment feels and listen to what the patient says. If the recommended pressure or temperature causes undue discomfort to the patient, stop the treatment. It is not used over high fluid areas or acute fractures. Additional contraindications include infection, pulmonary edema, and congestive heart failure.

Intermittent compression treatments generally last for 15 to 30 minutes. Other modalities can also be added to the intermittent compression treatments; for example, an electrical stimulating current can be used to help pump fluid from the injured area during the compression treatments.

Traction

traction

the distraction, or pulling, of a body part or segment for rehabilitative purposes.

Traction is the rehabilitative distraction, or pulling, of a body part or segment (see Figure 23-19). Cervical and lumbar traction is used to relieve joint pain and muscle spasms and to treat conditions such as degenerative joint disease, herniated disks, spinal nerve impingement or inflammation, joint hypomobility, and spondylolisthesis. Different effects can be achieved by altering the treatment variables, including the load of traction, the position of the patient, and the duration of the treatment. Traction can be applied in various ways: continuously, intermittently, manually, or gravitationally. The amount of weight varies according to the type of traction used. For example, cervical traction weight

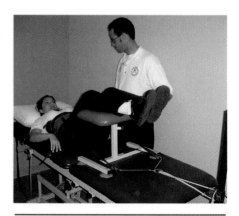

FIGURE 23-19 Traction can be applied continuously, intermittently, manually, or gravitationally. Continuous lumbar traction is shown here.

may range from 10 to 20 pounds, and lumbar traction weight may range from 65 to 200 pounds. As with all modalities, it is also important to follow manufacturers' guidelines in the use of equipment and to listen to what the patient says. Always avoid causing undue discomfort.

Continuous traction is applied for several hours with low weight. Static traction treatments can range from a few minutes up to 30 minutes without a rest cycle, depending on the physician's or therapist's recommendation. Intermittent traction is applied and released periodically during the course of the treatment, and may occur as often as 16 times per minute. Gravitational traction uses a portion of the patient's body weight as a source of pull. If the pain spreads to surrounding areas, traction treatments should be discontinued.

The use of traction should be avoided for three to five days following an acute injury such as a sprain and in cases of pregnancy, unstable vertebrae, fractures, decreased circulation, bone cancer, osteoporosis, possible tumors, bone diseases, and some joint diseases. If pain increases or radiates during or after treatment, stop the treatment and consult a physician.

Massage Therapy

Massage is the systematic manipulation, methodical pressure, friction, and kneading of the soft tissues of the body. It is used to stimulate muscles, decrease muscle spasms, increase circulation, decrease edema, and promote relaxation (see Figure 23-20). There are five types of massage: effleurage, pétrissage, deep friction, tapotement, and vibration. Lubricants, such as oil, lanolin, powder, analgesic balms, or special massage lotions, may be used with any of these forms of massage to decrease the skin friction.

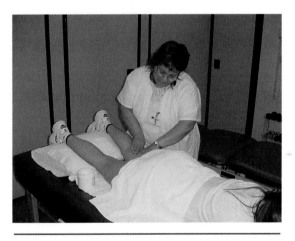

FIGURE 23-20 Massage therapy is used to stimulate muscles, decrease muscle spasms, increase circulation, decrease edema, and promote relaxation.

massage
the systematic manipulation, methodical pressure, friction, and kneading of the soft tissues of the body to increase circulation, decrease pain, and promote relaxation.

Effleurage: Consists of strokes that glide over the skin without attempting to move the deep muscle group. This form of massage is done with either the palms or the fingers. Usually, effleurage is used to either begin or end a massage treatment; it may also be used to detect muscle tightness.

Pétrissage: Done by kneading the soft tissues between the thumb and forefinger or with the palm of the hand. The rolling and twisting motion of the tissue stimulates fluid drainage. Fluid drainage is beneficial to the patient because it eliminates cellular waste from the tissues.

Deep Friction: Massage performed primarily on joints and areas with little soft tissue. The thumbs and fingers are rotated on the skin in a circular pattern, applying enough pressure to contact the underlying tissue. An alternative to the circular pattern of deep friction massage is transverse friction. In transverse friction massage, the strokes are applied in a transverse pattern over a tendon. The effects of friction massage are to increase circulation and decrease scar tissue.

Tapotement: Also called percussion; involves "beating" the hands or fingers upon the skin. This form of massage can be done using clenched hands, the palms of the hand, the ulnar borders of the palms, or the fingertips. Care is taken to avoid inducing pain by contacting the person too harshly.

Vibration: Massage that makes use of a vibrating machine or quick motions of the fingers to produce therapeutic benefits. The benefits of vibration are increased circulation and lymphatic drainage. Vibration massage also provides a mild stretch of the superficial tissues, which is beneficial because it increases the elasticity of those tissues.

Massage is contraindicated over acute contusions, sprains, strains, fractures, open wounds, or areas of infection or malignancy. Patients with acute phlebitis, thrombosis, cellulitis, synovitis, arteriosclerosis, and severe varicose veins are also contraindicated. Although beneficial to overall healing of tissues, massage does not strengthen muscles, increase muscle tone, cause nerve growth, or remove adipose tissue.

General guidelines for performing a massage follow:

1. Expose the area to be massaged and drape the patient to provide warmth and maintain professional standards of modesty, making sure to have good access to the area. (Never massage an infected area or over a recent injury.)

2. Position the patient as comfortably as possible.

3. Apply a light lubricant to the body area.

4. Begin with light massage strokes (effleurage). Deeper, heavier massage may follow, depending upon the client's comfort level and therapeutic needs. Watch the patient's face and/or body movements to monitor the client's tolerance to different levels of massage pressure. Avoid harsh massage strokes that cause undue discomfort to the patient.

5. Keeping one hand on the patient's body at all times, lets the patient know where the therapist is in relation to the body. It also helps to avoid startling the patient with an unexpected touch.

6. When reduction of edema is the goal, stroke from below the injury site toward the heart.

7. Maintain a steady rhythm during the massage and end the session with light massage strokes. The last step in giving the treatment is to remove the massage lubricant. This is done with a clean, dry towel.

8. Leave the treatment area clean when finished. Discard used towels in the place designated by the facility.

Figure 23-21 provides some guidelines on effects and uses of therapeutic modalities.

Guidelines for Effects and Uses of Therapeutic Modalities

Modality	Therapeutic Effect	Indications	Contraindications
Cryotherapy	decreases circulation; relieves pain; controls swelling; decreases muscle spasms	acute/chronic pain; muscle spasms	decreased sensation or circulation; diabetes; cardiac condition; Raynaud's phenomenon; uncovered wounds
Ice Pack	decreases circulation; relieves pain; controls swelling; decreases muscle spasms	acute/chronic pain; muscle spasms; first-degree burns	redness and swelling associated with a rash; see cryotherapy
Ice Massage	decreases circulation, then increases bloodflow to the area once the treatment has ended; decreases muscle soreness; decreases pain	chronic tendonitis and bursitis; muscle strains	not for acute injuries; pressure of massage may irritate some injuries; see cryotherapy
Vapo-Coolant Spray	increases ROM; decreases muscle spasms and pain	muscle spasms; decreased ROM; lumbar and cervical strains; hamstring injuries	can cause frostbite; allergy to spray; open wounds; eyes
Ice Water Immersion	used on extremities; reduces temperature quickly; reduces edema; decreases circulation, inflammation, pain and muscle spasms	acute injuries of extremities	redness and swelling associated with a rash; see cryotherapy
Whirlpool Bath	cold: decreases circulation, pain, muscle spasms, and edema hot: increases circulation and flexibility; decreases pain and muscle spasms	cold: edema; muscle spasms; pain hot: muscle stiffness; pain; muscle spasms	cold: temperature regulating deficiency, areas of malignancy; see cryotherapy hot: see thermotherapy
Thermotherapy	increases circulation; decreases pain and muscle spasms; promotes tissue healing; fights infection	subacute or chronic injuries; edema; muscle spasms; some infections; joint stiffness	acute injuries; inflammation; impaired circulation or sensation; areas of malignancy; reduced thermal regulation; diabetes; open wounds; some infections; over eyes, genitalia, or pregnant abdomen
Moist Heat Pack	increases circulation and flexibility; decreases muscle spasms and pain; relaxes muscles	subacute to chronic pain	see thermotherapy
Fluidotherapy	increases circulation and flexibility; decreases edema and muscle spasms	subacute injuries; edema; muscles spasms; can only be used on certain areas of the body	open wounds (cover first); extremely poor local circulation; see thermotherapy

FIGURE 23-21 Guidelines for Effects and Uses of Therapeutic Modalities

Modality	Therapeutic Effect	Indications	Contraindications
Paraffin Bath	increases circulation and flexibility; decreases pain; for hands, feet, and elbows	chronic inflammation; bursitis; tendonitis; epicondylitis; arthritis; deep muscle spasms; subacute sprains and strains; loss of ROM	extremely poor local circulation; see thermotherapy
Ultrasound Therapy	increases circulation and flexibility; decreases pain; decreases muscle spasms	subacute pain, inflammation, and muscle spasms	areas of acute injury; hemorrhages; areas of infection, extremely poor circulation, or suspected malignancy; stress fracture sites; epiphyseal growth plates; over high fluid areas (eyes, ears, brain, heart, spine, or genitals)
EMS or NMS	re-educates injured muscles; strengthens healthy muscles; slows atrophy	muscle atrophy, decreased mobility	over a cardiac pacemaker or the carotid arteries; over high fluid areas (eyes, ears, brain, heart, spine, or genitals)
Medical Galvanism	regulates circulation; decreases pain, edema, and muscle spasms	pain; decreased circulation; edema; muscle spasms; contusions, sprains, and strains	over a cardiac pacemaker or the carotid arteries; over high fluid areas (eyes, ears, brain, heart, spine, or genitals)
IFS	regulates circulation; strengthens muscle tissue; increases flexibility; decreases pain, edema, and muscle spasms	decreased or increased circulation; pain; muscle spasms; contusions; sprains; strains; edema	over a cardiac pacemaker or the carotid arteries; over high fluid areas (eyes, ears, brain, heart, spine, or genitals); undiagnosed pain; pregnancy; prolonged use
Iontophoresis	reduces edema, pain, and inflammation; drives medications into damaged tissue	inflammation; tendonitis; bursitis	over a cardiac pacemaker, the carotid arteries, unhealed wounds, or new scar tissue; pregnancy; over high fluid areas (eyes, ears, brain, heart, spine, or genitals)
TENS	decreases pain	pain	over a cardiac pacemaker, the carotid arteries, or metal implants; over high fluid areas (eyes, ears, brain, heart, spine, or genitals); undiagnosed pain; pregnancy; hypertension; diabetes; allergic reaction from tape, gel, or electrodes
Diathermy	increases circulation and flexibility; decreases pain and muscle spasms	subacute inflammation; bursitis; tendonitis; epicondylitis; arthritis; deep muscle spasms; arthritis; chronic sprains and strains; limited ROM	over internal or external metal objects, open wounds, or epiphyseal plates; pacemakers; over high fluid areas (eyes, ears, brain, heart, spine, or genitals); areas of hemhorrage, malignancy, acute inflammation, moisture, or extremely poor circulation; hemophilia; pregnancy

FIGURE 23-21 Guidelines for Effects and Uses of Therapeutic Modalities *(Continued)*

Modality	Therapeutic Effect	Indications	Contraindications
Intermittent Compression	decreases edema	edema	infection; over high fluid areas (eyes, ears, brain, heart, spine, or genitals); over acute fractures; pulmonary edema; congestive heart failure; pressures above patient's diastolic blood pressure
Traction	increases the amount of separation between bones, easing pain and nerve impingements	muscle spasms; joint pain; degenerative joint disease; herniated disks; spinal nerve impingement or inflammation; joint hypomobility; spondylolisthesis	unstable vertebrae; fractures; decreased circulation; osteoporosis; bone cancer; increased or radiating pain during or after treatment; pregnancy; acute injuries; possible tumors; bone diseases; some joint diseases
Massage	increases circulation; decreases pain, edema, and muscles spasms; promotes relaxation	edema; pain; tension muscle fatigue or weakness; muscle spasms; decreased circulation	acute contusions, sprains, or strains; fracture sites; open wounds; infections; acute phlebitis; thrombosis; severe varicose veins, cellulitis; synovitis; arteriosclerosis; areas of malignancy

FIGURE 23-21 Guidelines for Effects and Uses of Therapeutic Modalities *(Continued)*

THINKING IT THROUGH

It was the second half of the North versus Poly girls' basketball game. While grabbing a rebound, Lea's foot landed on Emilee's foot, causing Leah to fall. Vic, the athletic trainer, went to Lea's aid immediately. Still on the floor, Lea was rocking back and forth in pain and holding her ankle. Vic decided to take her to the training room for a thorough evaluation, away from all the spectators.

After helping her to the training room, Vic took off both of Lea's shoes and performed an evaluation. The involved ankle had already started to swell and Lea was still in a lot of pain. Suspecting a sprain, Vic made immediate use of the appropriate therapeutic modality to begin Lea's treatment. He also called the team physician, Dr. Wall, for a diagnosis and to make sure there was no fracture.

Dr. Wall came in and examined the ankle. He suspected a sprain, but ordered x-rays to rule out a fracture. So, they transported Lea to the clinic for x-rays. After looking at her films, Dr. Wall concluded that the injury was, indeed, a sprain—somewhere between first- and second-degree. He said that Lea would probably be out for up to two weeks.

Lea immediately freaked out. Play-offs were in two weeks and she intended to play. Coach Harris was also concerned; she wanted what was best for Lea, but Lea was very important to the team's success. Both Lea and the coach relayed their concerns to Dr. Wall and to Vic.

What type of modality would Vic have used immediately in the training room? Why did Vic take off both shoes, rather than just the one on the involved foot? What modalities should be used on Lea for the first three days? When would you change modalities, and what would you use? Discuss what you would do to get Lea back on the court as quickly as possible without causing more injury.

CHAPTER SUMMARY

Therapeutic modalities are methods of applying physical agents to create an optimal environment for healing and reduce an individual's pain and discomfort following injury or recognition of certain disease processes. These modalities, which include cryotherapy, thermotherapy, and electrical and mechanical modalities, are used to ease the patient's pain and promote tissue healing. They are the primary tools of rehabilitation.

Cryotherapy chills the tissues, decreasing bloodflow to the area as well as reducing edema and pain. Cryotherapeutic methods include ice packs, ice massage, vapo-coolant sprays, ice water immersion, and cold whirlpool baths. Thermotherapy is the application of heat to certain body tissues. It is used to increase bloodflow and flexibility to those tissues as well as to reduce pain and muscles spasms. Thermotherapeutic methods include heat packs, fluidotherapy, paraffin baths, and warm whirlpools. Electrical modalities, such as ultrasound, EMS, IFS, galvanic stimulation, iontophoresis, TENS, and diathermy, stimulate the body's tissues using an electrical current to promote healing and reduce pain. Mechanical modalities promote healing through the application of pressure to the soft tissues, increasing circulation and/or distracting (pulling) bony structures. Such modalities include intermittent compression, traction, and various forms of massage therapy.

Some modalities are easy to use, but most require formal training or application by a licensed professional. Laws regulating the use of therapeutic modalities vary from state to state. Therefore, anyone who works in a rehabilitative environment should check the laws of that state to see what one may legally do.

STUDENT ENRICHMENT ACTIVITIES

Complete the following sentences.

1. Cryotherapy causes the tissues to vasoconstrict, which causes _____ bloodflow to the area.

2. Thermotherapy causes vasodilation, which causes _____ bloodflow to the area.

3. The idea behind the use of therapeutic modalities is to _____, slow down, or _____ the muscle spasm/pain cycle.

4. Most commonly, a vapo-coolant is used on _____ injuries, and _____ and _____ strains.

5. Treatment time for a whirlpool bath is _____ to _____ minutes.

6. Ultrasound therapy utilizes a high-frequency _____ _____ that is converted to heat.

7. A whirlpool bath combines the heat transfer methods of _____ and _____ to produce therapeutic effects in the tissues.

8. _____ is the systematic manipulation, methodical pressure, friction, and kneading of the soft tissues of the body.

Write T for true, or F for false. Rewrite the false statements to make them true.

9. T F Regulations concerning the use of therapeutic modalities vary from state to state.

10. T F Keeping records on the use of modalities isn't necessary.

11. T F Cryotherapy should not be used on a patient for more than 30 minutes at one time.

12. T F Ice massage is used most often for relief in the treatment of chronic tendonitis, muscle strains, and chronic bursitis.

13. T F It's best not to apply heat treatments for muscle spasms and joint stiffness.

14. T F Heat applied immediately on an injury will keep the swelling down.

15. T F Because of the high temperature and the swirling action of the water, whirlpool baths do not require maintenance.

16. T F A paraffin bath is a mixture of six parts wax to one part mineral oil.

17. T F Unless it is applied under water, ultrasound therapy requires the use of a coupling medium.

Match the terms in Column A with the appropriate description in Column B.

Column A	Column B
18. radiation	**A.** heating through direct contact with a hot medium (heating pads)
19. conversion	
20. conduction	**B.** heating indirectly through another medium (whirlpool bath)
21. convection	
22. electrical muscle stimulation (EMS)	**C.** heating transferred through space from one object to another (infrared light)
23. ultrasound	**D.** heating through other forms of energy (ultrasound)
24. paraffin bath	
25. massage	**E.** heat modality that uses wax to warm distal extremities
26. traction	
	F. high-frequency sound wave; one of the deepest penetrating heat sources available
	G. uses electrical stimulation to re-educate injured muscles, strengthen healthy muscles, and slow the effects of atrophy in a given area
	H. continuous, intermittent, manual, or gravitational weight application
	I. effleurage, pétrissage, deep friction, tapotement, and vibration

Match the following modalities with the appropriate classification.

27. ice water immersion	**A.** cryotherapy
28. fluidotherapy	**B.** thermotherapy
29. hydrocollator pack	**C.** electrical modality
30. ice pack	**D.** mechanical modality
31. interferential stimulation	
32. intermittent compression	
33. galvanic stimulation	
34. tapotement	
35. paraffin bath	
36. TENS	
37. traction	
38. ultrasound therapy	
39. vapo-coolant spray	

Define the following terms, explaining the circumstances under which they are used and precautions that must be taken.

40. thermotherapy

41. cryotherapy

42. mechanical modality

43. electrical modality

Complete the following exercise.

44. Identify which modalities would be used on an acute knee sprain, and explain your choices.

CHAPTER 24

Physical Rehabilitation

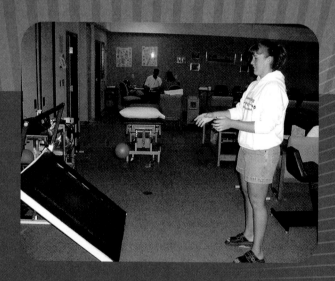

OBJECTIVES

After completing this chapter, you should be able to do the following:

1. Define and correctly spell each of the key terms.

2. Compare different phases of the rehabilitation process.

3. Describe at least five ways to make rehabilitation an enjoyable and productive experience.

4. Explain what "SOAP notes" are and how they are used.

5. Discuss the effects of proper and improper posture as they relate to physical therapy.

6. Demonstrate how to use a goniometer to measure range of motion.

KEY TERMS

* ADLs

* ambulation

* asymmetry

* body mechanics

* crutches

* exercise modality

* goniometer

* motivation

* patient history (Hx)

* perpendicular

* posture

* progress notes

* rehabilitation

* SOAP notes

THE GOALS OF REHABILITATION

Physical **rehabilitation** is the process of recovering from an injury. Also known as "rehab," rehabilitation consists of treatment and education designed to help injured patients regain maximum function, a sense of well-being, and the highest level of independence possible. True rehabilitation consists of both a psychological and a physical recovery. Psychological recovery requires that the patient experience the stages of psychological adjustment discussed in Chapter 22. This chapter focuses on the physical aspects of rehabilitation, but it is important to realize that physical recovery hinges greatly on certain aspects of psychological recovery (see Figure 24-1).

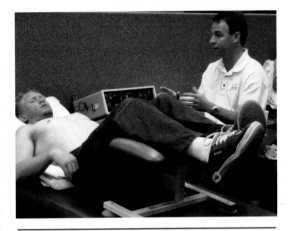

FIGURE 24-1 Assisting in the process of rehabilitation can be very rewarding.

rehabilitation

the process of recovering from an injury through treatment and education designed to assist injured patients in regaining maximum function, a sense of well-being, and the highest level of independence possible.

Because success is measured by the degree to which the patient can return to preinjury activities, the therapeutic goals are determined by the individual's level of activity prior to injury. Assisting a patient in the process of reaching those goals is rewarding, but it can also be difficult—for the patient and the rehabilitation staff. Thus, work in this field requires patience, empathy, and an optimistic and encouraging attitude. It also requires a thorough understanding of the processes, tools, and procedures that are used to promote physical recovery in the patient. Some of the tools and procedures used in rehabilitation have already been discussed, so this chapter will focus on the rehabilitative process: who is involved, the optimal environment, the phases of rehabilitation, and the importance of patient education.

THE REHABILITATION TEAM

Successful rehabilitation is a result of the combined efforts of the rehabilitation team, consisting of several key staff members with a wide range of responsibilities and training. Depending on individual needs or specific settings, the rehabilitation team may be large or small.

Physician

The physician, as the captain of the rehabilitation team, determines the rehabilitation program's goals and orders medications and physical therapy treatments. Possessing a medical degree, the physician has the most extensive training of all the members of the rehabilitation team (see Figure 24-2).

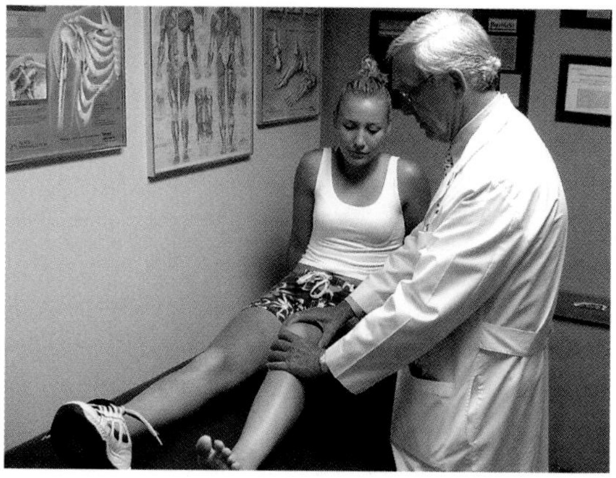

FIGURE 24-2 The physician is the captain of the rehabilitation team; all physical therapy is done in accordance with the physician's recommendations.

Physical Therapist

The physical therapist is responsible for evaluating patients, initiating treatment plans, and performing treatments and procedures. The physical therapist also assesses patient progress and the effectiveness of therapeutic methods. In addition to their four-year degrees, physical therapists hold post-graduate degrees and must be licensed or registered by the state in which they practice.

Athletic Trainer

As previously discussed, the athletic trainer's role in the rehabilitation process may sometimes be based on time restraints, number of athletes, number of teams, amount of help, accessibility to other allied health care practitioners, equipment, supplies, and available facilities. Many times the athletic trainer or the athletes will not have access to a physical therapist, or insurance will not provide adequate rehabilitation, so the rehabilitation will be performed by the athletic trainer. State laws may also dictate what the athletic trainer may and may not do. Although the athletic trainer's most general responsibilities center around the prevention and treatment of athletic injuries, the athletic trainer's scope of duties also includes rehabilitation strategies, education regarding nutrition, and the assessment of an individual's physical condition.

Strength and Conditioning Specialist

Strength and conditioning specialists frequently can become involved in the final phase of rehabilitation. At this point, the patient has typically regained most of the strength and function lost in the injury and is ready to return to an active lifestyle. Strength and conditioning specialists can help physicians, physical therapists, athletic trainers, and other therapists in transitioning the patient back to the activities of daily living.

Physical Therapist Assistant

The role of the physical therapist assistant is to assist the physical therapist with treatments, procedures, and patient assessments. Physical therapist assistants receive their training through to two-year associate degree programs and then must work under the direction and supervision of a licensed physical therapist.

Physical Therapy Aide

Physical therapy aides are responsible for nontechnical, but essential, duties associated with physical therapy, such as transporting patients, answering telephones, helping to apply some modalities, and assisting in making patients comfortable. These aides are usually trained in occupational education programs, vocational schools, or on-the-job training programs, and work under the direction and supervision of a licensed physical therapist.

The Patient's Family

Often the biggest source of support, the patient's family is a vital part of the rehabilitation team (see Figure 24-3). Family members can help in obvious ways by assisting the patient with exercises, furnishing transportation to appointments, and helping with the management of recommended home therapies. But often, the most significant contribution the family members can make to the patient's recovery is the simple reassurance that the patient is not alone. Depending on the situation, empathy, encouragement, or a "get-tough" attitude may all be appropriate responses to a patient's needs, as is the assurance of unconditional love in the face of potential disability.

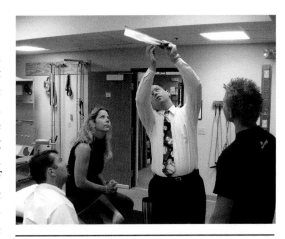

FIGURE 24-3 The support of the patient's family is important to the success of many rehabilitative efforts.

The Teammates

Often considered members of the athlete's extended family, the teammates may also play a valuable role in rehabilitation. Teammates can offer sympathy and encouragement to the patient. Even more important than these forms of emotional support, however, is the incentive to heal. Teammates who help the patient still feel a valuable part of the team whose presence is missed will help provide the motivation to heal.

The Patient

The patient must always be considered a member of the rehabilitation team. Physical therapy is not something that is "done to" a person; it is a process that requires the individual's active participation. Without a properly motivated patient, even the most skilled professionals cannot succeed. Successful rehabilitation hinges on a patient's belief that recovery is possible. Equally important is recognizing the importance of compliance in adhering to the program throughout all phases of rehabilitation. Rehabilitation is a seven-day-a-week commitment.

Additional members of a rehabilitation team may include a recreational therapist, a recreational therapy aide, an exercise physiologist, an occupational therapist, a nutritionist, a coach, a psychologist, and/or a social worker.

THE REHABILITATION ENVIRONMENT

As discussed in the previous section, successful physical rehabilitation requires more than quality medical care. Whether it takes place in a clinic, hospital, school, gym, or at home, successful physical rehabilitation requires belief in a positive outcome, particularly when the injury is severe. Formed by a combination of experiences, information, feelings, and observations, beliefs and attitudes are often the driving force behind our actions. If a patient believes that recovery is possible, that belief will serve as motivation to work hard at getting better. Much of the belief in the success of a patient's own rehabilitation program will be based on the information the physician provides when the diagnosis is made. That belief is then either bolstered or undermined by the patient's observations and feelings. For this reason, the rehabilitative environment should reflect a sense of competence and optimism, encouraging the patient to believe that healing is possible and to place trust in the rehabilitative team (see Figure 24-4).

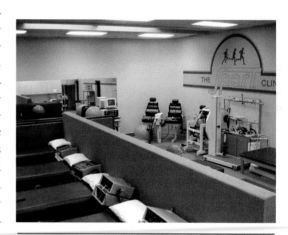

FIGURE 24-4 The rehabilitation environment should reflect professionalism and promote patient trust.

To create an optimal environment for healing, address these considerations:

* Patient safety
* Patient needs
* Patient comfort
* Staff conduct

Patient Safety

Professional rehabilitative settings such as hospitals, clinics, schools, and gyms should be safe for all who enter. This means such places must be clean and organized; there should be no clutter for patients or staff to fall over. Equipment should be cleaned and maintained on a regular basis, spills cleaned up immediately, and proper treatment procedures followed. Furthermore, work areas should be well-lit, areas in which chemicals are used should be well-ventilated, and safety inspections should be made regularly.

Patient Needs

The setting in which therapy is performed must have the personnel and equipment necessary to meet the physical and psychological needs of the patient (see Figure 24-5). Facilities with a large staff of trained therapists and a wide variety of therapeutic and exercise equipment have the most to offer their patients throughout all phases of rehabilitation. However, the size of the facility is not what is most important; what counts is the degree to which the facility can match the patient's needs.

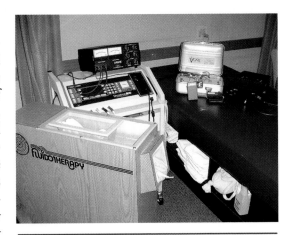

FIGURE 24-5 The proper equipment is vital to the success of many rehabilitation programs.

Access to appropriate therapy is vital to successful rehabilitation. Health insurance will determine where, how often, and how long rehabilitation will take place. Adequate insurance is important to the rehabilitation of an injury. Different settings offer different advantages for the patient: clinics and hospitals often have sophisticated medical equipment for use in therapy, whereas schools and gyms can offer a variety of exercise equipment. For example, a patient who needs ultrasound therapy will likely require a clinic or hospital for therapy. A patient who needs therapeutic exercise will probably require a gym of some kind. But a patient in the final phase of rehabilitation may benefit most from a home exercise program and a return to activities of daily living (**ADLs**).

Patient Comfort

Comfort is a key issue in creating an optimal therapeutic environment. Without being comfortable while in therapy, a patient is unlikely to follow through with the program given. Patient comfort can be influenced greatly by some simple adjustments of the therapeutic environment.

The first step in increasing patient comfort is making sure the facility is bright, clean, and organized. Chrome should be well-polished, surfaces dusted, desktops clean, and weights arranged neatly. If equipment or other essentials are stored under the table, they should be well-organized and accessible. Everything in the clinic should look as if it has a place.

Second, make sure every patient is welcomed with a smile and made to feel like an important part of the rehabilitation team. Medical environments can be intimidating to some people. It is important to remember that patients may feel vulnerable while in therapy. They are usually in pain or dealing with some sort of loss of function; they hear words they do not always understand; they are often uncertain about their recovery; and they are probably aware that they will have the medical professional's attention only for a limited time. A pleasant, upbeat, and courteous

ADLs

activities of daily living: everyday actions, such as self-care, communication, and mobility skills, required for independent living.

attitude that affirms the patient's importance as an individual will help put the patient at ease.

Third, provide patients with a sense of privacy. Cubicles that partially screen patients and curtains that can be drawn to increase privacy during treatment will help patients feel less like they are "on display" (see Figure 24-6). Such arrangements will also facilitate discussions of a private nature, and decrease the potential for suggestions of impropriety that, unfortunately, are easier to make when in a fully enclosed room. In facilities with separate rooms for patients, doors should be closed once the patient enters the room, and staff should knock before entering.

Fourth, whenever possible, the therapeutic atmosphere should reflect the mindset of the patients it serves. Although this is not always possible because of the wide variety

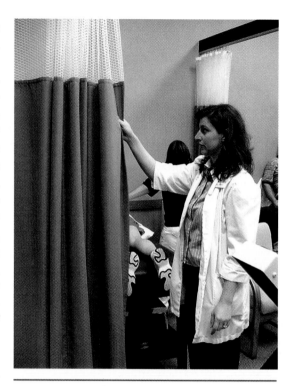

FIGURE 24-6 Curtains can often be drawn around cubicles to increase patient privacy.

of patients served in many clinics, it is a worthy goal. For example, a school clinic might provide stimulation suitable to the students who use it. Music would be popular and upbeat, colors trendy, and posters and pictures would reflect the general interests of that age group. Similarly, a clinic that serves the residents of a retirement community might best serve their patients by using music, colors, and artwork that are calming in nature, to avoid overstimulation. These examples are somewhat generalized, but many clinical environments, whether by design or by chance, tend to have patients with similar needs. In such cases, patient comfort and participation can be increased by some gentle tweaking of the environment.

Well-planned stimulation of the senses can be very effective in producing desired responses from people. Anyone who has ever been to an amusement park or a shopping mall has, no doubt, had their behavior influenced by such use of sounds, colors, and fragrances. With this in mind, it should be easy to think of a variety of ways in which the senses can be used to promote a sense of well-being in the rehabilitative setting. Some examples are listed below.

Sight: The visual displays on the walls and around the clinic should illustrate the services the clinic promotes (see Figure 24-7). For example, a work area that has posters of athletes on the walls indicates it specializes in treating athletes. If the facility offers outdoor rehabilitative activities, a picture or an announcement of those activities posted for the patients to read would be a good idea. Plants or flowers always brighten up the reception area; color can perk up a patient's mood.

Smell: The clinical environment should always smell clean, healthy, and fresh. Offensive odors can be prevented by cleaning the workout equipment regularly. The workplace should not smell like mildew. Avoid any "hostile" smells like medicine or tobacco smoke. No-smoking laws have all but eliminated smoke smells. Excessive cologne or perfume can also be offensive to patients.

Sound: Background sounds should be positive, upbeat, and comforting. Music can be played in the background to affect the patient's mood and provide motivation through the session.

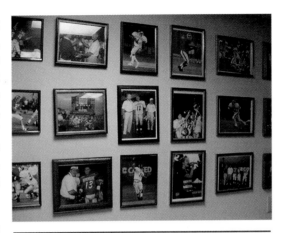

FIGURE 24-7 Photo displays can be used to illustrate the populations served by a given facility.

Touch: Appropriate physical contact, such as a handshake, at the first meeting will help put the patient at ease. In addition, chairs and exam tables should be as comfortable as possible to patients, and the temperature should be set to a comfortable range. Setting the thermostat to maintain a temperature range of 68 to 72°F will create a comfortable work environment for most people.

Staff Conduct

From the physicians to the aides, the members of the rehabilitative team must conduct themselves appropriately. The keys to proper conduct in the rehabilitative environment are professionalism and compassion. The patients are the staff's top priority, and professional, compassionate behavior from the staff will reflect that concern. Such conduct requires efficiency, a cheerful outlook, good communication skills, knowledge of and adherence to proper procedures, a strong work ethic, and general behavior that reflects respect and concern for others (see Figure 24-8).

Appropriate conduct also includes dressing professionally. The way the staff looks and dresses

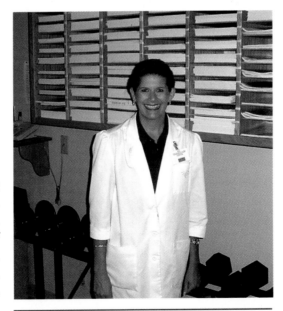

FIGURE 24-8 A cheerful outlook is as important to the staff's image as professional clothing.

makes an important impression on patients and visitors. The clothing worn should be clean, wrinkle-free, and in accordance with facility policy. Because of the active nature of the work, clothing should also allow movement without restriction.

One of the most important, and often overlooked, behavioral considerations in health care is learning to restrict certain types of conversation while at work. Workplace conversations should be moderate in volume, positive in nature, geared to the work at hand, and respectful of the patient and privacy. The use of excessive slang and offensive language should always be avoided. Discussions with coworkers that are not work-related should be kept for breaks, lunch hours, or after work; plans for the evening, what was for lunch, or watercooler gossip are not suitable topics for discussion with other staff members while providing treatment to a patient. Such conversations have nothing to do with the patient, and only indicate that the focus is not on the patient as it should be. Except for short, necessary work-related questions, conversations during a treatment session should be directed to the patient and, like all other behavior, should reflect concern for that person's well-being. Some conversations are not appropriate for anyone but a physician to have with a patient. If the patient or the patient's family requests a diagnosis or prognosis, the question should always be tactfully referred to the supervising physician.

Similarly, discussion of a patient's treatment, condition, or progress with someone who is not a member of the rehabilitation team—or even within earshot of such a person—is not appropriate. With HIPAA regulations a top concern, patient confidentiality is an important concept and should be taken seriously. More information about patient confidentiality can be found in Chapter 4. All of these behaviors will work toward creating the sense of trust and belief that is vital to successful rehabilitation.

Always respect the patient. Avoid a compromising situation with a patient during a treatment or an evaluation. If at anytime a sensitive part of the body may need to be evaluated or treated, bring in a second person and use the situation as an educational opportunity; however, keep the patient's feelings or concerns in mind.

THE FIRST SESSION

Patient History

Before beginning any rehabilitation program, the clinician(s) responsible for the therapy must read the patient's record. The chart will state a physician's diagnosis (Dx), the name of the doctor who referred the patient, the patient's contact information, and the patient's history. The **patient history (Hx)** consists of age, past illnesses, inherited conditions, previous therapies, and information about prescribed medications. The history will also list any precautions associated with the patient's condition. In other words, any existing information that relates to the injury and/or the patient's recovery is a part of the patient's history (see Figure 24-9).

The patient history contains facts that are important considerations in the rehabilitation process, as they can affect the design of the rehabilitation plan. Reading the patient's chart in advance gives the person in charge of the rehab session the opportunity to obtain the proper equipment and supplies for the session. Such planning will help ensure that the appropriate physical therapy is performed in a timely manner.

When looking at a patient's chart, various symbols and abbreviations will be noted. Medical staff members use such medical shorthand to help communicate information about the patient's condition and treatment in a universal and concise

> **patient history (Hx)**
>
> a form that describes the patient's medical history and chief medical complaint.

KNEE EVALUATION

HISTORY

NAME _Tran Nguyen_
ADDRESS _2111 Maple St._
OCCUPATION _Route Sales_
DIAGNOSIS _s/p menisectomy med/lat. Ⓡ_
REFERRING PHYSICIAN _D. L. Jackson, M. D._

DATE _4/11/xx_
PHONE _(909) 555-4376_
AGE _42_
WORK STATUS _Off work_
PHONE _(909) 555-6600_

DOI _11/17/xx_　　　　　DOS _4/05/xx_

MECHANISM OF INJURY _Up and down on knees at work & one day began to have knee p̄n –_
No specific incident that pt. can remember.

PAIN LEVEL/PRESENT SYMPTOMS _No resting pain, just stiffness & tenderness ove medial jt. line._
Reports some pain at end range of flexion.

WHEN WORSE _at end of day – knee becomes swollen_

WHEN BETTER _"Getting off it"_

DIAGNOSTIC TESTS _X-ray, MRI_

MEDICATION _None_

PAST MEDICAL HISTORY _Previous P. T. at Brecklin P. T. prior to Surg. until 1/01, Good health_
Recreational Activities:　Coaches Pony League Baseball

EVALUATION

GAIT _Amb. c̄ mild limp on Ⓡ, ✓'d hip flexion in Swing phase._

FUNCTIONAL TESTS
(4=NORMAL 3=MILD COMPROMISE 2=DIFFICULT 1=WITH AIDE 0=UNABLE N/A=NONAPPLICABLE NT=NOT TESTED)
(*=MIN PAIN **=MOD PAIN ***=SEVERE PAIN)

1. WALK ON TOES _4_
2. WALK ON HEELS _3_
3. STAND ON ONE LEG _4_

4. SQUATTING _NT_
5. KNEELING _↓_
6. STAIRS _3_

A/prom

AROM	(RIGHT)	LEFT	STRENGTH	(RIGHT)	LEFT
EXTENSION	-10° / -8°	0°	QUAD/VMO	NT	5/5
FLEXION	107° / 110°	122°	HAMSTRINGS	↓	↓

Sitting at edge of table

FIGURE 24-9 Sample Patient Chart with History

manner. Never guess at what an abbreviation or symbol might mean; if there are any doubts, ask someone with more experience. Learning the accepted medical abbreviations is vital for anyone who has the authority to read or update a patient's chart. Accurate communication among health care staff members is vital to quality patient care. Therefore, make sure to only use abbreviations and symbols that are acceptable to the rehabilitation facility. Otherwise, no one will be able to understand the information.

Figure 24-10 is a partial list of common medical abbreviations and symbols used in the rehabilitative environment. Please note that some abbreviations may have additional meanings that do not relate to the rehabilitative environment. These additional meanings are not listed.

Common Abbreviations and Symbols

Body Area

ACL: anterior cruciate ligament.
ant: anterior.
BE: below elbow.
BLE: both lower extremities.
BUE: both upper extremities.
CNS: central nervous system.
CV: cardiovascular.
ext: external.
GH: glenohumeral joint.
HS: hamstrings.
int: internal.
LA: left arm.
lat: lateral.
LCL: lateral collateral ligament.
LE: left extremity.
LLE: left lower extremity.
Lt: left.
LUE: left upper extremity.
MCL: medial collateral ligament.
PCL: posterior cruciate ligament.
RA: right arm.
RLE: right lower extremity.
Rt: right.
RUE: right upper extremity.
sup: superior.
TIB-FIB: tibia-fibula.
UE: upper extremity.
VMO: vastus medialis oblique.

Range of Motion and Exercise

ADL: activities of daily living.
AROM: active range of motion.
CWI: crutch-walking exercise.
ex: exercise.
FWB: full weight-bearing.
NWB: no weight-bearing.
PNF: proprioceptive neuromuscular facilitation.
PRE: progressive resistance exercises.
PROM: passive range of motion.
PWB: partial weight-bearing.
ROM: range of motion.
ROT: rotate, rotational.
RROM: resistive range of motion.
SLR: straight-leg raise.
WFL: within functional limits.

Dosages

ac: before meals.
ad lib: as desired.
BID or **bid:** twice daily.
/d: per day.
meds: medication.
od: once daily.
pc: after meals.
PRN: whenever necessary or as needed.
Q or **q̄:** every.

FIGURE 24-10 Common Abbreviations and Symbols

Dosages (Continued)

QD or qd: every day; daily.

qh: every hour.

q2h: every 2 hours.

q4h: every 4 hours.

QID or qid: four times per day.

qn: every night.

QOD or qod: every other day.

TID or tid: three times daily.

W/cm²: watts per centimeter squared.

x: times (3x means 3 times).

Modalities and/or Treatments

CWP: cold whirlpool.

EMS: electrical muscle stimulation.

ES: electrical stimulation.

HP: heat pack.

HVPGS: high-voltage pulsed electrogalvanic stimulation.

HVGS: high-voltage electrogalvanic stimulation.

HWP: hot whirlpool.

ICE: ice, compression, elevation.

IF: interferential.

IFS: interferential stimulation.

MENS: microcurrent electrical neuromuscular stimulation.

MWD: microwave diathermy.

RICE: rest, ice, compression, elevation.

SWD: shortwave diathermy.

TENS: transcutaneous electrical nerve stimulation.

tx: traction (also treatment, transmit).

US or Uz: ultrasound.

UV: ultraviolet.

WP: whirlpool.

Measurements and Time

+ or pos: positive.

− or neg: negative.

⊂: less than.

⊃: greater than.

=: equals.

am: before noon; morning hours.

am: before noon; morning hours.

C: Centigrade or Celsius.

d: day.

F: Fahrenheit.

h: hour.

noc: night.

pm: afternoon or evening.

sos: when necessary; if necessary.

stat: at once; immediately.

s̄s̄: one-half.

wk: week.

WNL: within normal limits.

Vital Signs

BP: blood pressure.

P: pulse (also, phosphorous).

R: respirations (also, rectal).

T or temp: temperature.

TPR: temperature, pulse, and respiration.

VS: vital signs.

Conditions/Diseases

AIDS: acquired immune deficiency syndrome.

Fx or Fr: fracture.

HBV: hepatitis B virus.

Hep B: hepatitis B.

HIV: human immunodeficiency virus.

HTN: hypertension.

Personnel/Specialties

ATC: certified athletic trainer.

CSCS: certified strength and conditioning specialist.

Dr: doctor.

MD: medical doctor.

ortho: orthopedics.

OT: occupational therapist/therapy.

PMD: primary medical doctor.

PT: physical therapist/therapy.

PTA: physical therapist assistant.

surg: surgical; surgery.

FIGURE 24-10 Common Abbreviations and Symbols (Continued)

General Note Taking

↑: up; increase.

↓: down; decrease.

♀ : female.

♂: male.

Δ: change.

1°: primary.

2°: secondary.

ā: before.

c̄ : with.

CC: chief complaint.

co or **c/o**: complaining of.

comp: complete.

cont: continue.

dc: discontinue.

dept: department.

DOI: date of injury.

DOS: date of surgery.

Dx: diagnosis.

ea: each.

eval: evaluation.

HEP: home exercise program.

ht: height.

Hx: history.

med: medical.

no: number.

NT: not tested.

OP: outpatient.

p̄: after; post.

per: by or through.

PH: past history.

PMH: past medical history.

post: posterior; after.

post-op: after the surgery.

pre-op: before the surgery.

p̄n̄: pain.

pt: patient.

re: regarding; relating to; pertaining to.

rxn: reaction.

RR: respiratory rate (also, recovery room).

R.O.: rule out.

Rx: prescription; take; treatment.

s̄ : without.

Sig: give the following directions.

SOB: short of breath.

Sx: symptoms.

tol: tolerates or tolerance.

VO or **vo**: verbal order.

w/c: wheelchair.

wt: weight.

XR: x-ray.

NOTE: It is recognized that sources differ regarding the use of periods with abbreviations. In this book, we have elected to follow the guidelines set forth by the *American Medical Association Manual of Style*, 9th Edition, which states that periods in abbreviations are to be omitted.

FIGURE 24-10 Common Abbreviations and Symbols *(Continued)*

Motivating the Patient

One of the most important things anyone can do to assist in a patient's recovery is to be a source of **motivation**. The patient should feel confident about completing the physical therapy session, and trust that such an achievement will assist in the recovery process. The patient must commit to being in the driver's seat for much of the rehabilitation program; recovery always depends on patient participation and commitment. Here are some ideas that can help to motivate a rehab patient:

1. Greet the patient with a smile and keep that smile throughout the treatment period (see Figure 24-11).

2. Dress professionally to suit the work environment.

3. Use the patient's name frequently throughout the treatment session.

4. Express an understanding of the nature of the patient's injury and knowledge of why the patient is in physical therapy.

motivation

the reason for performing an action; the stimulus for behavior.

5. Make sure the patient understands what is causing the condition.

6. Convey confidence about the physical therapy procedure to the patient.

7. Explain the objectives of the physical therapy to the patient.

8. Point out improvements the patient can watch for while going through the physical therapy sessions.

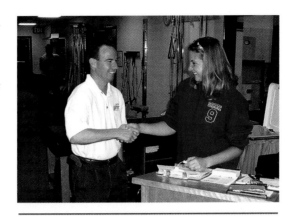

FIGURE 24-11 Patients should always be greeted by name and with a smile.

9. Suggest and/or organize group activities for the patient; this helps some patients through tough times.

10. Always provide the patient with clear and simple directions about the physical therapy exercises.

11. Maintain a positive attitude about the techniques used.

12. Provide a clean, organized, and pleasant rehabilitative environment.

13. Always give the patient full attention.

14. Present a professional attitude.

15. Stay in good health in order to display a positive example to the patient and co-workers.

POSTURE AND JOINT ASSESSMENT

Proper body alignment is vital to the functioning of the body's muscles and joints. Patients with poor body alignment are eventually limited in their normal movements because the joints and tissues surrounding them become stressed when the joints are not properly aligned. This stress leads to tissue breakdown. Active participants in the rehabilitative process must be able to assess a patient's ability to move and the ways in which body alignment may be affecting that movement.

Body alignment is assessed and ROM is measured with the following objectives in mind:

* Establish a guide for rehabilitative exercise programs.

* Provide a record for future evaluations of the patient's progress.

* Motivate the patient as measurements improve.

* Educate the patient in understanding the health concepts related to posture.

Posture Assessment

A person's **posture** is a visual guide to body alignment and is assessed on the lateral and anterior planes. To assess posture, ask the patient to stand on both feet,

posture

the position or alignment of the body.

with the arms relaxed at the sides of the body. The patient should not focus attention on the way the body is aligned. Observe the alignment of the following anatomical points, from head to toe, on the lateral and anterior planes. Record these assessments on the patient's chart. If a change for the worse during the course of treatment is noted, refer the patient to a physician.

Observing the patient from both lateral views, make the following observations:

1. Is the patient's spine straight?

   * Does the patient's neck tilt the head forward, or does this cervical portion of the spine continue in a vertical line with the superior portion of the thoracic spine so the lobes of the ears are directly over the clavicles of the shoulders? A forward tilt of the cervical spine may be caused by a weakness in the splenius muscles.

   * Is there an increase in the posterior protrusion of the thoracic curve (kyphosis)? Does it change when the patient bends over (see Figure 24-12)? This may be caused by a congenital condition, disease, malignancy, or a compression fracture.

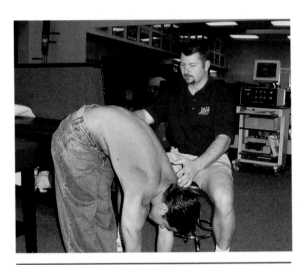

FIGURE 24-12 A Lateral Posture Assessment

   * Is there an exaggeration of the normal anterior convex curve of the lumbar spine (lordosis)? Does it change when the patient bends over? This may be caused by spondylolisthesis (the slipping forward of one lumbar vertebra on top of the one below), or achondroplasia, (the abnormal conversion of cartilage into bone that results in dwarfism). Additional causes may include congenital abnormalities, injury to the lumbar spine, and other diseases.

   * Does the abdomen protrude anteriorly? This may be caused by weak abdominal muscles or tight hamstrings.

2. Are the patient's knees aligned properly?

   * Are the knees hyperextended (genu recurvatum)? This may be caused by a weakness in the hamstrings or quadriceps muscles or excessive joint laxity, or it could be a hereditary condition.

Observing the patient from an anterior view, assess the following anatomical landmarks. While doing this, look for signs of **asymmetry** between the right and left sides of the patient's body (see Figure 24-13).

asymmetry

lacking correspondence in shape, proportion, and relative position between opposing body parts.

3. Is the neck straight?

* Is the patient's neck **perpendicular** to the shoulders?

4. Are the shoulders even?

* Is the distance from the patient's ear lobes to the shoulders equal on both sides?

5. Is the spine straight?

* Does it change when the patient bends over?

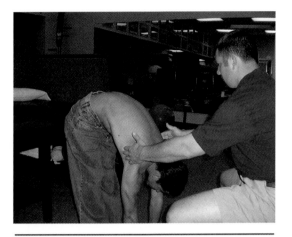

FIGURE 24-13 An Anterior Posture Assessment

perpendicular

forming right angles to a given plane.

6. Is the chest normal, or irregular in shape?

* Is the sternum sunken or depressed? This is a hereditary condition, called a funnel chest (pectus excavatum).

* Is the sternum displaced anteriorly? This is a hereditary condition, called a pigeon chest (pectus carinatum).

7. Are the hips even?

* Are the superior aspects of the iliac crests the same height?

8. Are the knees aligned?

* Are the knees knocked-kneed (genu valgum), or bowlegged (genu varum)?

Additional factors can influence adult posture: heredity, disease, habit, mood, energy level, joint mobility, skeletal abnormalities, laxity of ligaments, hamstring or hip flexor tightness, poor muscle tone in the trunk, and injury to spinal nerves. Poor alignment caused by heredity and some diseases may not be correctable, but, in most cases, the other causes of poor posture can be eliminated or reduced. These treatable irregularities are addressed in the patient's rehabilitation program. Even some inherited and disease-related conditions can be corrected with braces or surgery combined with rehabilitation.

If the patient was sent by a physician for rehabilitation of an injury, it is likely that the physician is already aware of any irregularities that exist. However, if any irregularities are detected in a person who is not under a doctor's care, or if the observed irregularities are unrelated to the patient's prescribed course of treatment, refer the patient to a physician before beginning any type of rehabilitation program. If the patient has already seen a physician, use the preceding assessments as a baseline for future evaluations. Make sure to include this baseline information in the progress reports that are sent back to the physician.

Joint Measurements

The instrument used for joint motion measurements is called a **goniometer**. A goniometer is a protractor-type instrument with two arms that attach at one end

goniometer

an instrument used to measure the movements and angles created by joints.

of each arm to form a moveable angle. Goniometers are available in 180° (half-circle) and 360° (full-circle) models, with the 180° model being the most common. Goniometers are marked with easy-to-read 1° increments.

Accuracy is most important when measuring with a goniometer. Accurate measurements depend on many things: training, repeatability, and experience. Because there are a variety of goniometers on the market, it is up to supervisors to train the proper personnel in the use of the particular goniometer(s) used in the facility. The instruction sheet sold with the goniometer may also be useful in learning how to use the instrument.

Although goniometer techniques vary, accurate tracking of patient progress depends on consistent and repeatable measurements from one session to the next. Therefore, everyone in the facility should use the same technique or procedure for goniometric measurements. Such consistency should produce no more than a 5° variation between each staff member's results. Equally important as consistent technique is consistent patient positioning. Whenever goniometers are used, the patient's position must be noted next to the measurement on the patient's chart. Making such notations will allow staff members involved in the next session to obtain a result that can be accurately compared to the previous measurement. If varied techniques or positions are used, inaccurate conclusions about the patient's progress will be made, possibly leading to unnecessary or inappropriate changes to the patient's rehabilitation program.

Accuracy in the use of goniometers is assisted by experience. It is common to feel a bit clumsy the first few times using a goniometer, so practice is important to becoming confident in its use. Take advantage of every opportunity to practice this technique. Remember: practice makes perfect!

Before taking the measurement, explain what is going to happen and what the patient will need to do. The part of the patient's body that is to be measured should be exposed (if possible), relaxed, and unrestricted from movement.

Place the goniometer so that the pivot point of the goniometer is on the joint, and each arm is over one of the two body segments creating the joint (see Figure 24-14). The placement of the instrument's arms for the majority of the tests should be along the central aspect of the body segments being measured. In some cases it may be necessary to adjust the patient's position to get the body segments in alignment. If this is the case, it will be necessary to double check the placement of the goniometer to make sure it is placed properly. The first measurement will be for passive ROM. Move the patient's joint through its range of motion until resistance is met, either due to the patient's pain or an anatomical endpoint. The arms of the goniometer must follow the motion of the two body segments being measured and remain aligned with the bones of those segments. Repeat this procedure for the active ROM. Write the results of each measurement on the patient's chart.

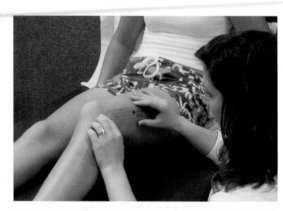

FIGURE 24-14 A goniometer may be used to measure either the PROM or AROM of a joint.

Range-of-Motion Norms

Cervical		Wrist	
Type of Joint: Pivot		**Type of Joint: Gliding**	
Flexion	0°–80°	Flexion	0°–90°
Extension	0°–70°	Extension	0°–70°
Lateral Flexion	0°–45°	Radial Deviation	0°–25 to 30°
Rotation	0°–80°	Ulnar Deviation	0°–45°
Lumbar		**Hip**	
Type of Joint: Cartilaginous		**Type of Joint: Ball & Socket**	
Forward Flexion	0°–60°	Flexion	0°–115 to 125°
Extension	0°–35°	Extension	0°–10 to 15°
Lateral Flexion	0°–20°	Abduction	0°–45°
Rotation	0°–50°	Adduction	0°–10 to 15°
		Internal Rotation	0°–45°
Shoulder		External Rotation	0°–45°
Type of Joint: Ball & Socket			
Flexion	0°–180°	**Knee**	
Extension	0°–60°	**Type of Joint: Hinge**	
Abduction	0°–180°	Flexion	0°–120 to 130°
Internal Rotation	0°–90°	Extension	130 to 120°–0°
External Rotation	0°–90°		
Horizontal Abduction/		**Ankle**	
Adduction	0°–135°	**Type of Joint: Hinge**	
		Dorsiflexion	0°–20°
Elbow		Plantar Flexion	0°–45°
Type of Joint: Hinge		Inversion	0°–35°
Flexion	0°–150°	Eversion	0°–25°
Extension	0°–10°		
Forearm			
Type of Joint: Pivot			
Pronation	0°–90°		
Supination	0°–90°		

FIGURE 24-15 Range-of-Motion Norms

Figure 24-15 shows range-of-motion norms for goniometer readings on specific joints. Ideally, a patient should be able to perform the full range of motion (from 0° to the upper value) both passively and actively by the end of Phase III (see "The Phases of Physical Rehabilitation" later in this chapter).

To provide the most complete progress notes possible, and to ensure proper continuity of care, additional notations are necessary on the patient's chart (see Figure 24-16). As mentioned previously, to ensure the accuracy of future comparisons, the patient's position during the measurement should be noted. Such notes might read: standing; sitting, with legs extended on table; or sitting, with feet resting on the floor. Also record whether the range of motion was passive or active and the date and time of

GIRTH MEASUREMENTS

NAME _Tran Nguyen_

	RIGHT	LEFT
12 CM ABOVE SUPRAPATELLA	49.8 cm	51.0 cm
SUPRAPATELLA	42.8 cm	39.6 cm
MID-PATELLA	42.0 cm	39.7 cm
INFRAPATELLA	41.0 cm	37.3 cm
12 CM BELOW INFRAPATELLA	38.0 cm	38.0 cm

QUAD SET: RIGHT - GOOD / FAIR / (POOR)   LEFT (GOOD) FAIR / POOR
STRAIGHT-LEG RAISE: RIGHT - GOOD (FAIR) POOR   LEFT - (GOOD) FAIR / POOR
EXTENSION LAG: RIGHT _–10°_   LEFT _0°_
HAMSTRINGS: (MIN) / MOD / SEVERE   (TIGHT)   BILATERALLY
EDEMA: 1--(2)--3
SENSATION _Intact_

REFLEXES   RIGHT KNEE _NT_   RIGHT ANKLE _NT_   LEFT KNEE _NT_   LEFT ANKLE _NT_
PALPATION _Mild point tenderness in medial jt. line_

SPECIAL TESTS

	RIGHT	LEFT	COMMENTS
VALGUS STRESS TEST	NT	NT	N/A
VARUS STRESS TEST			
ANTERIOR DRAWER			
POSTERIOR SAG SIGN			
PIVOT SHIFT TEST			
McMURRAY'S			
BOUNCE HOME TEST			
LACHMAN'S			
FABERE'S TEST			
THOMAS TEST			
OBER'S TEST			
ELY'S TET			
APLEY'S COMPRESSION			
APLEY'S DISTRACTION			

PATELLAR POSITION

SUPERIOR VIEW   INFERIOR VIEW OF PATELLA

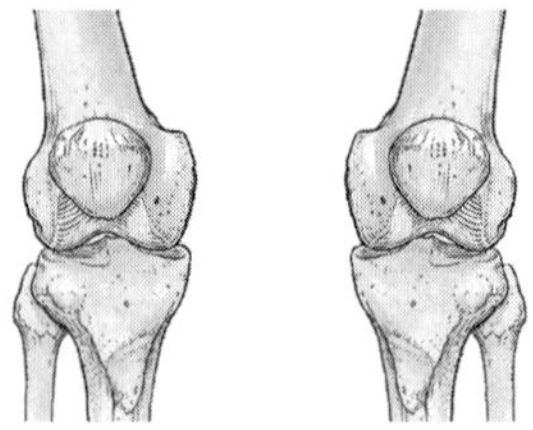

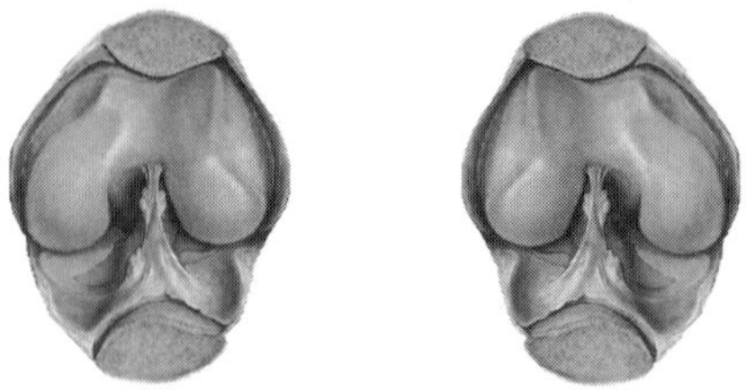

RIGHT   LEFT   RIGHT   LEFT

RIGHT PATELLAR ALIGNMENT IMPRESSION _no significant deviations_

LEFT PATELLAR ALIGNMENT IMPRESSION

FIGURE 24-16 Documentation of a Knee Assessment

the measurement, noting whether the measurement was taken before, during, or after the treatment. If any difficulty arises when using the goniometer, ask for assistance.

SOAP NOTES IN DOCUMENTATION

"SOAP" is an acronym for *subjective findings, objective findings, assessment,* and *plan*. **SOAP notes** are a concise, easy-to-read method of documenting the patient's health status (see Figure 24-17). This technique is also an efficient means of recording the patient's progress as well as any difficulties encountered along the way. SOAP notes improve charting by providing an organized method of communication to other members of the rehabilitation team. Such documentation is the basis for consistent patient care by the various members of the rehabilitation team. An athletic training student may document the SOAP notes, but the notes must be reviewed and approved by the supervising certified athletic trainer or physical therapist. Please note that HOPS (history, observation, palpation, and stress tests) (see Chapter 9) or HIPS (history, inspection, palpation, and stress tests) notes may be used as alternate methods of documentation to SOAP notes. However, the most predominantly used method of documentation is SOAP notes.

> **SOAP notes**
>
> an organized method of documenting a patient's status on his or her chart that includes subjective findings, objective findings, assessments, and plans for each problem experienced by the patient.

Subjective Findings

The "S" in SOAP is for *subjective findings*. These notes report anything the patient, the patient's family, nurse, physical therapist, teammate, or anyone else says about the patient or the patient's treatment. Notes under this heading would also include information about an injury, or signs or symptoms the patient may have, and what the patient has done prior to seeking treatment. To make this clearer, the subjective statements should be able to be prefaced with words such as, "Patient states . . ." or "Patient's family thinks . . ." Use the patient's own words, set off by quotation marks, whenever possible. The following are examples of subjective findings:

1. Patient states that his "right leg hurts while working."

2. Family states that patient was unmotivated at home.

3. Patient complains of feeling "sick to her stomach."

4. Patient discussed wanting to go home throughout the session.

5. Patient feels the coach is pushing him too hard to return to play.

6. Family says she seems "depressed."

Objective Findings

The "O" in SOAP is for *objective findings*. Objective findings document things that are observable and/or measurable during the patient's treatment. Another person can be used to verify this information. Therefore, other staff members involved in the treatment will often confirm the objectivity of observations. These notes will include information taken from the observation, palpation, and stress test portions of the HOPS procedure. The following are examples of objective findings:

1. Patient ambulates with walker 150 feet.

2. Patient refused treatment the past three days.

NAME *Tran Nguyen*

2/11/02	S: Pt is a 42 y/o ♂ c̄ DX: s/p ®menisectomy med / lat. DOI: 11/17/00, DOS: 4/05/01
	O: Initial eval completed, see forms for details. Instr. & Issued written HEP of HS stretches,
	wall slides, quad sets, and SLR's; See flow sheet.
	A: See eval, tol. ex's well.
	P: Cont. P.T. 3 X 4 wks for HEP, then ex, neuromuscular Re-ed, and modalities PRN.
	B. Ryann P.T.
2/16/02	S: No Pain Reported. "Sure!"
	O: Rx per Flow sheet. Re-eval completed. Review HEP.
	A: Tol rx in full s̄ adverse rxns. VMO Function Fair
	Good effort c̄ all ex's
	P: Cont. to progress C. Sidney P.T.
2/20/02	S: No c/o pain. "Just Tightness"
	O: Rx per Flow sheet. AROM ✓ = 118°, Ext = 6°
	A: Tol rx in full s̄ adverse rxns. Improved AROM, strength, VMO Function.
	Good effort c̄ ex.'s
	P: Cont. to progress C. Sidney P.T.
2/20/01	Addendum: PR to MD (2/23 appt.)
2/25/02	S: no new c/o
	O: Rx per Flow sheet.
	A: Tol rx in full s̄ adverse rxns. Endurance improving. No noted antalgic gait.
	P: Cont. as tol. B. Ryann P.T.
2/30/02	S: No c/o
	O: Rx per Flow sheet. Re-eval completed.
	A: Tol rx in full s̄ adverse rxns. Progressing well c̄ advanced protocol
	P: Cont as tol. C. Sidney P.T.
3/4/02	S: No c/o reported.
	O: Rx per Flow sheet.
	A: Tol rx in full s̄ adverse rxns. Good effort in all ex's
	P: Cont. to progress C. Sidney P.T.
3/11/02	S: No new c/o
	O: Rx per Flow sheet.
	A: Tol rx in full s̄ adverse rxns. Posture, gait, WFL Good compliance noted.
	P: Cont. to progress C. Sidney P.T.
3/16/02	S: No new reports of pain.
	O: Rx per Flow sheet.
	A: Tol rx in full s̄ adverse rxns. Improved balance and coordination c̄ lat. hopping drill.
	P: Cont. to progress. B. Ryann P.T.

FIGURE 24-17 SOAP Notes

3. Patient keeps knees bent during **ambulation**.

4. Patient keeps head and trunk forward during ambulation, but will correct it with cuing (when prompted).

5. Patient becomes tired while walking, or requires frequent rests.

6. Patient is capable of 30° of shoulder flexion.

ambulation

the ability to move about from place to place.

Assessment

The "A" in SOAP is for *assessment*. Assessment notes document a licensed professional's opinions of the patient's condition, progress, or potential obstacles to rehabilitation. These notes may also include explanations of observations recorded in the objective statement. Some examples of assessment notes are as follows:

1. Patient still has difficulty getting his weight forward when rising from a seated position.

2. Patient's balance has improved and is now fair.

3. Range of motion has increased in patient's right shoulder this week.

4. Patient seems depressed.

5. Patient seems anxious about going home.

6. Patient has developed soreness from the custom brace.

Plan

The "P" in SOAP is for *plan*. Plan notes state what the rehabilitation team wants to accomplish with the patient in terms of both short- and long-term goals. The plan should include ways of addressing the concerns presented in the other three portions of the SOAP notes. Examples of plan notes are as follows:

1. Advance the patient to the use of a cane this week (as able).

2. Continue to encourage patient's participation in exercises.

3. Make arrangements to go to a local gym.

4. Talk to the coach to discuss potential flaws in athletic skill techniques.

5. Schedule re-evaluation.

Once a plan has been established to fill the patient's needs, the initial SOAP notes are complete. However, this is not the end of note taking over the course of the patient's treatment. **Progress notes** are written after each treatment session and, at times, may follow the SOAP format. Flow sheets and other forms may also be used to help chart the patient's progress. The main purpose of these notes is to track the changes, both good and bad, in the patient's progress. Careful examination of progress notes may also reveal some equally important information not expressly stated in the notes. For example, the notes may reveal an improving attitude as the patient reaches long-term goals outlined in the plan. Progress notes may also provide the staff with information as to which treatments work better for certain types of injuries.

progress notes

notes on the patient's chart that document patient progress in rehabilitation and that may follow the SOAP format.

Detailed records about patient progress will protect the rehabilitation team from potential litigation. The more detail provided in the progress notes, the better. Information gathered during the treatment sessions is much more reliable than trying to remember specific details after the fact.

Progress notes will vary in length and detail. For instance, notes on a long-term patient with a chronic condition that shows little change will tend to be short; progress is minimal, so the progress notes are likely to be brief. However, for patients with acute injuries, the notes may be longer and more detailed. Progress notes should be concise, but should provide enough detail to allow a staffperson who has never worked with that patient to understand the treatment and progress up to that point and continue with the treatment plan.

Outcomes

Finding out what will increase the chances of an injury, what might bring that injury back to health sooner, along with ways to prevent injuries in the future can be important. This can be done by recording outcomes. This information will also help coaches keep their players participating, the administration ensure it is doing everything to prevent injuries, and the clinician make sure the rehabilitation process is effective.

Keeping records with information such as when the athlete was injured (in practice or game), the environment on which the athlete was injured (on grass or turf), even the type of shoes worn during preconditioning workouts compared to the shoes worn in the off-season is important. Much can be learned through good record-keeping that provides statistical information.

THE PHASES OF PHYSICAL REHABILITATION

Successful rehabilitation is a complex process that may be short or long, depending on the severity of the injury and the degree of function that must be regained. Other variables such as the type of health insurance, access to care, speed and quality of care, degree of motivation, and preexisting conditions may also influence the length and success of the rehabilitation program. Although each rehabilitation program is unique, the healing process is universal. Three phases of healing must take place in order for the patient to resume preinjury activities: the pain and damage resulting from the injury must first be controlled; then the damage must be repaired; and finally, the now-healthy tissue must be built up again. Nearly all physical rehabilitation programs can be thought of in terms of these phases.

Phase I begins immediately after the injury has occurred. The main purposes of Phase I are to prevent additional injury, decrease pain, and control inflammation. Phase II begins the process of repairing the damaged tissues. Strength and ROM are increased under controlled conditions to prevent reinjury. Ideally, Phase III involves returning the patient to the activity (sport, work, and activities of daily living) that as enjoyed prior to the injury. The patient learns how to reuse the injured area to its maximum potential without fear of reinjury. Full return to the former activities is not always possible. Sometimes the severity of the injury makes it necessary to teach the patient how to compensate for losses in strength or motion by modifying the way in which ADLs are performed, with the understanding that full recovery is not always likely.

These three phases represent a somewhat simplified way of looking at a complex process. The objectives of the phases are interlinked, so the end of one phase can easily become blurred with the beginning of another phase. It may also be necessary to regress a phase during rehabilitation. For example, if during range-of-motion exercises (Phase II) the patient experiences an increase in swelling or pain, it may be necessary to return to the PRICE procedure (Phase I) for a few days to get the pain and swelling under control. Depending on the severity of the injury, these phases may take a year or more to complete. Progression from one phase to the next, like all changes in treatment, is always based on recommendations by the supervising physician or therapist.

As prescribed by the supervising physician or therapist, therapeutic modalities are used in each of the phases of rehabilitation to help the patient achieve goals. These modalities are discussed in Chapter 23.

Safety Guidelines for All Phases of Rehabilitation

Certain precautions must always be observed as the patient progresses through each phase of rehabilitation:

1. Monitor any type of increase in edema or pain.

2. Advise each patient of the need to regain strength, but emphasize the importance of building up slowly; be sure that patients work to a level just below their capacity to avoid additional pain and injury.

3. Review the limitations of daily activities with each patient.

4. Make sure each patient understands how to perform home exercises properly.

PHASE I: CONTROL INFLAMMATION

The first phase of rehabilitation takes place just after the injury has happened. It often lasts two to three days, but may last longer, depending on the nature of the injury and the patient's adherence to the rehabilitation program. The primary goal is to decrease inflammation, thereby reducing pain and swelling. In the case of open wounds, the prevention of infection is also of primary importance. The secondary goals are to prevent additional loss of function by protecting the injury, establishing a baseline from which to assess functional improvement, and maintaining existing levels of fitness (Figure 24-18). In addition, patient

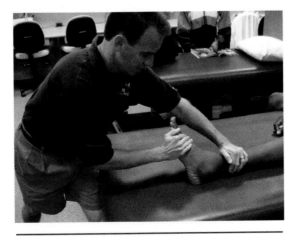

FIGURE 24-18 In Phase I, existing strength is maintained in the involved area with isometric exercise.

motivation and education must be addressed in every phase of rehabilitation.

Phase I Plan

1. Decrease bloodflow to the tissues to control inflammation as well as resulting pain and swelling. In the case of open wounds, prevent infection.

    * Use the PRICE procedure (see Chapter 14).

    * Additional Phase I therapeutic modalities may include: cold whirlpools, vapo-coolant sprays, galvanic stimulation, interferential stimulation, intermittent compression, and/or massage.

    * Use Universal Precautions in the case of contact with blood or other body fluids.

    * Prevent infection in the patient's wound with proper cleansing and the application of appropriate dressings (see Chapter 14).

2. Protect the injured area to prevent further damage.

    * Consider bracing (Figure 24-19), splinting, or taping the area (see Chapter 21).

    * Suggest use of supportive or assistive devices, such as slings or crutches (see "Crutches" later in this chapter).

3. Evaluate strength, ROM, and amount of edema.

    * Evaluate strength using an appropriate strength test, taking care to avoid causing additional injury in the process (see Chapters 16 and 18).

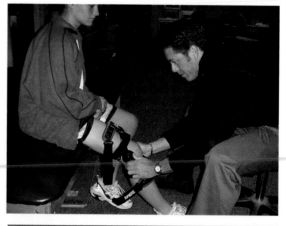

FIGURE 24-19 In some cases, protective braces can prevent additional injury.

    * Evaluate ROM using a goniometer, taking care to avoid causing additional injury in the process.

    * Evaluate the amount of swelling present by performing a girth measurement. Locate a landmark on the uninvolved extremity, such as the epicondyle, and measure the girth, or circumference, of the extremity about 5 centimeters above or below that landmark, depending on the location of the injury. Record this measurement; then compare the same point on the involved extremity. These measurements will be taken in each phase and used to assess the patient's progress.

4. Maintain strength and flexibility in the injured area as well as the rest of the body to prevent additional loss of function.

* Strengthen the injured area using isometric exercises (strengthening without motion) to maintain strength; non-weight-bearing pool therapy to maintain strength while decreasing the stress on the injured area; electrical muscle stimulation (EMS) to teach the muscles how to contract (muscle education).

* Strengthen the uninvolved areas of the body and perform aerobic exercises that do not cause pain to increase fitness in the rest of the body.

* Maintain flexibility in the injured area using stretching exercises, continuous passive motion (CPM) equipment, and overhead pulleys.

5. Educate the patient in safe and effective methods of strengthening that can be done at home, and caution the patient against specific activities of daily living that might lead to further injury.

   * Design an isometric home exercise program for the patient, demonstrating proper technique for each exercise.

   * Explain how ADLs may need to be modified during recovery and how, in some cases, continuing with normal ADLs will help enhance mobility.

6. Bolster the patient's confidence and self-esteem using motivation techniques.

   * Express confidence in the patient's ability to overcome the physical and psychological setbacks created by the injury.

   * Provide assurance that the patient is not alone in his or her efforts.

   * Encourage the patient by setting one or two achievable, short-term goals that are reachable by the next therapy session.

   * When possible, use the strength, ROM, and girth measurements to illustrate the patient's success to date.

PHASE II: REPAIR

Once the inflammation is decreased, the second phase of a patient's rehabilitative physical therapy begins. This phase consists of repairing damaged tissue by increasing strength and range of motion and by decreasing pain (see Figure 24-20). This phase also includes the promotion of self-sufficiency in terms of rehabilitation and a return to sports and activities of daily living.

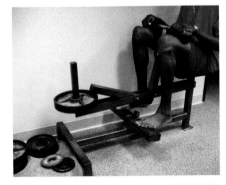

FIGURE 24-20 In Phase II, strength and ROM are increased with isotonic exercises.

Safe manipulation of the injured areas requires sufficient bloodflow to the area. Therefore, modalities that increase bloodflow are used prior to treating the injured area. To decrease the possibility of swelling and edema, modalities that decrease bloodflow are used at the end of the session.

Phase II Plan

1. Evaluate strength, girth, and ROM. Then compare results with previous Phase I measurements to assess progress.

   * See Phase I.

2. Increase the functional use of the injured area once pain and swelling are reduced, in preparation for return to play or normal activities.

   * Change the home exercise program to include isotonic (strengthening with motion) or variable resistance (strengthening with variable weight and speed) exercises (see Figure 24-21).

   * Begin working appropriate muscle groups to achieve balance of strength in the injured area.

   * Increase ROM in the injured area over that achieved in Phase I.

3. Increase bloodflow prior to strengthening.

   * Use any of the following modalities (if indicated): hot packs, hot whirlpools, galvanic stimulation, ultrasound, phonophoresis, iontophoresis, massage, or interferential stimulation.

4. Continue to decrease pain and edema.

   * See Phase I modalities (cryotherapy).

5. Begin gait training (walking without a limp) and improve weight-bearing abilities for patients with lower-extremity injuries.

   * Discontinue the use of supportive or assistive devices (if used in Phase I). However, use of braces and tape may continue.

6. Increase the patient's activities of daily living as appropriate, taking care to avoid causing additional injury. (See "Activities of Daily Living" later in this chapter.)

   * Add walking up and down stairs to the home exercise plan.

   * Add over-the-head lifting exercises to the home exercise plan.

7. Continue to increase the patient's confidence and self-esteem.

   * Enlist the help of individuals close to the patient to provide encouragement and support.

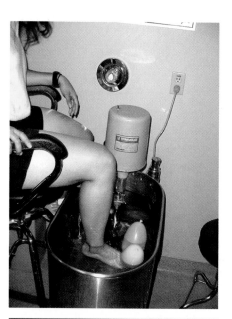

FIGURE 24-21 Be creative! This strengthening exercise makes use of a balloon filled with air and tied in the middle. The patient grasps the middle of the balloon with the toes and pushes the balloon down against the resistance of the water to strengthen the gastrocnemius and soleus complex.

* Continue to provide encouragement during therapy sessions.

* Continue to set short-term, achievable goals for the patient.

* Continue to use the strength, ROM, and girth measurements to illustrate the patient's success to date.

PHASE III: REMODEL

Remodeling refers to the retraining of the muscles to function in their normal capacity or as near normal as possible. This phase begins when the supervising physician or therapist believes that sufficient repair of the injured tissues has taken place. The primary objective in this phase is to prepare the patient to go back to daily life, including athletics or work. Because this phase requires the patient to take more control over his or her own physical therapy needs, the use of therapeutic modalities is decreased. Instead, the sessions are used to assist the patient in finding other methods of rehabilitation that can be done outside of the rehab center.

Because this phase prepares the patient to return to preinjury levels, **exercise modalities** are used more than therapeutic modalities. Therapeutic exercise is the movement of injured or debilitated muscles as a means of relieving weakness, pain, and/or stiffness (see Figure 24-22). Additionally, exercise modalities may be used in rehabilitation to improve the condition of muscle tissue. All of the conditioning exercises presented in Chapter 7 can be used as exercise modalities in rehabilitation. They can be done using any of the following methods, depending on the severity of the injury and the phase of rehabilitation:

* Isotonics

* Variable resistance

* Isokinetics

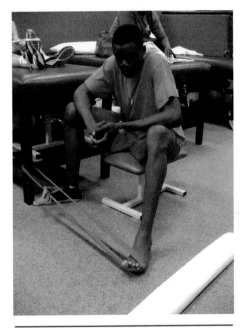

FIGURE 24-22 In Phase III, the strengthening exercises are often increased to variable resistance exercises, as shown here, or isokinetics.

> **exercise modality**
>
> a rehabilitative treatment involving the use of physical activity to increase strength and flexibility.

Phase III Plan

1. Increase endurance, strength, and flexibility in the injured area to, or as near as possible to, preinjury levels. In some cases, the patient will need to accept the fact that some former abilities may not be fully restored.

    * Progress both the clinical and home exercise programs. In a clinic, patients can do isokinetic (strengthening with variable resistance and

constant speed). In both places, they can do variable resistance exercises (strengthening with variable weight and speed)—preferably using motions and forces that mimic activities of daily living or sports-specific skills—as well as isotonic exercises (free weights).

* Help redefine the patient's concept of "normal" through instruction in new techniques for accomplishing tasks that were once simple, but now difficult, by reinforcing the positive aspects of life that have not changed.

2. Teach the patient how to use the therapeutic effects of heat and cold at home in continued treatment.

* Typically in Phase III, the patient can warm up the injured area prior to exercise with a hot shower, warm-water bucket, or a heat pack, and then ice it down following the activity to decrease any swelling.

3. Prepare the patient to return to work and/or sports.

* Minimize protective bracing, if it is possible to do so.

* Encourage self-confidence in the patient's physical and mental abilities to resume former pursuits.

4. Evaluate strength, girth, and ROM. Do comparisons with previous phases to assess progress.

* See Phase I.

5. Enhance coordination and balancing skills that are appropriate to the patient's sport or career through the use of exercise modalities (see Figure 24-23).

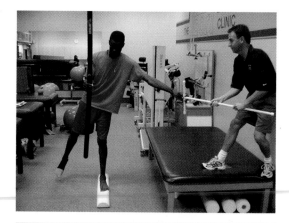

FIGURE 24-23 Exercise modalities can be combined to improve coordination and balancing skills.

* Add balancing exercises that use the lower extremities to the exercise program (e.g., standing on one foot or walking on a balance beam).

* Add balancing exercises that use the upper extremities to the exercise program (e.g., leaning against a basketball with one hand and balancing on it against the floor or a wall).

* Use functional activities and equipment relating to the patient's sport or job to begin to regain coordination in required movements (e.g., swinging motions with a baseball bat or tennis racquet, or set-like arm extensions with a volleyball).

6. Assist in organizing and developing a plan to meet the patient's fitness and nutritional needs.

* Advise the patient regarding good eating habits, and refer the patient to a nutritionist if necessary.

* Develop a new conditioning program for the client.

At the end of Phase III, the patient may be released from physical therapy by a physician or, in some cases, by the athletic trainer. This release should be a sign of the patient's ability to go forward with daily activities or a sport with limited precautions or restraints. In Phase III, the patient should also be psychologically ready to go back to work, or to return to an alternative job if not able to return to the previous job. Always make sure that the patient knows and understands that additional instruction or rehabilitation will still be available if the patient feels the need for help.

THE IMPORTANCE OF PATIENT EDUCATION

Beginning in Phase I, patients must be educated about their rehabilitation. At all times, they must be kept informed about what they should be doing to speed their recovery, how they can protect the injury, and what kind of progress they should expect (see Figure 24-24). Patients must understand the injury and how it affects their abilities and limitations. For example, it may be necessary to restrict participation in throwing activities and other overhead motions until the shoulder pain goes away. Educating patients shows them how they can get better and gives them a sense of control over their progress.

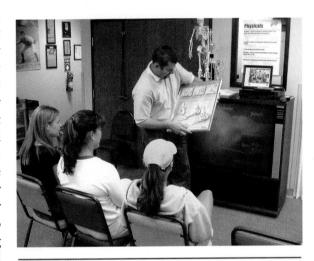

FIGURE 24-24 Patients must be kept informed about what they can do to speed their recovery, how they can protect themselves from reinjury, and what kind of progress they should expect.

Ongoing communication is vital to patient education. The results of periodic assessments, such as strength tests or range-of-motion evaluations, should be shared with the patient. Such information can be used as a source of motivation. Information on progress must always be shared with the patient. Such information is vital to rehabilitation as the patient progresses from one phase to another. For instance, in Phase I, the patient will need to understand the nature of the injury, how to protect it, and how to prevent additional loss of function. In Phase II the patient will need to know how to alter exercises to accommodate repair of the injured tissue. In Phase III, the patient will require instruction regarding the safe return to activities of daily living and may need education in the use of heat and cold to produce desired therapeutic effects.

The above examples are far from a complete listing of the information that must be supplied to patients; patient education depends on the type and severity of the injury, as well as any questions the patient may have. Patients need much information during the rehabilitative process. Do not expect them to search for the information—they may not even realize they need it. It is the responsibility of every member of the rehabilitation staff to make sure patients understand what they need to do, how to do it, and who to ask if they have questions.

Activities of Daily Living (ADLs)

Activities of daily living is a program composed of specific activities to mobilize patients and to help them regain the ability to function in their daily lives using their own capabilities. These activities, which build upon one another, should be designed to fit the needs and abilities of each patient. Being able to complete or perform each activity without pain or discomfort is critical before moving on to the next step. In all, the ADL program is designed to get patients back into action and help them lead pain-free lives.

An important aspect of the ADL program is the provision of pain-free alternatives to daily living activities. For example, if the patient finds it painful to walk for any distance greater than 200 yards, the patient might be advised to walk in a pool. The buoyancy of the water decreases pressure on the joints, reducing the pain. If it hurts the patient to lift things above the head, the patient should be advised to get a step ladder to assist in reaching high objects. If it hurts the patient to type, voice-recognition software could be utilized. Make sure the patients understand how to use proper body mechanics in their daily activities to avoid additional injuries.

Proper **body mechanics** is the safe and efficient use of all parts of the body in exercise and in daily activities. Using good body mechanics will lower the risk of injury and greatly reduce back fatigue and strain (see Figure 24-25). Tasks such as lifting, pulling, and pushing are much easier to do when the muscles are used properly. Over time, poor body mechanics can lead to disc, muscle, and nerve damage.

For example, instruct patients to keep their backs healthy by following these guidelines.

> **body mechanics**
>
> the efficient and safe use of the body during activity.

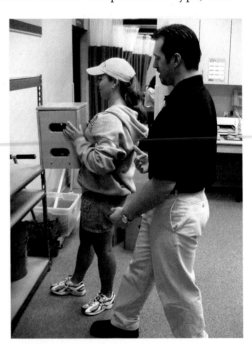

FIGURE 24-25 The use of good body mechanics can help prevent injuries.

* Maintain a broad base of support with the feet, approximately shoulder width. This keeps the natural curves of the back in proper alignment.

* Always bend at the knees, keep the back straight, and use the largest muscles of the legs (the thighs, buttocks, etc.) to do the work. Bending and reaching from the waist forces the back to support the upper body as well as the load. Avoid bending over for a prolonged time.

* Keep the load close to the body to reduce the strain on the lower back and provide the proper leverage. This keeps the back in proper alignment and distributes the weight evenly throughout the spine.

* Whenever possible, push or pull an object instead of lifting it. Use body weight to push or pull.

* Instead of twisting and turning, turn the entire body while keeping the feet, hips, and upper body pointed in the same direction. Position the body so that after the load has been lifted, there is a direct path to where the object is being taken. Remember to let the arms and legs do the work—not the back!

* Assess the weight of the object before attempting to lift it. If the object is too heavy, reduce the amount of weight or get assistance from another person before attempting to lift it.

Nutritional Needs

Patients will need to understand that their nutritional needs may change as a result of injury or illness. For instance, because they have an injury, they almost certainly will have a decrease in activity level. As a result, they will not burn as many calories. It's not unusual for injured individuals to gain weight. When this happens, the patient has two problems: an injury and unwanted pounds. Weight gain and the health problems that accompany it can be avoided by educating patients about the relationship between activity and nutritional needs. The best solution for this scenario would be to recommend the patient see a nutritionist for information on diet. If this is not possible, recommend a modest reduction in the patient's caloric intake until the injury has healed, reducing the amount of possible weight gain.

Crutches

Crutches are often used in the rehabilitation of injuries to the lower extremities. To be of good use, they must be properly fitted for each patient (see Figure 24-26). The crutch tips are placed 6 inches from the outer margin of the patient's shoes and 2 inches in front of the shoes. The underarm crutch brace position is approximately 1 inch below the underarm. The hand braces are placed even with the patient's hands, with the elbows flexed at approximately 30°. Before the patient leaves the facility for the first time with the crutches, have the patient test the fit of the crutches to see how they feel. If the patient thinks it feels awkward, check the crutches again for proper fit.

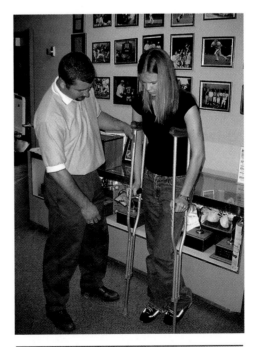

FIGURE 24-26 Crutches must be fitted to the patient to be used properly.

> **crutches**
>
> devices used to assist injured or weak patients with walking.

Tell the patient never to rest the weight on the underarm crutch brace. Excessive pressure on this area can lead to arterial and nerve damage, causing numbness in the arms and hands. This condition can also be caused by improperly fitted crutches.

There may be times when a patient must be taught how to use crutches. At such times, explain to the patient that the body movements involved in walking with crutches are similar to those involved in walking without crutches. There are many different methods of using crutches and other ambulation devices. The following are some methods that are commonly taught to patients who have suffered a mild to severe injury to one or both of the lower extremities.

A swinging method may be used if there is an injury to both the lower extremities and the patient is in good physical shape otherwise. This method involves placing the crutch tips in front of the feet a short distance, one to two paces. Both feet are then swung through and past the crutch tips another one or two paces. While the feet are swinging forward, the body weight is supported on the crutch handles. This method is then repeated by placing the crutch tips ahead of the feet again, and so on.

The tripod, or three-point-gait, method is used for patients who have injured one lower extremity. Using this method, both crutch tips and the involved leg are moved forward approximately 12 to 15 inches. After the patient has recovered balance and is supporting the body weight with the crutches, the uninvolved leg is moved forward and brought to a rest in line with the crutch tips. This method is used primarily during Phase I of rehabilitation.

During the later phases of rehabilitation, partial weight-bearing on the involved limb may be prescribed. However, a physician should be consulted before the patient begins partial weight-bearing. If there still is considerable pain or discomfort when placing weight on the limb, have the patient return to whatever method used previously.

When going down stairs, the crutch tips and the involved limb are moved down one step, followed by the uninvolved leg. To help the patient remember which leg to lead with, say, "down with the bad, up with the good." If handrails are available, the patient puts both crutches under the outside arm and does a similar pattern using the handrail for support. The handrail will provide a more stable support than the second crutch can offer.

When going up stairs, the good limb is moved up one step while the hands support the body weight on the crutches. The full weight of the body is then transferred to the good leg so the crutches and the involved limb can be brought up to the step together.

Make sure the patient gets an opportunity to practice using the crutches before leaving the facility with them for the first time. Do not allow the patient to leave without demonstrating the ability to use them safely. Assistive devices like crutches are used to help patients heal from injuries, but improperly used, they can cause injury.

THINKING IT THROUGH

It is halfway through the swimming season and Molly can't take the pain in her shoulder anymore. It is her junior year and she has been doing okay, but not as well as everyone expected after such a great sophomore year. Since she has started high school she has not had a break: she goes from water polo right into swimming, and the off-seasons are filled with club teams. This relentless pace has given her terrible shoulder pain, making it impossible to keep up with the workouts despite her best efforts. After admitting to Chip, the high school's athletic trainer, that the pain is more than she can manage, they decided that it was time to see Dr. Mirich.

Dr. Mirich says that Molly has an impingement in her shoulder that has resulted in a slight tearing of the supraspinatus. This means she will have to be out of the water for a while—maybe even as long as nine months. Molly hasn't been out of the water for more than a week since she entered high school. Her only break was a week-long family vacation. She is devastated. Dr. Mirich told her to keep working with Chip, but he also recommended some formal physical therapy. He believes she will benefit from intensive one-on-one therapy sessions that Chip cannot provide, because of the number of students under his care.

Molly made an appointment with Gina, a physical therapist at the SPORT clinic. Gina noticed right away that Molly was feeling down. So, right after their first session concluded, Gina called Chip to see how the two of them could work together to get her motivated for the long rehabilitation she is about to enter.

What are some things Gina and Chip can do to get Molly motivated? Why is motivation important? How can Gina explain the phases of rehabilitation to Molly in a way that she will understand?

CHAPTER SUMMARY

A patient's goal in physical rehabilitation is to regain the ability to return to normal life at an effective level of performance. To help patients meet this goal, the rehabilitative environment should reflect a sense of professionalism, motivate the patient, and promote patient confidence in a positive outcome. An optimal healing environment can be created by assessing and making any necessary adjustments to the following areas: patient safety, patient needs, patient comfort, and staff conduct.

Many people contribute to the success of a patient's physical rehabilitation. They may include the physician, the physical therapist, the athletic trainer, the strength and conditioning specialist, the physical therapist assistant, the physical therapy aide, the patient's family, the patient, and other therapists. The staff members communicate with each other regularly about the patient's condition and progress—primarily via the patient's chart. This valuable file provides all of the patient's medical information necessary to develop an effective therapy program.

During rehabilitation, SOAP notes and progress notes are used by staff members to communicate with one another about the patient's progress. All of these notes are recorded on the patient's chart to ensure consistent and quality care by the rehabilitation team. Since abbreviations are commonly used on patient charts, all members of the rehabilitation staff must learn the abbreviations accepted for use by their facility. Proper communication among health care staff is vital to quality patient care.

The body's muscles and joints work best when the body's parts are properly aligned. For this reason, posture and range of motion are assessed at the beginning of the program, and then periodically thereafter to determine progress. Assessment of the patient's posture and ROM is done to meet four objectives: to establish a guide for the rehabilitation program; to provide a record for future progress evaluations; to motivate the patient; and to educate the patient in the ways posture may reflect, or even affect, physical health.

Although every patient's rehabilitation is unique, there are three phases of healing that must take place before former activities can be safely resumed. Understanding these phases will help in guiding the patient to a successful recovery. Phase I begins immediately after injury. The primary goal of this phase is to control inflammation. Additional loss of function is prevented through isometric strengthening and, in some cases, with supportive devices.

In Phase II the focus is on repairing damaged tissues. Strength and ROM are increased by changing to isotonic exercises and by increasing the patient's ADLs. Therapeutic modalities are also used in Phases I and II to produce desired therapeutic effects such as the reduction of pain and edema. Phase III is devoted to remodeling. The patient is prepared to return to normal life and to take responsibility for continuing physical therapy outside of the rehabilitation center. Exercise modalities, which increase strength and flexibility, generally replace the use of therapeutic modalities in Phase III. These exercises can take the form of isokinetic and/or variable resistance exercises. If full return to the former activities is not possible, the patient is taught to compensate for the loss of function by modifying the way in which activities of daily living are performed.

Finally, it is impossible to overstate the importance of patient education in the rehabilitative process. Patients must be kept informed of their health status, what to expect in terms of future progress, and how to prevent reinjury in all phases of rehabilitation. As injuries improve, a patient must be taught how to safely resume activities of daily living through the use of proper body mechanics and other preventive measures. Additional information about proper nutrition and the use of crutches or other assistive devices may also be necessary to help the patient in the return to normal life.

STUDENT ENRICHMENT ACTIVITIES

Complete the following sentences.

1. Rehabilitation consists of _____ and _____ designed to help disabled patients regain maximum function, a sense of _____, and the highest level of _____ possible.

2. The athletic trainer's role in the rehabilitation process corresponds to the_____ of injury, intensity of therapeutic goals, and state _____.

3. The keys to proper conduct in the rehabilitative environment are _____ and _____.

4. "SOAP" is an acronym for _____ findings, _____ findings, _____, and _____.

5. A person's _____ is a visual guide to his or her body alignment.

Complete the following exercises.

6. List two examples of subjective findings.

7. List two examples of objective findings.

8. List two examples of assessment notes.

9. List two examples of plan notes.

10. List four considerations that should be addressed in creating an optimal environment for healing.

11. List the four safety guidelines that must be followed in all phases of rehabilitation.

12. List three subjects about which a patient might need to be educated.

Write T for true, or F for false. Rewrite the false statements to make them true.

13. T   F   The athletic trainer's role is always supplemental to the physician's course of action.

14. T   F   For Phase I, the therapeutic modalities used generally will be ones that decrease bloodflow.

15. T   F   Patients who believe they will get better are more likely to work hard to make it happen than patients who do not have this confidence.

16. T   F   The purpose of Phase II in rehabilitation is to control inflammation.

17. T   F   Remodeling is done in Phase III.

18. T   F   In Phase III, the patient can often warm up the injured area prior to exercise and then ice it down after the activity to decrease subsequent swelling.

19. T   F   Phase I strengthening is isotonic.

20. T   F   In Phase II, the functional use of the injured area is increased, whether or not pain and swelling have been reduced.

Define the following abbreviations.

21. **ACL**

22. **BLE**

23. **GH**

24. **FWB**

25. **/d**

26. **Q** or **q̄**

27. **x**

28. **CWP**

29. **HP**

30. **US** or **Uz**

31. **Fx** or **Fr**

32. **PT**

33. ↑

34. **Δ**

35. **1°**

36. **c̄**

37. **Dx**

38. **Hx**

39. **pt**

40. **Sx**

Complete the following exercises.

41. Explain why strengthening exercises in a rehabilitation program should begin with isometrics. Then explain what types of exercises should be used in subsequent phases and why.

42. Explain why both cryotherapy and thermotherapy might be used in Phases II and III. Be sure to include the circumstances under which cold and heat may be used in your answer.

CHAPTER 25

The Selling Point: Promoting Fitness Products and Services

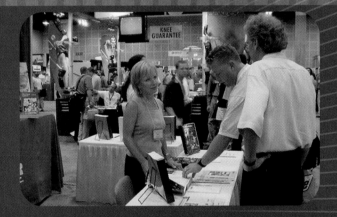

OBJECTIVES

After completing this chapter, you should be able to do the following:

1. Define and correctly spell each of the key terms.

2. List five types of sales presentations.

3. Describe techniques for creating a good impression over the telephone, in person, and in written correspondence.

4. Develop an effective resumé and cover letter.

5. List the key elements of an employment plan.

6. List the key elements of a business plan.

7. Name three sources of information about continuing education and related opportunities in the field of sports medicine.

KEY TERMS

* business plan
* cover letter
* demographics
* employment plan
* entrepreneur
* self-promotion
* resumé

THE HEALTH PROFESSIONAL AS A SALESPERSON

Sports medicine is a business. It's the business of taking care of athletes and others who are fitness-minded. Athletic trainers, strength and conditioning specialists, and others with similar educational backgrounds will benefit from viewing themselves as businesspeople. Regardless of whether such a person is an employee of a company or self-employed, a successful career depends on the realization that good sales technique is one of the most important talents a person can possess.

Success in business depends on establishing a need, then providing the service or product to fit that need. Athletes and fitness enthusiasts have many needs and desires; therefore, all are potential clients. One aspect of the health professional's job is to allow them the opportunity to access services or products being sold that will help them meet their goals. Products and services may include physical fitness instruction, athletic training services, physical therapy, and/or health care supplies and equipment (see Figure 25-1). Knowing the products and services inside and out is essential to good sales technique. Without an understanding and appreciation of all the benefits you have to offer as a sales professional, you won't be able to effectively explain to your clients why they need your products and services.

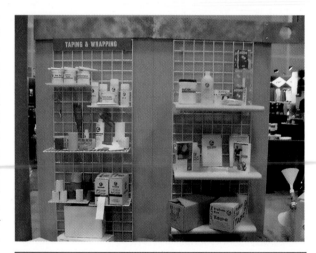

FIGURE 25-1 With the knowledge you have gained, you may have the opportunity to sell a wide variety of fitness or health-related products.

This chapter outlines the fundamental concepts of **self-promotion** and some basic rules of selling. Self-promotion is simply a matter of selling others on *you*. To do that, you must present your best qualities with a specific purpose in mind. For example, you may be an excellent cook and a capable soccer coach; however, if your purpose is to demonstrate your coaching skills to someone, showing them a press release about your team's recent victory would be more effective than offering your favorite recipe. Likewise, if you are selling your own fitness services or products, you would emphasize your own good physical health, or that of your

self-promotion

the presentation of one's self or company to buyers for acceptance through advertising and publicity.

other clients, rather than try to impress a potential customer with the fact that your success has allowed you to purchase a luxury car. While there are no absolute rules for a successful sale, this chapter offers strategies that are easily adapted to the widest possible range of situations.

> *The answers to three questions will determine your success or failure. 1. Can people trust me to do my best? 2. Am I committed to the task at hand? 3. Do I care about other people and show it? If the answers to these questions are "yes," there is no way you can fail.*
> Lou Holtz
> Football Coach

TYPES OF SALES PRESENTATIONS

Sales presentations can take many different forms. They can range from face-to-face meetings, to telephone conversations, to Internet or postal transactions, to mass-media promotions. Some forms of presentation are adaptable to a variety of situations. For instance, face-to-face meetings can take place in a store, a boardroom, a trade show, a restaurant, or numerous other places, whereas an online catalog must be viewed in a computerized environment to access the information. Choosing the best sales method for you will depend on your qualifications, your product or service, your customers, and your budget. A brief discussion of some different forms of sales presentations follows.

Face-to-Face Meetings

Face-to-face presentations usually take place in brick-and-mortar (retail) stores. A brick-and-mortar store is a building where you sell products and services to clients who come in to look for specific merchandise or just to browse. These face-to-face encounters are excellent opportunities to get familiar with your client's needs. Product knowledge, well-developed conversation and memory skills, intuition, a good sense of humor, and the ability to make the client feel comfortable are the keys to successful face-to-face meetings (see Figure 25-2). These skills and personal qualities can be adapted to any sales situation and will enhance the client's impression of your business.

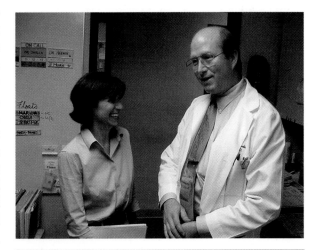

FIGURE 25-2 A good sense of humor is an excellent asset in face-to-face presentations.

Internet-Based Presentations

Several types of sales presentations can be done using the Internet. These include e-commerce, click-and-mortar presentations, and educational Web sites. E-commerce refers to selling items through the Internet. Often this method of presentation is driven by links that provide consumers with access to information about your products and services through other sites and searches, making this information available to the widest possible range of potential clients. E-commerce also makes use of online catalogs that list products, descriptions, and prices for customers to view using their computers. Click-and-mortar sales refer to a combination of e-commerce and a physical building. An example of a click-and-mortar sales presentation would be the online introduction and marketing of a custom knee brace that must be purchased at a brick-and-mortar store so that the brace can be properly fitted to the customer. Educational Web pages may also be used to demonstrate your commitment to continuing education. While these pages are not used overtly to sell products, they can enlighten consumers in a way that will focus their attention—and their business—on your click-and-mortar sales presentation.

Telephone Sales

Using the telephone to promote products and services is called *telemarketing*. Excellent conversation skills, a good sense of humor, no fear of rejection, self-motivation, and a clear focus on obtaining results are the key elements that will help make this a positive and rewarding presentation method. Telemarketing can be done from an office, from home, or from the road using a cell phone. However, like all sales presentations, it is best to plan the sales call for a time when interruptions and distractions are unlikely. You want your customer's undivided attention, and you owe that customer the same degree of attention.

Educational Materials for Handouts, Trade Shows, and Direct Mail

Educational material can take the form of informative brochures, descriptive flyers, event announcements, broadcast faxes, newsletters, seminars, infommercials, and, as already mentioned, Web pages. Well-researched, up-to-date educational material will help to identify you as a knowledgeable and reliable source of information, and will establish your expertise in a particular market area. Trade shows and conventions that promote related equipment and/or services are excellent opportunities to distribute educational material and get to know other professionals in your field (see Figure 25-3). You should also make a point to be aware of and attend relevant organizational events, such as play-offs or championship series, off-season training camps, and open-door wellness clinics.

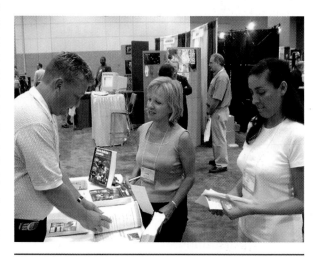

FIGURE 25-3 Trade shows are excellent opportunities to get to know other professionals in your field and distribute educational materials.

Direct mail is another great way to generate business

once your target **demographics** have been firmly established. As with all sales presentations, understanding what type of consumer will have the most interest in your services is the key to a successful direct mail campaign. Make sure your solicitation goes out to people who are most likely to be interested in your products and not to people who have no interest at all. When determining your target demographics, you will want to consider things like age, marital status, geographic location, income, common interests, and related leisure activities of your potential clients. A clear understanding of your target consumer will help you to access appropriate mailing lists and labels. There are many agencies that can provide these services to you.

> **demographics**
> statistical characteristics of given populations used to define business markets.

Mass Media Promotions (Television/Radio/Print)

Sales promotions using the more traditional mass media are yet another method of attracting customers who may be interested in your products and services. These traditional media include television, radio, and print advertising. Again, knowledge of your target demographics both regionally and financially is essential to this type of sales strategy. Media presentations can be costly and ineffective if you have the wrong or misinterpreted demographic data. Additionally, a clear understanding of "hooks" or "tag lines" that will capture consumers' interest in your services is a vital component of any successful media promotion. Finally, an understanding of contracts and negotiations associated with this type of marketing can be an invaluable business tool; take the time to fully research this or any other presentation method to make sure that you are using it to your best advantage.

Each of these sales presentation methods has its own benefits and drawbacks. Further, we have not even attempted to list all the variations on these basic principles of sales technique and strongly encourage you to consult several other sources that may provide additional details or information on alternate sales strategies. Once you have thoroughly researched what others have to say, you must evaluate each method with respect to your professional goals, taking the best elements of each suggestion to develop a strategy that will work best for you.

MAKING A GOOD FIRST IMPRESSION

The old saying is true: "You never get a second chance to make a good first impression." First impressions tend to be lasting ones. Whether you are applying for a position with a company or making a sales call, make the most of every opportunity to make a good first impression by preparing in advance and always remembering your manners.

Meeting Someone in Person

Meeting someone in person is always the best opportunity to present yourself and your services. Only in a face-to-face meeting are you virtually guaranteed of having the listener's undivided attention. When seeking employment, picking up an application is often the first impression; be aware that the receptionist will be passing on his or her first impression to the appropriate person. The same rules apply to individuals making sales calls. A smile and a pleasant, respectful attitude to all you meet will pay off in ways you might not imagine. Do not just reserve your good manners for the person you intend to meet; you never know who else might have influence over your potential customer. Guidelines for effective face-to-face meetings are presented in "Techniques for Interviews and Other Face-to-Face Presentations" later in this chapter.

Using the Telephone

As seen in the telemarketing sales method, telephones are an important method of communication (see Figure 25-4). If you choose to contact a potential employer by telephone, or if you need to speak with or leave messages for your clients over the phone, use your best telephone etiquette! The following are some general guidelines and suggestions to help you courteously conduct business using the telephone.

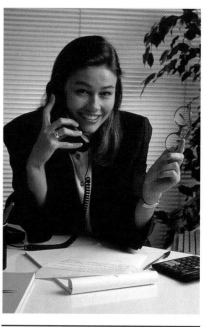

FIGURE 25-4 Always use your best manners when using the telephone.

1. Prepare yourself in advance by knowing what questions you want to ask and what information you want to provide *before* you dial the number. Write this information down in advance and keep it in front of you during the call. Mark each question off as it is asked and write down the answers. Always make sure that you have paper and something to write with before placing a call.

2. Speak clearly and maintain a positive frame of mind. No one wants to receive a call from someone who seems to be in a bad mood. Attitude is projected through your voice: If you smile while you speak, your attitude will be evident to the person on the other end of the line.

3. Speak at a moderate volume, as if the listener were across a large desk from you. Shouting can be as irritating to the listener as mumbling.

4. Introduce yourself and ask to "please" speak with the appropriate person. If you know the person's name, ask for him or her by name. If you are inquiring about a job opening, or if you don't know the person's name, give the person answering the phone the simplest, most direct purpose for your call. For example, "I'm calling about the position advertised" (always name the position and say where you saw the ad); or "I am returning Susan's call." Keep in mind that opportunities are not always advertised—especially in large companies. Don't hesitate to call companies and organizations that are relevant to your services or career goals and introduce yourself to the human resources or personnel department.

5. Always thank the person answering the phone for transferring your call, taking a message, or providing information.

6. Ask if you may follow up the telephone call by presenting the company or client with your resumé and/or filling out an employment application.

7. Always thank the listener for his or her time.

8. When receiving telephone calls, always answer in a courteous and professional tone. This applies to outgoing messages on voicemail as well.

Written Introductions

Most employment opportunities will require a **resumé** and a **cover letter** (see Figure 25-5). Designed to provide potential employers with selected information, a resumé is a summary of your professional work experience, personal attributes, and education. Only the information you choose to reveal about yourself should be included. The goal of the resumé is to grab the interest of the person who is doing the hiring. Writing a resumé that persuades a potential employer to contact you for an interview is a time-consuming project. An important aspect of writing an effective resumé is to do it when you are in a positive frame of mind. Positive thinking will project a positive attitude about you through your resumé.

Some other helpful suggestions for resumé and cover letter submissions are addressed in the following section. Additional forms of written introduction for those who are involved in sales are discussed in the promotional materials section of "Techniques for Interviews and Other Face-to-Face Presentations," later in this chapter.

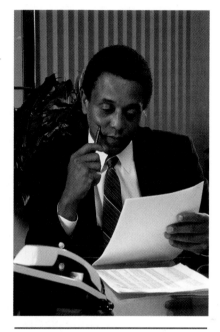

resumé

a brief, written account of personal and professional qualifications and experience prepared by an applicant for a position.

cover letter

a letter that accompanies a resumé to explain or introduce its contents.

FIGURE 25-5 Written introductions often consist of a resumé and a cover letter.

CREATING EFFECTIVE WRITTEN INTRODUCTIONS

There is no one correct way to format your resumé or to word your cover letter. Be creative, but do not go overboard. Employers may be turned off if too much is happening on the resumé or if a letter is unprofessional in appearance or content. The look of your resumé and the words you use in your cover letter should reflect your personality. However, professionalism generally dictates that certain stylistic guidelines be followed in all business-related written correspondence. Following are some guidelines to consider.

General Guidelines for Correspondence

1. Store your resumé and cover letter electronically on your computer's hard drive or a storage device such as a CD-ROM or USB flash drive. Never make a change to a printed copy and send it out; always make the correction electronically and then print a new, error-free copy. Neatness counts!

2. Print the document on a high-quality printer.

3.   Use plain, white, resumé-quality paper.

4.   Side margins should always be consistent. (If you use a 3/4-inch right margin then try to use a 3/4-inch left margin too.) Generally, the top and bottom margins should also be consistent on resumes.

5.   The spacing of each section should also be consistent. For example, double spaces between each category and single spaces between the paragraphs in each section may be appropriate.

6.   Use a simple font style to make it easy to read.

7.   Use correct grammar and punctuation, and do a spell-check as well as a thorough proofread. Spell-checkers don't catch all errors! Proofreading the documents at least twice will help avoid any errors or typos the computer did not catch. If you have the time, it is a good idea to put it away for a day or two and then come back to it. If you try to edit it right after you finish, there is a tendency to overlook careless mistakes. Having someone else proofread it is also a good idea.

8.   Use words and phrases common to the industry, but make sure you use them correctly. Don't fake knowledge or experience you don't have. Most employers are unimpressed with long words, and are quick to spot inaccurate use of medical or fitness jargon!

9.   Make sure your sentences are short, specific, and truthful. Statements that are too general or vague can waste space and are not effective if they obscure your meaning.

10. A resumé should not exceed one or two 8½ × 11-inch sheets of paper in length. Your resumé will likely be read along with countless others, so you'll want to make it easy for the reader to locate the desired information. A concise resumé is easier to read than a lengthy one.

Resumés and other correspondence may be mailed, faxed, e-mailed, or hand-delivered. If you are contacted for an interview, always bring one clean (unmarked) copy for the interviewer and one for yourself. If you are e-mailing your resumé, try to find out what software the receiver is using and submit the resumé as an attachment to an e-mailed cover letter to preserve formatting.

Developing the Resumé

There are several different ways in which resumés may be organized and formatted. In general, you should organize the information in a manner that presents you and your qualifications in the best way possible. However, it is safe to assume that all employers will be looking for a contact heading at the top of the page and a summary of your background and qualifications. The heading should include three items: your first and last name; your complete address; and your complete telephone number(s), including the area code. If possible, avoid using a post office box number; employers associate box numbers with instability. Make yourself easy to contact; be sure to list any additional phone numbers where you want to be reached, such a work or a cell phone number.

When describing your background and qualifications for the job, the information should directly relate to the position for which you are applying. If you are applying for jobs with different titles and/or job descriptions, it is a good idea to customize your resumé. Remember to keep notes or use file names to keep track of which resumé you sent to each company. The following categories of information are generally included on resumés.

1. *Objective:* This statement describes your career goal. You should be able to achieve this goal with the position for which you are applying.

2. *Summary of Qualifications:* This section should include your employment history. The jobs should be listed in reverse chronological order. This means that your current or most recent job is listed first, then the one you held before it, etc. Consider listing your responsibilities and duties for your most recent job. Try to work in some of your strongest attributes in this section, and try to quantify your job accomplishments. Be sure to include the dates you worked for these previous jobs.

3. *Educational Background:* Start with your most recent educational experience and work backward. College education, vocational training, and seminars all are important to potential employers. You should list the dates you attended, the name of the institution, and any degrees, diplomas, or certifications you received. High school information may be omitted from the resumé five years after graduation.

The following is a list of additional categories that may be included in the resumé. These items may be left off the resumé if the document is becoming too lengthy. If there is information you would like to pass along regarding any of these sections but are limited on space, state it in the cover letter that accompanies the resumé.

1. *Community Involvement:* Membership in professional organizations and volunteerism indicate a desire for continuous self-improvement and a willingness to help others.

2. *Offices Held:* Official positions can indicate leadership abilities and respect from peers.

3. *References:* Only provide names if they are specifically requested. Otherwise state, "References available upon request" at the bottom of the resumé. Be sure to have a list of references and their complete contact information with you during the interview.

4. *Salary Range:* Include your salary history only if it is requested.

5. *Miscellaneous:* Use this section to indicate your willingness to travel or relocate and the date you would be available to start work. This section also should include any professional achievements, such as professional certifications and titles.

Sell yourself as you develop the resumé! You are your own marketing department. Emphasize your positive aspects. Your career is an important part of your life so take the time to put together a well-crafted resumé. Use the sample resumé shown in Figure 25-6 as an example. A resumé is a special kind of sales presentation in itself—if done with care and thought it can be the first of many presentations.

Writing a Cover Letter

Your resumé should be accompanied by a cover letter. A cover letter serves as an introduction and communicates your desire to be considered for a particular position. Keep the letter short and simple. It is not necessary to provide details of your qualifications or personal attributes in the cover letter; these will be reflected in the resumé. When writing a cover letter, or a letter of inquiry, try to incorporate words and phrases used in the announcement, taking care to address the needs of the client or employer. A sample cover letter is shown in Figure 25-7. The letter should be formatted in business style, spaced as shown in the sample, and have equal margins.

TECHNIQUES FOR INTERVIEWS AND OTHER FACE-TO-FACE PRESENTATIONS

Interviews and other in-person meetings can be deal-makers or deal-breakers. The way in which you present yourself will greatly influence a potential customer or employer's willingness to listen to what you have to say. The following guidelines will help you make any face-to-face presentation a positive experience. Never miss an opportunity to make a good first impression. Remember this when preparing for job interviews, client conferences, public events, or any other professional appointments.

1. Be aware of the importance of personal hygiene to a first impression. First impressions take place before any word is said. Therefore, properly groomed hair, clean hands, manicured nails, brushed teeth, and fresh breath are all important parts of any first impression. Perfume or cologne may be used, but it should be pleasant—not too strong. Never use fragrance to compensate for a missed shower day.

2. Dress in a professional style that will offer a good impression and that does not make people uncomfortable in your presence. If in doubt about what to wear, remember that it is usually better to be overdressed than underdressed. Shoes should always be clean and well-shined.

3. Be punctual. If you have an appointment, arrive at least 5 minutes early. Be ready and eager when the time comes. If something happens that causes you to be late, call and let your client know when you expect to be there. This gives the client the opportunity to do other work or reschedule for another time. Don't make a habit of being late. The client or employer may accept it this once but may not accept it twice.

4. Look the client or employer in the eyes and provide a firm handshake with a sincere greeting. Ask for his or her name, and repeat it in your head at least four times to help you to remember it. Try to associate the name with something about the person. For example, if the person's name is Jim try to connect the name with the idea that he works in a gym. This may sound

Tasha Smith
1234 Main Street
Options, CA 00000-0000
Telephone: (123) 555-5678
e-mail: TS198@misc.org

OBJECTIVE
A full-time position as a certified athletic trainer in a high school setting.

SUMMARY OF QUALIFICATIONS
January (year) to Present
Athletic Training Student, ABC University, Anytown, MD
Assigned to football, soccer, swimming, and diving teams. Performed the following duties under the supervision of the certified athletic trainer:

- Evaluated, treated, and prevented athletic injuries
- Familiar with a variety of therapeutic modalities including: electrical muscle stimulation, ultrasound, fluidotherapy, hydrocollator packs, ice packs, whirlpools, and paraffin bath
- Assisted with athlete physicals and fitness testing
- Wrote and maintained individual athlete injury and rehabilitation reports

Summers, (year) – (year)
Athletic Training Student, Youth Cheer Camps and Youth Gymnastics, ABC University, Anytown, MD

September (year) – December (year)
Athletic Training Student, John Smith High School, Anytown, MD
- Assigned to football, volleyball, girls basketball, and wrestling teams

EDUCATIONAL BACKGROUND
Currently working toward NATA certification. Examination scheduled for December.
Teaching Credential in progress. Extension Courses, ABC University. Estimated completion date (year).
Certified, Sports Medicine First Aid and CPR, (year).
Bachelor of Science, Athletic Training, ABC University, (year).
Associate of Arts, General Education, Valley College, (year). Graduated with Honors.
Graduated, Valley High School, (year). Highest Honors.
Completed High School Athletic Training Course with Honors.

References: Available upon request.

FIGURE 25-6 A Sample Resumé

Tasha Smith
1234 Main Street
Options, CA 00000-0000
Telephone: (123) 555-5678
e-mail: TS198@misc.org

November 15, (year)

Ms. Rebecca Jackson
Director of Human Resources
Riverdale School District
2345 Education Lane
Wellness, CA 11111-2222

Dear Ms. Jackson:

I am responding to your advertisement in the _____
on _____ for the position of _____. I am a
recent honor graduate of ABC University and am pursuing a career as an athletic trainer.

Enclosed for your review is my resumé. I would appreciate consideration for
an interview for the above position. As my resumé reflects, I have six years of
experience as an athletic training student and I'm currently working on my
teaching credential. Now that I have graduated, I am eager to begin a full-
time career in the field of sports medicine.

If you desire additional information, or would like to schedule an interview,
please contact me by telephone at (123) 555-5678.

Thank you for considering my application.

Sincerely,

Tasha Smith
Tasha Smith

Enclosure

FIGURE 25-7 A Sample Cover Letter

silly, but it is very important to use and remember people's names. Use a cheat sheet if necessary. Once you leave, write down the person's name along with any important details and where the conversation left off. Some people have the ability to just remember these things; but there is nothing wrong with using memory aids if you are not among those endowed with that ability.

5. Listen to what others have to say. It is important for clients or potential employers to listen to your sales pitch, but even more important for you to listen to their needs. The information they give you will help you align your presentation to their interests.

6. Know your product. In any interview or presentation your confidence will be boosted by your knowledge of the subject you are presenting. Whether you are presenting yourself, a particular product, or a valuable service, it is essential that you understand what you are selling. Introduce your product, explain what it can do, and show how it will best suit the client's needs. Finally, show the client or employer how his or her goals can be met through you.

7. Research your product. Write out 20 questions about your product. Your product could be an ultrasound machine, a fitness program, or athletic training services for a basketball team. Remember, if you can't explain the product or service to yourself, you will not be able to explain it to anyone else. Practice with friends; see if they can come up with any questions you didn't answer in your practice presentation. You should feel good about your product and transfer that feeling to the client in your presentation (see Figure 25-8).

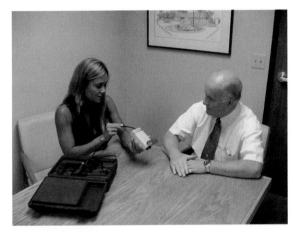

FIGURE 25-8 Thorough knowledge of your product will give you confidence in your presentation and provide your clients with the best service possible.

8. Be prepared to give the client any information that might be needed. Explain your product and if you don't have an answer to a question, assure the client you will get the information by a specific time and date. Then, be sure to deliver as promised. Never fake it; people will see right through phoniness. Never promise anything you can't do.

9. Be versatile in your presentations. Sales presentations can take place in a variety of settings: retail stores, social engagements, patient appointments, or corporate environments. This is why you must understand your product well—you must be able to explain it in any situation. If you have a chance to give your pitch in a boardroom, in a gym, or in a national meeting, become

familiar with the type of presentation the client prefers (see Figure 25-9). This can range from a computer presentation to an outline and notes written in pencil on a lined pad.

10. Always use the client or potential employer's name when saying good-bye. Regardless of the outcome of the meeting, look the person in the eyes and thank him or her sincerely for spending time with you, because you know how valuable that person's time is.

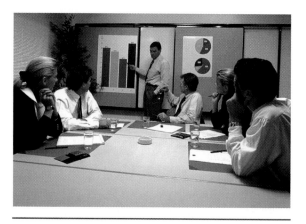

FIGURE 25-9 If possible, find out what type of sales presentation your client prefers, and design your presentation to suit those preferences.

Promotional Materials

For practical purposes, clients need to feel that you are accessible to them and that they can reach you easily. At the very least, make sure you always leave a potential client with your business card. A business card should include the standard information: your name, your title, the business name, the address, telephone and fax numbers (with area codes), an e-mail address, and a Web site address. There is nothing wrong with making your business card into a small, concise brochure about your product. This can be done on the front, on the back, or using a folded format. Folded cards offer twice as much room for information. Some people like to keep the back of the card partially blank to provide a place for the client to write notes about the meeting.

As a sales representative, providing your clients with an opportunity to get to know you will help to establish a mutually beneficial relationship. You can assist clients in getting to know you by providing them with an opportunity to read about you and your product or service. Well-designed brochures, handouts, and Web sites provide important information about you, your company, or your product/service that can be studied at the client's leisure. Remember, if you are self-employed, *you* are the company. Your professional brochure, Web site, or promotional handout should contain the following information:

* The products and/or services you are offering

* The needs met by these products and services

* The company name and logo

* Pictures of products

* A hook—the aspect of your product or service that will draw in clients and distinguish you from the competition

* Your name and location; provide mailing, physical, and/or Web addresses, as appropriate

* How to contact you; provide telephone, cell, and fax numbers as well as e-mail addresses

* Your certifications and other licensing qualifications, such as CPR and first aid certification or teaching licenses

* Memberships in, or affiliations with, pertinent professional organizations

* The company's history, accomplishments, and goals

Promotional materials are not effective unless they are used, opened, read, and acted upon, or at least kept for future reference. An attractive exterior will help assure that the brochure is opened; a clear message will make sure that it gets read; and a hook (e.g., 10% off coupon) or a clever tag line will make consumers want to take action. By including additional promotional items in your handouts, you can encourage consumers to keep your materials handy for future action. Examples of such items include a pad of sticky notes, a refrigerator magnet, or a mouse pad that has your business phone number and Web address on it. Using promotional items is a great way of keeping you, your business, and your message fresh in the consumer's mind (see Figure 25-10). Remember to put your complete business information on everything you hand or send out.

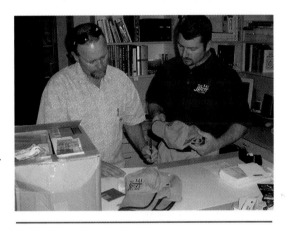

FIGURE 25-10 Your company's name and logo can be put on many items for promotional purposes.

Other methods of sending promotional information include e-mail, faxes, and informative answering systems. These do not always have the same effect as eye-catching brochures and Web sites; the nature of these information systems limits their visual appeal and, sometimes, their ability to get the client's attention. However, these methods can be very effective in getting basic information to those who need it in a timely manner.

* E-mail: This allows you to contact people efficiently. Don't send junk mail; this will turn the client off about your product. Treat all clients as if their time is very, very valuable. This doesn't mean you can't ask if they want to be informed about any new products or service that you may have.

* Faxes: This is another way to contact people efficiently. The recommendations pertaining to e-mail, especially about not wasting client's time, apply to faxes as well. Some software programs can assist with the organization and transmission of faxes.

* Informative Answering Systems: These can be used for answering frequently asked questions automatically, such as directions, hours, and upcoming events.

PLAN FOR SUCCESS

"Plan to succeed; or don't plan and don't succeed."

Bill Gates
Microsoft Corporation

To make the most of your career, you must plan for success. Success doesn't just happen—it requires hard work and careful planning, but it does not mean the same thing for everyone. Success is defined by what is important to you or what you hope to achieve. Your goals should be the driving force behind every aspect of finding a job, starting a business, or selling products and services. Remember, goals are not set in stone; they can be modified. As your priorities change, so will your goals.

In order to set goals, you need to know what you want. What do you want to be doing in one year? What about five years? How about 10 years? For some people, the answers to these questions are easy, but for others they are not. The Career Path Self-Assessment test (Figure 25-11) will help you explore whether self-employment might be right for you, or whether you might be happier as an employee of a company. Of course, no two companies are exactly alike, so being an employee of Company A may be totally different from being an employee of Company B; however, some generalizations can be made about employment that can help you decide upon an appropriate career path.

Once you have answered these questions, look at the number of blue answers you gave and compare them to the number of red answers you chose. A majority of

Career Path Self-Assessment		
Do I think I want to be an employee?	yes	no
Do I think I want to own my own business?	yes	no
Do I want regular raises?	yes	no
Do I want to set my own direction each day?	yes	no
Am I a self-starter?	yes	no
Am I a leader?	yes	no
Am I a follower?	yes	no
Am I willing to go through the proper licensing, permit, and tax procedures to start my own business?	yes	no
Do I want someone else to take care of my withholding tax?	yes	no
Do I want regular vacations?	yes	no
Do I want to work more than 8 hours a day?	yes	no
Do I like to make decisions?	yes	no
Do I like challenges?	yes	no
Do I have the resources to start my own business?	yes	no
Am I good at managing my money?	yes	no
Would I feel more secure financially as an employee of an organization than as an entrepreneur?	yes	no

FIGURE 25-11 Career Path Self-Assessment

blue answers may indicate a predisposition toward self-employment, or being an **entrepreneur**, whereas a majority of red answers may indicate characteristics that make an employee situation more desirable.

Deciding on a career path can be difficult. At times, your options may seem overwhelming and you may find yourself wishing you had fewer options to choose from. But by researching the choices available to you, you have the opportunity to make an informed decision about what is best for you (see Figure 25-12). To assist in this process, talk to people you know, both employed and self-employed, about your options, and listen to any advice they may offer as well as what they say about their own experiences. Some people will have good information, and some will not. You don't have to act on everything, but do take the time to listen—sometimes you will be surprised at what you learn. Individuals who have found success in what they do may have some valuable advice for you. It is also important to discuss your

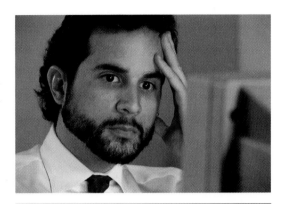

FIGURE 25-12 Take the time to research your career options and really think about what is important to you.

ideas with people who will play the role of "devil's advocate" for you. Encouragement is great, but the real world is very competitive, so you must prepare yourself properly. Bounce ideas off people who won't just tell you what you want to hear.

Talk with those who are closest to you about the information you obtain. They may be able to help you determine which steps may help you reach your goals and which ones are better left untried. Then, make your own decision based on the information obtained from the self-assessment, the information you obtain from your discussions, and your gut instincts. Ultimately, it will not be the answer to any one of these questions, but a cumulative response to these and other questions that should guide your decision.

Once you've decided on a career path—even if it is only a tentative decision, a plan for achieving your goals must be established. It is vital to have the plan in writing; a written plan helps you stay focused and communicates thought, effort, and sincerity, whereas a plan that you keep in your head can shift and become vague, jeopardizing key elements. Remember—if it is not in writing, the chances of it happening decrease immensely.

The Employment Plan

If you are leaning toward applying your skills to a more traditional employer-employee relationship, you will need an **employment plan**. An employment plan is a set of steps that you intend to take to achieve your career goals (see Figure 25-13). Your employment plan should be specific, but flexible. Know what you are looking for, but be open to any unexpected opportunities that may arise. Like all plans, your employment plan should consist of long- and short-term goals. A realistic and effective plan should acknowledge existing obstacles, describe expected rewards, contain motivating statements that help you envision your success, and list any other comments you believe helpful. The plan should also include scheduled dates for

entrepreneur

an individual who organizes, manages, and assumes the responsibility for a business.

employment plan

a detailed description of an individual's strategy for finding employment and advancing in a career.

Employment Plan

Long-term Goal: A permanent position as a head ATC for football, soccer, and swimming at the high school level

Short-term Goals: Check want ads; Call every high school within a 60 mile radius of home; Complete education and certification process

Obstacles: Competition; Still working toward certification

Rewards: Job security; Rewarding job; It's what I like to do; I like working with kids.

Reasons I Will Succeed: I have the basic education to get an entry-level position; I'm getting the education I need for the advanced position.

Comments: I have the support of my family.

Dates Plan Reviewed: March 12, April 12

FIGURE 25-13 A Sample Employment Plan

review and/or modification of the plan. As time goes on, you may find it necessary to make revisions.

In forming your plan, you might first want to consider the type of position you would most like to have. In doing so, you should also assess your salary requirements. Do you have the skills necessary for the position you desire? If not, do you know how you can obtain those skills? How much money do you need to make each month in order to pay your bills and to set some money aside for the future? Check current salary ranges for the positions you are considering. Do they match your immediate financial needs and desires? If not, you may need to consider another type of position, or reassess your financial needs. Sometimes it can be worthwhile to trim a budget temporarily in order to get started on a career you will find fulfilling.

Everyone has to start somewhere; entry-level positions often provide ample room for advancement.

Next, you might want to identify the types of businesses, organizations, or institutions that offer the kinds of opportunities you have targeted. Schools, community sport leagues, fitness centers, medical supply companies, fitness equipment companies, and health clinics are just a few examples of sources for career opportunities relating to sports medicine. Once you have identified such general sources for employment opportunities, locate the specific businesses, institutions, and/or organizations in your areas that may be able to offer you such opportunities. Check Internet, professional magazine, and newspaper job postings, too, but don't rely solely on posted job openings. Seek out and create your own opportunities using the sales techniques previously discussed in this chapter.

The planning doesn't end with employment. Once you've obtained a position, you will need to create a new plan that reflects your new goals. What do you want to do next? Do you want to progress beyond the position you've just obtained? What opportunities for advancement exist within the company? Do you want a higher position, or simply more money as time goes on? Do you view your new position as a steppingstone to a more desirable position with another company, or do you see yourself staying with the new company for years to come? Answers to all of these questions and any others you feel are important should be reflected in your written employment plan.

The Business Plan

A **business plan** is an employment plan for the self-employed. The purpose of a business plan is to define your goal and outline a plan for achieving it. A well-written business plan can simplify the potentially intimidating task of starting a new business by breaking the entrepreneurial process down into small steps. A business plan also communicates your vision to individuals you would like to include in your business, such as investors, vendors, customers, employees, friends, and family. Simply put, a business plan is a story of your business that you want investors and partners to read to win their endorsement of the concept. This is particularly important if you are seeking outside financing; if you are seeking a loan, the bank will require a business plan.

Business plans vary in design and content, but there are four subjects that must be addressed: a business description; the marketing strategy; the management strategy; and the financial strategy. Additional items of concern often include: a statement of purpose; an industry and market analysis; a description of the competition; operating procedures; business insurance; personnel; budgets; financial reports; assumptions; trends; comparatives; cash-flow statements; income statements; balance sheets; sources and uses of funds; and an executive summary. Depending on your business, these considerations may serve as an excellent outline for a business plan. However, there are still more details that must be considered before launching your own business venture. What are your time commitments to family and other current obligations? What can you give up? What must you keep? Do you intend to form a partnership, corporation, or sole proprietorship? Must you file a fictitious business name with the city? What licenses and/or permits will you need to do business in that city? Do you need the protection of a patent, copyright, or trademark? All of these questions and more should be answered in the business plan.

Developing a plan that effectively describes such key information can be a difficult task; however, there are many software programs and business services that

business plan

a detailed description of the business strategy for an established or start-up business.

provide assistance in the formation of a business plan. Check the Internet by doing a search on the phrase "business plan" and see what looks to be worth your time. Figure 25-14 outlines the key elements of a business plan.

ELEMENTS OF A BUSINESS PLAN

Statement of Purpose

Description of the Business (location, products, and services)

Industry and Market Analysis

Description of the Competition

Marketing Strategy (Pricing, Advertising, and Public Relations)

Operating Procedures

Business Insurance

Management Strategy
    Personnel

Financial Strategy
    Start-up Budget
    Operating Budget

Appendices (supporting documents and financial projections such as financial reports; assumptions, trends, and comparatives; cash-flow statements; income statements; balance sheets; sources and uses of funds)

Executive Summary

FIGURE 25-14 Elements of a Business Plan

Once you have addressed these considerations and analyzed your responses to the issues presented in this chapter, you might be ready to step into action. Or, you may find that you simply have more questions. Only when you are finally satisfied with your answers and confident in your solutions (which may include a backup plan) should the process begin. Having said this, don't be overly afraid of making mistakes. Learn from the mistakes you make and keep trying. Nothing will happen if you don't try. Fear can be paralyzing.

Taking Action (Playing the Option)

As you begin to outline your career goals, the decision to become a member of an organization or go solo with your own business will probably top your list of considerations, because each option offers a distinct path to different goals (see Figure 25-15). If you choose to become an employee, educational requirements, work environments, and salaries may top your list of concerns. On the other hand, if you decide to go it alone, even more decisions must be made regarding location, inventory, funding, competition, logos, copyrights, trademarks, accounting, and legal implications. Many excellent reference guides are available for establishing and growing a small business.

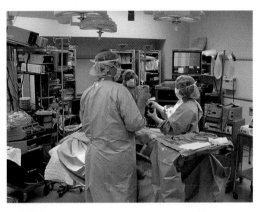

FIGURE 25-15 Don't limit yourself. With the knowledge you've acquired, you can sell all kinds of health care equipment and supplies: surgical equipment, taping supplies, orthopedic aids, etc.

Search online, or consult your local library or bookstore for appropriate titles.

No matter which path you choose, this is an extremely important stage in your life. It really doesn't matter if you decide to change your mind later; having a well-thought-out, clearly established plan at the outset will also help you to recognize when your objectives and methods need to be revised as time goes on. Discussing the experiences and opinions of others can help make this initial planning a lot easier than worrying in the dark.

> *If you decline to take risks early—you'll decline in the market later. But if you bet big—only a few of these risks have to succeed to provide for your future.*
>
> Bill Gates
> Microsoft Corporation

CONTINUING YOUR EDUCATION

Further education and certification significantly increase job opportunities. As discussed in Chapters 2 and 3, advanced degrees and certifications are available from a wide variety of sources, depending on your specialization. The National Athletic Trainers' Association (NATA), the National Strength and Conditioning Association (NSCA), and the American College of Sports Medicine (ACSM) are all excellent sources of information on approved programs, accredited colleges, available certifications, and upcoming workshops and exams. Other sources of continuing education include local colleges, hospitals, and clinics.

Even with certification, the learning never stops (see Figure 25-16). Sports medicine is an exciting field—one that is constantly changing. New products, theories, and jobs are emerging all the time. To stay up-to-date, you will need to make a conscious effort to get educated about these changes. Attend conferences and workshops on new products, emerging techniques, and changing laws whenever possible. Read everything you can get your hands on. Regardless of your path, careers in sports medicine can always be enhanced by information that can be obtained from books and articles on health, health care, fitness, sports, physical therapy, occupational therapy, marketing, advertising, business, accounting, personnel, time management, investing, and business or medical law.

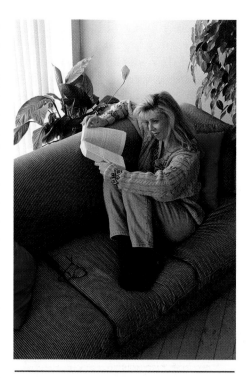

FIGURE 25-16 Add to your knowledge by reading everything you can find that relates to your career.

Use your spare time to learn. If you think you don't have any spare time, think again. Find creative ways to squeeze in a little extra time to gain more knowledge. Use the time spent in your car to listen to educational and/or motivational audio tapes. Before you shut down your computer at the end of the day, visit one educational or competitive Web site to learn about the latest trends, or new research, or to keep your eye on the competition. Networking can also be a valuable means of getting information you need; contact friends and/or colleagues who are knowledgeable in a given area and ask questions. Just remember to be respectful of their time.

Regardless of the career path you choose, staying in charge of your future means never taking anything for granted. Take advantage of every opportunity to gain new information and skills in the subjects that affect your career. As you do this, strive to maintain a healthy balance of work and relaxation in your life. This requires effective time-management skills and the ability to prioritize. Achieving the proper balance between your career and the rest of your life is one of the most important lessons you can learn. Know what is important to you and concentrate on the things that will put your goals within reach. The knowledge you've obtained from this book has given you a great start on your education. Continue your quest for knowledge by exploring the aspects of the field that interest you most and by pursuing the options that seem the most compelling. Stay curious and you will find endless opportunities for a rewarding career and a fulfilling life.

There's really no secret about our approach. Keep moving forward. Open new doors and keep doing new things, because we are curious and curiosity keeps leading us down new paths.

Walt Disney

THINKING IT THROUGH

Lisa has been an athletic training student for a year. Now that she has graduated, she wants to go to work in the business world. She has spent the past year learning all about injuries and how to take care of them. But she is so good at sales and service, she is considering a career in the sales of fitness equipment.

Her education and experience has given Lisa a basic understanding of electrical modalities, but she would really like to learn more. She saw an advertisement in the paper for a sales associate for TEAM Rehabilitation and responded to the ad with a resumé and cover letter as requested. TEAM Rehabilitation is an established company with a good track record. Lisa has seen their representatives around and is impressed with their professionalism.

After a week of waiting, Lisa received a phone call from Nancy, the CEO of TEAM Rehabilitation. Nancy asked Lisa to come in for an interview. In addition to the expected information such as references, a driver's license, and a clean copy of her resumé, Lisa was also asked to prepare a few additional items for the meeting. Nancy asked Lisa to make up a sales presentation for the interview. She specifically requested the following items: a business card; sales demographics of the local area; a daily work schedule if she were to get the job; and a list of Lisa's strengths and weaknesses as she sees them.

Nancy isn't that interested in Lisa's knowledge of the product yet—she can teach Lisa that. Her primary concerns are Lisa's character, which she will judge from the letters of recommendation, and Lisa's understanding of sales techniques, which she will assess in the interview. Additional characteristics Nancy is hoping to see include punctuality, communication skills, organization skills, and a professional appearance.

Besides assembling the requested materials, what else should Lisa do in preparation for the interview? How might she go about obtaining the sales demographics Nancy requested? If you were Nancy, what would you expect Lisa to bring to the interview? Are your own letters of recommendations in order and is your resumé ready to hand out?

CHAPTER SUMMARY

Careers in sports medicine require good sales skills. Extensive education, solid experience, and exceptional clinical skills are vital tools of the trade, but they are no longer enough. Today's competitive job market requires good sales technique too. Sales skills are used everywhere—in every profession, and at every level. Regardless of the career path you travel in sports medicine, the most important thing you can market or promote is yourself. Your success hinges greatly on recognition of this simple fact.

Success means different things to different people; but in business, success generally means meeting the needs of customers better than anyone else. In the business of sports medicine, potential clients and employers must be able to trust you with their time, their money, and often with their health. To provide these people with the best care and service possible, you must exhibit genuine concern for them, possess a thorough understanding of their needs, and demonstrate the ability to meet those needs with your products or services. You can present yourself, your product, or your services in the following ways: face-to-face meetings, Internet-based presentations, telephone sales, educational materials, or traditional mass media.

You may have the best technical skills of anyone in your graduating class, but without the ability to present yourself in a professional manner, you will never get a chance to prove your skills. Whether it is done by telephone, written correspondence, or in person, a professional image is established by creating a positive, capable first impression. This professional image is then bolstered by a thorough understanding of your product or service and the ability to effectively communicate how you can benefit your listener.

As you go about your business, always remember that although you are in a sales position, the bottom line is not the money that you make or don't make. What counts is how you perform your job. If you are good at what you do, the money will come. As a sports medicine professional, you are in the business of caring for people. By caring for your athletes' or clients' needs, you will find your own success. Stay consistent, keep learning, and aim for quality in everything you do.

See you on the sidelines!

STUDENT ENRICHMENT ACTIVITIES

Complete the following sentences.

1. Success in business depends on establishing a need, then providing the _____ or _____ to fit that need.

2. Choosing the best sales method for you will depend on your qualifications, your product or service, your customers, and your _____.

3. Product knowledge, well-developed conversation and memory skills, intuition, a good sense of humor, and the ability to make the client feel comfortable are the keys to successful _____ meetings.

4. Click-and-mortar sales refer to a combination of _____ and a physical _____.

5. Using the telephone to promote products and services is called _____.

6. _____ shows and _____ that promote related equipment and services are excellent opportunities to distribute educational material and get to know other professionals in your field.

7. The traditional mass media include _____, _____, and _____.

8. Meeting someone _____ is always the best opportunity to present yourself and your services.

9. To make the most of your career, you must _____ for success.

10. A business card should include your _____, your title, the business name, the address, _____ and _____ numbers, your _____ address, and your Web site address.

Complete the following exercises.

11. List eight techniques for courteous use of the telephone.

12. List 10 guidelines for effective written introductions.

13. List 10 techniques for effective face-to-face presentations.

14. Using the guidelines presented in this chapter, create a resumé for yourself.

15. Using the guidelines presented in this chapter, create a sample cover letter for an advertised position.

16. Explain how you might alter the cover letter you just wrote if you wanted to use it as a written introduction for an unadvertised position.

17. Develop a detailed employment plan for yourself, or create an outline of a potential business plan, addressing as many considerations as you can think of.

18. List three sources of information for continued education in sports medicine.

Glossary

abrasion (14) an open wound, road burn, or rug burn in which the outer layer of skin has been scraped off.

acceptance (22) coming to terms with the outcome of one's prognosis.

acromioclavicular (AC) sprain test (16) downward distraction of the humerus to assess stability, or the possibility of a sprain, of the AC joint.

active range of motion (9) AROM; movement of a joint though a range of motion produced by muscle contraction (i.e., without assistance).

adipose tissue (17) fatty tissue that stores energy, insulates, and cushions.

ADLs (24) activities of daily living: normal, everyday actions, such as self-care, communication, and mobility skills, required for independent living.

AIDS (11) acquired immune deficiency syndrome; a viral disease caused by the human immunodeficiency virus (HIV), which destroys the immune system and renders the patient susceptible to other infections. It is contracted through blood and other body fluids, and is incurable.

alveoli (17) microscopic air sacs within the lungs responsible for the exchange of oxygen and carbon dioxide.

ambulation (24) the ability to move about from place to place.

anaphylactic shock (14) a severe, sometimes fatal allergic reaction that causes a sharp drop in blood pressure and breathing difficulties.

anaphylaxis (19) a severe and life-threatening type of allergic reaction.

anatomy (14) the study of the structure of the body (how the body is put together).

anger (22) frustration, bitterness, or hostility.

anterior compartment syndrome (18) swelling of the tissues between the tibia and fibula that requires rapid treatment to prevent permanent neural and vascular damage.

anterior drawer test for the ankle (18) application of posterior force to the heel to assess the stability of the ankle joint.

anterior drawer test for the knee (18) application of anterior force to the proximal posterior aspect of the tibia to assess the stability of the ACL.

aorta (17) the main artery in the body.

apathy (22) lack of interest or concern.

Apley compression test (18) compression of the meniscus of the knee combined with internal and external rotation on a patient who is face-down to assess the integrity of the meniscus.

appendicitis (20) inflammation of the appendix, producing sudden onset of abdominal pain and other flu-like symptoms.

apprehension test (16) movement of a joint while observing the patient for signs of pain and increased joint laxity, to assess joint stability.

arteries (17) blood vessels that carry oxygen-enriched blood away from the heart to the tissues.

articulation (14) a joint; the point at which two or more bones meet.

aseptic (11) sterile; preventing infection.

ashen (9) a gray skin color seen in shock patients.

assessment (9) evaluation of a patient's physical condition.

assumption of risk (2) acceptance of responsibility for the risks involved in the participation in a given activity.

asthma (20) a lung disorder that causes breathing difficulty, wheezing, and coughing, and that can lead to airway obstruction.

asymmetry (24) lacking correspondence in shape, proportion, and relative position between opposing body parts.

athlete's foot (18) a fungal infection of the foot.

athletic adhesive tape (21) cloth tape backed with adherent used in preventing and supporting athletic injuries.

athletic trainer's injury report (10) a report given to the coach explaining the nature of an athlete's injury or illness, treatment protocols, and suggestions for allowable activities.

athletic training (1) the division of sports medicine that deals with the care and prevention of athletic injuries and the management of the training methods used by professional or amateur athletes and the active population.

athletic training student/aide (2) an individual who is studying the skills necessary for the prevention, assessment, treatment, and rehabilitation of athletes. Athletic training students follow a detailed curriculum and are supervised and assigned duties by certified athletic trainers. Athletic training aides are exploring interest in the profession and assist the athletic trainer or athletic director at their schools.

atria (17) the upper chambers of the heart, also known as the receiving chambers.

ausculate (9) to listen.

automated external defibrillator (AED) (13) small, portable device that can accurately identify need, analyze rhythm, alert the rescuer, and provide the necessary shock through electrode pads adhered to the victim's chest.

avulsion (14) a painful soft tissue injury in which a flap of tissue is torn loose or pulled off completely.

backcloth (21) the cloth layer of the athletic tape.

bargaining (22) attempting to make a deal with an authority figure in an attempt to change the outcome of a situation.

basic first aid kit (10) a first aid kit appropriate for most sports activities.

battery (4) the unlawful touching of an individual without consent.

blister (14) a bubble-like collection of fluid beneath or within the epidermis of the skin.

blood pressure (12) the pressure exerted by the circulating blood against the walls of the arteries.

Board of Certification (BOC) (1) the certifying organization for the athletic trainer. The mission of the BOC is to certify athletic trainers and to identify for the public quality health care professionals through a system of certifications, adjudication, standards of practice, and continuing competency programs.

body composition (3) the ratio between lean body mass and fat. Generally read as % body fat.

body mechanics (24) the efficient and safe use of the body during activity.

bony prominences (21) protrusions of bone, such as the lateal malleoli.

bursitis (14) inflammation of a bursa.

business plan (25) a detailed description of the business strategy for an established or start-up business.

buttonhole deformity (16) abnormal contracture of a phalange in which the proximal joint flexes and the distal joint hyperextends because of tendon rupture.

callus (14) a thickened, usually painless area of skin caused by friction or pressure.

calorie (6) a unit of heat.

capacity (8) maximum capability.

carbohydrate (6) a complex sugar that is a basic source of energy for the body.

cardiac arrest (13) asystole; the absence of a heartbeat.

cardiac muscle (14) the muscle of the heart, adapted to continued rhythmic contraction.

cardiopulmonary resuscitation (CPR) (13) a lifesaving procedure involving artificial ventilation and chest compressions that is done for cardiac arrest.

cardiovascular endurance (3) the ability of the heart, blood vessels, and lungs to perform efficiently during sustained physical activities.

cell (14) the basic unit of life.

central nervous system (CNS) (15) the body system composed of the brain and the spinal cord.

certified athletic trainer (ATC) (1) allied health care professional educated and trained in the prevention, assessment, treatment, and rehabilitation of injuries.

chest compressions (13) controlled and repeated application of pressure to the sternum of a victim of cardiac arrest to keep the supply of oxygen moving throughout the body.

chondromalacia patellae (CMP) (18) abnormal softening of the cartilage beneath the patella.

clammy (9) moist.

clean technique (11) the removal or destruction of infected material or organisms.

coma (9) a state of unconsciousness or deep stupor.

competitive fitness (5) the strength, endurance, and mental well-being required to be competitive in sports activities.

compression test (16) compressing above and below an injury site to assess the possibility of a fracture.

concentric contraction (7) the shortening of a muscle during contraction.

concussion (15) injury to the brain or spinal cord, accompanied by loss of neural function, resulting from a blow to the head or a fall.

conditioning (7) the process of preparing the body for optimized performance.

congenital (5) a condition present at birth.

contact sports (15) sports in which physical contact between players is expected during the normal course of play.

contusion (14) a soft tissue injury caused by seepage of blood into tissue; a bruise.

convection (19) a method of heat loss in which the layer of heated air next to the body is constantly being removed and replaced by cooler air, such as by a fan.

coping mechanisms (22) defense mechanisms; the psychological or physical methods by which an individual adjusts or adapts to a challenge or stressful situation.

core temperature (12) the internal body temperature.

coronary circulation (17) the flow of blood through the muscular tissue of the heart.

cover letter (25) a letter that accompanies a resumé to explain or introduce its contents.

crepitation (14) a crackling or grating sound heard upon movement of a damaged bone or joint.

crutches (24) devices used to assist injured or weak patients with walking.

cryotherapy (23) rehabilitative treatments involving the use of cold to decrease circulation in order to decrease pain, muscle spasms, inflammation, and edema.

cyanosis (9) a bluish tint to the skin and mucous membrane caused by a decrease in oxygen.

dehydration (6) the loss of water from a body or substance; to become dry.

demographics (25) statistical characteristics of given populations used to define business markets.

denial (22) refusal to believe that which is true or real.

depression (22) extreme feelings of sadness or hopelessness.

diabetes mellitus (20) excess urine production caused by high blood glucose (sugar) levels.

diabetic coma (20) coma induced by a lack of insulin in the body, resulting from diabetic ketoacidosis.

diagnosis (22) identification of the nature of a disease or condition based on scientific assessment.

diathermy (23) the therapeutic use of high-frequency electrical current to increase circulation and flexibility as well as to decrease pain and muscle spasms in a given area of the body.

dietary fiber (6) material in food that resists digestion and adds bulk to the diet.

Dietary Guidelines for Americans (6) recommendations for good health made by the U.S. Department of Agriculture and U.S. Department of Health and Human Services.

Dietary Reference Intakes (DRIs) (6) a set of nutrient reference values used to plan and evaluate diets for good health.

direct axial load (18) direct pressure applied to the long axis of a body or limb.

disc (15) acts as shock absorber for the spine.

dislocation (14) the separation of a joint and malposition of an extremity.

distended (9) expanded or swollen.

drop arm test (16) abduction of the arm followed by controlled lowering to assess the possibility of injury to the rotator cuff.

duration (8) the length of time an activity is performed.

eccentric contraction (7) the lengthening of a muscle during contraction.

ecchymosis (14) ruptured blood vessels in the subcutaneous tissue, noticeable by a purple discoloration of the skin.

edema (9) swelling because of excess fluid in the tissues.

electrical modality (23) rehabilitative treatment that uses electrical current to achieve therapeutic results.

electrical muscle stimulation (EMS) (23) also known as neuromuscular stimulation (NMS); the use of electrical stimulation to re-educate injured muscles, strengthen healthy muscles, and slow the effects of atrophy in a given area.

Emergency Action Plan (9) a written plan that describes procedures and rolls that must be in place for emergency situations.

emergency medical services (EMS) (9) mobile emergency health care providers.

employment plan (25) a detailed description of an individual's strategy for finding employment and advancing in a career.

empty can test (16) flexion of the shoulder followed by resistance to observe for weakening of the supraspinatus muscle.

energy expenditure (6) the total calories used for all activities over a given period of time.

energy intake (6) the sum of the caloric content in food ingested.

entrepreneur (25) an individual who organizes, manages, and assumes the responsibility for a business.

epicondylitis (16) inflammation of the medial or lateral epicondyle of the humerus and its surrounding tissues.

epilepsy (20) a group of nervous system disorders that involve disturbed rhythms of the electrical impulses that fire throughout the cerebrum, resulting in seizure activity or abnormal behavior.

epistaxis (15) a nosebleed.

essential body fat (5) the minimum amount of body fat necessary for the proper protection of internal organs.

ethics (4) morals; a set of principles or values that influence behavior.

evaporation (19) a method of heat loss in which a liquid changes from a liquid to vapor, as with perspiration.

exercise modality (24) a rehabilitative treatment involving the use of physical activity to increase strength and flexibility.

expiration (9) exhalation; the act of breathing out.

fasciitis (21) inflammation of a sheet of connective tissue covering or binding together body structures (fascia).

fat (6) a substance made up of lipids or fatty acids that is a source of energy and is vital to growth and development.

fat weight (5) the weight of a body after the lean body weight has been subtracted; the weight of the adipose tissue of the body.

Finkelstein's test (16) stretching or lengthening of the thumb tendon to assess the possibility of de Quervain's disease, or tenosynovitis of the thumb tendon.

flail chest (17) a condition in which two or more fractures on a given rib cause the chest wall to become unstable, resulting in respiratory movements of the chest opposite to those desired.

flash-to-bang method (19) manner of estimating the proximity (miles away) of dangerous lightning by counting the seconds between a flash of lightning and the bang of thunder. Dividing the number of seconds by five gives the miles away.

flexibility (3) the ability to stretch a muscle through its full range of motion (ROM) without causing pain or muscle tearing.

fluidotherapy (23) a "dry" whirlpool in which cellulose particles are dispersed in a whirlwind of heated air to decrease pain and muscle spasms as well as to increase flexibility and circulation in the treated area.

Food Guide Pyramid (6) educational tool that enables incorporating dietary guidelines into daily use.

fracture (14) a crack or break in a bone.

frequency (8) the number of times an activity is performed within a specific time frame.

full arrest (13) respiratory and cardiac arrest.

galvanic stimulation (23) the use of a direct electrical current to regulate circulation as well as to decrease pain, edema, and muscle spasms in a given area of the body.

gamekeeper's thumb test (16) application of a valgus stress to the medial joint line at the base of the thumb to assess the possibility of injury to the ulnar collateral ligament.

ganglion cyst (16) a cystic tumor rising from a tendon, often on the back of the wrist, that creates a knot beneath the skin.

general fitness (5) the ability to perform daily activities with vitality and energy, to withstand stress without undue fatigue, and to maintain physical health without medical intervention.

goniometer (24) an instrument used to measure the movements and angles created by joints.

grimace (22) a facial expression that reflects discomfort; a frown.

hamstrings (5) the muscles on the posterior aspect of the femur.

Hawkins-Kennedy test (16) compression of the supraspinatus tendon against the coracoacromial ligament to assess the possibility of impingement of the subcromial bursa.

head injury and concussion information sheet (10) instructions for care given to an athlete or the athlete's parents/guardian when a head injury is suspected.

head-tilt, chin-lift maneuver (13) a procedure for opening a blocked airway in which a patient's head is tilted back and the chin is lifted.

Health Insurance Portability and Accountability Act (HIPAA) (4) a federal regulation establishing national standards for health care information to protect personal health information.

Health Maintenance Organization (HMO) (1) group health care plan that provides a predetermined, prepaid medical care benefit package.

heat cramps (19) muscle spasms resulting from dehydration.

heat exhaustion (19) a physical reaction to heat exposure resulting from dehydration and characterized by profuse sweating and extreme weakness or fatigue; can lead to heatstroke.

heatstroke (19) elevated body temperature such that the body's internal organs begin to shut down because of excessive heat.

hematoma (14) a blood-filled swollen area; a goose-egg mass caused by bleeding under the tissues.

hemorrhage (15) the severe, abnormal internal or external discharge of blood.

hemothorax (17) blood within the pleural cavity.

hepatitis A (11) inflammation of the liver caused by a virus and spread by the fecal-oral route either from poor handwashing or contaminated food.

hepatitis B (11) inflammation of the liver caused by a virus and spread through contact with infected blood and body fluids. It is the most common form contracted by health care workers.

hernia (17) the protrusion of an organ or part of an organ through a wall of a cavity normally containing the organ.

homeostasis (12) a state of equilibrium within the body maintained through the adaptation of body systems to changes in either the internal or external environment.

HOPS (9) a system of medical evaluation based on history, observation, palpation, and stress tests.

humidity (19) a measurement of moisture in the air based on the difference between the amount of water vapor in the air and the maximum amount the air could contain at the same temperature.

hydrated (2) possessing water or fluid, especially in the tissues.

hydrocollator pack (23) a moist heat pack used to increase circulation and flexibility as well as decrease pain and muscle spasms in the treated area.

hyperventilation (17) prolonged, deep, and rapid breathing, resulting in decreased levels of CO_2 in the blood.

hypothermia (19) an unusually low body temperature capable of causing cardiac arrest and problems with the central nervous system

ice massage (23) direct application of ice to the body to obtain a therapeutic numbing effect; used to decrease circulation, inflammation, muscle spasms, and pain in a local area.

ice pack (23) ice, placed in a plastic bag, applied to an injury to decrease circulation, pain, edema, muscle spasms, and inflammation.

ice water immersion (23) the cooling of tissues through submersion in ice cold water; used to decrease circulation, inflammation, muscle spasms, edema, and pain in the treated area.

impingement (16) compression of soft tissue between the ends of two or more bones because of tissue inflammation or bone displacement.

incision (14) a clean, straight, knife-like cut.

ingrown toenail (18) a toenail that has grown into the skin of the toe.

injury report (10) a legal document containing information about the nature and treatment of injuries that is used in the evaluation of treatment procedures.

inspiration (9) inhalation; the act of breathing something into the lungs.

insulin shock (20) shock caused by an overdose of insulin.

intensity (8) the degree of effort required to complete a physical activity.

interferential stimulation (IFS) (23) the uses of interfering electrical currents to increase circulation and flexibility as well as to decrease muscle spasms in a given area of the body.

intermittent compression (23) the periodic application of compression to a part of the body to reduce edema in that area.

iontophoresis (23) the administration of ionized medications to the tissues through the use of an electrical current.

ischemia (21) reduced or obstructed blood circulation.

isokinetic contraction (7) a muscle contraction produced by a variable external resistance at a constant speed.

isolated injury assessment (9) a thorough examination of a specific part of the body to determine the extent of injury that may have occurred.

isometric contraction (7) a muscle contraction with no motion that results in no change in the length of the muscle.

isotonic contraction (7) a muscle contraction produced by a constant external resistance.

joint laxity (14) joint play; motions occurring between the ends of two or more bones that form a joint as it moves through its range of motion.

kidney (17) one of a pair of organs located in the dorsal cavity of the body that are responsible for filtering blood and producing urine.

laceration (14) a jagged tear in the flesh.

Lachman test (18) application of anterior and posterior force to the proximal posterior tibia to determine the stability of the ACL and PCL.

lean body weight (5) the weight of a body after the fat weight has been subtracted.

liability (2) legal responsibility to perform duties in a reasonable and prudent manner.

ligament (14) a band of white, fibrous connective tissue that helps hold bone to bone.

log roll (9) the method used to turn a patient with a spinal injury, in which the patient is moved to the side in one motion.

lungs (17) the two organs of respiration contained within the thorax.

mallet finger (16) flexion of the distal interphalangeal joint of the finger caused by damage to the extensor tendon.

malpractice (4) professional misconduct or lack of professional skill that results in injury to the patient; negligence by a professional, such as a physician, nurse, certified athletic trainer, or coach.

massage (23) the systematic manipulation, methodical pressure, friction, and kneading of the soft tissues of the body to increase circulation, decrease pain, and promote relaxation.

McMurray test (18) compression of the meniscus of the knee combined with internal and external rotation while the patient is face-up to assess the integrity of the meniscus.

mechanical modality (23) rehabilitative treatment that uses external force to increase or decrease circulation and reduce pain.

mechanism of injury (9) how the injury occurred.

meniscal tear (18) a partial or complete tear of the meniscus.

metabolism (6) the sum of all physical and chemical processes that take place in the body; the conversion of food into energy.

minerals (6) inorganic compounds that are essential to body function.

mode (8) the equipment and exercises used in an exercise program.

motivation (24) the reason for performing an action; the stimulus for behavior.

mucus (9) fluid secreted from the nose.

multitasking skills (3) skills that enable a person to competently perform more than one task at a time.

muscle contraction (5) the tensioning of the muscle during shortening (concentric), lengthening (eccentric), or no motion (isometric).

muscle endurance (3) the ability of a muscle or a group of muscles to apply repeated force over a period of time until fatigue prevents the lifting or moving of the resistance.

muscle mass (7) the girth or size of the muscle.

muscle rupture (16) a complete tear of a muscle.

muscle spasm/pain cycle (23) a debilitating syndrome in which pain caused by injury produces muscle spasms that increase pain and spasms in a cyclical manner.

muscle tone (7) the shape of a muscle in its resting state.

myositis ossificans (14) a condition in which bone forms in and replaces muscle tissue as a result of trauma.

National Athletic Trainers' Association (NATA) (2) a not-for-profit organization that is committed to the advancement, encouragement, and improvement of the athletic training profession.

negligence (4) the failure to give reasonable care or to do what another prudent person with similar experience, knowledge, and background would have done under the same or similar circumstances.

nutrients (6) substances that provide nourishment.

obstructed airway maneuver (13) quick upward thrust performed against a patient's abdomen while standing behind a patient to remove an obstruction and open free passage of air from the mouth or nose to the lungs.

optimal support (21) when half of the first anchor is taped to the underwrap and half directly to the skin.

organ (14) a structure within the body made up of tissues that allow it to perform a particular function.

orientation (9) the ability to comprehend one's environment regarding time, place, situation, and identity of persons.

Osgood-Schlatter disease (18) inflammation or irritation of the tibia at its point of attachment with the patellar tendon.

overload principle (7) the application of greater than normal stress to a muscle, resulting in increased capacity to do work. Gradually the muscle will adapt to increased demand, making it necessary to increase the stress again.

pain threshold (22) the point at which pain affects performance.

pancreas (17) the organ in the abdominal cavity that produces insulin and aids in digestion.

paraffin bath (23) the immersion of a body part in melted paraffin to increase circulation and flexibility as well as to decrease pain and muscle spasms.

parallel (5) extending in the same direction and remaining separated by the same distance along the entire length, never crossing paths.

paralysis (9) loss of sensation and movement over an area of the body because of nerve damage.

paresthesia (14) an abnormal sensation of the skin, such as numbness, tingling, prickling, or burning, with no apparent cause.

passive range of motion (9) PROM; movement of a joint through a range of motion produced by an outside force (i.e., with assistance).

patella grind test (18) application of inferior force to the superior aspect of the patella as the quadriceps are flexed to assess the condition of the cartilage beneath the patella.

patellar tendon rupture test (18) extension of the lower leg to assess the integrity of the patellar tendon.

pathogen (11) a disease-causing microorganism.

patient history (Hx) (24) a form that describes the patient's medical history and chief medical complaint.

percussion test (16) tapping a bone to assess the possibility of a fracture.

PERL (9) abbreviation for pupils equal and react to light.

perpendicular (24) forming right angles to a given plane.

personal kit (10) the first aid kit that is kept with sports medicine professionals at all times and contains the most essential emergency supplies. These will vary with athletes' medical needs.

Phalen's test (16) compression of the median and ulnar nerves to assess the possibility of impingement of those nerves at the wrist.

physical capabilities (3) physical health characteristics that increase one's physical abilities and that must be considered in the development of a fitness program.

physical fitness (3) the ability to perform daily tasks vigorously and alertly, with energy left over for enjoying leisure-time activities and meeting emergency demands.

physical fitness program (1) a method of exercise designed to prepare an individual to become physically able to do the activities he or she wishes to do in daily life, without causing undue physical stress.

physical limitations (3) physical health characteristics that inhibit one's physical abilities and that must be considered in the development of a fitness program.

physical therapy aide (1) an individual who is not licensed but is able to perform clerical tasks under the direct supervision of a physical therapist or physical therapy assistant.

physical therapy assistant (1) an individual who has earned a two-year associate's degree and is involved in clinical tasks, such as patient care and recording treatments, under the direct supervision of a physical therapist.

physician's kit (10) items the team physician uses for advanced medical care and treatment the athletic trainer cannot provide.

physician's report (10) a report prepared by the physician that describes the extent of the injury or illness, the course of treatment, and recommended activities. This report also provides the written authorization for the athlete's return to play, if applicable.

physiology (14) the study of the function of the body (how the body works).

pivot shift test (18) internal rotation of the ankle combined with medial force to assess the stability of the ACL.

placebo effect (6) a false sense of benefit felt by a patient caused by the psychological belief that the treatment is effective.

plantar fasciitis (18) inflammation of the fibrous membranes, or connective tissue, in the sole of the foot.

plateau (22) a period in the process of rehabilitation in which no significant improvement or progress is shown.

pneumothorax (17) the presence of air in the thoracic cavity resulting from the perforation of the chest wall or the visceral pleura.

posterior drawer test for knee (18) application of posterior force to the proximal anterior aspect of the tibia to assess the stability of the PCL.

posttraumatic amnesia (15) loss of memory for events immediately following a trauma.

posture (24) the position or alignment of the body.

power (7) the ability to apply force with speed.

PRICE procedure (14) systematic steps taken to mitigate or minimize injury: protect, rest, ice, compress, and elevate.

primary survey (9) an examination of the patient to determine the presence of any life-threatening emergencies; the initial assessment of airway, breathing, and circulation on a patient.

proactive (22) acting in advance to avoid or manage an anticipated difficulty.

prognosis (22) an estimate of a chance for recovery; a prediction of the likely outcome of a disease or injury.

progress notes (24) notes on the patient's chart that document patient progress in rehabilitation and that may follow the SOAP format.

prophylactic strapping (21) taping that helps to prevent or decrease the severity of injuries.

proprioception (7) the ability to sense the location, position, orientation, and movement of the body and its parts.

protein (6) any of a class of complex, nitrogenous, organic compounds that function as the primary building blocks of the body.

psychological fitness (22) the mental and emotional ability to perform in competition without undue strain on other aspects of one's life.

psychrometer (19) an instrument used to measure relative humidity.

pulmonary circulation (17) the flow of oxygen-depleted blood form the right ventricle of the heart to the lungs for reoxygenation and then on to the left atrium of the heart.

pulse (12) a vital sign; a quantitative measurement of the heartbeat using the fingers to palpate an artery or a stethoscope to listen to the heartbeat.

puncture wound (14) a soft tissue injury caused by the penetration of a sharp object.

radiating pain (15) pain that spreads from a central point, such as the point of injury.

radiation (19) the release of rays in different directions from a common point; the transfer of loss of heat by or from its source to the surrounding environment in the form of heat waves or rays.

range of motion (ROM) (14); the maximum range through which a joint can move.

rapport (3) good relationships and communication with clients.

recovery heart rate (5) the number of times the heart beats in 1 minute 60 seconds after completion of 3 or more minutes of exercise.

referred pain (15) pain at a location other than the injured organ or site.

rehabilitation (24) the process of recovering from an injury through treatment and education designed to assist injured patients in regaining maximum function, a sense of well-being, and the highest level of independence possible.

relative humidity (19) a measurement of moisture in the air based on the difference between the amount of water vapor in the air and the maximum amount the air could contain at the same temperature.

repetition (5) the completion of a designated movement through the entire range of motion.

resistance (7) counterforce.

respiration (12) breathing; the process of bringing oxygen into the body and expelling carbon dioxide from the body.

resting heart rate (5) the number of times the heart beats in 1 minute when no physical activity is taking place.

restricted participation (22) engaging in athletic activity while injured, but in a restricted manner that prevents an injury from becoming worse.

resumé (25) a brief, written account of personal and professional qualifications and experience prepared by an applicant for a position.

risk management (4) reduction of the potential for injury.

secondary survey (9) a head-to-toe physical assessment; an additional assessment of a patient to determine the existence of any injuries other than those found in the primary survey.

second-impact syndrome (SIS) (15) a second concussion received before the signs and symptoms of the first concussion have been resolved: a life-threatening emergency.

self-esteem (22) pride in oneself; self-respect.

self-promotion (25) the presentation of one's self or company to buyers for acceptance through advertising and publicity.

set (7) a group of repetitions.

shin splints (medial tibial stress syndrome) (18) pain in the lower leg following strenuous or repetitive lower-extremity exercise.

shock (17) a condition that occurs when an inadequate amount of blood flows through the body, causing extremely low blood pressure, a lack of urine, and other disorders; a potentially fatal condition.

skeletal or striated muscle (14) voluntary muscles that can be consciously controlled, unlike involuntary muscles, which work whether the body is conscious or unconscious.

smooth or visceral muscle (14) muscle tissue that contracts without voluntary control; contracts slowly and sustained over a longer time; found in internal organs and blood vessels.

SOAP notes (24) an organized method of documenting a patient's status on his or her chart that includes subjective findings, objective findings, assessments, and plans for each problem experienced by the patient.

special populations (8) individuals with special physical capabilities or limitations that make adjustments necessary to a standard fitness program.

specificity principle (7) the way in which an exercise relates to the activity for which performance enhancement is sought.

Speed's test (16) stretching or lengthening of the biceps tendon to assess the possibility of tenosynovitis.

splint (14) a rigid device that holds parts of the body together and limits motion.

sports medicine (1) the branch of health care that deals with evaluating athletes and preventing and treating injuries. These athletes will range from wheelchair basketball players to the extreme skier.

sprain (14) a stretching or tearing of the ligaments, characterized by the inability to move, deformity, and pain.

standard of care (4) the degree of care, skill, and diligence an equally qualified caregiver in the profession would provide in similar circumstances.

sterile technique (11) the procedure used by health care workers when performing or assisting with sterile procedures.

sternoclavicular (SC) sprain test (16) application of posterior force to the clavicle to assess stability, or the possibility of a sprain, of the SC joint.

stirrup (21) a general term describing strips of tape applied from one side of the ankle to the other, passing beneath the heel.

stoma (9) surgically constructed opening in throat used for breathing.

strain (14) a pulled muscle.

strength (3) the ability of a muscle to exert a maximum force against a resistance.

strength and conditioning specialist (SCS) (1) a professional member of the sports medicine team who evaluates existing levels of fitness and athleticism, along with helping increase the strength and endurance of an individual or team while promoting a healthier lifestyle.

stretching (7) gently forcing the muscle to lengthen.

striated muscle (14) see **skeletal muscle.**

subluxation (14) a partial dislocation.

sudden cardiac arrest (13) a sudden stopping of the heartbeat, which may cause death.

sulcus test (16) downward distraction of the humerus to assess stability, or the possibility of a sprain, of the glenohumeral joint.

synovitis (14) inflammation of the synovial membrane in a joint, characterized by pain, swelling, localized tension, and increased pain with movement.

systemic circulation (17) the flow of oxygen-enriched blood from the left ventricle of the heart to all parts of the body (except the lungs) and the return of oxygen-depleted blood to the heart through the right atrium.

systemic reaction (14) a reaction that involved the whole body rather than just a part of it.

talar tilt test (18) inversion of the foot to determine the stability of the ankle joint.

target heart rate range (8) the lower and upper limits of the rate in which the heart should beat to achieve significant cardiovascular benefits; used to access intensity of exercise.

target zone (8) the desired level of fitness.

tendon (14) fibrous connective tissue around a joint that connects muscle to bone.

tendonitis (14) inflammation of a tendon.

tendon rupture (18) a complete tear of a tendon.

tenosynovitis (16) inflammation of the tendon sheath.

tensile strength (21) the ability of fabric or tape to resist tearing, based on thread count.

tension (21) the degree to which tape is stretched.

therapeutic modality (1) the use of heat, cold, or electrical stimulation to produce an increase or decrease in blood flow.

thermotherapy (23) treatments involving the use of heat to increase circulation in order to improve flexibility and decrease pain and muscle spasms.

30/30 rule (19) If the flash-to-bang calculation is 30 seconds or less, people should seek shelter and not resume outdoor activity until 30 minutes after the last audible thunder.

Thompson test (18) compression of the calf muscle while observing for plantar flexion to assess the stability of the Achilles tendon.

Tinel's sign (16) a tingling sensation produced by percussion of the ulnar nerve.

tissue (14) a collection of similar cells and their intercellular substances that work together to perform a particular function.

tort (4) a wrongful act resulting in injury to another's person, property, or reputation, for which the injured party is entitled to seek compensation.

traction (23) the distraction, or pulling, of a body part or segment for rehabilitative purposes.

Trainer's Angel (9) a device made specifically to cut off the side tabs of the face mask to hinge it back or remove it.

transcutaneous electrical nerve stimulation (TENS) (23) the use of electrical current to block the sensation of pain to a given area of the body.

treatment record (10) a legal document used to track the course of care for an injured athlete and to evaluate various treatment methods.

trunk (5) the torso; the area of the body on either side of and including the spine, but excluding the arms and legs.

ultrasound therapy (23) the application of sound waves to a body area to increase circulation and flexibility as well as to decrease pain and muscle spasms in that area.

Universal Precautions (11) guidelines developed by the Centers for Disease Control and Prevention (CDC) for protecting health care workers from exposure to blood-borne pathogens in body secretions.

valgus stress test (16) application of a medial force to the lateral aspect of a joint in an attempt to create a gap in the medial joint line, thereby testing the stability of the medial aspect of the joint.

vapo-coolant spray (23) an aerosol coolant used to quickly lower the temperature of superficial body tissues and decrease pain.

variable resistance (7) a resistance exercise that varies through the range of motion.

variation principle (7) the alteration or modification of exercises to work an entire muscle or group of muscles and to combat boredom.

varus stress test (16) application of a lateral force to the medial aspect of a joint in an attempt to create a gap in the lateral joint line, thereby testing the stability of the lateral aspect of the joint.

veins (17) blood vessels that carry oxygen-depleted blood to the heart.

ventricles (17) the pumping chambers of the heart, located inferior to the atria.

vertebrae (15) the individual bone segments of the spine.

vital signs (12) assessments of pulse, respiration, blood pressure, and temperature; body functions essential to life.

vitamins (6) organic substances, other than proteins, carbohydrates, fats, and organic salts, that are essential in small quantities for normal body function.

Volkmann's contracture (16) contracture and damage to the muscles of the forearm because of injury to their blood supply.

water (6) H_2O; the odorless and tasteless fluid that is the principle chemical constituent of the human body.

whirlpool bath (23) a therapeutic bath of heated or cooled water in which all or part of the body is exposed to forceful, massaging currents in the water.

winged scapula test (16) flexion of the serratus anterior to observe for weakening of that muscle as indicated by a protruding scapula.

Bibliography

Alter, Michael J. *Science of Flexibility.* 3rd ed. Human Kinetics, 2004.

Anderson, Marcia K. *Fundamentals of Sports Injury Management.* 2nd ed. Lippincott, Williams & Wilkins, 2002.

Anderson, Marcia K., Susan J. Hall, and Malissa Martin. *Foundations of Athletic Training.* 3rd ed. Lippincott Williams & Wilkins, 2005.

Andrews, James R., Gary L. Harrelson, and Kevin E. Wilk. *Physical Rehabilitation of the Injured Athlete.* 3rd ed. Saunders, 2004.

Andrews, James R., William G. Clancy, and James A. Whiteside. *On-Field Evaluation and Treatment of Common Athletic Injuries.* Mosby, 1997.

Arnheim, Daniel D., and William E. Prentice. *Essentials of Athletic Training.* 6th ed. McGraw-Hill, 2005.

Austin, Karin, Kathryn Gwynn-Brett, and Sarah Marshall. *Illustrated Guide to Taping Techniques.* Mosby, 1994.

Blauvelt, Carolyn Taliaferro, and Fred R.T. Nelson. *A Manual of Orthopaedic Terminology.* 6th ed. Mosby, 1998.

Boissonnault, William G. *Primary Care for the Physical Therapist.* Elsevier Saunders, 2005.

Brotzman, S. Brent, and Kevin E. Wilk. *Clinical Orthopaedic Rehabilitation.* 2nd ed. Mosby, 2003.

Coleman, Ellen. *Eating for Endurance.* 4th ed. Bull Publishing, 2003.

Cotton, Richard T. *Personal Trainer Manual: The Resource for Fitness Professionals.* 3rd ed. ACE, 2003.

DeCarlo, Mark, and Kathy Oneacre. *Current Topics in Musculoskeletal Medicine.* Slack, 2001.

Denegar, Craig R. *Therapeutic Modalities for Musculoskeletal Injuries.* 2nd ed. Human Kinetics, 2006.

Donatelli, Robert, and Michael J. Wooden. *Orthopaedic Physical Therapy.* Churchill Livingstone, 2001.

Dwyer, Gregory B., and Shala E. Davis. *ACSM's Health-Related Physical Fitness Assessment Manual.* Lippincott, Williams & Wilkins, 2005.

Ehlich, Ann, and Carol L. Schroeder. *Medical Terminology for Health Professions.* 5th ed. Thomson Delmar Learning, 2005.

Ellenbecker, Todd S. *Knee Ligament Rehabilitation.* Churchill Livingstone, 2000.

Garrick, James G., and David R. Webb. *Sports Injuries Diagnosis and Management.* 2nd ed. Saunders, 1999.

Hillman, Susan Kay. *Introduction to Athletic Training.* 2nd ed. Human Kinetics, 2005.

Hoeger, Werner W.K., and Sharon A. Hoeger. *Principles and Labs for Fitness and Wellness.* 6th ed. Wadsworth, 2006.

Houglum, Joel, Gary Harrelson, and Deidre Leaver-Dunn. *Principles of Pharmacology for Athletic Trainers.* Slack, 2005.

Incidental Contact. Incidental Contact, LLC. March 2007. <http://www.incidentalcontact.com>.

Jones, Betty. *Comprehensive Medical Terminology.* 2nd ed. Thomson Delmar Learning, 2003.

Kaminsky, Lenard A. *ACSM's Resource Manual for Guidelines for Exercise Testing and Prescription.* 5th ed. Lippincott, Williams & Wilkins, 2006.

Kolt, Gregory S., and Lynn Snyder-Mackler. *Physical Therapies in Sport and Exercise.* Churchill Livingstone, 2003.

Konin, Jeff. *Clinical Athletic Training.* Slack, 1997.

Konin, Jeff G., and Margaret A. Frederick. *Documentation for Athletic Training.* Slack, 2005.

Konin, Jeff G. *Practical Kinesiology for the Physical Therapist Assistant.* Slack, 1999.

Loudon, Janice, Stephania Bell, and Jane Johnston. *The Clinical Orthopedic Assessment Guide.* Human Kinetics, 1998.

Low Back Exercise Program. The Nicholas Institute of Sports Medicine and Athletic Trauma (NISMAT). March 2007. <http://www.nismat.org/orthocor/programs/lowback.html>.

MacDonald, Rose. *Taping Techniques: Principles and Practice.* 2nd ed. Butterworth-Heinemann, 2004.

Maffetone, Philip. *Complementary Sport Medicine.* Human Kinetics, 1999.

Matheson, Gordon O. *Preparticipation Physical Evaluation.* 3rd ed. McGraw-Hill, 2005.

Mullin, Bernard J., Stephen Hardy, and William A. Sutton. *Sports Marketing.* 2nd ed. Human Kinetics, 2000.

Myers, Thomas W. *Anatomy Trains.* Churchill Livingstone, 2001.

Norman, Wesley, PhD, DSc. *The Anatomy Lesson.* March 2007. <http://mywebpages.comcast.net/wnor/homepage.htm>.

Norris, Christopher. *Sports Injuries; Diagnosis and Management.* 3rd ed. Butterworth Heinemann, 2004.

O'Connor, Francis G., and Richard Birrer. *Sports Medicine for the Primary Care Physician.* 3rd ed. Saunders, 2004.

Perrin, David H. *Athletic Taping and Bracing.* 2nd ed. Human Kinetics, 2005.

Pfeiffer, Ronald P., and Brent C. Mangus. *Concepts of Athletic Training.* 4th ed. Jones & Bartlett, 2005.

Potts, Keri A. *The National Collegiate Athletic Association Sports Medicine Handbook.* 13th ed. National Collegiate Athletic Association, 2000.

Prentice, William E. PhD. *Arnheim's Principles of Athletic Training.* 11th ed. McGraw-Hill, 2003.

Prentice, William E. *Therapeutic Modalities for Physical Therapists.* 2nd ed. McGraw-Hill, 2001.

Ray, Richard. *Management Strategies in Athletic Training.* 3rd ed. Human Kinetics, 2005.

Rizzo, Donald C. *Fundamentals of Anatomy & Physiology.* 2nd ed. Thomson Delmar Learning, 2006.

Rubin, Aaron. *Sports Injuries & Emergencies.* McGraw-Hill, 2003.

Safran, Marc, David A. Stone, and James Zachazewski. *Instructions for Sports Medicine Patients.* Saunders, 2003.

Sallis, Robert E. *Essential of Sports Medicine.* Mosby, 1997.

Scott, Ann Senisi, and Elizabeth Fong. *Body Structures & Functions.* 10th ed. Thomson Delmar Learning, 2004.

Scuderi, Giles R., and Peter D. McCann. *Sports Medicine: A Comprehensive Approach.* 2nd ed. Mosby, 2005.

Sharp, Richard M., and Vicki F. Sharp. *WebDoctor Your Online Guide to Health Care and Wellness.* Quality Medical Publishing, 1997.

Shields, Clarence L. *Manual of Sports Surgery.* Springer-Verlang, 1987.

Spencer, John W., and Joseph J. Jacobs. *Complementary Alternative Medicine.* Mosby, 1999.

Standring, Susan. *Gray's Anatomy.* 39th ed. Elsevier Churchill Livingstone, 2005.

Starkey, Chad. *Therapeutic Modalities for Athletic Trainers.* 2nd ed. F.A. Davis, 2004.

Sullivan, J. Andy, and Steven J. Anderson. *Care of the Young Athlete.* AAOS, 2000.

Thibodeau, Gary A., and Kevin T. Patton. *Anatomy & Physiology.* 16th ed. Mosby, 1999.

Waddell, Gordon. *The Back Pain Revolution.* 2nd ed. Churchill Livingstone, 2004.

Wilksten, Denise, and Carolyn Peters. *The Athletic Trainer's Guide to Strength and Endurance Training.* Slack, 2000.

Woodrow, Ruth. *Essentials of Pharmacology for Health Occupations.* 5th ed. Thomson Delmar Learning, 2007.

Index